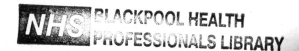

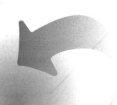

Progress in

Obstetrics and Gynaecology

Progress in Obstetrics and Gynaecology
Edited by John Studd

Contents of Volume 16

First published 2005

ISBN 0 443 07422 4

ISSN 0261 0140

Progress in

Obstetrics and Gynaecology

VOLUME 17

Edited by

John Studd
Professor of Gynaecology, Imperial College, London University
Chelsea and Westminster Hospital, London, UK

Seang Lin Tan
James Edmund Dodds Professor and Chairman
Department of Obstetrics and Gynaecology, McGill University
Royal Victoria Hospital, Montreal, Canada

Frank A. Chervenak
Given Foundaton Professor and Chairman
Department of Obstetrics and Gynaecology
New York Weill Cornell Medical Center, New York, USA

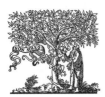

ELSEVIER

EDINBURGH LONDON NEW YORK OXFORD PHILADELPHIA St LOUIS SYDNEY TORONTO 2006

ELSEVIER

First published 2006

ISBN-10: 0 443 10313 5
ISBN-13: 978–0–443–10313–1

British Library Cataloguing in Publication Data
A catalogue record for this book is available from the British Library

Library of Congress Cataloging in Publication Data
A catalog record for this book is available from the Library of Congress

Note
Knowledge and best practice in this field are constantly changing. As new research and experience broaden our knowledge, changes in practice, treatment and drug therapy may become necessary or appropriate. Readers are advised to check the most current information provided (i) on procedures featured or (ii) by the manufacturer of each product to be administered, to verify the recommended dose or formula, the method and duration of administration, and contraindications. It is the responsibility of the practitioner, relying on their own experience and knowledge of the patient, to make diagnoses, to determine dosages and the best treatment for each individual patient, and to take all appropriate safety precautions. To the fullest extent of the law, neither the Publisher nor the Editors assumes any liability for any injury and/or damage to persons or property arising out or related to any use of the material contained in this book.

Commissioning Editor – Timothy Horne
Development Editor – Gill Haddock
Senior Designer – Sarah Russell
Editorial and Typesetting services – BA & GM Haddock
Printed in UK

The
publisher's
policy is to use
paper manufactured
from sustainable forests

Contents

GYNAECOLOGY

Contributors

Alok Ash MBBS MD(Cal) FRCOG
Consultant Obstetrician, Guy's and St Thomas's Hospital NHS Foundation
Trust, and Honorary Senior Lecturer, King's College London, London, UK

Louise Ashelby MB ChB
Specialist Obstetric Registrar, Maternity Unit, Taunton & Somerset NHS
Trust, Taunton, UK

Tom Bourne PhD MRCOG
Consultant Gynaecologist and Head of Unit, Early Pregnancy, Gynaecological
Ultrasound and MAS Unit, St George's Hospital Medical School, London, UK

Richard N. Brown MBBS MRCOG
Assistant Professor of Obstetrics and Gynecology, McGill University,
Women's Pavillion, Royal Victoria Hospital, Montreal, Quebec, Canada

Irina D. Burd MD PhD
Department of Obstetrics and Gynecology, Jefferson Medical College of Thomas
Jefferson University, Division of Maternal-Fetal Medicine, Philadelphia, USA

Sue M. Calvert MRCOG
Consultant in Obstetrics and Gynaecology, Bradford Royal Infirmary, Bradford, UK

Jerry Chan MB BCh BaO MA MRCOG
Assistant Professor, Department of Obstetrics and Gynaecology, Yong Lu Lin
School of Medicine, National University of Singapore and National
University Hospital, Singapore

Frank A. Chervenak MD
Given Foundation Professor and Chairman, Department of Obstetrics and
Gynecology, Weill Medical College of Cornell University, The New York
Presbyterian Hospital, New York, USA

Wayne R. Cohen MD
Chairman of Obstetrics and Gynecology, Jamaica Hospital Medical Center
and Professor of Clinical Obstetrics and Gynecology, Weill-Cornell Medical
College, New York, USA

George Condous MRCOG FRANZCOG
Clinical Research Fellow, Royal North Shore Hospital, University of Sydney,
Department of Obstetrics and Gynaecology, St Leonards, NSW, Australia

Charlotte L. Deans MBBS MRCOG
Maternal Medicine Clinical Fellow, Chelsea and Westminster Hospital,
London, UK

Gian Carlo Di Renzo MD PhD
Head, Department of Obstetrics and Gynaecology, Monteluce Hospital,
University of Perugia, Italy/Italian Representative of the New European
Surgical Academy (NESA)

Alaa A. El-Ghobashy MD MRCOG
Specialist Registrar in Obstetrics and Gynaecology, St James's University
Hospital, Leeds, UK

Diaa M. El-Mowafi MD
Professor, Obstetrics and Gynecology Department, Benha Faculty of
Medicine, Egypt; Educator & Researcher, Wayne State University, Detroit,
Michigan, USA; Fellow, Geneva University, Geneva, Switzerland; Consultant
& Head of Obstetrics and Gynecology Department, King Khalid General
Hospital, Hafr El-Batin, Saudi Arabia

Nicholas M. Fisk PhD FRCOG
Experimental Fetal Medicine Group, Institute of Reproductive and
Developmental Biology, Division of Surgery, Oncology, Reproductive Biology
& Anaesthesia, Imperial College London and Centre for Fetal Care, Queen
Charlotte's and Chelsea Hospital, London, UK

Robert Fox MD MRCPI MRCOG
Consultant Obstetrician, Maternity Unit, Taunton & Somerset NHS Trust,
Taunton, UK

Ruth C. Fretts MD MPH
Assistant Professor, Harvard Medical School, Harvard Vanguard Medical
Associates, Boston, Massachusetts, USA

Sandro Gerli MD
Senior Gynaecologist, Department of Obstetrics and Gynaecology, Monteluce
Hospital, University of Perugia, Italy

Thomas Murphy Goodwin MD
Professor and Chief, Maternal-Fetal Medicine, University of Southern
California, Women's and Children's Hospital, Los Angeles, California, USA

Kavita Goswami BSc MBBS MRCOG MMedSci Dip Obs & Gynae USS
Consultant Obstetrician and Gynaecologist, University Hospitals of Coventry
and Warwickshire, Coventry, UK

Amos Grunebaum MD
Department of Obstetrics and Gynecology, New York Weill Cornell Medical
Center, New York, USA

Gerald Gui MS FRCS FRCS(Ed)
Consultant Surgeon, The Department of Academic Surgery (Breast), Royal Marsden Hospital, London, UK

Sebastian Illanes MD MSc
Clinical Fellow, Fetal Medicine Research Unit, University of Bristol, St Michael's Hospital, Bristol, UK

Sharif I.M.F. Ismail MSc MBA MA MMedSci(Ed) LLM MD MRCOG
Locum Consultant Obstetrician and Gynaecologist, Royal Bournemouth Hospital, Bournemouth, UK

Margaret Johnson MD FRCP
Consultant in Thoracic/HIV Medicine and Medical Director, Royal Free Hospital, London, UK

Khalid Khan MRCOG
Professor of Obstetrics and Gynaecology and Clinical Epidemiology, University of Birmingham, Birmingham, UK

Aradhana Khaund MRCOG
Specialist Registrar in Obstetrics and Gynaecology, South Glasgow University Hospitals NHS Trust, Southern General Hospital, Glasgow, UK

Mark D. Kilby MD MRCOG
Professor of Maternal and Fetal Medicine, Fetal Medicine Centre, Birmingham Women's Hospital, Edgbaston, Birmingham, UK

Mary Ann Lumsden MD FRCOG
Professor of Reproductive and Maternal Medicine, Division of Developmental Medicine, Glasgow Royal Infirmary, Glasgow, UK

Laurence B. McCullough MD
Professor of Medicine and Medical Ethics, Center for Medical Ethics and Health Policy, Baylor College of Medicine, Houston, Texas, USA

Suneeta Mittal MD FAMS FICOG FIMSA FICMCH
Professor and Head, Department of Obstetrics and Gynaecology, All India Institute of Medical Sciences, New Delhi, India

R. Katie Morris MRCOG
Clinical Research Fellow, University of Birmingham, Birmingham, UK

Farr Nezhat MD FACOG
Professor of Obstetrics and Gynecology and Director, Gynecologic Minimally Invasive Surgery, Department of Obstetrics, Division of Gynecologic Oncology, Mount Sinai Medical Center, New York, USA

Jillian Noble MBChB MRCP(UK)
Specialist Registrar Medical Oncology, The Department of Academic Surgery (Breast), Royal Marsden Hospital, London, UK

Keelin O'Donoghue PhD MRCOG
Experimental Fetal Medicine Group, Institute of Reproductive and Developmental

Biology, Division of Surgery, Oncology, Reproductive Biology & Anaesthesia, Imperial College London and Centre for Fetal Care, Queen Charlotte's and Chelsea Hospital, London, UK

Anna Marie O'Neill MD
Instructor, Department of Obstetrics and Gynecology, Jefferson Medical College of Thomas Jefferson University, Division of Maternal-Fetal Medicine, Philadelphia, Pennsylvania, USA

Jorma Paavonen MD
Professor, Department of Obstetrics and Gynecology, University of Helsinki, Helsinki, Finland

Nicholas Panay BSc MRCOG MFFP
Consultant Obstetrician & Gynaecologist, Specialist in Reproductive Medicine & Surgery, Queen Charlotte's and Chelsea Hospital & Chelsea and Westminster Hospital, London

Tanja Pejovic MD PhD
Department of Obstetrics and Gynecology, Oregon Health & Science University, Portland, Oregon, USA

Norma Pham MD
Senior Resident, Department of Obstetrics, Gynecology and Reproductive Sciences, Yale University School of Medicine, New Haven, Connecticut, USA

Juan Carlos Sabogal MD
Department of Obstetrics and Gynecology, Jefferson Medical College of Thomas Jefferson University, Division of Maternal-Fetal Medicine, Philadelphia, Pennsylvania, USA

Peter E. Schwartz MD
John Slade Ely Professor, Department of Obstetrics, Gynecology and Reproductive Sciences, Yale University School of Medicine, New Haven, Connecticut, USA

Jolene Seibel-Seamon MD
Department of Obstetrics and Gynecology, Jefferson Medical College of Thomas Jefferson University, Division of Maternal-Fetal Medicine, Philadelphia, Pennsylvania, USA

Abeer M. Shaaban PhD MRCPath
Consultant Histopathologist/Honorary Senior Lecturer, Leeds General Infirmary, Leeds, UK

Sapna Shah BSc MBBS DFFP
Clinical Research Fellow in HIV & Women's Health, Royal Free and University College Medical School, London, UK

Jai B. Sharma MD DNB MRCOG MFFP MAMS FICOG
Assistant Professor, Department of Obstetrics and Gynaecology, All India Institute of Medical Sciences, New Delhi, India

Gordon C.S. Smith MD PhD MRCOG
Professor and Head, Department of Obstetrics and Gynaecology, Cambridge University, Rosie Maternity Hospital, Cambridge, UK

Peter Soothill BSc MD FRCOG
Professor of Obstetrics and Gynaecology, Fetal Medicine Research Unit, University of Bristol, St Michael's Hospital, Bristol, UK

Olanrewaju Sorinola MRCOG MMedSc
Consultant Obstetrician and Gynaecologist, South Warwickshire General Hospitals NHS Trust and Honorary Senior Lecturer, University of Warwick, Warwick Hospital, Warwick, UK

Michael Stark MD
President, The New European Surgical Academy (NESA) and Chairman of the Gynaecological Departments, HELIOS Hospitals Group, Berlin, Germany

Philip J. Steer BSc MB BS MD FRCOG
Professor of Gynaecology, Chelsea and Westminster Hospital, London, UK

John Studd DS MD FRCOG
Professor of Gynaecology, Imperial College, London University, and Chelsea and Westminster Hospital, London, UK

Yatin Thakur MD DNBE MRCOG
Specialist Registrar, Basildon University Hospital, Basildon, Essex, UK

Steven Thornton MD FRCOG
Professor of Obstetrics and Associate Dean (Research), Warwick Medical School, University of Warwick and Associate Medical Director (Research), University Hospitals of Coventry and Warwickshire, Coventry UK

Anselm Uebing MD
Fellow in Adult Congenital Heart Disease, Royal Brompton Hospital, London, UK

Rajiv Varma FRCOG
Consultant Obstetrician and Gynaecologist, Basildon University Hospital and Honorary Senior Lecturer University College London, Basildon University Hospital, Basildon, Essex, UK

Chloe Vera MD
Department of Obstetrics and Gynecology, Brigham and Women's Hospital, Boston, Massachusetts, USA

Stuart Weiner MD
Associate Professor of Obstetrics and Gynecology, Division of Maternal-Fetal Medicine, and Director, Division of Reproductive Imaging and Genetics, Jefferson Medical College of Thomas Jefferson University, Philadelphia, Pennsylvania, USA

Cathy Winter RCM
Specialist Midwife, Maternity Unit, Taunton & Somerset NHS Trust, Taunton, UK

Preface

It is 25 years since the first volume of *Progress in Obstetrics and Gynaecology* was published. It was an immediate success. Although a new volume appeared almost every year, Volume 1 was reprinted seven times until 1990. The contents remain relevant today: *The epidemiology of peri-natal loss, First trimester haemorrhage, Pre-eclampsia, Management of stage 1 cancer of the cervix, Management of stage 1 cancer of the ovaries, Hirsutism, Tubal microsurgery, Surgery of urinary incontinence* and two iconoclastic chapters on *Second thoughts on stopping labour* and *Second thoughts on routine monitoring of labour*. They could be written today.

However, it is time for a change. Although it has become one of the best selling annual publications in the English language with a truly international authorship, its influence in North America is insignificant. It is vital that we broaden the appeal of this series and continue to commission chapters from the senior stars in our specialty as well as ambitious, bright trainees. As my practice is entirely gynaecological with merely a remote memory of obstetrics, it seemed important that I share the editorship with two distinguished friends and colleagues. In future, the co-editors will be Professor Seang Lin Tan of McGill University, Montreal, and Professor Frank Chervenak at Cornell University, New York.

I am most grateful for their assistance in taking on this task with me. I have no doubt that the series will continue to be a major component of postgraduate training all over the English-speaking world. Who knows, the new editorship and format might even increase sales in North America! The present volume, number 17 demonstrates the exciting developments in our specialty with chapters ranging from: *Stem cell therapy, HIV in gynaecology, Fibroid embolisation, Intra-uterine surgery, Modern pelvic floor surgery, Fetal therapy, Doppler ultrasound and laparoscopic surgery*. None of these subjects were on the horizon 25 years ago.

It clearly is a very exciting period in medical developments which we should be able to capture in subsequent editions of *Progress in Obstetrics and Gynaecology*.

At the moment we have no policy concerning etiology or aetiology, estrogens or oestrogens, gynecology or gynaecology, or pg, or pmol/l but are content to have authors write in the style with which they feel comfortable. If the problems of the two nations separated by common language is no more controversial than medical terminology, there should be no great concern.

John Studd
June 2006

Frank A. Chervenak Laurence B. McCullough

Ethical issues in obstetric and gynaecological practice

Ethics have become an essential dimension of obstetrics and gynaecology.[1-3] In this chapter, we present a framework for clinical judgement and decision-making about the ethical dimensions of obstetric and gynaecological practice. We will emphasize a preventive ethics approach. Preventive ethics appreciates the potential for ethical conflict and adopts ethically justified strategies to prevent those conflicts from occurring. Preventive ethics helps to build and sustain a strong physician–patient relationship. We begin by defining ethics, medical ethics, and the fundamental ethical principles of medical ethics, beneficence and respect for autonomy. Second, we explain how these two principles should interact in gynaecological clinical judgement and practice. Third, we explain how these two principles should interact in obstetric judgement and practice, with emphasis on the core concept of the fetus as a patient.

DEFINITIONS

Medical ethics

The concept of ethics has been understood for centuries in global culture to be the disciplined study of morality. Medical ethics have been understood to be the disciplined study of morality in medicine. Medical ethics concern the obligations of physicians and healthcare organizations to patients as well as the obligations of patients.[4] It is important not to confuse medical ethics with

Frank A. Chervenak MD (for correspondence)
Given Foundation Professor and Chairman, Department of Obstetrics and Gynecology, Weill Medical College of Cornell University, The New York Presbyterian Hospital, 525 East 68th Street, M-7, New York, NY 10021, USA. E-mail: fac2001@med.cornell.edu

Laurence B. McCullough MD
Professor of Medicine and Medical Ethics, Center for Medical Ethics and Health Policy, Baylor College of Medicine, Houston, TX 77030, USA

the many sources of morality in modern pluralistic societies and global cultures. These include, but are not limited to, law, the world's religions, ethnic and cultural traditions, families, the traditions and practices of medicine (including medical education and training), and personal experience. Medical ethics since the 18th century European and American enlightenments has been secular.[5] By 'secular', we mean that medical ethics do not need to make reference to God or revealed tradition, but only to what rational discourse produces. As a result, ethical principles and virtues become accessible to all physicians, regardless of their personal religious and spiritual beliefs, and can be reliably applied in clinical practice in diverse global cultures.[6]

The traditions and practices of medicine constitute an important and enduring source of morality for physicians. These traditions and practices provide a reference point for medical ethics because they are based on the obligation to protect and promote the health-related interests of the patient. This obligation instructs physicians on what morality in medicine ought to be, but in very general, abstract terms. Providing a more concrete, clinically applicable account of physicians' obligations in clinical practice is a central task of medical ethics, using ethical principles.[4]

The medical ethical principle of beneficence

In general, the ethical principle of beneficence requires one to act in a way that is expected reliably to produce the greater balance of benefits over harms in the lives of others.[6] To put this ethical principle into clinical practice requires making it specific to clinical practice. Specifying the general ethical principle of beneficence requires a reliable account of the benefits and harms relevant to the care of the patient and of how those goods and harms should be reasonably balanced against each other when not all of them can be achieved in a particular clinical situation, such as a request for an elective caesarean delivery.[7] In medicine, the ethical principle of beneficence requires the physician to act in a way that is reliably expected to produce the greater balance of clinical benefits over harms for the patient.[4] Physicians have no special competence to address the many other benefits and harms that are of concern to human beings.

Beneficence-based clinical judgement has ancient roots, with its first expression found in the Hippocratic Oath and accompanying texts.[8] It makes an important claim to interpret reliably the health-related interests of the patient from medicine's perspective. This perspective is provided by accumulated scientific research, clinical experience, and reasoned clinical responses to uncertainty. This perspective should not be understood to be the function of an individual physician's clinical perspective and, therefore, should not be based merely on the clinical impression or intuition of an individual physician. Beneficence-based clinical judgement should be the function of a rigorous clinical perspective that appeals to the best available evidence and its clinical application to a particular case. Beneficence-based clinical judgement identifies the benefits that can be achieved for the patient in clinical practice based on the competencies of medicine. The benefits that medicine is competent to seek for patients are the prevention and management of disease, injury, handicap, and unnecessary pain and suffering and the prevention of premature or unnecessary death. Pain and suffering should be judged clinically unnecessary when they do not result in achieving the other goods of medical care, *e.g.* allowing a woman to labour without effective analgesia.[4]

Non-maleficence means that the physician should prevent causing harm and is best understood as expressing the limits of beneficence. This is commonly known as *Primum non nocere* or 'first do no harm'. This widely invoked dogma is really a Latinized misinterpretation of the Hippocratic texts which emphasized beneficence while avoiding harm when approaching the limits of medicine.[4] We caution that there is an inherent risk of paternalism in beneficence-based clinical judgement. By this we mean that beneficence-based clinical judgement, if it is mistakenly considered to be the sole source of moral responsibility and, therefore, moral authority in medical care, invites the unwary physician to conclude that beneficence-based judgements can be imposed on the patient in violation of her autonomy. Paternalism can be a dehumanizing response to the patient and, therefore, should be avoided in the practice of obstetrics and gynaecology.

The preventive ethics response to this inherent paternalism is for the physician to explain the diagnostic, therapeutic, and prognostic reasoning that leads to his or her clinical judgement about what is in the health-related interest of the patient so that the patient can assess that judgement for herself. In clinical practice, the physician should disclose and explain to the patient the major factors of this reasoning process, including matters of uncertainty. In neither medical law nor medical ethics does this require that the patient be provided with a complete medical education.[9] The physician should then explain how and why other clinicians might reasonably differ from his or her clinical judgement. The physician should then present a well-reasoned response to this critique. The outcome of this process is that beneficence-based clinical judgements take on a rigor that they sometimes lack, and the process of their formulation includes explaining them to the patient. Beneficence-based clinical judgement usually results in the identification of a continuum of clinical strategies that protect and promote the patient's health-related interests, such as the choice of preventing and managing the complications of menopause. Awareness of this feature of beneficence-based clinical judgement provides an important preventive ethics antidote to paternalism by increasing the likelihood that one or more of these medically reasonable, evidence-based alternatives will be acceptable to the patient.

One advantage for the physician in carrying out this approach to communicating with the patient would be, we believe, to increase the likelihood of compliance.[10] This is especially pertinent to gynaecological practice, where the patient often must monitor herself for clinical changes (*e.g.* a woman at risk for ectopic pregnancy) and take an active role in preventive medicine (*e.g.* breast self-examination) as well as to obstetric practice (*e.g.* self-observation for unusual weight gain or bleeding). Another advantage would be to provide the patient with a better-informed opportunity to make a decision about whether to seek a second opinion. This should make such a decision less threatening to her physician, who has already shared with the patient the limitations on clinical judgement.

The medical ethical principle of respect for autonomy

In contrast to the principle of beneficence, there has been increasing emphasis in the global literature of medical ethics on the principle of respect for autonomy.[6] This principle requires one always to acknowledge and carry out the value-based preferences of the adult, competent patient. Female and pregnant patients bring to their medical care their own perspectives on what is in their health-related and other interest. The principle of respect for autonomy translates this fact into autonomy-based clinical judgement. Because each patient's perspective on her interests is a function of her values and beliefs, it is impossible to specify the benefits and harms of autonomy-based clinical judgement in advance. It would be inappropriate for the physician to do so, because the definition of her benefits and harms and their balancing are the prerogative of the patient. Autonomy-based clinical judgement is strongly antipaternalistic in nature.[4]

To understand the ethical implications of this principle for clinical practice, we need an operationalized concept of autonomy. We, therefore, identify three sequential autonomy-based behaviours on the part of the patient: (i) absorbing and retaining information about her condition and alternative diagnostic and therapeutic responses to it; (ii) understanding that information (*i.e.* evaluating and rank-ordering those responses and appreciating that she could experience the risks of treatment); and (iii) expressing a value-based preference. The physician has a supportive role to play in each of these. They are, respectively: (i) to recognize the capacity of each patient to deal with medical information (and not to underestimate that capacity), provide information (*i.e.* disclose and explain all medically reasonable alternatives, supported in beneficence-based clinical judgement), and recognize the validity of the values and beliefs of the patient; (ii) not to interfere with but, when necessary, to assist the patient in her evaluation and ranking of diagnostic and therapeutic alternatives for managing her condition; and (iii) to elicit and implement the patient's value-based preference.[4]

In the common law of the US, legal obligations of the physician regarding informed consent were established in a series of cases during the 20th century. In 1914, Schloendorff v. The Society of The New York Hospital established the concept of simple consent, *i.e.* whether the patient says 'yes' or 'no' to medical intervention.[9,11] To this day in the medical and bioethics literature of the US, this decision is quoted: 'Every human being of adult years and sound mind has the right to determine what shall be done with his body, and a surgeon who performs an operation without his patient's consent commits an assault for which he is liable in damages'.[11] This principle of legal self-determination is not limited in its legal meaning and application to the US.

The legal requirement of consent further evolved to include disclosure of information sufficient to enable patients to make informed decisions about whether to say 'yes' or 'no' to medical intervention.[9] In the US, there are two legal standards for such disclosure. The professional community standard, adopted by the minority of states in the US, defines adequate disclosure in the context of what the relevantly trained and experienced physician tells patients. The reasonable person standard, which has been adopted by most states, goes further and requires the physician to disclose 'material' information, clinical information that any patient in the patient's condition needs to know and the lay person of average sophistication should not be expected to know.

This legal review has ethical significance because the reasonable person standard has emerged as the ethical standard, and we therefore urge obstetricians and gynaecologists to adopt it. On this ethical standard, the obstetrician, for example, should disclose to the patient her or the fetus's diagnosis (including differential diagnosis when that is all that is known), the medically reasonable alternatives to diagnose and manage the patient's condition, and the short-term and long-term benefits and risks of each alternative.

In the US, a particularly important dimension of informed consent in practice involves what have come to be known as 'advance directives'.[12] Spurred by the famous case of Karen Quinlan in New Jersey in 1976,[13] all states have enacted advance directive legislation.[14]

The basic clinical concept of an advance directive is that a patient, when autonomous, can make decisions regarding her medical management in advance of a time during which she becomes incapable of making healthcare decisions. The ethical dimensions of autonomy that are relevant here are the following:

1. A patient may exercise her autonomy in the present in the form of a request for, or refusal in the future of, life-prolonging interventions.

2. Autonomy-based requests for or refusals of treatment, expressed in the past and left unchanged, remain ethically authoritative for any future time during which the patient becomes non-autonomous.

3. Past autonomy-based requests or refusals should, therefore, translate into physicians' ethical obligations at the time the patient becomes unable to participate in the informed consent process.

4. Refusal of life-prolonging medical intervention should translate into the physicians' orders for the withholding or withdrawal of such interventions, including artificial nutrition and hydration.

The concept of a durable power of attorney or medical power of attorney is that any autonomous adult, in the event that that person later becomes unable to participate in the informed consent process, can assign decision-making authority to another person. The clinical advantage of the durable power of attorney for healthcare is that it applies only when the patient has lost decision-making capacity, as judged by her physician. Court review is not required. It does not, as does the living will or directive to physicians, also require that the patient be terminally or irreversibly ill. However, unlike the living will or directive to physicians, the durable power of attorney does not necessarily provide explicit direction, only the explicit assignment of decision-making authority to an identified individual or 'agent'. Obviously, any patient who assigns durable power of attorney for healthcare to someone else has an interest in communicating her values, beliefs, and preferences to that person. The physician can play a facilitating role in this process. Indeed, in order to respect the patient's autonomy, the physician should play an active role in encouraging this communication process so that there will be minimal doubt about whether the person holding durable power of attorney is faithfully representing the wishes of the patient.

The main clinical advantages of these two forms of advance directives are that they encourage patients to think carefully in advance about their request for or refusal of medical intervention and that these directives, therefore, help to prevent ethical conflicts and crises in the management especially of terminally or irreversibly ill patients who have decision-making capacity. Unfortunately, the use of advance directives in the US is not as wide-spread as it should be.[15] The reader is encouraged to think of advance directives as powerful, practical strategies for preventive ethics for end-of-life care and to encourage patients to consider them carefully, especially patients with gynaecological disease – particularly gynaecological cancers – that could become or are life-threatening.

BENEFICENCE AND RESPECT FOR AUTONOMY IN GYNAECOLOGICAL PRACTICE

Beneficence-based and autonomy-based clinical judgements in gynaecological practice are usually in harmony. For example, a woman may present with an ectopic pregnancy. The gynaecologist explains this diagnostic finding and the potential for maternal death and the unlikelihood of spontaneous resolution. In beneficence-based clinical judgement, evidence supports the clinical judgement that surgical management provides a clear-cut greater balance of clinical benefits over harms for the patient, whereas non-surgical management provides a clear-cut greater balance of clinical harms over benefits for the patient. Beneficence-based clinical judgement requires a careful explanation of these matters to the patient and supports a definitive recommendation for surgical management. Respect for the patient's autonomy also requires explanation of these matters but goes further and obligates the physician to elicit the patient's value-based priorities for the management of the newly diagnosed condition, which almost always coincide with beneficence-based clinical judgement. Synergy between beneficence and respect for autonomy occurs when the physician's clinical management plan is carried out in conjunction with the patient's informed consent.

Sometimes, beneficence-based and autonomy-based clinical judgements come into conflict in gynaecological practice. In such situations, neither beneficence nor respect for autonomy should be viewed as automatically over-riding the other. Instead, both principles should be understood as theoretically equally weighted. Thus, their differences must be negotiated in clinical judgement and practice. The competing demands of both principles must be balanced and negotiated in the specific clinical case to determine which management strategies protect and promote the patient's interests. In the technical language of ethics, medical ethical principles as *prima facie* or potentially over-ridable in nature.[4,6]

The process of negotiating conflict between medical ethical principles is a function of several factors involved in gynaecological clinical judgement: subject matter; probability of net clinical benefit; availability of reasonable alternatives; and the ability of the patient to participate in the informed consent process. When the subject matter is primarily technical in nature, such as the selection of an effective antibiotic regimen or intra-operative surgical technique, clinical judgement is justifiably beneficence-based. This is because technical matters largely concern the evidence-based benefits for the population of patients with a particular diagnosis and treatment plan. Such decisions are justifiably within the gynaecologist's purview. The individual values and beliefs of a particular patient cannot readily be taken into account in this process. By contrast, when the patient's basic values and beliefs are at stake, *e.g.* the work-up or treatment of infertility or elective abortion, clinical judgement is justifiably autonomy-based. This is because particular diagnostic or treatment interventions can directly and adversely affect the basic values and beliefs of a particular patient, a matter that only each individual patient can decide. Such decisions are justifiably within the patient's purview.

When the probability of net clinical benefit for the patient of diagnostic or therapeutic medical intervention is high, *e.g.* chemotherapy for some forms of gestational trophoblastic disease, or surgical correction of a prolapsed uterus, beneficence-based clinical judgement is dominant. This is because, in such circumstances, the net benefit is clear-cut. The gynaecologist is justified in recommending interventions that have a high probability of net clinical benefit. When that probability is low, *e.g.* experimental therapy for advanced ovarian malignancy or prophylactic oophorectomy at 40–45 years of age, clinical judgement is justifiably autonomy-based. This is because, when there is no clear-cut clinical benefit and significant risks of intervention exist, the female patient is in the best position to determine which trade-off makes the most sense. The gynaecologist is, therefore, justified in offering these alternatives but not in recommending one as indisputably the best.

When there is no reasonable alternative to manage the patient's condition (*e.g.* removal of a ruptured ectopic pregnancy or screening for cervical cancer by Pap smears), clinical judgement is appropriately beneficence-based: there is no other alternative that to any degree protects and promotes the health-related interests of the patient. The gynaecologist is, therefore, justified in strongly recommending the intervention in question. By contrast, when there are reasonable alternatives, such as surgery versus radiotherapy for stage 1A cervical cancer or a method of contraception versus tubal ligation, clinical judgement is appropriately autonomy-based. This is because reasonable alternatives all promote the patient's interests to a significant degree, and no one alternative can exclude any other as unreasonable. The gynaecologist is justified in presenting or offering the reasonable alternatives.

When the ability to implement the informed consent process is low, as for a patient with severe or profound mental retardation or in a life-threatening emergency without time for consent, clinical judgement is justifiably beneficence-based. It is impossible in such cases to identify the patient's relevant values and beliefs because of either significant irreversible cognitive impairment or urgent lack of time. The gynaecologist is, therefore, justified in basing clinical decision-making primarily on beneficence. By contrast, when the ability of the patient to participate in the informed consent process is not low, as in a speaker of a foreign language or the existence of a legally valid advance directive, then clinical judgement is justifiably autonomy-based. This is because the ability of the patient to participate in the informed consent process is presumed in the absence of compelling reasons to the contrary.

As a rule, the result of the informed consent process should be implemented. When the patient refuses to accept any of the alternatives supported in beneficence-based clinical judgement, the physician is ethically and, in the US legally, obligated to engage in what is known as 'informed refusal'. This legal and ethical obligation arises from the 1980 case of Truman v. Thomas from California.[9,16] Dr Thomas had delivered several of Mrs Truman's babies and, on the delivery of her last child, had recommended that she have a Pap smear. She refused to have this test until she could pay for it and did not accept Dr Thomas's offer to perform it without charge. Mrs Truman next presented to Dr Thomas with advanced cervical cancer, from which she died. In the malpractice action brought by her survivors, Dr Thomas stated that, although they were of clinical concern to him in the management of Mrs Truman, he did not tell Mrs Truman of the risks of having detectable presymptomatic changes in her cervix indicative of cervical cancer or that he was concerned that she could die from such disease. The California Supreme Court ruled that, because risks were of clinical salience to Dr Thomas – they were the motivation for his offering the Pap smear – he should have informed Mrs Thomas about these risks so that her refusal would be informed. This case changed practice and introduced the concept of informed refusal into medical law and ethics.

The ethical and legal obligation of the physician in the matter of informed refusal is very clear and not difficult to fulfil in clinical practice. The patient should be informed about the medical risks that she is taking in her refusal. The risks to be disclosed are those that are salient in clinical judgement: if they are important to the physician, that is, motivating the offering or recommending of the diagnostic test or therapy, they are salient. This discussion, especially the risks of refusal, should be thoroughly documented in the patient's chart. This is all that the law requires. Preventative ethics requires that this disclosure be followed by a recommendation that the patient reconsider her refusal. This preventive-ethics approach avoids the need to abandon the patient, keeps lines of communication open, and sends a powerful signal of concern by the physician to the patient about the medical folly of her refusal.

Patients sometimes demand clinically inappropriate management.[17] We suggest the following preventive ethics strategy in response:

1. Is the intervention reliably expected to have its intended, usual anatomical or physiological effect? If in reliable, evidence-based, beneficence-based clinical judgement it is not expected to do so, then the physician should not offer it. There is no obligation to offer or to perform medical interventions that are futile in this strict sense, such as providing a feeding tube for a patient with cancer cachexia.

2. Is the intervention reliably expected to have some minimal clinical benefit, defined as maintaining some minimal level of ability to interact with the environment and thus grow and develop as a human being? Is the patient in a persistent or permanent vegetative state? If, in reliable beneficence-based clinical judgement, it is not expected to do so, then the physician should offer the intervention and then recommend against it. We suggest this approach to respect a patient's or surrogate decision makers who are vitalists, *i.e.* who value the preservation of life at any cost. The physician should explain that this is not a value in medical ethics and never has been. Moreover, the intervention in question, whether it is initiated or continued, will just sustain a false hope of recovery.

3. If the patient or the patient's surrogate persists in the demand, then the physician should consult with colleagues and then the Ethics Committee, when one is available, which should have a clear policy on response to demands by patients or their surrogates for futile intervention.

BENEFICENCE AND RESPECT FOR AUTONOMY IN OBSTETRIC PRACTICE

The medical ethical principles of beneficence and respect for autonomy play a more complex role in obstetric clinical judgement and practice. There are obviously beneficence-based and autonomy-based obligations to the pregnant patient: the physician's perspective on the pregnant woman's health-related interests provides the basis for the physician's beneficence-based obligations to her, whereas her own perspective on those interests provides the basis for the physician's autonomy-based obligations to her. Because of an insufficiently developed central nervous system, the fetus cannot meaningfully be said to possess values and beliefs. There is, therefore, no basis for saying that a fetus has a perspective on its interests. There can, therefore, be no autonomy-based obligations to any fetus. This has a major implication: the language of fetal rights has no meaning and, therefore, no application to the fetus in obstetric clinical judgement and practice despite its popularity in public and political discourse in the US and other countries. Obviously, the physician has a perspective on the fetus's health-related interests, and the physician can have beneficence-based obligations to the fetus, but only when the fetus is a patient. Because of its importance for obstetric clinical judgement and practice, the ethical concept of the fetus as a patient requires detailed consideration.[4]

The ethical concept of the fetus as a patient

The ethical concept of the fetus as a patient is essential to obstetric clinical judgement and practice. Developments in fetal diagnosis and management strategies to optimize fetal outcome have become widely accepted in industrialised countries, encouraging the development of this concept. This concept has considerable clinical significance. When the fetus is a patient, directive counselling, that is, recommending a form of management, for fetal benefit is appropriate. When the fetus is not a patient, non-directive counselling, that is, offering but not recommending a form of management for fetal benefit, is appropriate. However, these apparently straightforward roles for directive and non-directive counselling are often difficult to apply in actual perinatal practice because of uncertainty about when the fetus is a patient.

One approach to resolving this uncertainty would be to argue that the fetus is or is not a patient in virtue of personhood, or some other form of independent moral status.

Independent moral status for the fetus means that one or more characteristics that the fetus possesses in and of itself and, therefore, independently of the pregnant woman or any other factor, generate and ground obligations to the fetus on the part of the pregnant woman and her physician. Many fetal characteristics have been nominated for this role, including moment of conception, implantation, central nervous system development, quickening, and the moment of birth. As a consequence, there has been considerable variation among ethical arguments about when the fetus acquires independent moral status. Some take the view that the fetus has independent moral status from the moment of conception or implantation. Others believe that independent moral status is acquired in degrees, thus resulting in 'graded' moral status. Still others hold, at least by implication, that the fetus never has independent moral status so long as it is *in utero*.[18,19]

There is a huge literature on this subject. However, there has been no closure on a single intellectually authoritative account of the independent moral status of the fetus. This is an unsurprising outcome because, given the absence of a single method that would be intellectually authoritative for all of the markedly diverse theological and philosophical schools of thought involved in this endless debate. To establish such an intellectual authority, debates about such a final authority within and between theological and philosophical traditions would have to be resolved in a way satisfactory to all, an inconceivable intellectual and cultural event. In its first sense, that of the independent moral status of the fetus, the fetus as a patient has no stable or clinically applicable meaning. We, therefore, abandon these futile attempts to understand the fetus as a patient in terms of independent moral status of the fetus and turn to an alternative approach that makes it possible to identify ethically distinct senses of the fetus as a patient and their clinical implications for directive and non-directive counselling.

Our explication of the ethical concept of the fetus as a patient begins with the recognition that being a patient does not require that one possess independent moral status. Rather, being a patient means that one can benefit from the applications of the clinical skills of the physician. A human being without independent moral status becomes a patient when two conditions are met: that a human being (i) is presented to the physician, and (ii) there exist clinical interventions that are reliably expected to be efficacious, in that they are reliably expected to result in a greater balance of clinical benefits over harms for the human being in question.[20] We call this the dependent moral status of the fetus.

The authors have argued elsewhere that beneficence-based obligations to the fetus exist when the fetus is reliably expected later to achieve independent moral status as a child and person.[4] That is, the fetus is a patient when the fetus is presented for clinical interventions, whether diagnostic or therapeutic, that reasonably can be expected to result in a greater balance of clinical goods over harms for the child and person the fetus can later become during early childhood. The ethical significance of the concept of the fetus as a patient, therefore, depends on links that can be established between the fetus and its later achieving independent moral status.

One such link is viability. Viability is not, however, an intrinsic property of the fetus because viability should be understood in terms of both biological and technological factors. Only by virtue of both factors is it the case that a viable fetus can exist *ex utero* and thus achieve independent moral status. Moreover, these two factors do not exist as a function of the autonomy of the pregnant woman. When a fetus is viable, that is, when it is of sufficient maturity to survive into the neonatal period and later achieve independent moral status given the availability of the requisite technological support, and when it is presented to the physician, the fetus is a patient.

Viability exists as a function of biomedical and technological capacities, which are different in different parts of the world. As a consequence, there is, at the present time, no world-wide, uniform gestational age to define viability. In the US and other industrialised countries, we believe, viability presently occurs at approximately 24 weeks of gestational age.[21]

When the fetus is a patient, directive counselling for fetal benefit is ethically justified. In clinical practice, directive counselling for fetal benefit involves one or more of the following: recommending against termination of pregnancy; recommending against non-aggressive management; or recommending aggressive management. Aggressive obstetric management includes interventions such as fetal surveillance, tocolysis, caesarean delivery, or delivery in a tertiary care centre when indicated. Non-aggressive obstetric management excludes such interventions. Directive counselling for fetal benefit, however, must take account of the presence and severity of fetal anomalies, extreme prematurity, and the obstetrician's beneficence-based an autonomy-based obligations to the pregnant woman.

In obstetric clinical judgement and practice, the strength of directive counselling for fetal benefit should vary according to the presence and severity of anomalies. As a rule, the more severe the fetal anomaly, the less directive counselling should be for fetal benefit. In particular, when lethal anomalies such as anencephaly can be diagnosed with certainty, there are no beneficence-based obligations to provide aggressive management. Such fetuses are dying patients, and the counselling, therefore, should be non-directive in recommending between non-aggressive management and termination of pregnancy, but directive in recommending against aggressive management for the sake of maternal benefit.[22] By contrast, third-trimester abortion for Down syndrome or achondroplasia is not ethically justifiable, because the future child with high probability will have the capacity to grow and develop as a human being.[23,24]

Directive counselling for fetal benefit in cases of extreme prematurity of viable fetuses is appropriate. In particular, this is the case for what we term just-viable fetuses, those with a gestational age of 24–26 weeks, for which there are significant rates of survival but high rates of mortality and morbidity. These rates of morbidity and mortality can be increased by non-aggressive obstetric management, whereas aggressive obstetric management may favourably influence outcome. Thus, it appears that there are substantial beneficence-based obligations to just-viable fetuses to provide aggressive obstetric management. This is all the more the case in pregnancies beyond 26 weeks of gestational age. Therefore, directive counselling for fetal benefit is justified in all cases of extreme prematurity of viable fetuses, considered by itself. Of course, such directive counselling is appropriate only when it is based on documented efficacy of aggressive obstetric management for each fetal indication. For example, such efficacy has not been demonstrated for routine caesarean delivery to manage extreme prematurity.

Directive counselling for fetal benefit should always occur in the context of balancing beneficence-based obligations to the fetus against beneficence-based and autonomy-based obligations to the pregnant woman. Any such balancing must recognize that a pregnant woman is obligated only to take reasonable risks of medical interventions that are reliably expected to benefit the viable fetus or child later. A unique feature of obstetric ethics is that the pregnant woman's autonomy influences whether, in a particular case, the viable fetus ought to be regarded as presented to the physician.

Obviously, any strategy for directive counselling for fetal benefit that takes account of obligations to the pregnant woman should be attentive to the possibility of conflict between the physician's recommendation and a pregnant woman's autonomous decision to the contrary. Such conflict is best managed preventively through the informed consent process as an on-going dialogue throughout a woman's pregnancy, augmented as necessary by negotiation and respectful persuasion.[25]

The only possible link between the previable fetus and the child it can become is the pregnant woman's autonomy, simply because technological factors cannot result in the previable fetus becoming a child. The link, therefore, between a fetus and the child it can become when the fetus is previable can be established only by the pregnant woman's decision to confer the status of being a patient on her previable fetus. The previable fetus, therefore, has no claim to the status of being a patient independently of the pregnant woman's autonomy. The pregnant woman is free to withhold, confer, or, having once conferred, withdraw the status of being a patient on or from her previable fetus according to her own values and beliefs. The previable fetus is presented to the physician as a function of the pregnant woman's autonomy.[4]

Counselling the pregnant woman regarding the management of her pregnancy when the fetus is previable should be non-directive in terms of continuing the pregnancy or having an abortion if she refuses to confer the status of being a patient on her fetus. If she does confer such status in a settled way, at that point beneficence-based obligations to her fetus come into existence, and directive counselling for fetal benefit becomes appropriate for these previable fetuses. Just as for viable fetuses, such counselling must take account of the presence and severity of fetal anomalies, extreme prematurity, and obligations owed to the pregnant woman.

For pregnancies in which the woman is uncertain about whether to confer such status, the authors propose that the fetus be provisionally regarded as a patient. This justifies directive counselling against behaviour that can harm a fetus in significant and irreversible ways, *e.g.* substance abuse, especially alcohol, until the woman settles on whether to confer the status of being a patient on the fetus.

Non-directive counselling is also appropriate in cases of what we term near-viable fetuses, that is, those that are 22–23 weeks of gestational age, for which there are anecdotal reports of survival. In our view, aggressive obstetric and neonatal management should be regarded as clinical investigation (*i.e.* a form of medical experimentation), not a standard of care. There is no obligation on the part of a pregnant woman to confer the status of being a patient on a near-viable fetus because the efficacy of aggressive obstetric and neonatal management has yet to be proven.

A subset of previable fetuses as patients concerns the *in vitro* embryo. It might seem that the *in vitro* embryo is a patient because such an embryo is surely presented to the physician. However, for beneficence-based obligations to a human being to exist, medical interventions must be reliably expected to be efficacious. In terms of beneficence, whether the fetus is a patient depends on links that can be established between the fetus and its eventual independent moral status. The reasonableness of medical interventions on the *in vitro* embryo, therefore, depends on whether that embryo later becomes viable. Otherwise, no benefit of such intervention can meaningfully be said to result. An *in vitro* embryo, therefore, becomes viable only when it survives *in vitro* cell division, transfer, implantation, and subsequent gestation to such a time that it becomes viable. The process of achieving viability occurs only *in vivo* and is, therefore, entirely dependent on the woman's decision regarding the status of the fetus(es) as a patient, should assisted conception successfully result in the gestation of the previable fetus(es). Whether an *in vitro* embryo will become a viable fetus, and whether medical intervention on such an embryo will benefit the fetus, are both functions of the pregnant woman's autonomous decision to withhold, confer, or, having once conferred, withdraw the moral status of being a patient on the previable fetus(es) that might result from assisted conception.

It is, therefore, appropriate to regard the *in vitro* embryo as a previable fetus rather than as a viable fetus. As a consequence, any *in vitro* embryo(s) should be regarded as a patient only when the woman into whose reproductive tract the embryo(s) will be transferred confers that status. Thus, counselling about pre-implantation diagnosis should be non-directive. Pre-implantation diagnostic counselling should be non-directive because the woman may elect not to implant abnormal embryos. These embryos are not patients, and so there is no basis for directive counselling. Information should be presented about prognosis for a successful pregnancy and the possibility of confronting a decision about selective reduction, depending on the number of embryos transferred. Counselling about how many *in vitro* embryos should be transferred should be rigorously evidence-based.[26]

CONCLUSIONS

In this chapter, we have provided an ethical framework for both gynaecological and obstetric clinical judgement and practice. Implementing this ethical framework in daily clinical practice is essential to creating and sustaining the physician–patient relationship in obstetrics and gynaecology. This ethical framework emphasizes preventive ethics, *i.e.* an appreciation that the potential for ethical conflict is built into clinical practice and the use of such clinical tools as informed consent and negotiation to prevent such conflict from occurring.

References

1 American College of Obstetricians and Gynecologists. Ethics in Obstetrics and Gynecology. Washington, DC: ACOG, 2002
2 Association of Professors of Gynecology and Obstetrics. Exploring medical-legal issues in Obstetrics and Gynecology. Washington, DC: APGO Medical Education Foundation, 1994
3 FIGO Committee for the Study of Ethical Aspects of Human Reproduction. Recommendations of Ethical Issues in Obstetrics and Gynecology. London:. International Federation of Gynecology and Obstetrics, 1997

TU05429

4 McCullough LB, Chervenak FA. Ethics in obstetrics and gynecology. New York: Oxford University Press, 1994

5 Engelhardt Jr HT. The foundations of bioethics, 2nd edn. New York: Oxford University Press, 1995

6 Beauchamp TL, Childress JF. Principles of biomedical ethics, 5th edn. New York: Oxford University Press, 2001

7 Chervenak FA, McCullough LB. An ethically justified algorithm for offering, recommending, and performing cesarean delivery and its application in managed care practice. Obstet Gynecol 1996; 87: 302–305

8 Hippocrates. Oath of Hippocrates. In Temkin O, Temkin CL. (eds) Ancient Medicine: Selected Papers of Ludwig Edelstein. Baltimore: Johns Hopkins University Press, 1976, 6

9 Faden RR, Beauchamp TL. A History and Theory of Informed Consent. New York: Oxford University Press, 1986

10 Wear S. Informed Consent: Patient Autonomy and Clinician Beneficence within Health Care, 2nd edn. Washington, DC: Georgetown University Press, 1998

11 Schloendorff v. The Society of The New York Hospital, 211 N.Y. 125, 126, 105 N.E. 92, 93, 1914

12 Lynn J, Teno JM. Death and dying: euthanasia and sustaining life: III. advance directives. In Reich WT. (ed) Encyclopedia of Bioethics, 2nd edn. New York: Macmillan, 1995, 572–577

13 In re Quinlan 355 A.2d 647 (1976), cert. denied sub nom

14 Meisel L. The Right to Die, 2nd edn. New York: John Wiley, 1995

15 SUPPORT Investigators. A controlled trial to improve care for seriously ill hospitalized patients. JAMA 1995; 274: 1591–1598

16 Truman v. Thomas 611 P.2d 902 (Cal. 1980)

17 Brett A, McCullough LB. When patients request specific interventions: defining the limits of the physician's obligations. N Engl J Med 1986; 315: 1347–1351

18 Callahan S, Callahan D. (eds) Abortion: Understanding differences. New York: Plenum, 1984

19 Annas GJ. Protecting the liberty of pregnant patient. N Engl J Med 1988; 316: 1213–1214

20 Chervenak FA, McCullough LB. Ethics in obstetrics and gynecology: an overview. Eur J Obstet Gynecol Reprod Med 1997; 75: 91–94

21 Chervenak FA, McCullough LB. The limits of viability. J Perinat Med 1997; 25: 418–420

22 Chervenak FA, McCullough LB. An ethically justified, clinically comprehensive management strategy for third-trimester pregnancies complicated by fetal anomalies. Obstet Gynecol 1990; 75: 311–316

23 Chervenak FA, McCullough LB, Campbell S. Is third trimester abortion justified? Br J Obstet Gynaecol 1995; 102: 434–435

24 Chervenak FA, McCullough LB, Campbell S. Third trimester abortion: is compassion enough? Br J Obstet Gynaecol 1999; 106: 293–296

25. Chervenak FA, McCullough LB. Clinical guides to preventing ethical conflicts between pregnant women and their physicians. Am J Obstet Gynecol 1990; 162: 303–307

26 Chervenak FA, McCullough LB, Rosenwaks Z. Ethical dimensions of the number of embryos to be transferred in *in vitro* fertilization. J Assist Reprod Genet 2001; 18: 583–587

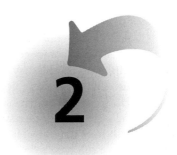

Jerry Chan   Keelin O'Donoghue   Nicholas M. Fisk

Developmental stem cell therapy

Stem cells are rare, primitive cells which can be defined by their capacity to self renew as well as to differentiate into one or more mature cell types. The archetypal example of a stem cell is the haemopoietic stem cell (HSC), which can divide to reproduce itself as daughter HSC and/or differentiate to form mature erythrocytes, leukocytes and platelets. Even though stem cells exist in the developing fetus, most of the current public and political spotlight is on embryonic stem (ES) cells or adult stem cells. However, fetal stem cells such as HSC found in umbilical cord blood, have been used clinically over the past 15 years to good effect[1] and transplantation of fetal mesencephalic tissue has resulted in clinical improvement in Parkinson disease.[2]

Totipotency, pluripotency and multipotency

Stem cells can be classified according to their differentiation potential. Totipotent cells have the ability to form all the cell types of the fetus and the placenta, and hence the entire organism. Cells which have this capacity are restricted to the zygote and its first few divisions. Pluripotent stem cells have the ability to form all the different cell types from the three germ layers – ectoderm, mesoderm and

Jerry Chan MB BCh BaO MA MRCOG (for correspondence)
Assistant Professor, Department of Obstetrics and Gynaecology, National University of Singapore and National University Hospital, 5 Lower Kent Ridge Road, Singapore 119074
E-mail: jerrychan@nus.edu.sg

Keelin O'Donoghue PhD MRCOG
Experimental Fetal Medicine Group, Institute of Reproductive and Developmental Biology, Division of Surgery, Oncology, Reproductive Biology & Anaesthesia, Imperial College London and Centre for Fetal Care, Queen Charlotte's and Chelsea Hospital, Du Cane Road, London W12 0NN, UK

Nicholas M. Fisk PhD FRCOG
Experimental Fetal Medicine Group, Institute of Reproductive and Developmental Biology, Division of Surgery, Oncology, Reproductive Biology & Anaesthesia, Imperial College London and Centre for Fetal Care, Queen Charlotte's and Chelsea Hospital, Du Cane Road, London W12 0NN, UK

endoderm – but not trophoblast cells. Examples include embryonic stem (ES) cells, embryonic germ (EG) cells[3] and embryonic carcinoma (EC) cells.[4] Multipotent cells have a more restricted ability to form only a few lineages, usually within one germ layer. Stem cells which fulfil this criteria include HSC,[5] neural and mesenchymal stem cells (NSC and MSC).[6,7] Though these cells are developmentally more restricted than ES cells, recent reports suggest that they may be able to cross canonical lineage boundaries and differentiate into a cell type from another germ layer.[8]

In this review, we discuss the range of stem cells found in the early embryo and throughout fetal development, their basic biology and potential therapeutic applications.

EMBRYONIC STEM CELLS

Embryonic stem (ES) cells were first isolated from the inner cell mass of pre-implantation murine embryos[9] in 1981 and, more recently, from the inner cell mass of human blastocysts derived from surplus *in-vitro fertilisation* (IVF) embryos.[10] ES cells fulfil the criteria of being a stem cell in the strictest sense: (i) they are clonogenic and undergo cell division symmetrically to form two identical daughter cells; and (ii) they can undergo asymmetrical division to form one daughter cell and cells which represent more differentiated derivatives of the primitive germ layers (ectoderm, mesoderm and endoderm). In addition, ES cells can differentiate into all three embryonic germ layers *in vitro* and contribute to chimera formation when injected into developing blastocysts.[11] ES cells can be expanded for over 300 population doublings without any evidence of senescence or ageing in culture, thereby escaping the Hayflick phenomenon[12] characteristic of non-stem cell types like fibroblasts. They express telomerase, an enzyme involved in the maintenance of telomere length at the end of chromosomes, believed to contribute to their level of immortality in culture, and maintain a stable karyotype in long-term culture. ES cells can also be characterised by their expression of 'embryonic markers' such as glycolipids and glycoprotein surface markers SSEA-3, SSEA-4, TRA-1-60 and TRA-1-81, originally identified on EG and EC cells. They express some antigens which are found on other stem cells such as CD133, CD117, CD135 (flt3) and CD9. They also express a range of transcription factors Oct-3/4 and their target genes Nanog and Rex-1. While EG and EC cells share some of these characteristics, they often have chromosomal abnormalities, and thus cannot be used clinically.

Therapeutic applications of ES cells

The potential of ES cells to form the 200 or so different cell types of the human body holds far reaching applications in the field of regenerative medicine. During evolution, the ability of higher vertebrates to regenerate tissues has become far more restricted than, for example, the intriguingly self-reparative flatworm or salamander. Hence, the promise of producing large quantities of specialised cell types from ES cells to treat degenerative diseases such as cardiac failure, Parkinson disease and diabetes has received considerable attention. Already, human ES cells have been coaxed to differentiate into cardiomyocytes,[13] neural stem cells,[14] insulin-producing cells,[15] and even germ cells,[16] all of which are applicable to common degenerative diseases without effective cures. However, before these cells can be used clinically, several issues need to be addressed.

Safety concerns

One of the main limitations with use of ES cells is their potential to form teratomas after transplantation. Indeed, some have argued that the ability to form tumours *in vivo* is an intrinsic property of ES cells. The essence of avoiding this complication will be manipulating ES cells to produce pure differentiated cells, uncontaminated by undifferentiated ES cells.

Another safety concern arises from the fact that most human ES cell lines have been derived using murine fibroblast feeder layers to sustain their proliferation. Such direct contact with mouse cells runs the risk of transfer of xenopathogens and excludes these cells from being used clinically. Strategies being addressed to overcome this include the use of human feeders and serum[17] and even feeder and serum-free conditions.[18,19]

Immunological barriers

The biggest hurdle to clinical use remains the risk of immune rejection of transplanted allogeneic cells. Rejection is mediated by class I major histocompatibility complex (MHC) antigens and by antigen presenting cells (APC) harbouring class II MHC antigens. This is supplemented by other immune defences including innate natural killer (NK) cell activity. ES cells typically express low levels of MHC class I, which increase during differentiation, while MHC class II antigens are not expressed in either differentiated or undifferentiated states.[20] Strategies to overcome this include the generation of large MHC homozygous ES cell banks, and the production of patient-specific ES cells via somatic cell nuclear transfer (SCNT), otherwise known as therapeutic cloning.

Therapeutic cloning and reproductive cloning

SCNT refers to the introduction of a nucleus from a mature differentiated somatic cell, such as a dermal fibroblast, into an enucleated ooctye. After electrofusion is performed, the ooctye cytoplasm reprogrammes the somatic nucleus back into its most undifferentiated state akin to a recently fertilised egg. This cloned embryo could then be grown in culture to blastocyst stage, when ES cells could be derived from the inner cell mass (ICM; Fig. 1). These ES cells would have identical nuclear genetic material to the donor, and thus would not be rejected. While this approach has been used in mice and cattle for some time, it is only recently that a Korean team has shown has shown that it can also be performed successfully in humans.[21] Two of the 11 lines generated were from a baby with congenital immune deficiency and a child with juvenile onset diabetes, respectively. This raises the exciting therapeutic possibility of correcting any genetic abnormality, by generating cell types for patient-specific treatment without rejection or the need for immunosuppression. Clearly, this strategy will need rigorous testing in animal models before translation into clinical practice. Yet, already the combination of gene therapy and SCNT strategies has been successfully applied to mice with immune deficiencies[22] and Parkinson disease.[23]

Therapeutic cloning should be distinguished from reproductive cloning, which is the generation of a cloned embryo via SCNT with the purpose of implanting it into a womb to generate a genetically-identical offspring (Fig. 1). This process is inefficient (< 4% success rates)[24] and is associated with numerous abnormalities in the offspring,[25,26] secondary to epigenetic errors created during SCNT.[27] Reproductive cloning, as opposed to therapeutic cloning,[28] is widely deemed unacceptable[29] by both the scientific community as well governments and the lay public.

Because current human ES cell lines are derived from left-over embryos, ES research has proved a hot-bed of ethical, political and religious contention from which varying legal restrictions have been imposed in different countries. For example, in the US, Federal funds can only be used for work on the 21 ES cell lines generated before 9 August 2001. Its suspect ethical and intellectual gymnastics apart, this decision substantially retards ES cell research in the world's leading biotechnology nation and, in particular, impedes therapeutic progress because these lines are contaminated by murine proteins. As a result, several groups have obviated this by obtaining private funding to generate new ES lines,[30] essential both for advancing understanding of ES cell biology and for developing clinical applications.

ES cells as a model for developmental biology

ES cells also represent a tremendous resource for studying embryonic events such as gastrulation and early embryonic differentiation, which was not previously possible in humans. In particular, the availability of ES cells from pre-implantation embryos with specific genetic diseases provides a developmental model for understanding their pathogenesis.[31]

However, the availability of surplus IVF embryos is limited and, accordingly, other methods of generating ES cells are required, such as deriving oocytes via directed differentiation of ES cells themselves, which would then be amenable for SCNT.[32] The surprising recent finding, that bone marrow cells may contribute to ooctye formation, raises the possibility of generating oocytes in a less ethically contentious manner.[33]

FETAL STEM CELLS

Haemopoietic stem cells

HSC are found in abundance during embryonic and fetal life and originate from haemangioblasts in the yolk sac and the aorto-gonado-mesonephros (AGM) region of the fetus.[34] These cells are characterised by their expression of CD34 and absence of any blood lineage markers such as CD38. They cycle slowly, differentiate down both myeloid and lymphoid lineages *in vitro*, and can repopulate the entire haemopoietic system when transplanted into xenogeneic recipients.[35]

First trimester fetal blood contains more CD34[+] cells than umbilical cord blood. These also have longer telomeres[36] and proliferate faster, producing colonies consisting of all haemopoietic lineages: CFU-GEMM, CFU-GM, CFU-ML, BFU-ML and BFU-e.[37] HSC frequency peaks during the second trimester

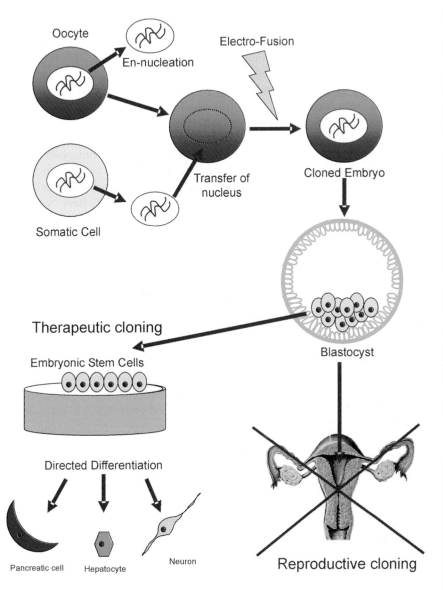

Fig. 1 Somatic cell nuclear transfer (SCNT) involves the transfer of a nucleus taken from a somatic cell such as a dermal fibroblast, and transferring it into an enucleated ooctye. Following electro-fusion, the cloned embryo progresses into a blastocyst within an *in-vitro* culture system. In therapeutic cloning, the inner cell mass of the blastocyst is harvested to generate ES cells which are genetically identical to the donor. These ES cells can then be expanded and differentiated into specialised cells for donor-specific cell replacement therapy. In reproductive cloning, the blastocyst is replaced into a primed uterus with the aim of producing a whole new organism with identical genetic make up as that of the donor; this is proscribed in most jurisdictions.

and gradually declines through the third trimester. This increase from first to second trimester is probably due to cells migrating from the fetal liver to establish haemopoiesis in the bone marrow, with the hepatic contribution declining on establishment of marrow haemopoiesis.[38] Among products of conception, fetal liver is an easily accessible source of HSC, but is compromised by the relatively small number of cells available and by their limited ability to expand in culture. A recent report, however, demonstrates *in vitro* generation of adequate numbers of fetal liver HSC for transplantation without affecting their lymphomyeloid repopulation potential.[39] Fetal HSC have a higher cloning efficiency and generate more progenitors than adult bone marrow (BM) HSC[40] and differ in both expression and activation of molecules involved in signal transduction and activation of other haemopoietic populations.[41] Fetal cells have a huge competitive engraftment advantage relative to adult BM in both fetal and adult recipients.[35,42,43] They also produce larger numbers and types of progeny after transplantation in mice than adult BM HSC. Moreover, only fetal HSC can repopulate a secondary recipient, demonstrating the utility of ontologically more primitive cells in cell transplantation therapy.[44] Already, fetal liver HSC have been used to treat human fetuses diagnosed with X-linked severe immune deficiency syndrome (SCID-X), leading to reconstitution of the immune system.[45,46]

Mesenchymal stem cells

MSC were first described by Friedenstein *et al.*[47] in 1968 who observed that non-haemopoietic cells which adhered to plastic could be isolated from bone marrow, but were not fully characterised until 1999 where strict culture techniques demonstrated their multilineage potential and ability to expand in culture.[7] Human fetal MSC (hfMSC) were first described by our group[48] in first trimester fetal blood, liver and bone marrow. In the presence of serum, these cells adhere to plastic and grow as spindle-shaped fibroblastic cells similar to adult BM MSC. They are non-haemopoietic, non-endothelial – consistently CD45$^-$, CD34$^-$, CD14$^-$ CD31$^-$ and vWF negative and express a number of adhesion molecules including CD44, VCAM-1 (CD106) and β_1-integrin (CD29). In their undifferentiated state, hfMSC stain positive for fibronectin, laminin, vimentin and mesenchymal markers such as SH2, SH3 and SH4. They demonstrate tremendous expansive capacity, and cycle faster than comparable adult BM-derived MSC, having a doubling time of 24–30 h over 20 passages (50 population doublings) without differentiating.[48,49] Like their adult counterparts, hfMSC possess the ability to differentiate into at least three different mesenchymal tissues – fat, bone and cartilage. More recent work demonstrates that skeletal muscle differentiation,[50] neuro-ectodermal differentiation into neurons and oligodendrocytes[51] and endodermal differentiation into hepatocytes and blood[52] may be possible (Fig. 2).

hfMSC are present in the fetal circulation from early gestation and then progressively decline in frequency in fetal blood during the late first trimester, suggesting that they may play an important role in establishing first trimester haemopoiesis.[48] Their presence before initiation of bone marrow haemopoiesis, their ability to support haemopoiesis in co-culture, and their decline in frequency as haemopoiesis is established is consistent with the hypothesis that fetal MSC are migrating to the definitive site of haemopoiesis in the bone marrow where they adhere, in preparation for HSC engraftment and haemopoiesis.[53] Other sources of fetal MSC have now been identified in a wide anatomical distribution including amniotic fluid,[54,55] pancreas,[56] lung[57] and kidney.[58] While demonstrating similar properties, they differ somewhat in their replicative and differentiation capacity, and in expression of various extracellular matrix proteins and cytokines, suggesting they have different roles depending on the organ of origin.[59,60]

hfMSC have intermediate levels of HLA class I antigens and do not express class II antigens. Like their adult counterparts, they do not elicit alloreactive T-cell proliferative responses to adult donors and inhibit mitogen-induced lymphocyte proliferation.[49,61] Thus, hfMSC possess at least the same degree, if not more, of immunomodulatory advantage as adult MSC[62] and, because of their higher proliferative and differentiative potential, should have significant advantages over adult sources of cells for transplantation and therapy.

Neural stem cells

Neural stem cells (NSC) have been found in many areas of the fetal brain[63] as well as the hippocampus and subventricular zone in the adult central nervous system (CNS).[64] Fetal NSC have the ability to self renew and differentiate into the three predominant cell types of the CNS – neurons, astrocytes and oligodendrocytes. When transplanted into immunodeficient newborn mice, they show engraftment, migration and site-specific neuronal differentiation up to 7 months later.[65] Adult NSC, on the other hand, are more difficult to isolate, are found in smaller numbers, and have a more limited proliferative and differentiation capacity.

Fetal neural tissue is one of the main sources of cells for replacement therapy in degenerative CNS injury. Preclinical rodent models demonstrated fetal graft survival and improvement of function after injury, while experience already exists with human fetal neural tissue transfer in patients with Parkinson disease. These grafts, were able to re-innervate the striatum, restore dopamine release and give symptomatic relief. However, a significant number of patients experienced unacceptable dyskinesia.[2] Also, there are problems with harvesting enough fetal tissue for transplantation, which requires multiple donors. One solution might be the large-scale expansion of NSC and transplantation after directed differentiation into dopaminergic neurons.

Potential applications of fetal stem cells

The potential applications of fetal stem cells are vast, and here we will consider those of relevance to fetal medicine.

Non-invasive prenatal diagnosis

It is well known that fetal stem cells traffic across the placenta into the maternal bloodstream during pregnancy, and this raises the possibility of isolating these cells for non-invasive prenatal diagnosis. Progress in this area had been hampered by the lack of a cell type unique to fetal blood, and the low frequency of fetal cells crossing into the maternal circulation.[66] Isolation of fetal haemopoietic progenitors by selecting an antigen predominantly expressed in the fetus, such as CD71, has been successfully demonstrated, but they are difficult to distinguish from maternal cells and most groups have been unable to expand such fetal cells sufficient for clinical use.[67,68]

We evaluated hfMSC as a target for non-invasive prenatal diagnosis, as they circulate in first trimester fetal blood and have no counterpart in maternal blood. Enrichment for fetal cells in maternal blood was performed via depletion of maternal blood cells and hfMSC successfully grown to produce a pure source of cells for pre-natal diagnosis.[69] Although we established the highest sensitivity of any candidate cell type reported in model mixtures, we were unable to isolate MSC in intact pregnancies, and could find hfMSC in maternal blood in only 1 of 20 pregnancies evaluated after a clinical paradigm of fetomaternal haemorrhage. Hence, stem cell approaches to non invasive prenatal diagnosis are unlikely to be used clinically.[69]

Microchimerism

The apparent low frequency of hfMSC circulating in maternal blood can be explained by rapid engraftment of these cells into maternal tissues, such as bone marrow. Expression of cell-adhesion molecules and the lack of expression of HLA II antigens suggest that hfMSC engraft and persist in maternal tissues. We recently identified male hfMSC in post-reproductive female bone marrow up to 50 years after the index pregnancy in a group of women who had sons.[70] This is the first report of a particular fetal cell type being implicated in microchimerism, a condition which has been implicated in autoimmune diseases through graft-versus-host like responses.[71]

Intra-uterine transplantation

Intra-uterine stem cell transplantation is a novel approach in the treatment of several genetic diseases. An intra-uterine approach has several potential advantages over a post-natal approach. First, stem cells may be delivered in time to prevent irreversible end-organ damage. Second, it obviates the considerable treatment-associated morbidity of postnatal bone marrow transplantation. Third, the fetal environment is highly conducive to expansion of stem cell compartments; indeed large-scale migration of stem cells occurs naturally only in fetal life. Fourth, there is a huge stoichiometric advantage – the human fetus is only about 30 g in size at 13 weeks, allowing delivery of proportionately more cells than can be given postnatally. Next, fetal cells have a competitive engraftment advantage over adult cells.[35,72] Finally, the immunological naiveté of the early gestation fetus produces tolerance to foreign antigens if presented before a critical window, around 12–14 weeks' gestation.[73]

Intra-uterine transplantation has only been evaluated in the mid-trimester using HSC with the rare successes limited to immunodeficient fetuses.[46,74,75] This might be due to inadequate cell dose or, more likely, transplantation during the second trimester, when the fetus acquires the ability to reject allogeneic cells. In contrast, MSC have immunomodulatory activities, they engraft widely after intra-uterine transplantation in animal models regardless of gestational age or immune competence at transplantation.[76] Similarly, hfMSC engraft into multiple organ compartments after intra-uterine transplantation into fetal sheep with evidence of site-specific differentiation.[52] Recently, hfMSC have been used for transplantation in a fetus with osteogenesis imperfecta, resulting in long-term chimerism in the bone and bone marrow, and a lack of alloreactivity to donor MSC.[77] Although further reports are awaited regarding the clinical progress of this child, this case report indicates proof of principle for intra-uterine hfMSC transplantation approaches.

Gene therapy

Stem cells have considerable utility as targets for gene therapy because they can self renew, thus precluding the need for repeated administration of the gene vector. *Ex vivo* gene therapy uses autologous stem cells which are then transduced by an integrating vector before re-infusion back into the patient. While this approach has already been validated in post-natal clinical trials with HSC,[78–80] the occurrence of leukaemia in 3 of 11 children treated in the French trial from insertion of the transgene near a proto-oncogene has raised serious concerns about such an approach.[81] Several strategies are being investigated to

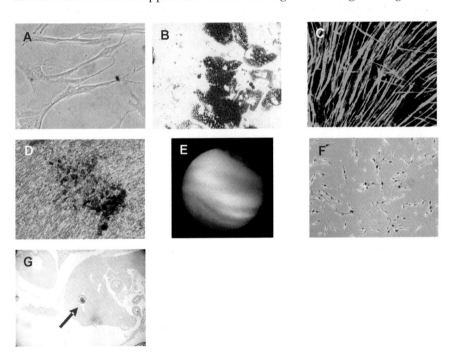

Fig. 2 Human fetal mesenchymal stem cells (hfMSC) grow as spindle shaped cells in culture (A) and can differentiate down multiple lineages such as adipocytes (B – oil-red O staining, x10), muscle (C – desmin immunostaining in green, x10) and osteoblasts (D – von Kossa staining of extracellular calcium, x10). These cells may be harvested from the umbilical vein in the first trimester of pregnancy via high-resolution ultrasound-guided or fetoscopic (E – umbilical vessels of a 12-week fetus via a 1-mm fibre-optic endoscope) approaches. They are readily transducible with integrating vectors (X-Gal staining of hfMSC transduced with a lentivirus containing a nuclear localising *LacZ* transgene, x10) and thus seem useful for *ex-vivo* gene therapy followed by re-infusion back into the fetus (G – human vimentin staining [brown] revealing a ball of human cells [red arrow] within the liver of a fetal mouse 2 days after intraperitoneal delivery of hfMSC, x4).

reduce this risk, such as the use of insertional site screening prior to re-infusion, the use of safer and/or site-specific vectors and the use of regulatable vectors which could be switched off should an adverse event arise.[81] The use of hfMSC as vehicles for gene delivery would be applicable to a number of diseases such as osteogenesis imperfecta, the muscular dystrophies and various enzyme deficiency syndromes. hfMSC are readily transduced with integrating vectors without affecting their stem cell properties of self renewal and multilineage differentiation (Fig. 2).[82] Transduced hfMSC can be clonally expanded and work is now underway clonally to select those where integration occurred at 'safe' regions of the human genome, in order to minimise the risk of any oncogenic event.

Collection of autologous stem cells in ongoing pregnancies

The development of autologous gene therapy necessitates collection of stem cells in on-going pregnancies. While the harvest of fetal bone marrow or brain is unlikely ever to be feasible in continuing pregnancies, the harvest of fetal liver has been reported in fetal sheep, albeit with significant morbidity and mortality.[83] Fetal blood is also amenable for collection, as hfMSC are found in the circulation between 7–14 weeks of gestation.[48] Relatively safe techniques for assessing the fetal circulation have been developed over the last two decades for fetal diagnosis and therapy after 16 weeks, with a fetal loss rate of about 1%. Prior to this, procedures are limited by the small size of fetal vessels, with the umbilical vein, for instance, measuring only 2 mm at 12 weeks' gestation. Nevertheless, one group has applied ultrasound-guided fetal blood samplings in on-going pregnancies at risk of haemoglobinopathies with a loss rate of only 5% at gestations as early as 12 weeks.[84] More recently, thin gauge embryo-fetoscopes have become available that may also allow early fetal blood sampling from the umbilical vessels under direct visualisation (Fig. 2).

UMBILICAL CORD BLOOD STEM CELLS

The same two major populations of stem cells found in early fetal blood are also harvestable from umbilical cord blood (UCB). HSC from cord blood has been used clinically for over a decade, now while UCB-derived MSC have recently been characterised.

Mesenchymal stem cells

The frequency of MSC in UCB is far lower than that found in first trimester fetal blood or in the bone marrow.[48] As such, their presence has only recently been unequivocally demonstrated using new culture methods with high volumes of UCB and additional cytokines to stimulate cell proliferation.[85,86] However, even with these culture techniques, UCB-MSC were isolated in less than a third of samples collected. Thus, culture techniques need to be improved considerably before their clinical value can be realised.

Haemopoietic stem cells

Umbilical cord blood is a rich source of HSC and progenitor cells, and used extensively as an alternative to BM and peripheral blood stem cells for transplantation in situations of marrow failure, malignancy and genetic disease.[87] Since the first successful umbilical cord blood transplantation (UCBT) of a child with Fanconi anaemia from a HLA-identical sibling in 1989, more than 3700 children and adult patients have undergone UCBT from unrelated donors, with more than 200,000 units of cord blood banked, ready for clinical use (Netcord <https://office.de.netcord.org/inventory.gif>).

There are several advantages of using UCB stem cells over the more traditional BM or peripheral blood harvested stem cell. First, banked cord blood samples have already been HLA-typed, screened for infection and are ready to be used, resulting in tissue matches completed within days and transplants within weeks, compared to an average 4 months to find a BM donor and arrange donation.[88] Second, there is a lower incidence of graft-versus-host disease (GVHD) among recipients of UCBT, probably secondary to the presence of immature alloreactive T-lymphocytes found in cord blood. This has the added benefit of increasing the donor pool due to better tolerance of mismatched transplantation antigens such as HLA-I and HLA-II.[89] Finally, there is a lower risk of transmission of latent viruses such as Epstein-Barr and cytomegaloviruses which can have profound effects in immunosuppressed recipients.[90]

The disadvantages of UCBT over BM transplantation relate mainly to the lower haemopoietic stem and progenitor cell numbers found in cord blood[91] and hence a higher risk of graft failure as well as delayed haematopoietic engraftment. As the dose of progenitor cells required to generate a successful transplant ranges between $15–50 \times 10^6$ cells/kg body weight, cord blood collections have, at least until very recently, been considered insufficient to repopulate an adult.[92,93] For this and other reasons, cord blood is now regarded as only the third choice for UCBT, behind matched BM or cytokine-mobilised HSC, and behind haplo-identical HSC from a parent or sibling.

Umbilical cord blood banking

Altruistic UCB samples stored within public stem cell banks over the past 15 years have contributed to the generation of high-quality cord blood units stored in over 50 banks world-wide. This has increased the availability of donor HSC for ethnic groups under-represented in the bone marrow registries covering > 6 million registrants. Recently, commercial firms have been offering pregnant women the possibility of preserving their own child's umbilical cord stem cells for a fee. The service is marketed to parents at a vulnerable time, urging them to take this 'once-in-a-lifetime opportunity', 'to do something that one day may save their baby's life' as '50% will develop a disease that will be cured by cord blood'. While the validity of public altruistic UCB banking, and UCB storage in families at increased risk of genetic diseases treatable by HSC transplantation is clear, directed autologous UCB storage in 'low-risk' families has been widely challenged. In 2001, the Royal College of Obstetricians and Gynaecologists Scientific Advisory Committee concluded that directed collection in low-risk families cannot be justified, both scientifically and because of the logistic burden of collection on maternity service providers, and thus could not be recommended.[94] This viewpoint was echoed in the US by the American Academy of Pediatrics[95] and the American College of Obstetricians and Gynecologists[96] and in Europe by the French National Consultative Ethics

Committee for Health and Life Sciences[97] and the European Group on Ethics in Science and New Technologies.[98]

There are a number of concerns about the routine commercial directed cord blood storage.[99] First ,the probability of a child needing an autologous transplant is less than one in 20,000. Indeed, for acute leukaemia, the most likely indication, improvements in conventional therapy and allogeneic transplantation have rendered UCB transplantation less frequent, while the existence of pre-leukaemic mutations generally precludes autologous use. Next, some of the advertising borders on the immoral, particularly in relation to speculative future uses of MSC for degenerative diseases, when no mention is made of the low frequency with which MSC can be expanded from cord blood. Then there is the administrative burden at what is otherwise a busy time for the accoucheur of full specimen collection to ensure a high volume (~80 ml), and of completing the considerable paperwork and parental blood collection for a myriad of providers. This is in contrast to collection for public banks, where specimens are only stored if complete, and there are no obstetric distractions. Although there is nothing intrinsically wrong with directed storage with parents who can afford this biological luxury, they should be aware that storage relies on continued commercial viability of the company, and there has already been one bankruptcy. Finally, there is general concern that such facilities will undermine support for the more valuable and utilitarian public blood banks. Thus EU guidance on UCB banking recommends that patients be told that the likelihood of using stored UCB to treat their child is negligible and that future applications are only hypothetical.[98]

CONCLUSIONS

The isolation of human ES cells has spawned a new era of stem cell research, opening up novel avenues for understanding both developmental and disease processes as well as the possibility of treating many common diseases. Similarly, the identification of different populations of primitive fetal stem cells raises the possibility of using them as targets for cellular or gene therapy for a wide variety of conditions. Fetal stem cells are more primitive than adult stem cells and have longer telomeres and greater differentiative potential. Fetal cells also have an engraftment advantage over adult cells, while fetal recipients are more permissive to allogeneic grafts than adult recipients.

However, several hurdles need to be overcome in robust experimental models before these new stem cell populations can be used clinically. In addition to addressing ethical reservations regarding use of ES cells and abortal tissue, these include the ability to generate large numbers of pure cell types without xenogeneic contamination, control of rejection by the host immune system and understanding the correct cell type and delivery route to treat a specific condition.

References

1 Rubinstein P, Carrier C, Scaradavou A et al. Outcomes among 562 recipients of placental-blood transplants from unrelated donors. N Engl J Med 1988; 339: 1565–1577
2 Lindvall O, Bjorklund A. Cell therapy in Parkinson's disease. NeuroRx 2004; 1: 382–393

3 Shamblott MJ, Axelman J, Wang S et al. Derivation of pluripotent stem cells from cultured human primordial germ cells. Proc Natl Acad Sci USA 1998; 95: 13726–13731

4 Andrews PW. From teratocarcinomas to embryonic stem cells. Philos Trans R Soc Lond B Biol Sci 2002; 357: 405–417

5 Weissman IL. Stem cells: units of development, units of regeneration, and units in evolution. Cell 2000; 100: 157–168

6 Kennea NL, Mehmet H. Neural stem cells. J Pathol 2002; 197: 536–550

7 Pittenger MF, Mackay AM, Beck SC et al. Multilineage potential of adult human mesenchymal stem cells. Science 1999; 284: 143–147

8 Blau HM, Brazelton TR, Weimann JM. The evolving concept of a stem cell: entity or function? Cell 2001; 105: 829–841

9 Evans MJ, Kaufman MH. Establishment in culture of pluripotential cells from mouse embryos. Nature 1981; 292: 154–156

10 Thomson JA, Itskovitz-Eldor J, Shapiro SS et al. Embryonic stem cell lines derived from human blastocysts. Science 1998; 282: 1145–1147

11 Hoffman LM, Carpenter MK. Characterization and culture of human embryonic stem cells. Nat Biotechnol 2005; 23: 699–708

12 Hayflick L. The limited in vitro lifetime of human diploid cell strains. Exp Cell Res 1965; 37: 614–636

13 Kehat I, Kenyagin-Karsenti D, Snir M et al. Human embryonic stem cells can differentiate into myocytes with structural and functional properties of cardiomyocytes. J Clin Invest 2001; 108: 407–414

14 Kim JH, Auerbach JM, Rodriguez-Gomez JA et al. Dopamine neurons derived from embryonic stem cells function in an animal model of Parkinson's disease. Nature 2002; 418: 50–56

15 Assady S, Maor G, Amit M et al. Insulin production by human embryonic stem cells. Diabetes 2001; 50: 1691–1697

16 Clark AT, Bodnar MS, Fox M et al. Spontaneous differentiation of germ cells from human embryonic stem cells in vitro. Hum Mol Genet 2004; 13: 727–739

17 Richards M, Fong CY, Chan WK, Wong PC, Bongso A. Human feeders support prolonged undifferentiated growth of human inner cell masses and embryonic stem cells. Nat Biotechnol 2002; 20: 933–936

18 Xu RH, Peck RM, Li DS et al. Basic FGF and suppression of BMP signaling sustain undifferentiated proliferation of human ES cells. Nat Methods 2005; 2: 185–190

19 Xu C, Inokuma MS, Denham J et al. Feeder-free growth of undifferentiated human embryonic stem cells. Nat Biotechnol 2001; 19: 971–974

20 Drukker M, Katz G, Urbach A et al. Characterization of the expression of MHC proteins in human embryonic stem cells. Proc Natl Acad Sci USA 2002; 99: 9864–9869

21 Hwang WS, Roh SI, Lee BC et al. Patient-specific embryonic stem cells derived from human SCNT blastocysts. Science 2005; 308: 1777–1783

22 Rideout 3rd WM, Hochedlinger K, Kyba M, Daley GQ, Jaenisch R. Correction of a genetic defect by nuclear transplantation and combined cell and gene therapy. Cell 2002; 109: 17–27

23 Barberi T, Klivenyi P, Calingasan NY et al. Neural subtype specification of fertilization and nuclear transfer embryonic stem cells and application in parkinsonian mice. Nat Biotechnol 2003; 21: 1200–1207

24 Wilmut I, Beaujean N, de Sousa PA et al. Somatic cell nuclear transfer. Nature 2002; 419: 583–586

25 Rhind SM, Taylor JE, De Sousa PA et al. Human cloning: can it be made safe? Nat Rev Genet 2003; 4: 855–864

26 Eggan K, Akutsu H, Loring J et al. Hybrid vigor, fetal overgrowth, and viability of mice derived by nuclear cloning and tetraploid embryo complementation. Proc Natl Acad Sci USA 2001; 98: 6209–6214

27 Rideout 3rd W M, Eggan K, Jaenisch R. Nuclear cloning and epigenetic reprogramming of the genome. Science 2001; 293: 1093–1098

28 ESHRE Taskforce on Ethics and Law. IV Stem cells. Hum Reprod 2002; 17: 1409–1410

29 Vogelstein B, Alberts B, Shine K. Genetics. Please don't call it cloning! Science 2002; 295: 1237

30 Cowan CA, Klimanskaya I, McMahon J et al. Derivation of embryonic stem-cell lines from human blastocysts. N Engl J Med 2004; 350: 1353–1356

31 Verlinsky Y, Strelchenko N, Kukharenko V et al. Human embryonic stem cell lines with genetic disorders. Reprod Biomed Online 2005; 10: 105–110

32 Toyooka Y, Tsunekawa N, Akasu R, Noce T. Embryonic stem cells can form germ cells *in vitro*. Proc Natl Acad Sci USA 2003; 100: 11457–11462

33 Johnson J, Bagley J, Skaznik-Wikiel M *et al*. Oocyte generation in adult mammalian ovaries by putative germ cells in bone marrow and peripheral blood. Cell 2005; 122: 303–315

34 Medvinsky A, Dzierzak E. Definitive hematopoiesis is autonomously initiated by the AGM region. Cell 1996; 86: 897–906

35 Taylor PA, McElmurry RT, Lees CJ, Harrison DE, Blazar BR. Allogenic fetal liver cells have a distinct competitive engraftment advantage over adult bone marrow cells when infused into fetal as compared with adult severe combined immunodeficient recipients. Blood 2002; 99: 1870–1872

36 Lansdorp PM. Telomere length and proliferation potential of hematopoietic stem cells. J Cell Sci 1995; 108: 1–6

37 Campagnoli C, Fisk N, Overton T *et al*. Circulating hematopoietic progenitor cells in first trimester fetal blood. Blood 2000; 95: 1967–1972

38 Clapp DW, Freie B, Lee WH, Zhang YY. Molecular evidence that *in situ*-transduced fetal liver hematopoietic stem/progenitor cells give rise to medullary hematopoiesis in adult rats. Blood 1995; 86: 2113–2122

39 Rollini P, Kaiser S, Faes-van't Hull E, Kapp U, Leyvraz S. Long-term expansion of transplantable human fetal liver hematopoietic stem cells. Blood 2004; 103: 1166–1170

40 Tocci A, Roberts IA, Kumar S, Bennett PR, Fisk NM. CD34 cells from first-trimester fetal blood are enriched in primitive hemopoietic progenitors. Am J Obstet Gynecol 2003; 188: 1002–1010

41 Ren AH, Zhang Y, Zhao YL *et al*. [Comparative study of differentially expressed genes in mouse bone marrow and fetal liver cells]. Zhongguo Shi Yan Xue Ye Xue Za Zhi 2003; 11: 444–449

42 Harrison DE, Zhong RK, Jordan CT, Lemischka IR, Astle CM. Relative to adult marrow, fetal liver repopulates nearly five times more effectively long-term than short-term. Exp Hematol 1997; 25: 293–297

43 Rebel VI, Miller CL, Eaves CJ, Lansdorp PM. The repopulation potential of fetal liver hematopoietic stem cells in mice exceeds that of their liver adult bone marrow counterparts. Blood 1996; 87: 3500–3507

44 Holyoake TL, Nicolini FE, Eaves CJ. Functional differences between transplantable human hematopoietic stem cells from fetal liver, cord blood, and adult marrow. Exp Hematol 1999; 27: 1418–1427

45 Touraine JL. The fetal liver as a source of stem cells for transplantation into fetuses *in utero*. Curr Top Microbiol Immunol 1992; 177: 187–193

46 Westgren M, Ringden O, Bartmann P *et al*. Prenatal T-cell reconstitution after in utero transplantation with fetal liver cells in a patient with X-linked severe combined immunodeficiency. Am J Obstet Gynecol 2002; 187: 475–482

47 Friedenstein AJ, Petrakova KV, Kurolesova AI, Frolova GP. Heterotopic of bone marrow. Analysis of precursor cells for osteogenic and hematopoietic tissues. Transplantation 1968; 6: 230–247

48 Campagnoli C, Roberts IA, Kumar S *et al*. Identification of mesenchymal stem/progenitor cells in human first-trimester fetal blood, liver, and bone marrow. Blood 2001; 98: 2396–2402

49 Gotherstrom C, Ringden O, Westgren M, Tammik C, Le Blanc K. Immunomodulatory effects of human foetal liver-derived mesenchymal stem cells. Bone Marrow Transplant 2003; 32: 265–272

50 Chan J, O'Donoghue K, Kennea N *et al*. Galectin-1 induces skeletal muscle differentiation in human fetal mesenchymal stem cells and increases muscle regeneration in vivo. Stem Cells 2006; In Press [ePub doi 10-1634 (2006)]

51 Kennea NL, Fisk NM, Edwards AD, Mehmet H. Neural cell differentiation of fetal mesenchymal stem cells [Abstract]. Early Hum Dev 2003; 73: 121–122

52 MacKenzie TC, Campagnoli C, Almeida-Porada G, Fisk NM, Flake AW. Circulating human fetal stromal cells engraft and differentiate in multiple tissues following transplantation into pre-immune fetal lambs [Abstract]. Blood 2001; 98: 798

53 de la Fuente J, O'Donoghue K, Kumar S, Chan J, Fisk NM, Roberts IAG. Ontogeny-related changes in integrin and cytokine production by fetal mesenchymal stem cells (MSC) [Abstract]. Blood 2002; 100: 526a

54 In't Anker PS, Scherjon SA, Kleijburg-van der Keur C *et al*. Isolation of mesenchymal stem cells of fetal or maternal origin from human placenta. Stem Cells 2004; 22: 1338–1345

55 In't Anker PS, Scherjon SA, Kleijburg-van der Keur C *et al*. Amniotic fluid as a novel source of mesenchymal stem cells for therapeutic transplantation. Blood 2003; 102: 1548–1549

56 Hu Y, Liao L, Wang Q *et al*. Isolation and identification of mesenchymal stem cells from human fetal pancreas. J Lab Clin Med 2003; 141: 342–349

57 Noort WA, Kruisselbrink AB, in't Anker PS *et al*. Mesenchymal stem cells promote engraftment of human umbilical cord blood-derived CD34(+) cells in NOD/SCID mice. Exp Hematol 2002; 30: 870–878

58 Almeida-Porada G, El Shabrawy D, Porada C, Zanjani ED. Differentiative potential of human metanephric mesenchymal cells. Exp Hematol 2002; 30: 1454–1462

59 Fibbe WE. Mesenchymal stem cells. A potential source for skeletal repair. Ann Rheum Dis 2002; 61 (Suppl 2): ii29–ii31

60 O'Donoghue K, Fisk NM. Fetal stem cells. Best Pract Res Clin Obstet Gynaecol 2004; 18: 853–875

61 Gotherstrom C, Ringden O, Tammik C *et al*. Immunologic properties of human fetal mesenchymal stem cells. Am J Obstet Gynecol 2004; 190: 239–245

62 Ryan JM, Barry FP, Murphy JM, Mahon BP. Mesenchymal stem cells avoid allogeneic rejection. J Inflamm (Lond) 2005; 2: 8

63 Carpenter MK, Cui X, Hu ZY *et al*. *In vitro* expansion of a multipotent population of human neural progenitor cells. Exp Neurol 1999; 158: 265–278

64 Johansson CB, Momma S, Clarke DL *et al*. Identification of a neural stem cell in the adult mammalian central nervous system. Cell 1999; 96: 25–34

65 Uchida N, Buck DW, He D *et al*. Direct isolation of human central nervous system stem cells. Proc Natl Acad Sci USA 2000; 97: 14720–14725

66 Jackson KA, Majka SM, Wang H *et al*. Regeneration of ischemic cardiac muscle and vascular endothelium by adult stem cells. J Clin Invest 2001; 107: 1395–1402

67 Zimmermann B, Holzgreve W, Zhong XY, Hahn S. Inability to clonally expand fetal progenitors from maternal blood. Fetal Diagn Ther 2002; 17: 97–100

68 Little MT, Langlois S, Wilson RD, Lansdorp PM. Frequency of fetal cells in sorted subpopulations of nucleated erythroid and CD34+ hematopoietic progenitor cells from maternal peripheral blood. Blood 1997; 89: 2347–2358

69 O'Donoghue K, Choolani M, Chan J *et al*. Identification of fetal mesenchymal stem cells in maternal blood: implications for non-invasive prenatal diagnosis. Mol Hum Reprod 2003; 9: 497–502

70 O'Donoghue K, Chan J, De La Fuente J *et al*. Microchimerism in female bone marrow and bone decades after fetal mesenchymal stem-cell trafficking in pregnancy. Lancet 2004; 364: 179–182

71 Bianchi DW, Zickwolf GK, Weil GJ, Sylvester S, DeMaria MA. Male fetal progenitor cells persist in maternal blood for as long as 27 years postpartum. Proc Natl Acad Sci USA 1996; 93: 705–708

72 Fukada S, Miyagoe-Suzuki Y, Tsukihara H *et al*. Muscle regeneration by reconstitution with bone marrow or fetal liver cells from green fluorescent protein-gene transgenic mice. J Cell Sci 2002; 115: 1285–1293

73 Shields LE, Lindton B, Andrews RG, Westgren M. Fetal hematopoietic stem cell transplantation: a challenge for the twenty-first century. J Hematother Stem Cell Res 2002; 11: 617–631

74 Flake AW, Roncarolo MG, Puck JM *et al*. Treatment of X-linked severe combined immunodeficiency by *in utero* transplantation of paternal bone marrow. N Engl J Med 1996; 335: 1806–1810

75 Wengler GS, Lanfranchi A, Frusca T *et al*. *In-utero* transplantation of parental CD34 haematopoietic progenitor cells in a patient with X-linked severe combined immunodeficiency (SCIDXI). Lancet 1996; 348: 1484–1487

76 Liechty KW, MacKenzie TC, Shaaban AF *et al*. Human mesenchymal stem cells engraft and demonstrate site-specific differentiation after *in utero* transplantation in sheep. Nat Med 2000; 6: 1282–1286

77 Le Blanc K, Gotherstrom C, Ringden O *et al.* Fetal mesenchymal stem cell engraftment in bone following *in utero* transplantation in a patient with severe osteogenesis imperfecta. Transplantation 2005; 79: 1607–1614

78 Hacein-Bey-Abina S, Le Deist F, Carlier F *et al.* Sustained correction of X-linked severe combined immunodeficiency by *ex vivo* gene therapy. N Engl J Med 2002; 346: 1185–1193

79 Aiuti A, Slavin S, Aker M *et al.* Correction of ADA-SCID by stem cell gene therapy combined with nonmyeloablative conditioning. Science 2002; 296: 2410–2413

80 Gaspar HB, Parsley KL, Howe S *et al.* Gene therapy of X-linked severe combined immuno-deficiency by use of a pseudotyped gammaretroviral vector. Lancet 2004; 364: 2181–2187

81 Kohn DB, Sadelain M, Glorioso JC. Occurrence of leukaemia following gene therapy of X-linked SCID. Nat Rev Cancer 2003; 3: 477–488

82 Chan J, O'Donoghue K, de la Fuente J *et al.* Human fetal mesenchymal stem cells as vehicles for gene delivery. Stem Cells 2005; 23: 93–102

83 Surbek D, Schoeberlein A, Dudler L, Holzgreve W. *In utero* transplantation of autologous and allogeneic fetal liver stem cells in fetal sheep. Am J Obstet Gynecol 2003; 189: S75

84 Orlandi F, Damiani G, Jakil C *et al.* The risks of early cordocentesis (12–21 weeks): analysis of 500 procedures. Prenat Diagn 1990; 10: 425–428

85 Lee OK, Kuo TK, Chen W-M *et al.* Isolation of multipotent mesenchymal stem cells from umbilical cord blood. Blood 2004; 103: 1669–1675

86 Bieback K, Kern S, Kluter H, Eichler H. Critical parameters for the isolation of mesenchymal stem cells from umbilical cord blood. Stem Cells 2004; 22: 625–634

87 Rocha V, Sanz G, Gluckman E. Umbilical cord blood transplantation. Curr Opin Hematol 2004; 11: 375–385

88 Barker JN, Krepski TP, DeFor TE *et al.* Searching for unrelated donor hematopoietic stem cells: availability and speed of umbilical cord blood versus bone marrow. Biol Blood Marrow Transplant 2002; 8: 257–260

89 Rocha V, Wagner Jr JE, Sobocinski KA *et al.* Graft-versus-host disease in children who have received a cord-blood or bone marrow transplant from an HLA-identical sibling. Eurocord and International Bone Marrow Transplant Registry Working Committee on Alternative Donor and Stem Cell Sources. N Engl J Med 2000; 342: 1846–1854

90 Barker JN, Martin PL, Coad JE *et al.* Low incidence of Epstein-Barr virus-associated posttransplantation lymphoproliferative disorders in 272 unrelated-donor umbilical cord blood transplant recipients. Biol Blood Marrow Transplant 2001; 7: 395–399

91 Gluckman E. Hematopoietic stem-cell transplants using umbilical-cord blood. N Engl J Med 2001; 344: 1860–1861

92 Laughlin MJ, Barker J, Bambach B *et al.* Hematopoietic engraftment and survival in adult recipients of umbilical-cord blood from unrelated donors. N Engl J Med 2001; 344: 1815–1822

93 Rogers I, Sutherland N, Holt D *et al.* Human UC-blood banking: impact of blood volume, cell separation and cryopreservation on leukocyte and CD34(+) cell recovery. Cytotherapy 2001; 3: 269–276

94 Royal College of Obstetricians and Gynaecologists Scientific Advisory Committee. London: RCOG, 2001

95 American Academy of Pediatrics Work Group on Cord Blood Banking. Cord blood banking for potential future transplantation. Pediatrics 1999; 104: 116–118

96 American College of Obstetricians and Gynecologists ACOG Committee Opinion. Routine storage of umbilical cord blood for potential future transplantation. Number 183. Int J Gynecol Obstet 1997; 58: 257–259

97 French National Consultative Ethics Committee for Health and Life Sciences. Umbilical cord blood banks for autologous use or for research. Opinion number 74. 2002 <http://www.ccne-ethique.fr/english/start.htm>

98 European Group on Ethics in Science and New Technologies. Umbilical cord blood banking. Opinion of the European Group on Ethics in Science and New Technologies to the European Commission. 2004 <http://europa.eu.int/comm/european_group_ethics/docs/avis19_19.pdf>

99 Fisk NM, Roberts IA, Markwald R, Mironov V. Can routine commercial cord blood banking be scientifically and ethically justified? PLoS Med 2005; 2: e44

Amos Grunebaum

Periconception care

The care for pregnant women has changed dramatically over the last century since Williams,[1] in the first edition of his textbook of obstetrics, wrote: 'ordinarily the services of an obstetrician are engaged some months before the expected date of confinement'.

In the 21st century, optimal obstetric care would include that a woman engage the services of an obstetrician several months prior to conception for periconception care, as soon as the couple is planning to become pregnant.

There is an evolving science showing that seeing a doctor or other provider prior to pregnancy, when the couple starts thinking about a family, can improve pregnancy outcomes for both the mother and the baby. The US Public Health Service has underscored the importance of preconception care by including several recommendations promoting the health of women before pregnancy (<www.health.gov/healthypeople/>). Benefits of periconception care such as the early identification of potential problems and medical treatment before pregnancy seem apparent, yet only recently has evidence emerged supporting improved outcomes in many conditions (*e.g.* diabetes mellitus, phenylketonuria, and a previous pregnancy with a fetus with a neural tube defect).[2-4] De Weerd *et al.*[5] have shown that two of the major components of preconception care – smoking cessation and folic acid supplementation – can lead to a significant cost-saving balance.

Since up to 50% of pregnancies are unintended,[6,7] promoting health and healthy life-styles prior to pregnancy is crucial among all childbearing couples, especially as planned pregnancies have better outcomes than unplanned ones.[8]

Periconception care begins prior to pregnancy at a time when preparations for pregnancy can be made. It usually involves one or more meetings between

Amos Grunebaum MD
Department of Obstetrics and Gynecology, New York Weill Cornell Medical Center, 525 East 68th Street, New York, NY 10021, USA
E-mail: amos@grunebaum.net

Table 1 Key elements of periconception counseling

Medical history and medication review
 Diabetes – identify prior to pregnancy and optimize control
 Hypertension – avoid ACE inhibitors, angiotensin II receptor antagonists,
  thiazide diuretics
 Epilepsy –optimize control; folic acid, 1 mg per day
 DVT – switch from warfarin (Coumadin) to heparin
 Depression/anxiety – avoid benzodiazepines

Genetic history
 Review family history of genetic issues
 Carrier screening (ethnic background):
  sickle cell anemia, thalassemia, Tay-Sachs disease
 Carrier screening (family history):
  cystic fibrosis, non-syndromic hearing loss (connexin-26)

Reproductive and gynecological history
 Review prior pregnancy outcomes and counsel about recurrence
 Review prior gynecological history
 Review history of PID or other tubal issues

Living environment: diet, weight, food, and medications
 Folic acid supplement (400 µg routine, 1 mg diabetes/epilepsy,
  4 mg previous neural tube defect)
 Assess weight, calculate body mass index (BMI), advise optimal BMI
 Recommend regular exercise in moderation
 Avoid hyperthermia (hot tubs, overheating)
 Assess risk of nutritional deficiencies (vegan, pica, milk intolerance,
  calcium or iron deficiency)
 Avoid overuse of vitamin A (limit to 3000 IU/day) and vitamin D
  (limit to 400 IU/day)
 Limit caffeine to two cups of coffee or six glasses of soda per day
 Screen for domestic violence
 Household chemicals – avoid paint thinners and strippers,
  other solvents, pesticides
 Smoking cessation and avoidance of secondary smoking
 Screen for alcoholism and use of illegal drugs

Fertility review and optimization
 Assess for regular ovulation, signs of PCOS
 Discuss fertility after birth control
 Review frequency and timing of sexual intercourse
 Refrain from using lubricants

Medical examination and testing: immunization
 Test for infectious diseases (*e.g.* HIV, syphilis)
 Hepatitis B immunization for at-risk patients
 Preconception immunizations (rubella, varicella)
 Counsel about avoidance of infections (*e.g.* toxoplasmosis,
  cytomegalovirus, parvovirus B19)
 Suggest a dental examination

Male periconception counseling and assessment
 Medical history and review
 Review of potentially harmful exposure
 Avoid exposure to heat
 Avoid alcohol, smoking and other harmful substances
 Suggest sperm analysis

the couple trying to conceive and a doctor or another healthcare provider like a nurse[9] who is experienced in this area, as well as some tests. Any doctor with interest in this area can provide many aspects of periconception care, but the obstetrician and gynecologist is best trained to handle most aspects of periconception care.

The overall goal of periconceptional care is to ensure that:

1. *Women and men are in their best health and practice healthy life-styles before conception.*

2. *Couples become aware that preconception, conception, pregnancy, birth and child rearing are a continuum in which earlier events affect the present and the future.*

3. *Physicians and care providers are able to identify prior to conception any issues and resolve them without being concerned about the on-going pregnancy.*

4. *Tests are done prior to pregnancy so that any necessary interventions can begin before the woman is pregnant.*

The best example of how periconception care can improve pregnancy outcome is supplementation with folic acid. An increase in the intake of folic acid among women planning a pregnancy was shown to prevent most neural tube defects.[10,41] Key elements of periconception counseling are summarised in Table 1 and are discussed below.

MEDICAL HISTORY AND HEALTH ASSESSMENT

The first step

There are many medical problems which place the mother and fetus potentially at risk.[11] Answering pertinent questions in advance allows for enough time to consider all answers and helps the provider to focus only on the significant issues. So the first step in identifying potential issues is to obtain a good medical and social history and this can optimally be achieved by having patients first fill in a periconception questionnaire or health assessment form. This questionnaire can help in the counseling and care process and organizes the periconceptual approach.[12] Filling out this questionnaire is not only time-saving, but it also allows for a complete evaluation of the couple's medical and surgical history. For more efficient use, there are several websites which allow patients to register and fill in their own questionnaire that can be printed out and given to the doctor (*e.g.* <http://www.periconception.com>) A sample short questionnaire which can be individualized for each special circumstances is given in Appendix 1.

Selected medical conditions

Diabetes mellitus

Women with poorly controlled diabetes have a significantly higher risk of spontaneous abortion and increased risk of severe fetal anomalies compared with women who have good control. Preconception diabetic management is offered in many locations[13] and can decrease the risk of abortions and congenital anomalies and lessens the complications of pregnancy.[14] Preconception is the optimal time to identify, evaluate, and treat hypertension, nephropathy, retinopathy, and thyroid disease in these patients and provide counseling on risks of pregnancy, requirement for increased visits, and close monitoring.[15] In addition, periconception provides the opportunity to evaluate patients for relative contra-indications to pregnancy such as those with blood urea nitrogen greater than 30 mg/dl (10.7 mmol/l), low creatinine clearance, and coronary artery disease.

Hypertension

Most patients with chronic hypertension can expect an uncomplicated pregnancy but will require enhanced monitoring for the risks of pre-eclampsia, renal insufficiency, and fetal growth retardation. It is important that women with hypertension be evaluated before pregnancy to determine the severity of the hypertension and to recommend potential life-style modifications. Preconception is the best time to review and change medications for use during pregnancy. Methyldopa (Aldomet) and calcium channel blockers are commonly used during pregnancy. Drugs that should be avoided in the first and second trimesters of pregnancy are angiotensin-converting enzyme inhibitors, angiotensin II receptor antagonists, and thiazide diuretics, which are associated with congenital defects.

Epilepsy

The incidence of malformations in infants of mothers with epilepsy who are treated with anti-epileptic drugs is 2–3 times that of infants of mothers without epilepsy,[16] and they also have an increased risk of developing epilepsy. Preconception counseling should include optimizing seizure control, prescribing folic acid supplements, 1–4 mg/day, and offering referral to a genetic counselor. When possible, use of multiple anticonvulsants should be avoided. The best single agent for the seizure type at the lowest protective level is best, and there is no single drug of choice. If a patient has been seizure-free for 2 years or longer, drug discontinuation with a long taper period (3 months) may be successful in individual cases, and tapering should begin 6 months prior to conception.[17]

Thrombo-embolism

Women with a history of a deep venous thrombosis (DVT) have a 0–13% risk of recurrence during pregnancy,[18] and those with a personal or family history of venous thrombo-embolism should be offered testing for thrombophilia before pregnancy. Those on warfarin (Coumadin) as maintenance therapy for DVT should be switched to heparin before conception, because warfarin is teratogenic. Heparin (in regular or low-molecular-weight form) is indicated for prophylaxis and should be started as early in pregnancy as possible.

Depression and anxiety

About 10% of pregnant women have depression. Tricyclic antidepressants and selective serotonin re-uptake inhibitors have not been shown to cause any teratogenic effects and may be used before conception.[44] Rarely, maternal use of benzodiazepines has been associated with an increased risk of malformations or oral cleft,[42] as well as a withdrawal syndrome in the newborn.

Asthma

Asthma is one of the most common medical illnesses likely to occur in women of childbearing age, with about 1% of pregnancies complicated by asthma.

Optimizing preconceptional asthma control and reviewing use of the peakflow meter and personal best surveillance, and offering influenza vaccine ensures that the patient begin her pregnancy in optimal condition. The fewest medications needed to control symptoms of asthma should be recommended.

Cardiac diseases

Maternal morbidity from cardiac diseases is as high as 7% in combined New York Heart Association classes III and IV heart disease, compared to only 0.5% in combined classes I and II. Certain cardiac disorders, such as primary pulmonary hypertension, place women at very high risk during pregnancy. Maternal mortality approaches 50% and counseling prior to pregnancy may help couples decide on the best course. The preconception evaluation should, therefore, identify cardiac disease risk factors, determine the extent of disease, identify correctable problems, and provide the patient with detailed information about maternal and fetal risks. Close consultation before and during pregnancy with a cardiologist may help guide a patient though the pregnancy.

Autoimmune disorders

Autoimmune disorders such as lupus are common among women of childbearing age. Patients should be counseled that the best time to attempt conception is during periods of inactive disease. Even women with quiescent disease or a distant history of disease should be carefully evaluated and counseled about maternal and fetal risks.

OBTAINING A GENETIC HISTORY

Genetic issues

The woman's family history and ethnicity for genetic disorders (such as cystic fibrosis, sickle cell anemia, and Tay-Sachs disease) and malformations (such as neural tube defects) should be reviewed thoroughly during the periconception visit. The clinician should consider referring the patient to a genetic counselor or maternal–fetal specialist if there is a personal or family history of a child with a potential genetic disorder or if advanced maternal age is an issue.

Advanced maternal age

The periconception time period is the optimal time to educate patients about a woman's fertility 'biological time clock' and the purposes and techniques of prenatal diagnosis during pregnancy. Advanced maternal age is becoming more common and women becoming pregnant at more advanced ages are at increased risk for: (i) infertility; (ii) having fetuses with chromosomal abnormalities; (iii) an increased likelihood of chronic medical illness; and (iv) adverse pregnancy outcomes.

Older couples should be counseled about genetic risks and the availability of antenatal testing (amniocentesis and chorionic villus sampling), which may not be options if the first visit for prenatal care is delayed. The risk of infertility also increases with age, rising to 20% in couples older than 35 years.

Table 2 Carrier screening by ethnicity

Ethnic origin	Screening recommended	Test	Frequency (%)
Black	Sickle cell trait	Sickle cell smear	10%
	β-Thalassemia	MCV < 70	5%
European Jewish	Tay-Sachs disease carrier; Canavan, cystic fibrosis, familial dysautonomia	Hexosaminidase A	4%
French Canadian	Tay-Sachs disease carrier	Hexosaminidase A	> 5%
Mediterranean	α-, β-Thalassemia	MCV < 70	10–20%
Southeast Asian (Laotian, Thai, Cambodian, Hmong)	α-, β-Thalassemia	MCV < 70	20–40%
Indian, Middle Eastern	Sickle cell trait α-, β-Thalassemia	Sickle cell smear MCV < 70	Unknown Unknown

MCV = mean corpuscular volume.
Adapted from Cowchock FS, Johnson A, Jackson LG. Screening for genetic abnormalities. *Infertil Reprod Med Clin North Am* 1994; **5**: 177–195.

Carrier screening

Periconception is an optimal time to review whether genetic testing should be done. The ethnic background of either partner determines whether genetic screening should be recommended for certain genetic conditions like sickle cell trait, thalassemias, and Tay-Sachs disease carrier state (Table 2). A family history that is positive for certain diseases, such as cystic fibrosis and congenital hearing loss, indicates the need for additional screening. The American College of Obstetricians and Gynecologists recommends that screening for Tay-Sachs, Canavan disease, cystic fibrosis, and familial dysautonomia should be offered for couples of Ashkenazi Jewish ancestry.[19]

Family history of thrombo-embolic disease
A family history of thrombo-embolic disease may identify a woman at risk for pregnancy complications and requires a thorough work-up prior to pregnancy.

REPRODUCTIVE AND GYNECOLOGICAL HISTORY

The time prior to pregnancy and especially prior to *in-vitro* fertilization is the optimal time to review gynecological and prior pregnancy issues and counsel couples about improving health and future pregnancy outcomes. A review of the gynecological and obstetric history can identify possible signs of infertility or issues which may affect future pregnancies.

Patients with irregular periods may have hormonal and ovulation problems or may have polycystic ovarian syndrome. Treating these problems will improve the patient's chances of getting pregnant. Patients with a history of recurrent miscarriages may benefit from a work-up and baby aspirin prior to pregnancy.

Previous pregnancy complications such as a history of a preterm delivery, a baby with intra-uterine growth restriction, diabetes, hypertension or pre-eclampsia, have an increased risk of repeating in future pregnancies and should be assessed prior to the next pregnancy.

If the patient has had a history of PID, then testing for fallopian tube patency may save many months of futile attempts to get pregnant.

Patients with a history of prior ectopic pregnancies have a 20-fold increased risk and should be counseled to see a doctor as soon as they believe that they are pregnant.

LIVING ENVIRONMENT

Exposure to harmful agents

Drug or chemical exposure causes 3–6% of anomalies and periconception care is ideal to prevent potential teratogenic effects on the developing fetus by stopping harmful influences or switching to safer medications.

In a retrospective, register-based cohort study,[20] about one in five women purchased at least one drug classified as potentially harmful during pregnancy, and 3.4% purchased at least one drug classified as clearly harmful. The authors concluded that their study places emphasis on the need for careful prepregnancy counseling. Preconception care should review exposure to any potentially harmful drugs, review the need to take them and offer alternatives.

The US Food and Drug Administration (FDA) has defined risk factor designations A, B, C, D, and X to classify drugs used during pregnancy. X drugs should never be used during pregnancy and while trying to conceive. Category X drugs include folic acid antagonist, warfarin, isotretinoin, and valproic acid.

Periconception retinoic acid can lead to fetal embryopathy[21] and the American College of Obstetrics and Gynecology (ACOG) recommends that pregnant and preconceptional women avoid taking more than 5000 IU of vitamin A daily, though one study showed no association between periconceptional vitamin A exposures at doses of > 8000 IU or > 10,000 IU/day and malformations in general.[22]

Alcohol

Alcohol consumption during pregnancy can lead to adverse pregnancy outcome such as fetal alcohol syndrome and lower birth weight babies;[23,24] many women stop consuming alcohol once they know that they are pregnant. But there is also an adverse effect of alcohol on women who are trying to conceive as it decreases their fertility and increases their risk of having a miscarriage. Alcohol consumption prior to conception is a potential risk factor for adverse fetal outcome and an important consideration for those females planning to have children. In a study involving mice,[25] long-term alcohol exposure prior to conception resulted in lower fetal body weights. The authors showed that fetal growth and development can be affected by alcohol consumption even prior to the time of conception. However, even modest amounts of alcohol consumption during pregnancy can cause a negative impact on the fetus.[24]

The US Surgeon General has advised that: 'the best way to improve pregnancy outcome is to not drink any alcohol when you are trying to conceive and during pregnancy'.

Smoking

Approximately 18% of pregnant women in the US report smoking tobacco and their pregnancy is at increased risk for such complications as abruptio placenta, pre-eclampsia, and preterm labor.[26] Additionally, tobacco is associated with decreased fertility rates and increased oocyte depletion rates as well as ectopic pregnancy.[27] Periconception is thus the optimal time to inform women about the risks associated with smoking prior to and during pregnancy.

Environmental toxins and exposure

Environmental toxins to be avoided are summarized in Table 3. Women trying to conceive and pregnant women should minimize use of common household products, such as paint and paint removal products, bleaches, lye, and oven cleaners. A detailed occupational history, including household and hobby activities, occupational exposure to organic solvents, anesthetic gases, and antineoplastic agents can reveal potential teratogenic exposures. Women susceptible to toxoplasmosis should be advised to stay away from undercooked meat sources and have someone else change the cat litter.

Folic acid supplementation

A minimum of 400 µg folic acid supplementation with or without a multivitamin decreases the risk of fetal malformations such as neural tube defects, miscarriages, and cardiac malformations.[28,29] This positive effect can only be achieved when the supplement is taken prior to conception – at least 1–2 months before conception. In the US, the average woman receives about 100 µg of folic acid per day from fortified breads and grains. Women trying to conceive and beginning at least 1–2 months before conception and continuing through the first 3 months of pregnancy should take a daily vitamin supplement containing at least 400 µg of folic acid. Higher dosages are indicated for special-risk groups. A dosage of 1 mg per day is recommended for women with diabetes mellitus or epilepsy. Mothers who have given birth to children with neural tube defects should take 4 mg of folic acid per day for subsequent pregnancies. Studies have shown that addressing folic acid use even at a single periconception visit can significantly improve mean red cell folate levels.[30]

Diet

Women trying to conceive and pregnant women should have a diet rich in iron, calcium, vitamins B, and low in saturated fats.[31] There are even diets suggested for women to improve fertility.[32] Except for added calories during pregnancy, women trying to conceive should follow the same diet as if they were already pregnant. If a diet deficiency is identified, a visit with a dietician may help the woman understand the importance of a healthy diet.

Table 3 Environmental toxins

Hazard	Types	Associated outcomes	Sources of exposure
Metals	Lead	Abnormal sperm, menstrual disorders, miscarriages, stillbirths, mental retardation	Solder, lead pipes, batteries, paints, ceramics, smelter emissions
	Mercury	Impaired fetal motor and mental development	Thermometers, mirror coating, dyes, inks, pesticides, dental fillings, fish from contaminated waters
Solvents	Trichloro-ethylene, chloroform, benzene, toluene	Birth defects	Dry cleaning fluids, degreasers, paint strippers, drug and electronics industries
Plastics	Vinyl chloride	Decreased fertility, chromo-somal aberrations, miscarriages, stillbirths, birth defects	Plastic manufacturing
Pollutants	Polychlorinated biphenyl, polybrominated biphenyl	Low birth weight, stillbirths	Pesticides; carbonless copy paper; rubber, chemicals, and electronics industries; fire retardants; food chain
Pesticides	2,4,5-T and 2,4-D organo-phosphates	Birth defects, miscarriages, low birth weight	Farm, home, and garden insect sprays; wood treatment
Gases	Carbon monoxide	Low birth weight, stillbirths	Auto exhaust, furnaces, kerosene heaters, cigarette smoke
	Anesthetic gases	Decreased fertility, miscarriages, birth defects	Dental offices, operating rooms, chemicals
industries			
Radiation	Radiographs, radioactive materials	Sterility, birth defects	Medical and dental offices, electronics industries

From Cefalo RC, Moos MK. Preconceptional health promotion. In: Cefalo RC, Moos MK. (eds) *Preconceptional health care: a practical guide,*. 2nd edn. St Louis, MO: Mosby, 1995; 41–42.

Caffeine

A high caffeine intake delays conception[45] and increases the risk for a miscarriage.[43] Women, therefore, should be advised to not have more than 300 mg of caffeine per day. That is equal to two 5-oz cups of coffee, three 5-oz cups of tea, or two 12-oz glasses of caffeinated soda.

Fish

Mercury can have a deleterious effect on the developing fetus and there is evidence that especially large fish can contain excessive amounts of mercury. To prevent potential mercury toxicity on the fetus, the US FDA recommends the following for fish consumption before, during, and after pregnancy: fish to be avoided – shark, swordfish, king mackerel, tile fish; fish to be limited – no more than 12 oz total per week of shellfish, canned fish, canned tuna, or farm-raised fish.

Weight

Both extremes of a woman's weight can lead to decreased fertility and an increase in adverse pregnancy outcomes. Women who are underweight (BMI < 20) are less likely to ovulate, have amenorrhea, infertility, and a low-birthweight baby.[33] Obesity also has a negative effect on fertility and increases the risks for gestational diabetes, hypertension, pre-eclampsia, and cesarean section.[34] The optimal time to lose weight and try to reach an ideal weight (BMI 20–25) is before conception.

Exercise and nutrition

Regular, moderate exercise is generally beneficial and the current evidence continues to demonstrate marked benefit to both the mother and fetus for women who exercise during pregnancy. The current recommendation is for women to continue their prepregnancy activity level when they become pregnant. Hyperthermia in the first trimester has been associated with increases in congenital anomalies. Pregnant women should limit vigorous exercise to avoid an increase in core body temperature above 38°C (100.4°F). They should be adequately hydrated, wear loose clothing, avoid extreme environmental temperatures and not spent too long in saunas or hot tubs.

Social risk factors

Pregnancy can be adversely affected by a woman's mental and social health and there is an association between pregnancy and risk for domestic violence.[35] The physician can use a simple 4-question screening tool modeled after the CAGE questionnaire for alcoholism:

1. How often does your partner hurt you?
2. How often does your partner insult or talk down to you?
3. How often are you threatened with physical harm?
4. How often does your partner scream or curse at you?

Responses of 'often' or 'frequent' to any of these questions place the women at risk for domestic violence. The patient should receive information about community resources for battered women and emergency shelters.

Illegal drugs

Using illegal drugs during pregnancy can have deleterious effects on pregnancy outcome. Advising patients to stop these drugs prior to pregnancy and referring patients to drug treatment can improve their pregnancy outcome. Women using illegal drugs such as cocaine, marijuana, or heroin should be encouraged to quit before pregnancy. Cocaine use in pregnancy is associated with miscarriage, prematurity, growth retardation, and congenital defects, while marijuana use can cause prematurity and jitteriness in the neonate. Use of heroin may lead to intra-uterine growth restriction, hyperactivity, and severe neonatal withdrawal syndrome. Women who use illegal drugs may need a referral to a special withdrawal program to be completed before conception. A methadone maintenance program is an alternative if the patient is unable to complete the withdrawal.

FERTILITY REVIEW AND OPTIMIZATION

Fertility review and testing

Women often assume that conception will happen quickly as soon as birth control has been stopped. However, only 50% of couples get pregnant after trying for 4–5 months, and 15% do not get pregnant even after a year. Especially as women get older, they will encounter increased difficulties getting pregnant. Any advise on how to improve fertility and maybe shorten the time period to get pregnant is important. Counseling couples about the basics of getting pregnant including timing and frequency of sexual intercourse. Reviewing the mechanism of conception and the physiology of ovulation and the menstrual cycle is often crucial in helping them achieve a healthy pregnancy. Lubricants can decrease the chance of conceiving, and couples trying to conceive should be advised to not use any lubricants.

Unfortunately, many infertile couples are seen very late in their unsuccessful attempts of getting pregnant. A quick review of fertility issues (*e.g.* regular ovulation and menstrual cycles, a history of PID, and a review of the mother's age) can assess whether an infertility evaluation may be indicated early on. For example, a sperm analysis is an easy test which may be recommended before the attempt of trying to conceive. In about 50% of infertile couples, there is a 'male' problem and if there is a problem it should be addressed before spending a long time trying to conceive in vain.

Conception after birth control

'When can I get pregnant after stopping the pill?' is among the first questions women on the pill ask. There are several different ways this question can be answered. First, there is the safety of getting pregnant after stopping the pill. Women should be informed that there is no known fetal harm if conception happens right after the pill is stopped. So there is no medical need to wait for fetal reasons. However, it may take some time for regular fertility to begin after stopping the pill. Ovulation may happen as soon as 2 weeks after the pill has been stopped but can sometimes take longer. Women should be advised to seek consultation if ovulation and a the menstrual period have not returned within 2–3 months after the pill was stopped. Many physicians advise waiting for at least one cycle before getting pregnant after removal of the intra-uterine device, but there is little scientific evidence to support this suggestion.

MEDICAL AND GYNECOLOGICAL EXAMINATION

Examination

The periconception examination should include a full physical examination (*e.g.* lung, breast, heart, abdomen, skin, extremities) as well as a gynecological history and examination including a Pap smear and a culture for chlamydia and gonorrhea. The examination should focus on possible problems which may affect the pregnancy. If a mammogram is indicated, it is best done prior to conception.

Screening for infectious diseases

During the preconception evaluation, a history of high-risk behavior, including multiple sexual partners, sexually transmitted diseases, blood transfusions, or intravenous drug abuse should be obtained from both the patient and her sexual partner. In addition, safe sex for prevention of sexually transmitted diseases and early medical care for vaginal discharge should be discussed.[36] Testing a women and husband for infectious diseases prior to pregnancy allows for early interventions, before the developing fetus can be potentially affected. A history of sexually transmitted disease and a history of a prior ectopic pregnancy increases the risk of ectopic pregnancy.[37] Patients with those histories should be counseled to see their doctor as soon as they believe that they are pregnant. Depending on individual circumstances, clinicians may do immunity or past or present infection tests prior to pregnancy (Table 4). Women susceptible to any of these should be counseled about immunization and about prevention of infections. Any active infection should be treated as appropriate.

Human immunodeficiency virus

All sexually active women should be offered HIV testing. Most women who might transmit the human immunodeficiency virus (HIV) infection to their fetus are asymptomatic. Preconception testing for HIV is important because the Pediatric AIDS Clinical Trials Study Group has shown that treatment with zidovudine (Retrovir) reduces the risk of transmission to the fetus from 25.5% to 8.3%. Earlier treatment of HIV and other sexually transmitted diseases decreases the risk of transmission to the fetus. Vertical transmission results in approximately a 30% chance of fetal infection from an untreated HIV-positive mother, a risk that can be reduced substantially with preconception or early pregnancy treatment. During the preconception period, women should be educated about high-risk behavior and given advice on contraception.

Table 4 Tests prior to pregnancy

- Human immune deficiency virus (both in husband and wife)
- Syphilis (both in husband and wife)
- Hepatitis B antigen and antibody (both in husband and wife)
- Gonorrhea
- Chlamydia
- Parvovirus
- Cytomegalovirus
- Toxoplasma
- Herpes (both in husband and wife)
- Varicella
- Rubella

Syphilis

The time prior to pregnancy is optimal to identify and treat syphilis because at that time there is no fetus yet to be concerned about when giving appropriate medications.

Gonorrhea, chlamydia

Both of these infections can lead to adverse pregnancy outcomes and to infertility if not treated appropriately. Treatment of both partners prior to pregnancy is preferred as it prevents unnecessary exposure of the fetus.

Hepatitis B and other immunizations

All women should be screened for hepatitis B, and those at high risk should be tested for the presence of both hepatitis B surface antigen and hepatitis B e antigen. The preconception time period is optimal to provide immunization and women who have not received the hepatitis B vaccine should be considered for immunization if they are at risk of sexually transmitted disease or blood exposure. The vaccine may be given during pregnancy. Hepatitis B is the most common type of hepatitis in the US.

Influenza

Pregnancy is considered a high-risk condition for influenza. According to CDC guidelines, all women who expect to be pregnant during the influenza season (November to April) should be vaccinated against influenza. The specific guidelines for immunizations for adults can be found under 'Update on Adult Immunization Recommendations of the Immunization Practices Advisory Committee' at <www.cdc.gov/mmwr/preview/mmwrhtml/00025228.htm>.

Rubella and varicella

Preconception evaluation should include tests for immunity to rubella and varicella. Women who have no immunity to varicella are at risk for development of varicella pneumonia, which has a maternal mortality rate as high as 40%. Because immunization against these include live-virus vaccines, women should be advised to not get pregnant for at least one month after immunization.

Toxoplasmosis

Toxoplasmosis may cause congenital infections if the mother becomes infected during pregnancy and testing during pregnancy can sometimes yield confusing results. Preconception is the optimal time to test for past exposure to toxoplasma. Currently, no immunizations are available for these infections. Women who have not previously been exposed to toxoplasmosis should be counseled to avoid contact with cat feces in litter boxes, wear gloves while gardening, and avoid eating raw or undercooked meat.[38]

Cytomegalovirus (CMV), parvovirus B19 (fifth disease)

CMV and parvovirus exposure in susceptible women is especially risky for childcare and healthcare workers.[26] Periconception testing for CMV or toxoplasmosis may be advantageous in counseling women about infection prevention during pregnancy. Women with negative titers prior to pregnancy should receive extensive counseling on how to avoid infections during pregnancy. Persons at risk should wash their hands frequently and use gloves to prevent transmission.[39]

Dental hygiene

There has recently been scientific evidence that gum disease increases the risk of preterm delivery.[40] Therefore, every woman should have dental care and treatment prior to pregnancy and during pregnancy to prevent adverse outcomes.

MALE PERICONCEPTION CARE

There is expanding scientific evidence of an association between male-associated health issues and pregnancy outcomes. Optimally, a couple should attend the periconception visit together and the woman's partner should be encouraged to be included in periconception counseling and care. Seeing the couple together allows the clinician to educate men about risks, review their family history for genetic disorders, and screen for sexually transmitted diseases and sexual dysfunction or refer them to a specialist. Paternal smoking as well as alcohol consumption have been associated with decreased fertility and adverse neonatal outcomes such as low birth weight and an increased incidence of fetal malformations. It takes on average 10–11 weeks for sperm to be produced. To optimize male fertility, men should abstain from alcohol and tobacco, and exposure to potentially damaging substances for at least 3 months prior to conception. Other substances and chemicals may adversely affect spermatogenesis and male fertility. In addition, smoking by the father and passive smoking by the prospective mother can equally have a potential negative effect on pregnancy. Sperm production in the testes requires a temperature that is lower than the core body temperature. To maximize sperm production, men should, therefore, refrain from staying too long in saunas or hot tubs and prevent overheating of testes (*e.g.* not wear too tight pants).

SUMMARY

Every physician and healthcare provider, not just obstetricians and gynecologists, should focus on periconception care during each annual visit of women of childbearing age. Patients should be asked about conception plans and early prenatal care when a pregnancy is confirmed should be encouraged. Clinicians should encourage all women of childbearing age to receive periconception care, and some may require a periconception consultation with a maternal–fetal medicine or other specialist. Encourage women to eat a healthy diet, try to reach their optimal weight, not drink any alcohol and stay away from smoking, limit consumption of certain fish, and supplement their diet with folic acid (0.4 mg/day). Encourage couples to enhance their probability of conception with regular midcycle coitus, ovulation monitoring, and avoidance of lubricants that can decrease fertility. Suggest early evaluation if infertility is an issue, especially in women older than 35 years.

KEY POINTS FOR CLINICAL PRACTICE

- Obtain a thorough personal, medical, and family history of the potential mother and father and an assessment of the health of both potential parents, although a greater emphasis is usually placed on that of the mother.

- Obtain a genetic history about family members with genetic problems and congenital birth defects and conditions like hypertension, diabetes, mental retardation, blindness, and deafness; test if indicated.

- Review the reproductive and gynaecological history and prior pregnancies.

- Review the couple's daily living and environment, reviewing medications both prescription and over-the-counter, and screening for exposure to potentially harmful substances both at home or at work. Review weight, diet and food and provide specific nutritional and exercise counseling.

- Review and optimization of fertility.

- Medical and gynaecological examination, reviewing and screening for infectious diseases, and updating immunizations. Perform additional tests if indicated (*e.g.* blood samples, HIV, infectious diseases, genetic predisposition).

- Male periconception counseling

References

1 Williams JW. Obstetrics: a textbook for the use of students and practitioners. Chapter VIII. D. Appleton, 1903; 175
2 Cox M, Whittle MJ, Byrne A *et al*. Prepregnancy counseling: experience from 1075 cases. Br J Obstet Gynaecol 1992; 99: 873
3 Kitzmiller JL, Gavin LA, Gin GD *et al*. Preconception care of diabetes: glycemic control prevents congenital anomalies. JAMA 1991; 265: 731
4 Waisbren SE, Hanley W, Levy HL *et al*. Outcome at age 4 in the offspring of women with maternal phenylketonuria. JAMA 2000; 283: 756
5 De Weerd S, Polder JJ, Cohen-Overbeck TE *et al*. Preconception care: preliminary estimates of costs and effects of smoking cessation and folic acid supplementation. J Reprod Med 2004; 49: 338
6 Adams MM, Bruce FC, Shulman HB *et al*. Pregnancy planning and pre-conception counseling. Obstet Gynecol 1993; 82: 955
7 Henshaw S. Unintended pregnancy in the United States. Fam Plan Perspect 1998; 30: 24
8 Hellerstedt WL, Pirie PL, Lando HA *et al*. Differences in preconceptional and prenatal behaviors in women with intended and unintended pregnancies. Am J Public Health 1998; 88: 663

9 Postlethwaite D. Preconception health counseling for women exposed to teratogens: the role of the nurse. J Obstet Gynecol Neonat Nurs 2003; 32: 523–532

10 MRC Vitamin Study Research Group. Prevention of neural tube defects: results of the MRC vitamin study. Lancet 1991; 338: 132–137

11 Sablock U, Lindow S, Arnott PIE, Masson EA. Prepregnancy counseling for women with medical disorders. J Obstet Gynecol 2002; 22: 637–638

12 De Weerd S, van der Bij AK, Cikot RJ, Braspenning JCC, Braat DDM, Steegers EAP. Preconception care: a screening tool for health assessment and risk detection. Prevent Med 2002; 34: 505–511

13 Hawthorne G, Modder J. Maternity services for women with diabetes in the UK. Diabetic Med 2002; 19: 50

14 Gunton JE, Morris J, Boyce S et al. Outcome of pregnancy complicated by pre-gestational diabetes – improvement in outcomes Aust NZ J Obstet Gynaecol 2002; 42: 478

15 American Diabetes Association. Preconception care of women with diabetes, Diabetes Care 2004; 27: S76–S78

16 Delgado-Escueta AV, Janz D. Consensus guideline: preconception counseling, management, and care of the pregnant woman with epilepsy. Neurology. 1992; 42 (Suppl 5): 149

17 Pennel PR. Pregnancy in women who have epilepsy. Neurol Clin 2004; 22: 799

18 Ginsberg JS, Bates SM. Management of venous thromboembolism during pregnancy. J Thromb Haemost 2003; 1; 1435

19 American College of Obstetricians and Gynecologists. Committee Opinion: Prenatal and Preconceptional Carrier Screening for genetic Diseases in Individuals of Easter European Jewish Descent. August 2004; Number 298

20 Malm H, Martikainen J, Klaukka T et al. Prescription of hazardous drugs during pregnancy. Drug Safety 2004; 27: 899

21 Lammer EJ, Chen DT, Hoar RM et al. Retinoic acid embryopathy. N Engl J Med 1985; 313: 837

22 Mills JL, Simpson JL, Cunningham GC et al. Vitamin A and birth defects. Am J Obstet Gynecol 1997; 177: 1

23 Marbury MC, Linn S, Monson R et al. The association of alcohol consumption with outcome of pregnancy. Am J Public Health 1983; 73: 1165

24 Lundsberg LS, Bracken MB, Saftlas AF. Low-to-moderate gestational alcohol use and intrauterine growth retardation, low birthweight, and preterm delivery. Ann Epidemiol 1997; 7: 498

25 Livy DJ, Maier SE, West JR. Long-term alcohol exposure prior to conception results in lower fetal body weights. Birth Defects Res B Dev Reprod Toxicol 2004; 71: 135

26 Brundage SC. Preconception health care. Am Fam Phys 2002; 65: 2507

27 Saraiya M, Berg CJ, Kendrick JS et al. Cigarette smoking as a risk factor for ectopic pregnancy. Am J Obstet Gynecol 1998; 178: 493

28 Brent R, Oakley G, Mattis D. The unnecessary epidemic of folic acid-preventable spina bifida and anencephaly. Pediatrics 2000; 106: 825

29 Botto LD, Moore CA, Khoury MJ et al. Neural tube defects. N Engl J Med 1999; 341: 1509

30 De Weerd S, Thomas CMG, Cikot R et al. Preconception counseling improves folate status of women planning pregnancy. Obstet Gynecol 2002; 99: 45

31 Hindmarsh PC, Geary MP, Rodeck CH et al. Effects of early maternal iron stores on placental weight and structure. Lancet 2000; 356: 719

32 Wynn M, Wynn A. A fertility diet for planning pregnancy. Nutr Health 1995; 10: 219

33 Grodstein F, Goldman MB, Cramer DW. Body mass index and ovulatory infertility. Epidemiology 1994; 5: 247

34 Castro LC, Avina RL. Maternal obesity and pregnancy outcomes. Curr Opin Obstet Gynecol 2002; 14: 601

35 Curry MA, Perrin N, Wall E. Effects of abuse on maternal complications and low birth weight in adult and adolescent women. Obstet Gynecol 1998; 92: 530

36 Hanlin RB. Congenital infections and preconception counseling. J S C Med Assoc 2002; 98: 277

37 Chow WH, Daling JR, Cates W et al. Epidemiology of ectopic pregnancy. Epidemiol Rev 1987; 9: 70

38 Lopez A, Dietz VJ, Wilson M *et al*. Preventing congenital toxoplasmosis. MMWR 2000; 49: 59

39 Allaire AD, Cefalo RC. Preconceptional health care model. Eur J Obstet Gynecol Reprod Biol. 1998; 78: 163

40 Champagne CM, Madianos PN, Lieff S *et al*. Periodontal medicine: emerging concepts in pregnancy outcome. J Intern Acad Periodont 2000; 2: 9

41 Berry RJ, Li Z, Erickson JD *et al*. China–U.S. Collaborative Project for Neural Tube Defect Prevention. Prevention of neural-tube defects with folic acid in China N Engl J Med 1999; 341: 1485–1490

42 Dolovich LR, Addis A, Vaillancourt JMR, Power JDB, Koren G, Einarson TR. Benzodiazepine use in pregnancy and major malformations or oral cleft: meta-analysis of cohort and case-control. BMJ 1998; 317: 839–843

43 Cnattingius S, Signorello LB, Anneren G *et al*. Caffeine intake and the risk of first trimester spontaneous abortion. N Engl J Med 2000; 343: 1839

44. Hendrick V, Smith LM, Suri R, Hwang S, Haynes D, Altshuler L. Birth outcomes after prenatal exposure to antidepressant medication. Am J Obstet Gynecol 2003; 188: 812–815

45 Stanton CK, Gray RH. Effects of caffeine consumption on delayed conception. Am J Epidemiol 1995; 142: 1322

APPENDIX 1

Sample periconception patient questionnaire

	Yes	No
Are you taking any prescription drugs?		
Are you using birth control pills or other hormonal contraceptives?		
Do you use over-the-counter (non-prescription) drugs?		
Do you take any vitamins, minerals, herbal supplements or other food supplements?		
Do you take a multivitamin containing 0.4 mg of folic acid every day?		
Do you use any recreational or street drugs (*e.g.* marijuana, cocaine, crack, *etc.*)?		
Do you smoke cigarettes? If yes, how many per day?		
Do you breathe second-hand smoke?		
Do you drink beer, wine, or hard liquor?		
How many drinks does it take to make you feel high?		
Have people annoyed you by criticizing your drinking?		
Have you felt you ought to cut down on your drinking?		
Have you ever had a drink first thing in the morning to steady your nerves or get rid of a hangover?		
Have you recently seen a dentist?		
Are you over or underweight?		

Personal information: Tell us about you and your partner

Family and genetic history: Tell us about your family and your genetic history

Your daily living and the environment: Tell us about your daily routines and your environment. Are you exposed to any harmful agents?

Diet and food: Tell us about your diet and food

Trying to conceive history: Tell us about your attempts to conceive

Gynecological history: Tell us about your gynecological history

Medical history: Tell us about your medical history

Infections: Have you ever had an infection or a sexually transmitted diseases?

Immunizations: Are you immunized against common childhood diseases and against Hepatitis B?

Prior pregnancies: Tell us about your prior pregnancies

What is your ethnic background?   —

Have you or the baby's father ever been screened for special diseases related to your ethnic background?	Yes	No
Have you or your partner had a baby with a genetic (inherited) problem or have there been any birth defects or mental retardation in the family?	Yes	No
Does anybody in the family have a history of a genetic disease such as: cystic fibrosis, Tay-Sachs disease, hemophilia?	Yes	No
Do you have a close family member with a medical condition such as diabetes or a history of seizures?	Yes	No
Did your mother have toxemia or high blood pressure in any of her pregnancies?	Yes	No
Do you or a close family member have a history of blood clots?	Yes	No
Do you have a close family member with ovarian or breast cancer?	Yes	No

Please enter here and explain for any question where you checked a 'Yes'.

Thomas Murphy Goodwin

Hyperemesis gravidarum

Hyperemesis gravidarum is a significant but underappreciated illness of pregnancy. It is most commonly defined as: (i) persistent vomiting in pregnancy not due to other causes; (ii) an indicator of acute starvation (*e.g.* large ketonuria); and (iii) some discrete measure of severity, the most commonly accepted criterion being loss of 5% of pre-pregnancy weight. Since the weight loss criterion may not be accessible, a requirement for hospitalization for intravenous hydration is sometimes substituted as an indicator of severity. The reported incidence is 0.5–2.0%. It is the most common indication for admission to the hospital in the first half of pregnancy and second only to preterm labor as a cause of hospitalization overall. The estimated cost for hospital care alone is more US$500 million for the 59,000 women hospitalized with hyperemesis gravidarum in the US annually.[1]

ETIOLOGY

Hyperemesis gravidarum is clearly related to a product of placental metabolism since it does not require the presence of the fetus. It occurs commonly with advanced molar gestation and multiple gestation. More than 20 studies of non-thyroidal hormonal changes in nausea and vomiting of pregnancy (NVP) have been published. The only differences between hyperemesis gravidarum and control subjects that have been reported in more than one study are with hCG and estradiol. Although there is conflicting information, several lines of evidence point towards a role for these two hormones.

Hormones

There is a strong temporal association between hCG concentrations and the time course of NVP (Fig. 1).[2,3] In addition, the association of biochemical

Thomas Murphy Goodwin MD
Professor and Chief, Maternal-Fetal Medicine, University of Southern California, Women's and
Children's Hospital, Room 5L–40, Los Angeles, California 90033, USA. E-mail: tgoodwin:usc.edu

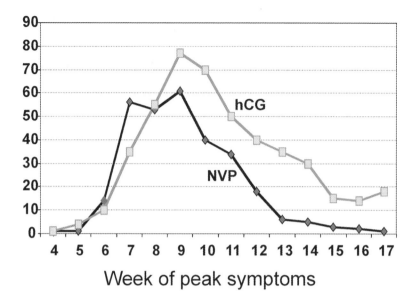

Fig. 1 Peak nausea and vomiting symptoms and hCG.

hyperthyroidism with the severity of NVP is strong. The thyroid stimulator of pregnancy is hCG.[4] It has been shown, in addition, that some of the variation in the relationship between total hCG concentrations and thyroid stimulation can be due to the fact that what is commonly called hCG is actually a family of isoforms which differ in half-life and potency at the LH (hCG) and TSH receptor. Forms lacking the carboxy-terminal portion, for example, are more potent stimulators of the TSH and LH receptors but have shorter half-lives. Hyperglycosylated hCG, on the other hand, has a longer half-life and has a longer duration of action.[5]

A link between the action of hCG and estradiol has been suggested by the finding that concentrations of hyperglycosylated hCG correlate with estradiol and the severity of nausea and vomiting. It is hypothesized that stimulation of maternal ovarian production of estradiol (and possibly fetal production) increases the estradiol concentration in the mother. Nausea and vomiting in women taking the combined oral contraceptive pill increases in direct correlation with the estradiol dose.[6] A history of nausea and vomiting while taking estrogens is a risk factor for development of hyperemesis gravidarum.

Cytokines

Recently, several groups have investigated the role of cytokines in hyperemesis gravidarum. The consistent finding has been an increased concentration TNF-α.[7] TNF-α is involved in regulation of the hCG production, suggesting a possible link to the hCG-hormone hypothesis. The normal shift in pregnancy to Th2 over Th1 dominance has been reported to be more exaggerated in women with hyperemesis gravidarum.[8] The increase in IL-4 secreting cells seen in this milieu also favors increased hCG production. Adenisone, which is

Table 1 Associations common to chemotherapy-induced nausea and vomiting, postoperative nausea and vomiting and nausea and vomiting of pregnancy

WORSE NAUSEA AND VOMITING
    Younger age
    History of motion sickness
    History of oral contraceptive sickness
    History of migraine
    Earlier in the day
    Female gender of patient

OTHER ASSOCIATIONS UNIQUE TO NAUSEA AND VOMITING OF PREGNANCY
    Family history
    Female gender of fetus
    History of migraine
    Multiple gestation
    Down syndrome
    Molar gestation

SMOKING DECREASES NAUSEA AND VOMITING OF PREGNANCY

thought to attenuate the oxidative burst of TNF-α, is also increased in hyperemesis gravidarum[9] as its is precursor catalytic enzyme 5'-nucleotidase.[10] These changes and the increase in hCG point to increased activity in the trophoblast cells at the maternal–fetal interface. Consistent with this is the finding of increased cell-free DNA in the plasma of women with hyperemesis gravidarum attributed to trophoblasts, damaged or destroyed by a hyperactive maternal immune response.[11]

Risk factors – common features with other vomiting syndromes

Epidemiological studies have, in general, identified some common threads between women with hyperemesis gravidarum and other common nausea and vomiting syndromes – postoperative nausea and vomiting, and chemotherapy-related nausea and vomiting. These are shown in Table 1. It is interesting to note that smoking is associated with decreased concentrations of hCG and estradiol while female gender of the fetus is associated with greater concentrations of hCG.[12]

In some instances, hyperemesis gravidarum can be due to an underlying maternal metabolic disorder. Nausea and vomiting are common manifestations of a number of disorders of fatty acid oxidation. Women who are carriers for recessive diseases of fatty acid transport and mitochondrial oxidation have been found to have increased risk for hyperemesis as well as other pregnancy complications.[13]

Genetics of hyperemesis gravidarum

Evidence in support of a genetic predisposition to nausea and vomiting of pregnancy includes: (i) the concordance in frequency of nausea and vomiting of pregnancy in monozygotic twins;[14] (ii) the fact that siblings and mothers of patients affected with nausea and vomiting of pregnancy are more likely to be affected than siblings of unaffected individuals; (iii)) the variation in the frequency of nausea and vomiting of pregnancy among different ethnic groups (Minturn and Weiher,[16] relying on data from the Human Relation Area Files, found that 8 of 30 societies with sufficient information on morning sickness reported none at all); and (iv) the occurrence of nausea and vomiting of pregnancy in women with inherited glycoprotein hormone receptor defects.[17]

Is there a role for psychopathology?

Apart from the epidemiological and biological associations that have accumulated over the years, one of the most enduring theories has been that NVP and hyperemesis gravidarum, in particular, are more likely to occur in women of a certain personality type or with a given psychopathological diathesis. The extensive literature on this subject is alternately confused and contradictory. Hyperemesis gravidarum has been characterized as a conversion or somatization disorder in psycho-analytical terms or as a result of the mother's inability to respond to life stresses. There are no controlled studies supporting these and related theories. Simpson and Buckwalter[18] applied validated psychological tests to women with hyperemesis and controls during pregnancy and postpartum. During pregnancy, women with severe nausea and vomiting scored significantly higher on three scales associated with a conversion disorder. However, there were no significant differences between subjects and controls postpartum. According to the authors, the changes were best explained as a response to the stress of being ill rather than as a reflection of a pre-existing personality disorder. The concept that women are, in a sense, responsible for their own hyperemesis gravidarum persists. In a recent survey study by Munch,[19] 93 of 96 women reported their own conviction that the condition had a biological basis and that psychological problems were secondary to the severe illness. Nevertheless, most of the same cohort reported that friends, family members and caregivers constantly implied that they were somehow in control of their disease state.

Part of the problem is due to the subjective nature of the condition. Like pain, nausea can only be understood by the person suffering it. Failure to appreciate the impact of pain on well-being has been epidemic in medicine. Only recently has this received specific attention. With nausea, especially in the absence of other objective findings of disease, there is still considerable skepticism. In addition, susceptibility to behavioral conditioning, something distinct from a personality type, may be related to NVP. In patients undergoing chemotherapy, anticipatory nausea and vomiting is well-described. This condition presents when visual or olfactory cues related to the initial episode of vomiting trigger a response. Unlike nausea and vomiting normally associated with chemotherapy, it is refractory to pharmacological intervention but does respond to behavioral therapy.[20] To what extent such a process of conditioned response may play a role in hyperemesis gravidarum is unknown. Uncontrolled case series have suggested a benefit of behavioral therapy or hypnosis in treatment of hyperemesis gravidarum. Interestingly, the food aversions in pregnancy are similar to those that develop with chemotherapy in that they do not generally persist after the acute course of the primary stimulus ends; this is distinct from conditioned responses otherwise which may persist for years.

Embryo protection hypothesis

The view that NVP is a mechanism preserved in evolution to protect the fetus from environmental teratogens and toxins has received considerable attention in recent years.[21] Central to the critique of this theory is an understanding of cause and effect that most obstetricians would find counter intuitive. For example, the fact that women with NVP are less likely to have spontaneous abortions is taken as evidence that vomiting and food aversions are protective for the fetus; other lines of evidence suggest that this reflects the fact that pregnancies destined to end in spontaneous abortions have deficient production of the placental factors responsible for NVP. Regrettably, some have interpreted the 'embryo-protection hypothesis' to mean that the large number of pregnant women with NVP who experience disability may not be worthy of serious attention or treatment.

NVP as a syndrome

NVP and hyperemesis gravidarum may be conceived of as a syndrome. The primary emetogenic stimulus arises from the placenta or is triggered by a placental product. The stimulus may be increased as in advanced molar gestation or multiple gestation or with other effects on placenta production such as with a female fetus or with Down syndrome. The response of the mother to this stimulus from the fetal genome is determined, in part, by her susceptibility to an emetogenic stimulus in general. These are patterns of susceptibility common to any postoperative nausea and vomiting and chemotherapy-induced nausea and vomiting and are mediated through vestibular, gastrointestinal and behavioral and central nervous system pathways. Susceptibility specific to hyperemesis gravidarum includes receptor abnormalities increasing sensitivity to the placental product. A strong genetic component probably influences more than one of these pathways.

CLINICAL PRESENTATION

Careful prospective studies show that virtually all women who develop NVP will have some symptoms by 9 weeks' gestation. Of pregnant women, 7% have symptoms before the time of the first missed period, 60% are symptomatic by 6 weeks, and 35% suffer NVP severe enough to miss work or to be unable to perform daily activities about the house. The importance of this observation in a discussion of hyperemesis gravidarum is that aggressive treatment of women at this stage of NVP appears to reduce the incidence and severity of subsequent hyperemesis gravidarum. For the subset of women with hyperemesis, there is a tendency for early onset of symptoms and much greater duration overall. Of women with NVP, 90% have no symptoms by 16 weeks but there is very little data on the duration of symptoms with hyperemesis. Of more than 1500 women with hyperemesis gravidarum responding to an internet survey, 67% reported symptoms beyond 20 weeks' and 41% had symptoms beyond 30 weeks' gestation.

In addition to nausea and vomiting, associated complaints include excess salivation (ptyalism), an increased olfactory and gustatory aversion and changes in test sensitivity. There are few systematically collected data on these complaints relative to NVP and hyperemesis gravidarum. Ptyalism is present in up to 60% of severe hyperemesis gravidarum.[22] Although there is a common perception that women with more severe NVP are most sensitive to olfactory stimuli, this has not been documented in objective studies. Rather, there is a change in the hedonic rating of odours, something similar to what is seen during chemotherapy-induced nausea.[23]

There is conflicting data as to whether hyperemesis gravidarum is more common in women with a higher or lower body mass index (BMI). Studies looking at all NVP have generally found it to be more common in women of higher body mass but a more recent study focusing just on those with vomiting severe enough to come to the hospital found a higher rate among women of lower BMI.[24] Oxygen consumption is decreased in hyperemesis gravidarum consistent with a state of metabolic suppression characteristic of starvation. This change, which links hyperemesis gravidarum to classic starvation experiences, is reversed promptly with re-feeding.[25]

Laboratory abnormalities

Women with hyperemesis gravidarum may present with a variety of biochemical abnormalities as listed in Table 2. The hyperthyroidism of hyperemesis gravidarum is transient and does not require specific treatment. Virtually all patients with this syndrome will have a normal TSH by 20 weeks' gestation. It may be distinguished from hyperthyroidism due to intrinsic thyroid disease by several points: no history of symptoms preceding pregnancy, absence of goiter, lack of other systemic signs of hyperthyroidism (except occasionally tachycardia), absence of thyroid antibodies.[26]

Changes in amylase, lipase and liver enzymes are transient and not indicative of pancreatic or liver disease *per se*. Occasionally, elevation in the bilirubin concentration may be much more dramatic than noted in Table 2. Several cases have been reported of marked jaundice and even hepatic dysfunction associated with hyperemesis gravidarum, one resolving only with termination of pregnancy.

Table 2 Laboratory abnormalities in hyperemesis gravidarum admitted to Los Angeles County Hospital

Test	Abnormal (%)	Typical range of abnormal
FT4 Index	60	13.2–40
FT3 Index	10	225–350
TSH suppressed	60	< 0.4 μU/ml
Na⁺ low	30	125–134 mmol/l
K⁺ low	15	2.3–3.1 mmol/l
Cl⁻ low	25	80–98 mmol/l
Bicarbonate high	15	27–35 mmol/l
ALT/AST high	40	41–350 U/l
Bilirubin high	20	1.1–5.0 mg/dl
Amylase high	15	131–400 U/l
Lipase high	30	61–240 U/l

Complications – Wernicke's encephalopathy

One of the most serious complications of hyperemesis gravidarum is Wernicke's encephalopathy.[27] This form of central nervous system dysfunction is due to a deficiency of thiamine (vitamin B_1). More than 30 cases have been reported in the last 20 years related to hyperemesis gravidarum. All patients presented after at least 3 weeks of pernicious vomiting. Most presented only with confusion and apathetic affect although other classic signs of Wernicke's encephalopathy including gait ataxia and nystagmus have been described. Some patients have presented with blindness. In the majority of cases, the patient either died or had permanent residual dysfunction. Cardiac dysfunction due to thiamine deficiency has also been reported. The condition may be precipitated by infusion of carbohydrate prior to thiamine replacement as the small amount of thiamine remaining may be consumed in the acute metabolism of a carbohydrate load.

The problem of Wernicke's encephalopathy is best addressed by prevention. All patients with hyperemesis gravidarum should at least receive the recommended daily amount (RDA) for thiamine, contained in most multivitamins (3 mg). When a patient is vomiting sufficient to require intravenous hydration, 100 mg thiamine should be administered parenterally on the presumption of thiamine deficiency. It is our practice to administer this daily for 3 days if a patient is in hospital for hyperemesis gravidarum.

Other reported complications of hyperemesis gravidarum include pneumothorax, Mallory Weiss tear of the esophagus, esophageal rupture, splenic avulsion, acute tubular necrosis, central pontine myelenolysis and peripheral neuropathy.

Psychological burden and long-term health consequences

In interviews with patients, one of the most crippling aspects of the disease is the sense of isolation that many patients have from suffering a disease of unknown etiology that is fundamentally subjective in nature. Many women are driven to seek termination of an otherwise wanted pregnancy, in part because of the physical suffering but also in part because of the sense of isolation. Testimony to the fact that hyperemesis gravidarum is often not taken seriously enough by care providers is the fact women who terminate pregnancy often have received no treatment for their hyperemesis gravidarum.[28] After pregnancy, women who have suffered from hyperemesis gravidarum often decide not to conceive again.

The long-term health consequences of hyperemesis gravidarum for the women who suffer from it are largely unknown. Two studies suggested an increased risk of breast cancer in these patients, based on a presumed hyperestrogenic milieu but this has not been confirmed in recent reports.[29] Reports of post-traumatic stress disorder, depression and a variety of neurological complaints are commonly mentioned by women but there has been no systematic follow-up.

Fetal consequences of hyperemesis

The long-standing dogma has been that women with NVP and even hyperemesis gravidarum have better pregnancy outcomes than women who have no NVP. This does appear to be true for NVP in general. With regard to hyperemesis gravidarum, it is clear that a mild form of hyperemesis gravidarum which may require intravenous hydration should be distinguished from more severe disease, generally distinguished by weight loss of more than 5%. In patients diagnosed with hyperemesis gravidarum who have lost weight, the incidence of SGA is clearly higher. In addition, there is evidence that, in this group, the rate of fetal death is higher, contrary to the prevailing dogma.[30] Interestingly, this increased rate of fetal death is seen after famine in early pregnancy.[31]

Major congenital anomalies appear to be less prevalent in women with NVP and hyperemesis gravidarum, although there is some conflicting data. Kulander and Kallen[32] found that hip dysplasia and Down syndrome were more common than expected in a population study of hyperemesis gravidarum in Sweden. But apart from these anomalies which appear to be related to the hormonal milieu in hyperemesis gravidarum, there is an overall lowering of the rate of birth defects.[33]

Long-term effects on offspring

The long-term consequences of hyperemesis gravidarum for the offspring are almost entirely unstudied. In general, practitioners have relied on the information from delivery data to re-assure patients that there are no adverse consequences. Nevertheless, a large body of information has now accumulated implicating calorie restriction in early pregnancy in the genesis of a number of adult disorders. Data from the Dutch famine cohort have shown that famine just in the first few months of pregnancy is associated with higher rates of pulmonary and cardiac disease as well as schizophrenia. This finding has been reported from other populations as well, most recently in an examination of Chinese who lived through the 'Great Leap Forward'.[34] An important link between classic starvation studies and NVP is the finding that vomiting during pregnancy was the only pregnancy-related event associated with schizophrenia in a case control study.[35]

A number of childhood cancers including testicular cancer and leukemia have been linked to hyperemesis although there is conflicting data.

DIFFERENTIAL DIAGNOSIS

The diagnosis of NVP is clinical in nature, based on its typical presentation and the absence of other diseases that could explain the symptoms. Although other causes of persistent nausea and vomiting are rarely encountered, failure to distinguish them from NVP can result in serious complications. The differential diagnosis of the patient with suspected NVP includes the conditions listed in Table 3.

History and physical findings

NVP begins before 9–10 weeks' gestation. Symptoms that start after this gestational age are due to other causes. It is important to note whether the patient has a history of pre-existing conditions associated with nausea and

Table 3 Differential diagnosis of hyperemesis gravidarum: classes of disorders and specific diseases reported to have presented as suspected hyperemesis gravidarum

Gastrointestinal
　　Gastroenteritis
　　Gastroparesis
　　Achalasia
　　Biliary tract disease
　　Hepatitis
　　Intestinal obstruction
　　Peptic ulcer disease
　　Pancreatitis
　　Appendicitis

Genito-urinary tract
　　Pyelonephritis
　　Uremia
　　Ovarian torsion
　　Kidney stones
　　Degenerating uterine leiomyoma

Metabolic
　　Diabetic ketoacidosis
　　Porphyria
　　Addison's disease
　　Hyperthyroidism
　　Hyperparathyroidism

Neurological disorders
　　Pseudotumor cerebri
　　Vestibular lesions
　　Migraine headaches
　　Tumors of the central nervous system
　　Lymphocytic hypophysitis

Miscellaneous
　　Drug toxicity or intolerance
　　Psychological

Pregnancy-related conditions
　　Acute fatty liver of pregnancy
　　Pre-eclampsia

vomiting (*e.g.* diabetes, porphyria, cholelithiasis, or migraine headaches). Abdominal pain is not a prominent feature of NVP; abdominal tenderness other than mild epigastric discomfort after retching is not seen with NVP. Pain that precedes or is out of proportion to the nausea and vomiting suggests an intra-abdominal or retroperitoneal cause for the vomiting. Fever is not present in NVP, but is characteristic of many other diseases associated with nausea and vomiting. Headache is not characteristic of NVP. An abnormal neurological examination suggests a primary neurological disorder as the cause of the nausea and vomiting, although it may rarely be encountered as a consequence of severe NVP (*e.g.* thiamine-deficient encephalopathy or central pontine myelinolysis). Although biochemical hyperthyroidism may be seen with moderate and severe NVP, a goiter is not found. If a goiter is present, primary thyroid disease should be suspected.

Laboratory tests

There are common laboratory abnormalities in hyperemesis gravidarum that may cause confusion. When primary hepatitis causes nausea and vomiting, the liver enzyme elevations are much higher, often in the thousands, and the bilirubin concentration is usually much higher also. Acute pancreatitis may cause vomiting and hyperamylasemia, but serum amylase concentrations are usually 5–10 times higher than the elevations associated with NVP. TSH is commonly suppressed in NVP. Because there is an inverse relationship between the severity of NVP and the TSH concentration, a non-suppressed TSH level suggests that the cause of the nausea and vomiting is something other than NVP. A TSH level greater than 2.5 µU/ml is rare with severe NVP, unless the patient has pre-existing hypothyroidism.

An ultrasound evaluation should be performed in cases of hyperemesis gravidarum as it may identify a predisposing factor such as multiple gestation or molar gestation.

MANAGEMENT

The best approach to hyperemesis gravidarum management is by prevention. To this end, there is evidence that women who are taking multivitamins at the time of conception and in early pregnancy are less likely to require intervention for hyperemesis gravidarum later in pregnancy.[36] The explanation is not clear but it has been shown in three populations. There is strong, albeit indirect, evidence that treatment of women who have NVP sufficient to interfere with their daily routine is associated with lower rates of hospital admission for hyperemesis gravidarum.[37] About one-third of pregnant women have complaints of this caliber. Historically, when Bendectin was available as a recommended treatment for NVP, 25–30% of all pregnant women were treated with it in the US (33 million between 1958 and 1983).

Diet and support

Once a decision has been made to treat a women with significant NVP, the key to the specific approach is an understanding of the safety (maternal and fetal) as well as the efficacy. There is very little firm data on the role of dietary modification to help with hyperemesis gravidarum. The most common recommendation (albeit unsupported scientifically) is to eat small portions of whatever seems palatable whenever symptoms allow. Some of the only analytic data correlated symptoms with electrogastrographic patterns.[38] It found that there is less nausea associated with protein meals compared to fat or carbohydrate and that liquid meals are better tolerated than solid.

As mentioned above, nausea and vomiting is correlated with food aversions and a change in hedonic scores for olfactory sensations. Advice to re-design the home environment to avoid sensory stimuli that provoke symptoms is based on science as well as common sense. Some women develop aversions to common sites and smells, which may include pets and even family members. Improvement in symptoms with a change in location or separation from the home and family often leads to the erroneous assumption that a conflict in the family is the basis for the hyperemesis gravidarum. Behavioral therapy, deconditioning and/or relaxation has been reported to be improve hyperemesis gravidarum in uncontrolled series.[39]

Pharmacological and alternative therapy

For women who continue to have problematic nausea and vomiting, vitamin B_6 10–30 mg tid is recommended. Three randomized, controlled trials (RCTs) suggest a benefit of vitamin B_6 in NVP in reducing nausea although the effect on vomiting is not clear.[40] Vitamin B_6 is safe for mother and fetus. Reports of vitamin B_6 toxicity with doses as low as 75 mg daily have been largely discounted. If symptoms persist, an antihistamine may be added. There is evidence of efficacy in treatment of NVP with antihistamines and there is a substantial body of safety evidence.[41]

The combination of vitamin B_6 and the first generation antihistamine doxylamine formed the basis of Bendectin which was used by about 25% of all pregnant women (33 million) women between 1958 and 1982. Several small RCTs attest to its efficacy.[42] Importantly, questions about its safety, which led to its withdrawal from the market, have not been substantiated. Because of the scrutiny brought on by litigation, Bendectin has been studied extensively. A meta-analysis of studies of Bendectin with more than 14,000 first trimester exposures found no increase in anomalies above the background rate.[43] Doxylamine itself is only available in the US in the form of Unisom sleep tablets, a formulation available over-the-counter. Vitamin B_6 (10–25 mg) plus half of a 25 mg Unisom sleep tablet 3–4 times daily approximates to the Bendectin regimen (10 mg vitamin B_6 and 10 mg doxylamine). The Bendectin formulation can also be obtained from compounding pharmacies and is available in Canada and several other countries as Diclectin. Other antihistamines may be substituted safely in this first level of pharmacological therapy.

For patients who receive no relief from this regimen or continue to progress in symptoms, a reasonable, well-attested next step is the herbal medication Ginger. Several RCTs attest to its efficacy. The main drawback to its use is that fetal safety data are limited. Nevertheless, problems have not been seen and theoretical concerns seem adequately addressed in a recent review.[44] Another alternative therapy, which has been studied extensively in NVP is acupuncture and acustimulation. Although there is some conflicting data, the weight of evidence suggests some benefit without significant risks.[40]

Other classes of anti-emetics include benzamides, phenothiazines, butyrophenones, 5-HT3 receptor antagonists and corticosteroids. While randomized trials of agents in most of these classes have shown some efficacy in NVP overall, There have only been 7 randomized trials in hyperemesis gravidarum, 4 involving steroids. Evidence for efficacy of any agent in hyperemesis gravidarum is inconclusive, perhaps due in part to methodology (see below). Nevertheless, because of their general effectiveness in relieving nausea and vomiting in other states, they have been commonly employed.

Safety data have been limited as well although in recent years there is some greater accumulation of data. Corticosteroids appear to increase the risk of facial clefts slightly when given in the first trimester. Other commonly used anti-emetics are not known teratogens although there is limited data on some agents.[40]

Since there is no good evidence for the efficacy of any one of the agents among the phenothiazines or benzamides, it is common practice to switch between agents or combine them. One of the principal dangers in this regard is the confluence of side-effects that may be seen. Several of these agents have similar side-effects and adverse reactions. There are few settings similar to hyperemesis in which anti-emetics may be employed for weeks and months consecutively. Thus, special care must be taken to limit adverse reactions. Anti-emetic agents which have been studied in NVP are shown in Table 4.

Ondansetron and other 5-HT3 receptor antagonists deserve special mention. Most women with hyperemesis gravidarum report that vitamin and herbal remedies and older anti-emetics bring little relief. Although these agents may be effective for less severe NVP, more potent interventions appear to be needed for established hyperemesis gravidarum. In this regard, ondansetron has become one of the most widely used anti-emetics, largely by analogy to its demonstrated superiority in chemotherapy-related nausea and vomiting. Although the only RCT of ondansetron for hyperemesis gravidarum showed that it was not more effective than phenergan, this may be due to selection of patients who were likely to improve with most interventions, a point discussed further below. More safety data have accumulated recently.[45]

Table 4   Anti-emetic medications studied in NVP

Drug class	Studied in NVP	Side effects
Antihistamines	Doxylamine Dimenhydrinate Diphenhydramine Promethazine Cetrizine Meclizine	Sedation, blurred vision, urinary retention, dry mouth, tachycardia
Phenothiazines	Prochlorperazine Chlorpromazine	Sedation, hypotension, extrapyramidal reactions, dry mouth, urinary retention, tachycardia, restlessness
Benzamides	Metaclopramide Trimethobenzamide	Drowsiness, restlessness, fatigue, anxiety, extrapyramidal reactions
5-HT3 antagonists	Ondansetron Dolasetron Granisetron	Headache, dizziness, mild drowsiness, constipation, arrhythmias (rare)
Corticosteroids	Methylprednisolone Prednisone	
Butyrophenones	Droperidol	Limited use – FDA warning re fatal arrhythmias

Corticosteroids are potent anti-emetics in the setting of chemotherapy-induced nausea and vomiting. They have been studied for their effect in hyperemesis gravidarum with conflicting results. Several series described significant diminution or complete resolution of nausea and vomiting with corticosteroid therapy. Randomized trials have failed to demonstrate a conclusive benefit, however. Safari and Goodwin[46] found that women discharged on corticosteroids were less likely to be re-admitted than those on phenergan but Yost and colleagues[47] did not find such a benefit. Moran and Taylor[48] asserted that the failure to show a benefit from the steroids is due to patient selection in that less ill patients (those without weight loss in their analysis) are likely to respond to a variety of treatments. The authors also review some of the particulars of dose adjustment including the remarkable recrudescence of symptoms with dose lowering which responds immediately to re-institution of therapy.

It is possible that there are different pathways to hyperemesis gravidarum such that specific therapeutic approaches are effective only in a subset of patients. There is ample evidence that short courses (6–8 weeks) of corticosteroids can be used safely in pregnancy from the maternal point of view. Fetal effects appear limited after the first trimester. Some studies have found an increase in facial clefts among those exposed to corticosteroids in early pregnancy. There may be a role for steroids for those patients who have not responded to other approaches and who now require nutritional supplementation with its attendant costs and adverse effects.

Nutritional support

For the patient who does not respond adequately to therapy and is unable to maintain her weight by oral intake, nutritional support is required. This recommendation is based on several points: higher rates of IUGR in this population, the probability of long-term adverse consequences for the fetus due to changes in programming and rare, life-threatening vitamin deficiency. Caloric support may be achieved either by enteral or parenteral nutrition. Probably because of a higher rate of patient acceptance, parenteral nutrition for women with hyperemesis gravidarum as been reported much more often the enteral nutrition. Serious complications can occur, however, including sepsis, thrombophlebitis, and death due to infection or pericardial tamponade. Peripheral placement of central access was thought to be associated with fewer complications but many of the same complications reported with central access have been reported.[49]

Enteral nutritional supplementation for hyperemesis gravidarum has been described using nasogastric, nasoduodenal and nasojejunal tubes as well as a percutaneous gastrostomy. While there is no doubt that these techniques are less expensive and subject to far fewer complications than parenteral nutrition, the reported experience is limited to case reports and small series. It is our experience that the nasal tubes are frequently declined by patients; once accepted, they may be difficult to place and are more subject to being vomited up than tubes placed for other reasons. This may be because few disorders requiring enteral nutrition are primarily disorders of vomiting *per se*. A recurring theme in reports of usage of enteral feeding is the presence of a

Preconception (for women with a history of HG)
Daily multivitamin

NAUSEA OR VOMITING INTERFERING WITH DAILY ROUTINE

Vitamin B6 10 – 30 mg tid-qid PO

Continued symptoms after 48 hours
Add doxylamine 12.5 mg tid – qid PO

Continued symptoms after 48 hours
Substitute doxylamine with other antihistamine:

Promethazine 12.5 – 25 mg q4h PO or PR
or
Dimenhydrinate 50 – 100 mg q4-6h PO or PR

Consider alternative therapies at any point in this sequence:
Acupuncture or acustimulation, Ginger tablets 250 mg qid

PERSISTENT SYMPTOMS, WITH OR WITHOUT DEHYDRATION

Prochlorperazine 25 mg q12h PR
or
Metaclopramide 5-10 mg q8h PO or IV
or
Trimethobenzamide 200 mg PR q6-8h

DEHYDRATION OR WEIGHT LOSS

Thiamine 100 mg IV daily for 3 days
Continue thiamine in MVI daily

Ondansetron 8 mg q8-12h IV or PO
or
Methylprednisolone up to 16 mg tid for three days
Taper over 2 weeks to lowest effective dose
Total duration of therapy 6 weeks

UNABLE TO MAINTAIN WEIGHT

INSTITUTE TOTAL ENTERAL OR PARENTERAL NUTRITION

Fig. 2 NVP/hyperemesis gravidarum treatment sequence at Los Angeles County Hospital/University of Southern California Medical Center.

skilled team for replacement and support that is capable of encouraging patients and anticipating their needs.

A schema for an overall approach to prevention and treatment of hyperemesis gravidarum is shown in Figure 2.

SUMMARY

Hyperemesis gravidarum is a complex syndrome that is a cause of significant morbidity for mother and fetus. Aggressive treatment and support can improve outcomes and improve quality of life.

References

1 Care of Women in U.S. Hospitals, 2000 AHRQ HCUP (Health Care Cost and Utilization Project) Fact Book No. 3

2 Braunstein GD, Hershman JM. Comparison of serum pituitary thyrotropin and chorionic gonadotropin throughout pregnancy. J Clin Endocrinol Metab 1976; 42: 1123–1126

3 Gadsby R, Barnie-Adshead AM, Jagger C. A prospective study of nausea and vomiting during pregnancy. Br J Gen Pract 1993; 43: 245–248

4 Yoshimura M, Hershman JM. Thyrotropic action of human chorionic gonadotropin. Thyroid 1995; 5: 425–434

5 Jordan V, Grebe SKG, Cooke RR et al. Acidic isoforms of chorionic gonadotropin in European and Samoan women are associated with hyperemesis gravidarum and may be thyrotrophic. Clin Endocrinol 1999; 50: 619–627

6 Goldzieher JW, Moses LE, Averkin E et al. A placebo-controlled double-blind crossover investigation of the side effects attributed to oral contraceptives. Fertil Steril 1971; 22: 609–623

7 Kaplan PB, Gucer F, Sayin NC et al. Maternal serum cytokine levels in women with hyperemsis gravidarum in the first trimester of pregnancy. Fertil Steril 2003; 79: 498–502

8 Yoneyama Y, Suzuki S, Sawa R et al. The T-helper 1/T-helper 2 balance in peripheral blood of women with hyperemesis gravidarum. Am J Obstet Gynecol 2002; 187: 1631–1635

9 Yoneyama Y, Shyunji S, Rintaro S et al. Plasma adenosine concentrations increase in women with hyperemesis gravidarum. Clin Chim Acta 2004; 342: 99–103

10 Yoneyama Y, Suzuki S, Sawa R et al. Increased plasma adenosine concentrations and the severity of preeclampsia. Obstet Gyencol 2002; 101: 1266–1270

11 Sugito Y, Dekizawa A, Farina A et al. Relationship between severity of hyperemesis gravidarum and fetal DNA concentration in maternal plasma. Clin Chem 2003; 49: 1667–1669

12 James WH. The associated offspring sex ratios and cause(s) of hyperemesis gravidarum. Acta Obstet Gynecol Scand 2001; 80: 378–379

13 Rinaldo P, Studinski AL, Matern D. Prenatal diagnosis of disorders of fatty acid transport and mitochondrial oxidation. Prenat Diagn 2001; 21: 52–54

14 Corey LA, Berg K, Solaas MH et al. The epidemiology of pregnancy complications and outcome in a Norwegian twin population. Obstet Gynecol 1992; 80: 989–994

15 Vellacott ID, Cooke EJA, James CE. Nausea and vomiting in early pregnancy. Int J Gynecol Obstet 1988; 27: 57–62

16 Minturn L, Weiher AW. The influence of diet on morning sickness: a cross-culture study. Med Anthropol 1984; Winter: 71–75

17 Rodien P, Bremont C, Raffin Sanson M et al. Familial gestational hyperthyroidism caused by a mutant thyrotropin receptor hypersensitive to human chorionic gonadotropin. N Engl J Med 1998; 339: 1823–1826

18 Simpson SW, Goodwin TM, Robins S et al. Psychological factors and hyperemesis gravidarum. J Women's Health Gender-Based Med 2001; 10: 471–477

19 Munch S. Women's experiences with a pregnancy complication: causal explanations of hyperemesis gravidarum. Soc Work Health Care 2002; 36: 59–76

20 Redd WH, Montgomery GH, Katherine N. Behavioral intervention for cancer treatment side effects. J Natl Cancer Inst 2001; 93: 813

21 Flaxman SM, Sherman PW. Morning sickness: a mechanism for protecting mother and embryo. Q Rev Biol 2000; 75: 113–148

22 Godsey RK, Newman RB. Hyperemesis gravidarum: a comparison of single and multiple admissions. J Reprod Med 1991; 36: 287–290

23 Hummela T, von Mering T, Huch R et al. Olfactory modulation of nausea during early pregnancy? Br J Obstet Gynaecol 2002; 109: 1394–1397

24 Ben-Aroya Z, Lurie S, Segal D et al. Association of nausea and vomiting in pregnancy with lower body mass index. Eur J Obstet Gynecol Reprod Biol 2005; 118: 196–198

25 Chihara H, Otsubo Y, Yoneyama Y et al. Basal metabolic rate in hyperemesis gravidarum: comparison to normal pregnancy and response to treatment. Am J Obstet Gynecol 2003; 188: 434–438

26 Goodwin TM, Hershman JM. Hyperthyroidism due to inappropriate production of human chorionic gonadotropin. Clin Obstet Gynecol 1997; 40: 32–44

27 Togay-Isikay C, Yigit A, Mutluer N. Wernicke's encephalopathy due to hyperemesis gravidarum: an under-recognised condition. Aust NZ J Obstet Gynaecol 2001; 41: 453–456

28 Mazzotta P. Factors associated with elective termination of pregnancy among Canadian and American women with nausea and vomiting of pregnancy. J Psychosom Obstet Gynaecol 2001; 12: 22–27

29 Erlandsson G, Lambe M, Cnattingius S et al. Hyperemesis gravidarum and subsequent breast cancer risk. Br J Cancer 2002; 87: 974–976

30 Bailit JL. Hyperemesis gravidarum: epidemiologic findings from a large cohort. Am J Obstet Gynecol 2005; 193: 811–814

31 Cai Y, Feng W. Famine, social disruption, and involuntary fetal loss: evidence from Chinese survey data. Demography 2005; 42: 301–302

32 Kallen B. Hyperemesis during pregnancy and delivery outcome: a registry study. Eur J Obstet Gynecol Reprod Biol 1987; 26: 291–302

33 Czeizel AE, Sarkozi A, Wyszynski DF. Effect of hyperemesis gravidarum for nonsyndromic oral clefts. Obstet Gynecol 2003; 101: 737–744

34 St Clair D, Xu M, Wang P et al. Rates of adult schizophrenia following prenatal exposure to the Chinese famine of 1959–1961. JAMA 2003; 294: 557–562

35 Ordonez AE, Bobb A, Greenstein D et al. Lack of evidence for elevated obstetric complications in childhood onset schizophrenia. Biol Psychiatry 2005; 58: 10–15

36 Kallen B, Lundberg G, Aberg A. Relationship between vitamin use, smoking, and nausea and vomiting of pregnancy. Acta Obstet Gynecol Scand 2003; 82: 916–920

37 Koren G, Maltepe C. Pre-emptive therapy for severe nausea and vomiting of pregnancy and hyperemesis gravidarum. J Obstet Gynaecol 2004; 24: 530–533

38 Jednak MA, Shadigian EM, Kim MS et al. Protein meals reduce nausea and gastric slow wave dysrhythmic activity in first trimester pregnancy. Am J Physiol 1999; 277: 855–861

39 Simon EP, Schwartz J. Medical hypnosis for hyperemesis gravidarum. Birth 1999; 26: 248–254

40 Jewell D, Young G. Interventions for nausea and vomiting in early pregnancy. Cochrane data base of systematic reviews: 2004

41 Seto A, Einarson T, Koren G. Pregnancy outcome following first trimester exposure to antihistamines: meta-analysis. Am J Perinatol 1997; 14: 119–124

42 Niebyl JR, Goodwin TM. Overview of nausea and vomiting of pregnancy with an emphasis on vitamins and ginger. Am J Obstet Gynecol 2002; 186: 253–255

43 Einarson TR, Leeder JS, Koren G. Method of meta-analysis of epidemiological studies. Drug Intell Clin Pharmacol 1988; 22: 813–824

44 Borrelli F, Capasso R, Aviello G et al. Effectiveness and safety of ginger in the treatment of pregnancy-induced nausea and vomiting. Obstet Gynecol 2005; 105: 849–856

45 Einarson A, Maltepe C, Navioz Y et al. The safety of ondansetron for nausea and vomiting of pregnancy: a prospective comparative study. Br J Obstet Gynaecol 2004; 111: 940–943

46 Safari HR, Alsulyman OM, Gherman RB et al. The efficacy of methylprednisolone in the treatment of hyperemesis gravidarum: a randomized, double-blind, controlled study. Am J Obstet Gynecol 1998; 179: 921–924

47 Yost NP, McIntire DD, Wians Jr FH et al. A randomized, placebo-controlled trial of corticosteroids for hyperemesis due to pregnancy. Obstet Gynecol 2003; 102: 1250–1254

48 Moran P, Taylor R. Management of hyperemesis gravidarum: The importance of weight loss as a criterion for steroid therapy. Q J Med 2002; 95: 153–158

49 Ogura JM, Francois KE, Perlow JH et al. Complications associated with peripherally inserted central catheter use during pregnancy. Am J Obstet Gynecol 2003; 188: 1223–1225

Sebastian Illanes   Peter Soothill

Fetal therapy

The last three decades have seen enormous scientific and technological advances in the wide variety of disciplines being applied to the study of the fetus. The use of this knowledge has led to the emergence of fetal medicine as a discipline and the possibility of fetal therapy. The development of tools such as ultrasound, allows inspection and examination of the unborn patient, and a wide range of invasive procedures can be used for diagnostic and therapeutic purposes. So, prenatal diagnosis of fetal problems or abnormalities is often only the preliminary step to fetal treatment or perinatal management.

The value of a fetal therapy relates to the balance between benefits (especially the avoidance of secondary effects) and risks while taking into account alternatives such as postnatal therapy. Since this balance is also determined by the natural history and prognosis of each condition, it is important that these are as clearly defined as possible. Several studies have shown that any problem diagnosed prenatally, usually has a worse prognosis than when the same diagnosis is made postnatally. This improvement of prognosis with time relates to the gestational age at diagnosis (the earlier the diagnosis the worse the prognosis because of early detection of the most severe cases and the non-detection of better prognosis cases). It also relates to complications occurring during the pregnancy such as the emergence of associated genetic syndromes resulting in the worst prognosis cases being excluded by for example miscarriage. Therefore, we should be very cautious

Sebastian Illanes MD MSc (for correspondence)
Clinical Fellow, Fetal Medicine Research Unit, University of Bristol, St Michael's Hospital, Southwell Street, Bristol BS8 4NE, UK
E-mail: s.illanes@bristol.ac.uk

Peter Soothill BSc MD FRCOG
Professor of Obstetrics and Gynaecology, Fetal Medicine Research Unit, University of Bristol, St Michael's Hospital, Southwell Street, Bristol BS8 4NE, UK
E-mail: peter.soothill@bristol.ac.uk

about counselling a pregnant woman at 20 weeks' gestation based on neonatal data and we need to adjust the prognosis given depending on the gestational age of the pregnancy.

We have classified the possible antenatal therapeutic interventions as transplacental treatment, invasive procedures, including transfusion and fetal surgery and future perspectives which we consider in an experimental stage but with clear possibilities of success.

TRANSPLACENTAL THERAPY

Fetal pharmacotherapy

Pharmacological therapy can be used to treat fetal disorders or improve the ability of the fetus to adapt to extra-uterine life. The transplacental route is the most commonly used way to administer drugs. However, transfer can be poor either because of the nature of the drug itself (*e.g.* digoxin) or if the condition requiring treatment reduces placental function (*e.g.* a hydropic placenta). Other approaches to drug therapy include direct fetal administration or by the intra-amniotic route but these have a very limited role at present because of the invasive nature of the procedures and because very little is known regarding the effects of fetal physiology on fetal drug distribution and effects.[1,2]

Therapies to improve the ability of the fetus to adapt to extra-uterine life
Several methods have been used to accelerate fetal maturation in fetuses at risk of preterm delivery, and the example most extensively studied and used is corticosteroids for lung maturity. Liggins[3] was the first to describe this effect in 1969, and 35 years later the administration of these drugs remains the most important step to prevent respiratory distress syndrome and also intraventricular haemorrhage in preterm infants.[4] The effect of treatment is optimal if the baby is delivered more than 24 h and less than 7 days after the start of treatment.[4] However, use of repeat corticosteroid courses every week should not be routinely used because this approach has not been shown to have any significant advantages[5] and there are growing concerns about the potential deleterious effects of repeated steroid exposure on the developing human brain.[6] The dose and administration route is well established and two doses of Betamethasone 12 mg given intramuscularly 24 h apart or four doses of Dexamethasone 6 mg given intramuscularly 12 h apart are equally effective.[7] However, the evidence that oral administration would not be just as effective is unclear. The addition of thyrotropin-releasing hormones (TRH) to corticosteroids has been suggested as a way of further improving fetal lung development, but five trials have failed to demonstrate any improvement in neonatal respiratory disease, chronic oxygen dependence, or fetal, neonatal or childhood outcome.[8]

Preventative therapies
A number of modalities have been studied over the years to try to prevent fetal serious disease that can lead to fetal death or serious long-term sequel in the child. One of the most successful strategies is supplementation with folic acid for the prevention of neural tube defects (NTDs), first proposed by Smithells *et*

al.[9] These conditions complicate 1.5/1000 pregnancies in the UK[10] and can include open spina bifida, anencephaly and encephalocele. Two randomised, placebo-controlled trials for primary prevention of NTD (with 400 µg/day folic acid) or prevention of recurrences (with 4 mg of folic acid) documented the ability to prevent these debilitating malformations in a majority of individuals.[11,12] This is the first congenital malformation to be primarily prevented by pharmacological fetal therapy.[13] In 1996, the US Food and Drug Administration initiated folic acid fortification of flour and mean folate levels in the population increased 2-fold to concentrations consistent with substantial decrease in the risk of NTD[1] and this policy has been implemented in many countries.[13] The successful prevention of serious fetal malformations by supplementing adequate amounts of an essential micronutrient highlights the tremendous potential of well-designed research followed by adequate public health policies.

Another successful strategy is the maternal administration of IVIg to prevent fetomaternal allo-immune thrombocytopenia (FMAIT). Bussel et al.[14] demonstrated that treatment with IVIg produced an increase in the platelet count of fetuses with allo-immune thrombocytopenia and observational studies have suggested an improvement in clinical outcome and reduction in the risk for intracranial haemorrhage when IVIg is administered to the mother throughout pregnancy.[15] Maternal therapy with IVIg may result in a fetal platelet count exceeding $50 \times 10^9/l$ in 67% of pregnancies with a history of sibling affected by FMAIT,[16] reducing the need of FBS and transfusions avoiding the complications of this technique.

Therapy for fetal disease

Fetal tachy-arrhythmias are good examples of a pathology which can be treated by therapeutic fetal drug therapy. When associated with hydrops fetalis these are associated with significant prenatal and postnatal mortality. Without hydrops, fetuses have a quite good prognosis and when the rhythm disturbance is severe enough, treatment can be very effective at preventing hydrops. When the patient presents with hydrops, most arrhythmias can often be controlled with transplacental treatment, but the mortality in this group remains quite high.[17] The goal of therapy is to achieve an adequate ventricular rate and optimal conversion to sinus rhythm and avoid or reverse cardiac failure.[1] Most anti-arrhythmic drugs used in adults and children have been tried in fetal arrhythmias with different levels of success but by far the most commonly used drugs are digoxin and Flecainide with different series showing equal rate of effectiveness.[1] Simpson and Sharland,[17] in one of the largest published series, show high rates of conversion to sinus rhythm using oral maternal digoxin or Flecainide treatment alone in non-hydropic fetus. However, use of Flecainide controlled the rhythm and caused resolution of hydrops more rapidly than digoxin even when the latter was combined with verapamil. Despite some reports that show increased incidence of arrhythmia-related deaths in patients treated with Flecainide compared with placebo,[18] Simpson and Sharland[17] did not find any serious effects in the mother and there is a large experience of its use in children without any problem. On this basis, treatment with Flecainide is generally now the preferred fetal arrhythmic when associated with hydrops or when there is therapeutic failure after digoxin. Some are using it as first-line treatment in non-hydropic cases as well and in our experience digoxin levels required to correct the fetal arrhythmia have been associated with significant maternal symptoms and, in one case, maternal arrhythmia.

INVASIVE PROCEDURES

Transfusion therapy

Red cell iso-immunisation

Intra-uterine blood transfusion of anaemic fetuses represents one of the great successes of fetal therapy. The first approach was intraperitoneal blood transfusion introduced in 1963 by Liley.[19] Subsequently, Rodeck et al.[20] described intravascular fetal blood transfusion (IVT) by needling of the chorionic plate or umbilical cord vessels under direct vision by fetoscopy. In 1982, Bang et al.[21] in Denmark started IVT by umbilical cord puncture under ultrasound guidance, a method now widely used by an increasingly large number of centres. IVT has produced a marked improvement in survival of the anaemic hydropic fetus and can also prevent this complication from developing by treating anaemic non-hydropic fetuses where moderate or severe anaemia is detected non-invasively by Doppler ultrasonography on the basis of an increase in the peak velocity of systolic blood flow or time-averaged mean velocity in the middle cerebral artery in fetus at risk.[22,23]

In preference, the umbilical vein is sampled because artery puncture may be a risk factors for bradycardia.[24] The haemoglobin concentration (Hb) is measured immediately and interpreted according to gestational age, classifying the severity on the basis of the deviation of the fetal haemoglobin from the normal mean for gestation into mild (haemoglobin deficit less than 2 g/dl), moderate (deficit 2–7 g/dl), and severe (deficit greater than 7 g/dl).[25] If the deficit is moderate or severe, the next step is the transfusion of blood. The volume of blood required to correct the fetal Hb can be determined by using the pre-transfusion Hb, the donor blood Hb (which is adult blood usually packed to a haematocrit of about 70–80%) and the gestational age.[26] The volume required is given as fast as possible without causing changes to the fetal heart rate and it seems that the feto-placental unit is able to handle the blood volume expansion much more easily than when transfusing neonates who are without the benefit of a placenta. Infusion of packed blood through a 15-cm long, 20-gauge needle at rates of 1–10 ml/min does not result in significant haemolysis.[26] After the volume calculated to correct the Hb deficit has been given, a post-transfusion Hb is measured to help time the next transfusion. After two or three transfusions, fetal blood production is suppressed and so adult blood cells predominant and then the fall of Hb becomes very predictable at about 1% haematocrit point per day.[2] We aim for the last transfusion at 35–36 weeks and then induce labour at 37 weeks to allow maturation of both the pulmonary and hepatic enzyme systems in the hope of avoiding neonatal exchange transfusions. In spite of the clear benefit of the treatment of this type of patients, the treatment of fetal anaemia is still a complicated area. The severely anaemic fetus at 18–24 weeks' gestation is less able to adapt to a complete correction of its anaemia and some recommend only partial transfusion the first time and then repeat of the procedure 7–10 days later.

Allo-immune thrombocytopenia

Fetomaternal allo-immune thrombocytopenia (FMAIT) may result from a maternal immunisation against fetal platelet antigens inherited from the father which are absent from the maternal platelets mostly anti-HPA-1a, or anti-HPA-5a.[27] When severe, this may result in intracerebral haemorrhage (ICH) leading to hydrocephalus and possible death of the fetus.[28] This disease often affects the first child and at the moment there are no screening tests available.[29] The antenatal management of fetal allo-immune thrombocytopenia is not an easy task and in many areas remains controversial. The only realistic approach at the moment is monitoring multiparous women with a history of giving birth to at least one allo-immune thrombocytopenic infant. Fetal therapy includes a combination of maternal intravenous gamma globulin (IVIgG) administration[14] (see above) and fetal blood platelet counts with intra-uterine platelet transfusions when necessary.

The timing of the fetal blood sampling (FBS) for platelet count is difficult to decide, and a background of sibling history of antenatal ICH or severe thrombocytopenia (platelet counts of $< 20 \times 10^9/l$) who are related with lower platelet counts[16] support early invasive assessment with platelet ready for transfusion by FBS at 21–22 weeks. If the history is milder, this may be delayed until 28–32 weeks and some have suggested even later. For fetal platelet transfusion, typed platelets from donors are used and last about 4–5 days in the fetal circulation. In very severe disease, platelets may need to be transfused every 7–10 days to maintain the platelet count at a safe level. In the European Fetomaternal Alloimmune Thrombocytopenia Study Group, none of the fetuses managed by serial platelet intra-uterine transfusions suffered ICH following treatment. However, some have estimated that serial weekly transfusion may be associated with a risk of about 6% per pregnancy, indicating the need to develop less invasive approaches.[30] The effectiveness of maternal therapy with IVIgG has led to management without an initial FBS, reserving this intervention for evaluation of the effectiveness of maternal therapy to indicate if more aggressive therapy is required.

Transient aplastic anaemia (parvovirus)

Parvovirus B19 accounts for about 25% of cases of non-immune hydrops fetalis in anatomically normal fetuses[31] as a result of fetal anaemia following tropism of B19 virus for erythroid precursor cells and the massive destruction of the infected erythroid cells and possibly myocarditis resulting in cardiac failure.[32,33] The mean gestational age of presentation of hydrops is 22 weeks but there are some reports of earlier presentation which might often be undiagnosed.[34,35] Also, some have suggested it may be a cause of apparently unexplained late still birth.[36] The highest risk for a fetus developing hydrops is when maternal infection is before 20 weeks' gestation probably due to the rapidly increasing red cell mass and short half-life of fetal red cells.[2] Diagnostic techniques aim at detecting maternal antibodies or either viral particles or DNA by polymerase chain reaction (PCR) in maternal serum, amniotic fluid or fetal blood.[33]

The fetal loss rate following maternal parvovirus infection is about 10%,[37] but this is much higher when hydrops develops, so management is by FBS for diagnosis of anaemia followed by transfusion if necessary.[38] In fact, the rates of death among those who receive an intra-uterine transfusion are significantly lower than among those who did not.[33,39] However, consideration should be given to the high fetal loss rate in cases of hydrops after fetal blood sampling.[40] Fetal blood results in these cases show a negative Coomb's test, anaemia, thrombocytopenia, and low reticulocyte count.[2] If the reticulocyte count is high at the first transfusion, this may indicate recovery already occurring and so a second transfusion may not be necessary. Usually, FBS is repeated if hydrops returns or more recently when Doppler studies suggest worsening anaemia.

In spite of some reports of hydrops due to fetal parvovirus infection resolving without treatment,[41,42] in our view if non-immune hydrops presents without obvious fetal malformations and anaemia is expected from the Doppler results, even if the mother does not give a clear history of parvovirus exposure, FBS should still be done urgently without waiting for maternal confirmatory tests and intra-uterine transfusion be done if there is evidence of severe fetal anaemia.

Amniotic fluid management

Amniotic fluid surrounds the fetus in intra-uterine life providing a protected, low-resistance space suitable for fetal movements, growth and development. Disturbance of the balance between amniotic fluid production and consumption leads to oligo- or polyhydramnios, both of which are associated with poor perinatal outcome related to the degree of fluid volume change.[43,44]

Severe polyhydramnios can cause maternal abdominal discomfort, respiratory embarrassment and preterm delivery.[45,46] Amniotic fluid reduction can relieve maternal symptoms with severe polyhydramnios and prolong the gestation in both singleton and multiple pregnancies and is one of the possible treatments for TTTS.[45,47] Abruption can be a complication of removal of large volumes of amniotic fluid and this risk has been estimated at about 3–4%.[48] Common criteria for amniotic fluid drainage are AFI > 40 cm or the deepest single pool of > 12 cm but many prefer to make the decision mostly on maternal discomfort.[2] Removal of a small volume can rapidly reduce amniotic fluid pressure but it usually re-accumulates quickly and approximately 1 1 needs to be removed for every 10 cm the AFI is elevated.[45,49] The procedure often has to be repeated in order to prolong gestational age until maturity allows delivery. The insertion of a tube to achieve chronic long-term drainage has been tried in the past but there is a high risk of infection and no evidence supporting this approach.

Oligohydramnios is found in 3–5% of pregnancies in the third trimester, but severe cases relating to impaired outcome are less common.[45] The significance of this finding relates mostly to the underlying cause, so the prognosis and the possibility of treatment depends on the aetiology. Attempts at therapy focus on restoring the amniotic fluid to allow continued development of the lungs during the canalicular phase. Quintero et al.[50] described effective re-sealing in cases of iatrogenic previable PPROM by intra-amniotic injection of platelets and cryoprecipitate although this approach has not been reported to work after spontaneous membrane rupture. Some reports have also shown that in pregnancies with preterm premature rupture of membranes (PPROM) with oligohydramnios at < 26 weeks' gestation, serial amnio-infusions improve the perinatal outcome when compared to those with persistent oligo-hydramnios.[51,52] Fisk *et al.* have recently described an amnio-infusion test procedure to try and pre-select cases of mid-trimester PPROM which may benefit from serial amnio-infusion. A quarter of patients who retained infused fluid went on to subsequent serial amnio-infusion and prolongation of pregnancy with decrease in the risk of pulmonary hypoplasia.[53] However, there are risks of procedure-related complications such as chorio-amnionitis, placental abruption and extreme prematurity, so ideally a large series in a prospectively randomised trial would be needed to assess the benefits.

Amnio-infusion has also been used to prevent or relieve variable decelerations from umbilical cord compression in cases of rupture of membranes and to dilute meconium when present in the amniotic fluid and so reduce the risk of meconium aspiration during labour. Two Cochrane reviews have been done, showing improvements in perinatal outcome[54] when it is used to dilute meconium and appears to reduce the occurrence of variable heart rate decelerations and lower the use of caesarean section due to cord compression in labour.[55]

Shunting

Pleuro-amniotic shunting

A pleural effusion may be an isolated finding or may occur in association with hydrops fetalis. When severe, this condition can produce hydrops, pulmonary hypoplasia by lung compression and polyhydramnios (caused by the pressure in the chest being above venous and so a reduction in venous return and generalised heart failure and oesophageal obstruction) with secondary risks of preterm delivery.[46] When due to a reversible cause such as chylothorax, the treatment of this condition by pleuro-amniotic shunting can be a very effective method[56] and can reverse the complications and prevent death. However, drainage does not help cases in which the pleural effusion is caused by an underlying progressive disease, or when the effusions are mild (and so will not produce secondary effects) or when the problem is diagnosed so late that pulmonary hypoplasia has already occurred and is irreversible. In fact, the survival of fetuses with severe pleural effusions after thoraco-amniotic shunting is only 50%.[57]

Vesico-amniotic shunting

Lower urinary tract obstruction has a significant impact on perinatal morbidity and mortality, related principally to pulmonary hypoplasia and renal impairment that produce at least a 40% of mortality.[58,59] Animal models of releasing obstruction have been very successful but these models are often different from human congenital urinary tract obstruction.[60] The insertion of a double pig-tailed vesico-amniotic catheter is the most commonly used method to relieve this obstruction *in vivo* but complications are quite common, including failure of drainage or migration of the shunt, premature labour, urinary ascites, chorio-amnionitis and iatrogenic gastroschisis.[61] The main concern about vesico-amniotic shunting is that by the time severe obstructive uropathy is detected, renal function may be already severely and irreversibly damaged.[59] Needle drainage has been used to obtain an assessment of renal function and identify fetuses with potential to benefit from *in utero* surgical intervention.[60] Sometimes, needle aspiration can appear to be therapeutic for megacystis in very early in the second trimester perhaps as a result of releasing urethral oedema secondary to pressure.[62] Amniofusion to correct oligohydramnios prior to shunt insertion is often necessary in order to make room for the catheter outside the fetus. In summary, we believe that vesico-amniotic shunting is a useful procedure but only in a few, well-selected cases and certainly women should be warned of the possibility of poor renal prognosis after the treatment.

Laser treatment

Twin–twin transfusion syndrome (TTTS) affects 10–15% of monozygous twin pregnancies with monochorionic placentation.[63,64] Without treatment, there is a very high risk of perinatal mortality and perinatal morbidity due to preterm delivery but also as a result of acquired brain injury *in utero*.[65] When TTTS is of early onset, the prognosis is even worse and interruption of the vascular anastomosis by fetoscopic laser ablation is a sensible treatment that has been used since the beginning of the 1990s.[66] With this treatment, in a third of pregnancies both twins survive, in another third one twin survives and in the remaining third both twins die.[67] The recently published Eurofetus study showed that laser therapy is associated with improved perinatal outcome compared with amnioreduction in women presenting with TTTS before 26 weeks' gestation.[68] To improve these results, we need better ways of identifying all arterial-venous (A–V) anastomoses before ablation, which will enable a true rendering into a DC placenta with minimal destruction of viable placental territory. There have been some attempts of delineating placental vascular anatomy *in utero* with contrast agents and power Doppler but without clear success.[69]

Laser ablation has also been used successfully to treat acardiac twin pregnancies that complicate 1% of monozygous twin pregnancies with monochorionic placentation[70] and are associated with congestive cardiac failure in the pump twin leading to polyhydramnios and preterm delivery with a reported perinatal mortality in untreated cases as high as 55%.[71] Laser or diathermy ablation is used to occlude the cord or the pelvic vessels within the abdomen of the acardiac twin.[72,73] A recent review suggests that intrafetal ablation is the treatment of choice for acardiac twins because it is simpler, safer and more effective when compared with the cord occlusion techniques.[71]

Open fetal surgery

Although most malformations diagnosed prenatally are best managed after birth, a few severe ones may be better treated before birth. The fetal malformations that warrant consideration for open surgical correction *in utero* are those that interfere with normal growth, development and are life-threatening, so that correction of the defect may prevent these effects. At present, only a few malformations have been successfully corrected, including fetal myelomeningocele (MMC) and congenital diaphragmatic hernia (CDH).

Fetal MMC can produce obstructive hydrocephalus in up to 85% of cases requiring ventriculoperitoneal shunting.[74] MMC can have other long-term sequelae such as motor impairment of the legs and loss of bowel and bladder control. The damage may be due to the defect in the bony spinal column exposing the spinal cord to the trauma from the amniotic fluid and the uterine environment[75] raising the possibility of covering the spinal cord in the uterus to avoid the damage. The accumulated experience with fetal MMC repair has been encouraging and suggests a decreased need for ventriculoperitoneal shunting, arrest or slowing of progressive ventriculomegaly, and consistent resolution of hindbrain herniation in the short-term follow-up.[74] However, further long-term follow-up is needed to evaluate neurodevelopment and bladder and bowel function.

Congenital diaphragmatic hernia has a high mortality rate, and many clinical and experimental efforts have been made in order to reduce it. Open fetal repair of the diaphragmatic defect was attempted but with an unacceptable high mortality rate and so has been abandoned.[75] Fetoscopic temporary tracheal occlusion has emerged as an alternative to open fetal surgery on the basis that the accumulation of lung fluid secretions can expand the lungs and so reduce the herniated viscera and avoid pulmonary hypoplasia. This approach may improve lung growth and development;[76] however, complications related to tracheal dissection, premature delivery and late morbidity are significant.[77] New techniques have been proven in the experimental stage with a less invasive approach but a recent randomised and controlled trial has failed to show any improvement of survival or morbidity rates when compared to the intra-uterine fetal endoscopic tracheal occlusion approach with optimal postnatal care.[78] The use of sonographic parameters to identify high- and low-risk groups of fetuses are needed in order to define the best management of CDH.

INTERVENTIONS IN EXPERIMENTAL STAGES

Ablation of tumours

Some tumours may grow to massive proportion in the uterus, inducing high-output failure leading to fetal hydrops which end usually in fetal demise. Fetal sacrococcygeal teratoma is a good example of this and surgery may have a role before the onset of hydrops in order to avoid this complication or after in order to resolve it. Ablation of the majority of the tumour tissue is not usually necessary and perhaps only ligation or coagulation of the vascular steal can reverse or avoid the high-output fetal heart failure.[79] Open fetal surgery with a high incidence of technique-related complications has been moving to less invasive approaches such as radiofrequency ablation and fetoscopic resection[80] but more studies are needed to assess the impact of these types of management and what groups of fetus benefit from them. With cervical teratomas, another possibility for tracheal obstruction can be the EXIT procedure where the fetus is partially delivered, maintaining the uteroplacental circulation in order to perform the surgery and achieve adequate ventilation.[81]

Stem cell transplantation

Bone marrow transplantation of normal haematopoietic stem cells can sustain normal haemopoiesis and be an alternative treatment of lethal haematological disease. In the case of congenital diseases like haemoglobinopathies, immunodeficiency disorders and inborn errors of metabolism that can be diagnosed prenatally and cured or improved by the engraftment of normal stem cells are theoretically an attractive alternative for the *in utero* transplantation of stem cells.[75] The unique characteristic of the haematological and inmunological system in the human fetus could circumvent the postnatal problems of transplantation, such as graft-versus-host disease; the remarkable abilities of stem cells to proliferate, differentiate and become tolerant to host antigens are encouraging

Gene therapy

The goal of gene therapy is to treat disease before damage secondary to the gene pathology is produce. Some reports show that using a percutaneous ultrasound-guided injection of gene transfers in the airway or in the amniotic cavity in animal, provided levels of gene expression in lung and intestine that could be relevant for a therapeutic application.[82,83] In spite of the large amount of experimentation already made in this field, we are still unsure if this technique will provide the desired therapeutic effect and if expression of the transferred genes will provide real clinical benefit.

References

1 Koren G, Klinger G, Ohlsson A. Fetal pharmacotherapy. Drugs 2002; 62: 757–773
2 Thein AT, Soothill P. Antenatal invasive therapy. Eur J Pediatr 1998; 157 (Suppl 1): S2–S6
3 Liggins GC. Premature delivery of fetal lambs infused with glucocorticoids. J Endocrinol 1969; 45: 515–523
4 Crowley P. Prophylactic corticosteroids for preterm birth (Cochrane Review). In: The Cochrane Library, Issue 1, 2004
5 Committee on Obstetric Practice. ACOG committee opinion. Antenatal corticosteroid therapy for fetal maturation. American College of Obstetricians and Gynecologists. Int J Gynecol Obstet 2002; 78: 95–97
6 Lamer P. Current controversies surrounding the use of repeated courses of antenatal steroids. Adv Neonat Care 2002; 2: 290–300
7 Royal College of Obstetrics and Gynaecology. Antenatal corticosteroid to prevent respiratory distress syndrome. Guideline No. 7. London: RCOG, 1999
8 Crowther CA, Alfirevic Z, Haslam RR. Prenatal thyrotropin-releasing hormone for preterm birth (Cochrane Review). In: The Cochrane Library, Issue 1, 2004
9 Smithells RW, Sheppard S, Schorah CJ. Vitamin deficiencies and neural tube defects. Arch Dis Child 1976; 51: 944–950
10 Abramsky L, Botting B, Chapple J, Stone D. Has advice on periconceptional folate supplementation reduced neural-tube defects? Lancet 1999; 354: 998–999
11. MRC Vitamin Study Research Group. Prevention of neural tube defects: results of the Medical Research Council Vitamin Study. Lancet 1991; 338: 131–137
12 Czeizel AE, Dudas I. Prevention of the first occurrence of neural-tube defects by periconceptional vitamin supplementation. N Engl J Med 1992; 327: 1832–1835
13 Royal College of Obstetrics and Gynaecology. Periconceptional Folic Acid and Food Fortification in the Prevention of Neural Tube Defects Scientific Advisory Committee Opinion Paper 4. London: RCOG, 2003

14 Bussel JB, Berkowitz RL, Lynch L *et al.* Antenatal management of alloimmune thrombocytopenia with intravenous gamma-globulin: a randomized trial of the addition of low-dose steroid to intravenous gamma-globulin. Am J Obstet Gynecol 1996; 174: 1414–1423

15 Rayment R, Brunskill SJ, Stanworth S, Soothill PW, Roberts DJ, Murphy MF. Antenatal interventions for fetomaternal alloimmune thrombocytopenia. Cochrane Database Syst Rev 2005; (1): CD004226

16 Birchall JE, Murphy MF, Kaplan C, Kroll H, European Fetomaternal Alloimmune Thrombocytopenia Study Group. European collaborative study of the antenatal management of feto-maternal alloimmune thrombocytopenia. Br J Haematol 2003; 122: 275–288

17 Simpson JM, Sharland GK. Fetal tachycardias: management and outcome of 127 consecutive cases. Heart 1998; 79: 576–581

18 Echt DS, Liebson PR, Mitchell B *et al.* Mortality and morbidity in patients receiving encainide, flecainide, or placebo. The cardiac arrhythmia suppression trial. N Engl J Med 1991; 324: 779–788

19 Liley AW. Intrauterine transfusion of fetus in haemolytic disease. BMJ 1963; ii: 1107–1109

20 Rodeck CH, Kemp JR, Holman CA, Whitmore CA, Karnicki J, Austin MA. Direct intravascular fetal blood transfusion by fetoscopy in severe Rhesus isoimmunisation. Lancet 1981; i: 625–627

21 Bang J, Bock JE, Trolle D. Ultrasound guided fetal intravenous transfusion for severe Rhesus haemolytic disease. BMJ 1982; 284: 373–374

22 Mari G, Deter RL, Carpenter RL *et al.* Noninvasive diagnosis by Doppler ultrasonography of fetal anemia due to maternal red-cell alloimmunization. Collaborative Group for Doppler Assessment of the Blood Velocity in Anemic Fetuses. N Engl J Med 2000; 342: 9–14

23 Abdel-Fattah SA, Soothill PW, Carroll SG, Kyle PM. Middle cerebral artery Doppler for the prediction of fetal anaemia in cases without hydrops: a practical approach. Br J Radiol 2002; 75: 726–730

24 Weiner CP, Wenstrom KD, Sipes SL, Williamson RA. Risk factors for cordocentesis and fetal intravascular transfusion. Am J Obstet Gynecol 1991; 165: 1020–1025

25 Nicolaides KH, Soothill PW, Clewell WH, Rodeck CH, Mibashan RS, Campbell S. Fetal haemoglobin measurement in the assessment of red cell isoimmunisation. Lancet 1988; 14(1) (8594): 1073–1975.

26 Nicolaides KH, Soothill PW, Rodeck CH, Clewell W. Rh disease: intravascular fetal blood transfusion by cordocentesis. Fetal Ther 1986; 1: 185–192

27 Kaplan C. Alloimmune thrombocytopenia of the fetus and the newborn. Blood Rev 2002; 16: 69–72

28 Montemagno R, Soothill PW, Scarcelli M, O'Brien P, Rodeck CH. Detection of alloimmune thrombocytopenia as cause of isolated hydrocephalus by fetal blood sampling. Lancet 1994; 343: 1300–1301

29 Murphy MF, Williamson LM. Antenatal screening for fetomaternal alloimmune thrombocytopenia: an evaluation using the criteria of the UK National Screening Committee. Br J Haematol 2000; 111: 726–732

30 Overton TG, Duncan KR, Jolly M, Letsky E, Fisk NM. Serial aggressive platelet transfusion for fetal alloimmune thrombocytopenia: platelet dynamics and perinatal outcome. Am J Obstet Gynecol 2002; 186: 826

31 Hall J. Parvovirus B19 infection in pregnancy. Arch Dis Child Fetal Neonat Edn 1994; 71: F4–F5

32 Yaegashi N, Niinuma T, Chisaka H *et al.* Parvovirus B19 infection induces apoptosis of erythroid cells *in vitro* and *in vivo*. J Infect 1999; 39: 68–76

33 von Kaisenberg CS, Jonat W. Fetal parvovirus B19 infection. Ultrasound Obstet Gynecol 2001; 18: 280–288

34 Yaegashi N, Niinuma T, Chisaka H *et al.* The incidence of, and factors leading to, parvovirus B19-related hydrops fetalis following maternal infection; report of 10 cases and meta-analysis. *J Infect* 1998; 37: 28–35

35 Sohan K, Carroll S, Byrne D, Ashworth M, Soothill P. Parvovirus as a differential diagnosis of hydrops fetalis in the first trimester. Fetal Diagn Ther 2000; 15: 234–236

36 Norbeck O, Papadogiannakis N, Petersson K, Hirbod T, Broliden K, Tolfvenstam T. Revised clinical presentation of parvovirus B19-associated intrauterine fetal death. Clin Infect Dis 2002; 35: 1032–1038

37. Public Health Laboratory Service Working Party on Fifth Disease. Prospective study of human parvovirus (B19) infection in pregnancy. BMJ 1990; 300: 1166–1170

38 Soothill P. Intrauterine blood transfusion for non-immune hydrops fetalis due to parvovirus B19 infection. Lancet 1990; 336: 121–122

39 Fairley CK, Smoleniec JS, Caul OE, Miller E. Observational study of effect of intrauterine transfusions on outcome of fetal hydrops after parvovirus B19 infection. Lancet 1995; 346: 1335–1337

40 Maxwell DJ, Johnson P, Hurley P, Neales K, Allan L, Knott P. Fetal blood sampling and pregnancy loss in relation to indication. Br J Obstet Gynaecol 1991; 98: 892–897

41 Pryde PG, Nugent CE, Pridjian G, Barr M, Faix RG Spontaneous resolution of nonimmunne hydrops fetalis secondary to human parvovirus B19 infection. Obstet Gynecol 1992; 79: 859–861

42 Rodis JF, Borgida AF, Wilson M et al. Management of parvovirus infection in pregnancy and outcomes of hydrops: a survey of members of the Society of Perinatal Obstetricians. Am J Obstet Gynecol 1998; 179: 985–988

43 Chamberlain PF, Manning FA, Morrison I, Harman CR, Lange IR. Ultrasound evaluation of amniotic fluid volume. II. The relationship of increased amniotic fluid volume to perinatal outcome. Am J Obstet Gynecol 1984; 150: 250–254

44 Chamberlain PF, Manning FA, Morrison I, Harman CR, Lange IR. Ultrasound evaluation of amniotic fluid volume. I. The relationship of marginal and decreased amniotic fluid volumes to perinatal outcome. Am J Obstet Gynecol 1984; 150: 245–249

45 Kyle PM, Fisk NM. Oligohydramnios and polyhydramnios. In: Fisk NM, Moise Jr KJ. (eds) Fetal therapy, invasive and transplacental. Cambridge: Cambridge University Press, 1997, 203–217

46 Phelan JP, Park YW, Ahn MO, Rutherford SE. Polyhydramnios and perinatal outcome. J Perinatol 1990; 10: 347–350

47 Wee LY, Fisk NM. The twin–twin transfusion syndrome. Semin Neonatol 2002; 7: 187–202

48 Leung WC, Jouannic JM, Hyett J, Rodeck C, Jauniaux E. Procedure-related complications of rapid amniodrainage in the treatment of polyhydramnios. Obstet Gynecol 2004; 23: 154–158

49 Abdel-Fattah SA, Carroll SG, Kyle PM, Soothill PW. Amnioreduction: how much to drain? Fetal Diagn Ther 1999; 14: 279–282

50 Quintero RA, Morales WJ, Allen M, Bornick PW, Arroyo J, LeParc G. Treatment of iatrogenic previable premature rupture of membranes with intra-amniotic injection of platelets and cryoprecipitate (amniopatch): preliminary experience. Am J Obstet Gynecol 1999; 181: 744–749

51 Locatelli A, Vergani P, Di Pirro G, Doria V, Biffi A, Ghidini A. Role of amnioinfusion in the management of premature rupture of the membranes at < 26 weeks' gestation. Am J Obstet Gynecol 2000; 183: 878–882

52 De Santis M, Scavo M, Noia G et al. Transabdominal amnioinfusion treatment of severe oligohydramnios in preterm premature rupture of membranes at less than 26 gestational weeks. Diagn Ther 2003; 18: 412–417

53 Tan LK, Kumar S, Jolly M, Gleeson C, Johnson P, Fisk NM. Test amnioinfusion to determine suitability for serial therapeutic amnioinfusion in midtrimester premature rupture of membranes. Fetal Diagn Ther 2003; 18: 183–189

54 Hofmeyr GJ. Amnioinfusion for preterm rupture of membranes (Cochrane Review). In: The Cochrane Library, Issue 1, 2004. Chichester, UK

55 Hofmeyr GJ. Amnioinfusion for meconium-stained liquor in labour (Cochrane Review). In: The Cochrane Library, Issue 1, 2004. Chichester, UK

56 Sohan K, Carroll SG, De La Fuente S, Soothill P, Kyle P. Analysis of outcome in hydrops fetalis in relation to gestational age at diagnosis, cause and treatment. Obstet Gynecol Scand 2001; 80: 726–730

57 Smith RP, Illanes S, Denbow ML, Soothill PW. Outcome of fetal pleural effusions treated by thoracoamniotic shunting. Ultrasound Obstet Gynecol 2005; 26: 63–66

58 Nakayama DK, Harrison MR, de Lorimier AA. Prognosis posterior urethral valves presenting at birth. J Pediatr Surg 1986; 21: 43–45

59 Freedman AL, Bukowski TP, Smith CA, Evans MI, Johnson MP, Gonzales R. Fetal therapy for obstructive uropathy: specific outcome diagnosis. J Urol 1996; 156: 720

60 Agarwal SK, Fisk NM. *In utero* therapy for lower urinary tract obstruction. Prenat Diagn 2001; 21: 970–976

61 Coplen DE. Prenatal intervention for hydronephrosis. J Urol 1997; 157: 2270–2277

62 Carroll SG, Soothill PW, Tizard J, Kyle PM. Vesicocentesis at 10–14 weeks of gestation for treatment of fetal megacystis. Ultrasound Obstet Gynecol 2001; 18: 366–370

63 Sebire NJ, Snijders RJ, Hughes K, Sepulveda W, Nicolaides KH. The hidden mortality of monochorionic twin pregnancies. Br J Obstet Gynaecol 1997; 104: 1203–1207

64 Carroll SG, Soothill PW, Abdel-Fattah SA, Porter H, Montague I, Kyle PM. Prediction of chorionicity in twin pregnancies at 10-14 weeks of gestation. Br J Obstet Gynaecol 2002; 109: 182–6

65 Denbow ML, Battin MR, Cowan F, Assopardi D, Edwards AD, Fisk NM. Neonatal cranial ultrasonographic findings in preterm twins complicated by severe fetofetal transfusion syndrome. Am J Obstet Gynecol 1998; 178: 479–483

66 De Lia JE, Cruikshank DP, Keye WR. Fetoscopic neodynium:YAG laser occlusion of placental vessels in severe twin-twin transfusion syndrome. Obstet Gynecol 1990; 75: 1046–1053

67 Ville Y, Hyett J, Hecher K, Nicolaides KH. Preliminary experience with endoscopic laser surgery for severe twin–twin transfusion syndrome. N Engl J Med 1995; 332: 224–227

68 Senat MV, Deprest J, Boulvain M, Paupe A, Winer N, Ville Y. Endoscopic laser surgery versus serial amnioreduction for severe twin-to-twin transfusion syndrome. N Engl J Med 2004; 351: 136–144

69 Denbow ML, Eckersley R, Welsh AW *et al. Ex vivo* delineation of placental angioarchitecture with the microbubble contrast agent Levovist. Am J Obstet Gynecol 2000; 182: 966–971

70 Moore TR, Gale S, Benirschke K. Perinatal outcome of forty-nine pregnancies complicated by acardiac twinning. Am J Obstet Gynecol 1990; 163: 907–912

71 Tan TY, Sepulveda W. Acardiac twin: a systematic review of minimally invasive treatment modalities. Ultrasound Obstet Gynecol 2003; 22: 409–419

72 Rodeck C, Deans A, Jauniaux E. Thermocoagulation for the early treatment of pregnancy with an acardiac twin. N Engl J Med 1998; 339: 1293–1295

73 Soothill P, Sohan K, Carroll S, Kyle P. Ultrasound-guided, intra-abdominal laser to treat acardiac pregnancies. Br J Obstet Gynaecol 2002; 109: 352–354

74 Johnson MP, Sutton LN, Rintoul N *et al.* Fetal myelomeningocele repair: short-term clinical outcomes. Am J Obstet Gynecol 2003; 189: 482–487

75 Evans MI, Harrison MR, Flake AW, Johnson MP. Fetal therapy. Best Pract Res Clin Obstet Gynaecol 2002; 16: 671–683

76 Sydorak RM, Harrison MR. Congenital diaphragmatic hernia: advances in prenatal therapy. Clin Perinatol 2003; 30: 465–479

77 Deprest J, Gratacos E, Nicolaides KH, FETO Task Group Fetoscopic tracheal occlusion (FETO) for severe congenital diaphragmatic hernia: evolution of a technique and preliminary results. Ultrasound Obstet Gynecol 2004; 24: 121–126

78 Harrison MR, Keller RL, Hawgood SB *et al.* A randomized trial of fetal endoscopic tracheal occlusion for severe fetal congenital diaphragmatic hernia. N Engl J Med 2003; 349: 1916–1924

79 Paek BW, Jennings RW, Harrison MR *et al.* Radiofrequency ablation of human fetal sacrococcygeal teratoma. J Obstet Gynecol 2001; 184: 503–507

80 Hirose S, Farmer DL. Fetal surgery for sacrococcygeal teratoma. Clin Perinatol 2003; 30: 493–506

81 Murphy DJ, Kyle PM, Cairns P, Weir P, Cusick E, Soothill PW. *Ex-utero* intrapartum treatment for cervical teratoma. Br J Obstet Gynaecol 2001; 108: 429–430

82 David A, Cook T, Waddington S *et al.* Ultrasound-guided percutaneous delivery of adenoviral vectors encoding the beta-galactosidase and human factor IX genes to early gestation fetal sheep *in utero*. Hum Gene Ther 2003; 14: 353–364

83 Garrett DJ, Larson JE, Dunn D, Marrero L, Cohen JC. *In utero* recombinant adeno-associated virus gene transfer in mice, rats, and primates. BMC Biotechnol 2003; 3: 16

R. Katie Morris   Khalid Khan   Mark D. Kilby

Congenital lower urinary tract obstruction and the efficacy of vesico-amniotic shunting

Lower urinary tract obstruction (LUTO) is a heterogeneous group of pathologies, most commonly urethral atresia and posterior urethral valves (PUVs),[1] that accounts for one-third of renal tract anomalies detected at autopsy following termination for ultrasound-diagnosed fetal anomaly.[2] The affected fetus is typically male. Posterior urethral valves account for about half of cases presenting with ultrasonic features of LUTO[3] in some case cohorts. Females may also be affected but often demonstrate more complex, morbid pathologies such as urethral atresia and cloacal plate anomalies, including megacystis microcolon syndrome (dysfunctional smooth muscle in bladder and distal bowel). Classically, the end-stage clinical situation is the 'Prune Belly syndrome' consisting of a triad of features including: (i) deficient or absent anterior abdominal wall musculature; (ii) dilation of the proximal and distal urinary tract (hydronephrosis, megacystis); and (iii) bilateral cryptorchidism, present in the neonatal period.

The importance of LUTO, in terms of perinatal outcome, lies in its clinical course with long-term urethral obstruction being potentially associated with cystic renal dysplasia, decreased abnormal renal (glomerular and tubular) function leading to severe oligohydramnios, pulmonary hypoplasia, and positional limb anomalies.[4] Animal studies have demonstrated a causal link between the distal renal tract obstruction in the fetus and these abnormalities. The fetal phenotype has been variously described, as has the effects of potential *in-utero* therapy.

R. Katie Morris MRCOG
Clinical Research Fellow, University of Birmingham, Birmingham, UK

Khalid Khan MRCOG
Professor of Obstetrics and Gynaecology and Clinical Epidemiology, University of Birmingham, Birmingham, UK

Mark D. Kilby MD MRCOG (for correspondence)
Professor of Maternal and Fetal Medicine, Fetal Medicine Centre, Birmingham Women's Hospital, Edgbaston, Birmingham B15 2TG, UK. E-mail: m.d.kilby@bham.ac.uk

Table 1 Summary of papers showing natural history of lower urinary tract obstruction (*Adapted with permission from* Anumba et al.[8] © John Wiley 2005)

Reference	Cases (n)	Mortality	Cystic renal disease/chronic renal failure in Anumba study	Pulmonary hypoplasia	Associated structural or chromosomal anomalies
Thomas et al. (1985)[67]	18	33%	56%	30%	56%
Mahoney et al. (1985)[68]	40	63%	45%	40%	–
Nakayama et al. (1986)[69]	11	45%	37%	48%	–
Hayden et al. (1988)[70]	14	64%	–	36%	43%
Reuss et al. (1988)[71]	43	72%	36%	10%	42%
Anumba et al. (2005)[8]	113	Prenatal detection 75% (includes TOP). Postnatal detection 53%	Detection before 24 weeks 67%. Detection after 24 weeks 40%	Without shunting 26%. With shunting 25%	23%
Total/mean values	239	58%	47%	31%	41%

Fetal LUTO, if untreated, carries a mortality rate of 45% mainly due to severe oligohydramnios in the mid-trimester[5] being associated with pulmonary hypoplasia. Even in those that survive the neonatal period, 25–30% develop end-stage chronic renal impairment necessitating dialysis and/or transplantation.[6] In fact, congenital obstructive uropathy accounts for up to 60% of all paediatric renal transplants.[7] It is, therefore, a morbid condition.

For this reason, prenatal *in-utero* therapy has been considered in 'selected' cases in an attempt to bypass the congenital urinary tract obstruction and attenuate the secondary developmental complications. Prenatal counselling in this situation is, however, difficult as the modalities used to assess fetal renal function have uncertain prognostic value and the effectiveness of therapy remains to be established.

Here, we shall discuss the epidemiology, pathophysiology, diagnosis and antenatal assessment of fetal LUTO and the potential *in-utero* treatment(s) utilised to improve outcome.

EPIDEMIOLOGY

There is only one study published in the medical literature giving population-based information and data from a Regional Congenital Anomaly Register (Northern Region). This identified 113 registered cases between 1984–1997, a 14-year period, and noted that the registry had a high notification rate with an ascertainment level of 95%. During the study period, an incidence of LUTO was calculated as 2.2 per 10,000 births (based upon total birth denominator data). The incidence of PUV, determined by postnatal investigations and autopsies, was 64%

(1.4/10,000 births), for urethral atresia 39% (0.7/10,000 births), and prune belly syndrome 4%. In 4 cases (4%), the primary cause could not be identified.[8]

NATURAL HISTORY AND PATHOPHYSIOLOGY

There have been several papers reviewing the natural history of LUTO, although most series are small they all agree that congenital urethral obstruction is a disease of high morbidity and mortality (Table 1).

Factors that most closely correlate with outcome are the timing of ultrasound detection, associated anomalies (structural or/and chromosomal) and degree of oligohydramnios (with the latter being the most important). In the series reported by Mahoney et al.,[68] a pregnancy associated with oligohydramnios had an overall mortality rate of 80%. This was predominantly due to the associated risks of pulmonary hypoplasia. Vergani et al.[9] also showed that the gestational age at which premature rupture of the membranes occurred and degree of oligohydramnios were independent predictors of the occurrence of pulmonary hypoplasia. However, this relates mainly to pregnancies complicated by amniorrhexis and, therefore, the data should be extrapolated with caution.

While the above studies can demonstrate the potential natural history of this condition, they may not explain the pathophysiology; for this, we have to look at animal models. Much of this work has been performed by Harrison and his group in San Francisco who identified the most successful model to be that of the fetal lamb.[10,11] With this model, the group assessed the effect of urethral obstruction and its subsequent correction on pulmonary and renal development (Fig. 1).

Such experiments demonstrated that complete urethral obstruction produced severe hydronephrosis, hydroureter, megacystis, and urinary ascites, as well as

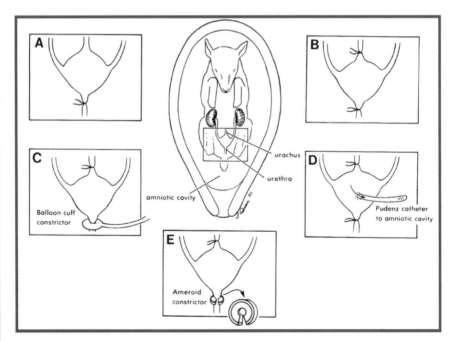

Fig. 1 Urethral ligation in sheep model. (*Reproduced with permission from:* Harrison MR, Golbus MS, Filly RA[72] Ch.31 © WB Saunders 1990)

Table 2 Lung volumes, alveolar, morphometrics and arterial morphometrics in fetal lambs following bilateral ureteral obstruction. (*Reproduced with permission from:* Harrison MR, Golbus MS, Filly RA[72] Ch.31 © WB Saunders 1990)

	Controls ($n = 4$)	Bilateral ureteral obstruction ($n = 3$)
Lung volume (ml)/body weight (kg)	50.2 ± 3.1	33.7 ± 11.3*
Radial alveolar count	5.41 ± 0.44	4.62 ± 0.23*
Mean linear intercept (μm)	34.9 ± 1.3	28.1 ± 0.7*
Intra-acinar arteries		
% muscularised	0.45	2.24#
% partially muscularised	2.01	4.32#
% non-muscularised	97.45	94.44#

*$P < 0.05$; #$P < 0.005$.

significant pulmonary hypoplasia, (measured by weight and volume). They could not, however, demonstrate that this caused cystic and dysplastic renal changes. It was also shown that with decompression *in utero*, some of the urinary tract dilatation resolved.[10,11]

Harrison postulated that pulmonary hypoplasia was secondary to compression from the massively dilated urinary tract or urinary ascites and not primary pulmonary malformation. The results of their studies showing that restoration of the amniotic fluid allows an increase in lung weight and a clinical improvement in respiratory function support this hypothesis. They have also shown the same results in rabbit models (Table 2, Fig. 2).[12]

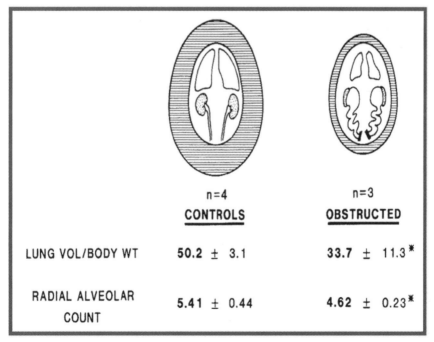

Fig. 2 Lung weight and alveolar count in lungs of lambs following bilateral ureteral obstruction. (*Reproduced with permission from:* Harrison MR, Golbus MS, Filly RA[72] Ch.31 © WB Saunders 1990)

Table 3 Effect of obstruction of fetal lamb kidney on renal function. (*Reproduced with permission from:* Harrison MR, Golbus MS, Filly RA[72] Ch.31 © WB Saunders 1990)

	Obstructed	Control
Renal weight (g)*	6.11 ± 0.96	11.26 ± 1.83
Output (ml/h)	2.64 ± 1.59	6.15 ± 4.63
Initial urinary Na+ (mEq/ml)*	105 ± 17	54 ± 15
Initial urinary Cl- (mEq/ml)*	75 ± 20	33 ± 0
Fractional Na+ excretion (%)	23.56 ± 8.29	3.48 ± 1.44
Creatinine clearance (ml/kg/h)	6.73 ± 3.80	45.18 ± 13.57
Iothalamate clearance (ml/kg/h)	5.89 ± 3.40	39.31 ± 12.06

*$P < 0.005$.

As mentioned earlier, these primary experiments failed to demonstrate a causative relationship with obstruction and cystic renal dysplasia. To address this, the group produced a complete unilateral ureteral obstruction in fetal lambs. They demonstrated that the kidney obstructed at 60 days was hydronephrotic and dysplastic (Table 3). The unobstructed contralateral kidney was unaffected.[13] The group then tried to address the question of whether decompression could prevent or reverse the renal dysplasia. The results showed there was significant correlation between the duration of *in-utero* ureteral decompression and urine output at birth; histological examination of the kidneys showed a correlation between severity of changes and length of time of obstruction.[14]

The applicability of animal models to human congenital disease, however, still remains controversial. Harrison *et al.*[72] could not reproduce the histological changes of renal dysplasia seen with urethral obstruction in the human fetus. Other authors, using an *in vitro* chick embryo experiment, have shown that obstruction of the ureter of the developing kidney caused only hydronephrosis and could not demonstrate renal dysplasia postulating that obstruction may not be the sole cause of the renal dysplasia seen in bladder outlet obstruction.[15]

DIAGNOSIS AND ASSESSMENT

Ultrasound

The detection of fetal lower urinary tract obstruction using ultrasound has a good accuracy,[16,17] partly because the anomalies of the renal tract and kidneys are also associated with secondary findings, such as oligohydramnios.

Assessment of the fetal genito-urinary tract forms a part of all routine ultrasound examinations; when abnormalities are detected, this should lead to a detailed assessment focusing on amniotic fluid volume, renal size, parenchyma, collecting system and bladder size. Dilatation of the renal pelvis and fluid-filled areas as small as 1–2 mm may be visualised *in utero* using high-resolution, real-time ultrasound scanning.[18] The types of abnormalities that can be detected are shown in Table 4.

Ultrasonography may help in the differentiation of obstructive and non-obstructive causes of megacystis, with the association of increased

Table 4 Urinary tract anomalies detectable by ultrasonography (*Reproduced with permission from* Coplen[60] © American Urological Association).

	Uropathy/renal failure	Bladder distension
OBSTRUCTIVE		
Ureteropelvic junction obstruction	Rarely if bilateral	No
Ureterovesical junction obstruction	Rarely if bilateral	No
Multicystic dysplastic kidney	Only if bilateral	No
Ureterocele/ectopic ureter	Rarely if bladder outlet obstructed (up to 50% of cases)	Possible
Posterior urethral valves	Always	Yes
Urethral atresia		Yes
NON-OBSTRUCTIVE		
Physiological dilatation (< 1 cm)	No	No
Vesico-ureteral reflux	No	Possible
Megacystis-mega-ureter-microcolon	No	Yes
Prune-belly syndrome	Yes with urethral atresia	Yes
Renal agenesis	Stillbirth if bilateral	No
Infantile polycystic kidneys	Depends on degree of penetrance	No

echogenicity and oligohydramnios in the presence of bladder distension being predictive of an obstructive aetiology in about 87% of cases.[17] It is, however, of limited value in differentiating PUV from other causes of LUTO.[17,19]

This has been further examined by Robyr et al.[28] In this study, detailed post-mortem examination was carried out on 24 male fetuses after termination of pregnancy who had presented prior to 25 weeks' gestation with ultrasound evidence of isolated severe LUTO. PUVs were suspected antenatally in 20 cases and urethral atresia in none. At post-mortem, urethral atresia was demonstrated in 6 cases and PUV in 9. Hydronephrosis was more frequent in cases with PUV (8/9) and urethral stenosis (6/8) than with urethral atresia (0/6). In LUTO presenting in the first and second trimester, hyperechogenic kidneys were predictive of renal dysplasia in 95% of cases. The association of a sagittal diameter of the bladder of at least 40 mm with hydronephrosis before 28 weeks was predictive of PUV with a positive (PPV) and negative (NPV) predictive value of 44.4% and 66.6%, respectively. Absence of hydronephrosis and a sagittal diameter of the bladder of less than 40 mm were predictive of urethral atresia or stenosis with a PPV and NPV of 100% and 47.6%, respectively. The absence of hydronephrosis was predictive of urethral atresia with a PPV and NPV of 66.6% and 100%, respectively.[16]

Detection of PUV varies with gestation with less than 50% being detected on routine second trimester scans performed before 24 weeks. Scanning after 28 weeks, however, can increase detection to 80%.[20,21]

The ultrasound findings of PUV include bladder distension with retrograde pressure in the ureters and renal pelvis resulting in dilated ureters and hydronephrosis . The bladder wall may also become thickened and appear echogenic due to muscular hypertrophy.[22] Oliveira et al.[23] performed a review of 148 cases of children with fetal hydronephrosis. A number of variables were assessed but only two were identified as independent predictors of fetal urethral obstruction –

oligohydramnios (odds ratio, OR = 5; 95% confidence interval [CI] = 1.3–15; P = 0.01) and megacystis (OR = 9; 95% CI = 2.0–40; P = 0.004). The sensitivity and specificity of the combination of both variables were 60% and 98.5%, respectively.[23]

It is important to differentiate true urethral obstruction from the megacystis-mega-ureter-microcolon syndrome (MMIHS), a rare disorder characterised by a functional intestinal obstruction/hypomobility and enlarged non-obstructed bladder. It is more common in females and has a very poor prognosis. As it can be difficult to differentiate on ultrasound, it is important to consider this diagnosis carefully in a female with LUTO but normal liquor volume. Animal experiments in transgenic mice have shown that lack of the $\alpha 3$ subunit or both $\beta 2$ and $\beta 4$ subunits of the nicotinic acetylcholine receptor subunit (nAChR) have a phenotype similar to that of MMIHS suggesting a basis for the condition.[24,25] In 2001, Richardson and his group[26] examined tissue from patients with MMIHS phenotypes and controls. They found that the MMIHS tissue gave negative staining for the $\alpha 3$ subunit.[26] Further work has looked at mutation analyses in the $\alpha 3$ and $\beta 4$ genes in MMIHS families enabling the human gene encoding the $\beta 4$ subunit to be fully characterised. Analysis of disease families and controls identified numerous genetic variants.[27]

While 3-D ultrasound has helped in the diagnosis of some fetal anomalies (such as facial clefts), it has not yet shown any advantages in the diagnosis of urinary tract anomalies.

Magnetic resonance imaging

More recently, due to the advent of single-shot fast-spin echo (SSFSE) techniques, MRI has been used in prenatal diagnosis. Most of the literature refers to its use in diagnosis of CNS anomalies as this is where it has been most successful. However, small studies have been done to assess its use in fetal urinary tract anomalies. Cassart *et al.*[28] looked at 16 third-trimester fetuses with suspected bilateral urinary tract anomalies following ultrasonography. The addition of MRI to sonography modified the diagnosis in 5 cases; in 4 of these cases, it led to a diagnosis that changed the decision to continue or terminate the pregnancy.[28] In the future, this imaging modality may improve the accuracy of diagnosis.

In-utero percutaneous cystoscopy

The group of Quintero[3] investigated 11 patients with sonographic findings of lower obstructive uropathy. Fetal cystoscopy was performed with a 0.7-mm fibre-optic endoscope, to assess urethral patency; a soft-tip wire guide was inserted through the endoscope in an attempt to cannulate the urethra. The endoscopic appearance of the proximal urethra was in agreement with the sonographic image in 10 of 11 fetuses. The combined sonographic/endoscopic technique allowed a diagnosis of prune belly syndrome in one fetus, megacystis-microcolon in another, and bladder-outlet obstruction in seven. It could not, however, distinguish between PUV and urethral atresia due to difficulty in negotiating the posterior urethra. In two cases, the group were able to extend the technique to allow the introduction of a urethral vesico-amniotic shunt; however, in the four other cases considered suitable for shunting, a standard vesico-amniotic shunt was inserted.[3]

More recently, the procedure has been performed in a European centre. Fisk's group from Queen Charlotte's Hospital performed cystoscopy in 13 fetuses and visualised the bladder wall in 12 and bladder neck in 11 cases. In 10 cases, the upper urethra was entered, the obstruction being visualised in 5 cases (4 PUV and one urethral atresia). There were, however, 5 cases of PUV which were not visualised. Therapeutic attempts (saline hydro-ablation and/or guide-wire passage) were successful in 60% of cases.[29]

Antenatal assessment

It is mandatory to perform a detailed anomaly scan, determine fetal sex and offer fetal karyotyping (due to the high incidence of karyotypic abnormalities) in cases of obstructive uropathy as demonstrated earlier (Table 5). Allocation of fetal gender may allow diagnosis to be further elucidated. Posterior urethral valves and urethral atresia having a very high prevalence in the male fetus. If there is severe oligohydramnios, then amnio-infusion may occasionally need to be utilised to allow accurate evaluation of fetal structures (Table 5).

If a normal karyotype is confirmed in a fetus with LUTO and no other congenital anomalies, then consideration may has to be given to *in-utero* treatment. Other prognostic indicators would be assessed from ultrasound such as kidney appearance and liquor volume. Consideration should also then be given to assessing kidney function. Several methods have been utilised including fetal urine, serum or amniotic fluid analysis and finally renal biopsy.

Fetal urine

Assessing fetal renal function in early pregnancy has been utilised in fetal triage prior to performing *in-utero* therapy. This is the most commonly used investigation to inform prognosis.

There are many published studies evaluating the use of fetal urine metabolites in determining fetal renal function but no consensus appears to have been reached as to the overall efficacy. Many of the studies are small-case, cohort series with different control groups. Normal ranges are also poorly defined in this group, measurement variation with gestational age is not often taken into account, and the outcome parameters also vary considerably.

Urinary sodium concentration has been used as an index of fetal renal tubular function, with values less than 90 mmol/l being normal at 20–30 weeks

Table 5 Non-urinary tract anomalies associated with lower urinary tract obstruction (*Adapted from* Anumba et al.[8] © John Wiley 2005).

Associated anomalies	Prenatal LUTO (*n* = 56)
Other renal	12 (21.4%)
Chromosomal	3 (5.3%)
Cardiac	2 (3.6%)
Rectal atresia	2 (3.6%)
CNS	1 (1.8%)
Multiple	2 (3.6%)
Cloacal dysgenesis	1 (1.8%)

of gestation, higher levels suggesting tubular dysfunction. Fetal urinary sodium or chloride values in excess of 100 mmol/l have also been shown to be highly predictive of fetal or perinatal death from terminal renal or pulmonary failure.[30,31] Other electrolytes (calcium, potassium and phosphate) mainly reflect tubular function.

β_2-Microglobulin has been suggested as being particularly important as it is a low molecular weight protein that is filtered by the glomeruli. In normal kidneys, > 99.9% is re-absorbed and metabolised in the proximal tubules; however, in renal disease with damage to this area, β_2-microglobulin is excreted in the urine. Lipitz et al.[32] reported that a β_2-microglobulin level > 13 mg/l was invariably associated with fatal outcome. It is important to point out that this pathophysiology has not been proven in the fetal kidney. Fetal serum β_2-microglobulin has been used as an index of fetal GFR and in the prediction of postnatal GFR.[33,34]

Two groups[35,36] have shown that electrolyte values drop when fetal urine is re-sampled after 24 h, and Johnson et al.[36] went on to show that sequential fetal urine analysis improves the discriminatory accuracy of identifying fetuses with severe underlying renal damage from those that may benefit from vesico-amniotic shunting. A summary of the results of some of the studies is shown in Table 6.

Fetal urine N-acetyl-B-glucosaminidase was examined by Lipitz et al.[32] and there was found to be no correlation with outcome. Other groups have found raised levels of cystatin C,[37] and insulin-like growth factor I (UIGF-1) and binding protein 3 (UIGFBP-3)[38] in cases of bilateral obstructive uropathy. UIGF-1 had a sensitivity of 90% and specificity of 88% for predicting serum creatinine > 50 µmol/l and UIGFBP-3 a sensitivity of 80% and specificity of 88%.

Fetal urinalysis has also been used to select suitable candidates for intra-uterine shunting and numerous studies have been published on its accuracy the more recent ones being.[33,38–41] These studies show that urinary sodium and calcium have the best accuracy (sensitivity 70–100%, specificity 60–80%) but that, for a single measure, urine β_2-microglobulin has the best accuracy.

Fetal serum

In the fetus, serum creatinine cannot be used to assess renal function as it crosses the placenta and is cleared by the mother.[42] This is, however, not the case for serum microglobulins such as α_1-microglobulin, retinol binding protein and β_2-microglobulin due to their molecular weight (MW < 40 kDa) which means they cannot cross the placenta but are still filtered by the glomerulus. Groups have also shown that serum β_2-microglobulin concentrations do not seem to vary with gestational age,[43–45] although this is disputed in one paper which found that levels seemed to decrease after the 31st week of gestation.[46]

A few groups have looked at α_1-microglobulin both in the serum and urine. Cagdas et al.[47] compared amniotic fluid obtained at amniocentesis and delivery with first urine obtained from neonates and found that microproteins in urine are of fetal origin and postulated that fetal maturation could be evaluated by measuring microproteins in the urine with the best indicator being α_1-microglobulin. Cobet et al.[48] looked at blood from nine fetuses with severe

Table 6 Summary of results of studies of urinalysis to predict renal dysplasia/CRF

	After data from Muller et al.[73] (n = 100). Prediction of serum creatinine > 50 µmol/l after 1 year		
Parameter	Threshold	Sensitivity	Specificity
Sodium (mmol/l)	> 50	82%	64%
Chloride (mmol/l)	> 50	70%	62%
Calcium (mmol/l)	> 0.95	53%	84%
β_2-Microglobulin (mg/l)	> 2	80%	83%
	After data from Johnson et al.[36] (n = 22–29). Sequential analysis, urine creatinine > 1 mg/dl at 2 years		
Parameter	Threshold	Sensitivity	Specificity
Sodium (mg/dl)	≤ 100		
First urine		70%	79%
Last urine		100%	79%
Chloride (mg/dl)	≤ 90		
First urine		60%	61%
Last urine		100%	72%
Calcium (mg/dl)	≤ 8		
First urine		75%	60%
Last urine		88%	47%
β_2-Microglobulin (mg/dl)	≤ 4		
First urine		33%	100%
Last urine		22%	100%
	After data from Anumba et al.[8] (n = 11). Prediction of renal dysplasia		
Parameter	Threshold	Sensitivity	PPV
Sodium	> 95% data interval	33%	100%
Calcium	> 1.2 µmol/l	66%	86%
β_2-Microglobulin	≥ 13 mg/l	63%	100%
	After data from Eugene et al.[39] (n = 56). Serum creatinine > 50 µmol/l after 1 year. Analysis via proton nuclear magnetic resonance spectroscopy		
Parameter	Threshold	Sensitivity	Specificity
Alanine/valine and valine/threonine ratio		88%	86%

bilateral renal dysplasia or agenesis and found elevated levels of α_1-microglobulin. The advantage of serum monitoring over fetal urine is that serial monitoring can occur even after placement of a shunt; however, this has to be weighed against the risks of serial cordocentesis (Table 7).

Fetal renal biopsy

This is rarely performed; however, in 1993, Greco et al.[49] reported three cases of renal biopsy. Bunduki et al.,[50] in 1998, then reported a series of 10 cases where fetal renal biopsy was compared with histological findings, ultrasound and fetal urinalysis, in fetuses with bilateral obstructive uropathy. Ultrasound-guided fetal renal biopsy was performed by fine needle aspiration. The success rate in

Table 7 Summary of papers looking at accuracy of fetal serum measurements in predicting renal dysplasia/CRF.

Parameter	Threshold	Sensitivity	Specificity
	After data from Berry et al.[43] (n = 15). Post-mortem and serum creatinine at birth		
β_2-Microglobulin (mg/l)	> 5.6 mg/l (control group)	80%	98.6%
	After data from Bökenkamp et al.[74] (n = 84) Serum creatinine at birth		
β_2-Microglobulin (mg/l)	Dynamic upper limit from control group	90%	85.5%
Cystatin C (mg/l)	Dynamic upper limit from control group	63.6%	91.8%
	After data from Dommergues et al.[34] (n = 61) Serum creatinine > 50 µmol/l postnatal		
β_2-Microglobulin (mg/l)	> 5 mg/l	67%	100%

obtaining fetal material was 50% with no maternal complications. Normal fetal renal histology was seen in 80%; in 4 out of the 11 cases renal histology added to the diagnosis and in 1 case changed the prognosis so that termination was not performed. The authors did, however, point out the limitations to this technique, the low rate of success at obtaining fetal tissue and that focal needle aspiration is not representative of the whole kidney parenchyma.[50]

In 2001, Nicolini and Spelzini[77] published a review of invasive methods of assessment of fetal renal abnormalities, they concluded that:

1. There were a number of potential biochemical markers, summarised in Table 8, but that their accuracy was far from perfect.

2. Fetuses with renal damage have hypertonic urine and increased urinary protein concentration.

Table 8 Predictors of poor renal function (*Reproduced with permission from* Nicolini and Spelzini[77] © John Wiley 2001)

Predictor	References
Increased urinary sodium	
100 mEq/l > 20 weeks	30, 31, 33, 75, 76
>95th data interval/centile	75, 76
Increased urinary calcium	
1.2 mmol/l	57
> 95th centile	58
Increased urinary β_2-microglobulin	
13 mg/l (perinatal death)	32
2 mg/l (postnatal renal failure)	73
95th centile	76
Increased serum β_2-microglobulin	
5.6 mg/l	43
> 4.9 mg/l	45

3. Serial urine samplings allow better definition of renal function.
4. Renal biopsy is still experimental and often fails to produce adequate samples.
5. Fetal blood sampling remains the only method where there is insufficient urine for urine sampling.

Chevalier[51] produced a review of biomarkers for congenital obstructive uropathy looking at future developments. New techniques were reviewed, such as immunohistochemical analysis and laser capture microscopy, to look at the cellular response of the developing kidney to urinary tract obstruction. These included components of the renin/angiotensin system, transforming growth factor-β, monocyte chemo-attractant protein-1 and epidermal growth factor. Microarray studies have also been used to look at the patterns of gene expression in the neonatal rat kidney subjected to ureteral obstruction.[51]

THERAPEUTIC OPTIONS

As discussed above, the experimental animal studies of Harrison and his group provide the theoretical basis for human fetal intervention. The basis for intervention is the relief of obstruction allowing optimisation of renal function, restoration of amniotic fluid volume and thus prevention of pulmonary hypoplasia.

Open fetal surgery

Open hysterotomy with direct fetal approach served as the initial model for access to the fetus. While these techniques were feasible, they were limited by the high complication rate associated with open surgery, the mother requires a laparotomy for the surgery and then one for delivery. There is also almost 100% complication by preterm labour immediately postoperatively requiring extensive tocolytic use.[52]

Harrison et al.[53-55] reported the first successful in utero decompression for hydronephrosis with open fetal surgery in 1981. Coplen,[60] in a review of prenatal intervention for hydronephrosis, discussed the results of 8 reported fetal surgeries (vesicostomies) performed at 17–24 weeks' gestation for obstructive uropathy (Table 9).

Reports have also shown an adverse effect on future reproductive outcomes for women with 35% having pregnancy complications including uterine

Table 9 Results of 8 reported fetal surgeries performed at 17–24 weeks of gestation for obstructive uropathy (*Reproduced with permission from* Coplen[60] © American Urological Association 1997)

	No./Total No. (%)
Neonatal survivors	4/8 (50)
Correction of oligohydramnios	4/8 (50)
Pre-term labour	8/8 (100)
Other maternal complications	0/8 (0)
Neonatal deaths from pulmonary hypoplasia	4/8 (50)
Survivors with end-stage renal disease	1/4 (25)

dehiscence/rupture (12%/6%), caesarean hysterectomy (3%) and antepartum haemorrhage requiring transfusion (9%).[56] Other groups have investigated the risk of neurological injury for the fetus that survives open fetal surgery, stating a risk of 21% and speculate that this may be due to sudden fluxes in cerebral blood flow, induced by maternal hypoxia or by the maternally administered tocolytic drugs used to prevent the postoperative preterm labour.[57]

There have been no new reports of open fetal surgery for obstructive uropathy since 1988[58] due to the complications and development of new fetoscopic techniques.

Minimal invasive therapy

Vesico-amniotic shunting: percutaneous, ultrasound-guided therapy

This is the most commonly used method to relieve urinary tract obstruction. It involves the placement of a double pig-tailed catheter under ultrasound guidance and local anaesthesia, with the distal end in the fetal bladder and the proximal end in the amniotic cavity to allow drainage of fetal urine.

Amnio-infusion is often recommended prior to shunt insertion in cases of severe oligohydramnios to allow space for insertion. The use of colour Doppler allows the umbilical arteries to be delineated as they course round the fetal bladder.

In 1986, the International Fetal Surgery Register audited 73 fetuses with ultrasound features of lower urinary tract obstruction that had been treated with in-dwelling vesico-amniotic shunts.[59] This audit demonstrated overall survival rates of 41%, with claims that perinatal mortality could at least be reduced to a figure as low as 30% with careful and appropriate patient selection using ultrasound and serial measurement of urinary analytes.

In 1997, Coplen[60] reviewed the five largest series of prenatal interventions comprising 169 cases of successful percutaneous shunt placements over 14 years (3 from a single institution, 1 fetal registry and 1 review). He found that overall survival rate was 47%, most fetuses had oligohydramnios and failure to restore amniotic fluid volume was associated with 100% mortality. Of survivors, 40% had end-stage renal disease. Patient selection was not, however, randomised nor were absolute indications for intervention and fetal ultrasound findings defined in the largest reports. Coplen[60] also concluded that limiting intervention to fetuses with good prognosis improved survival and resulted in a lower incidence of renal failure in survivors.

In Coplen's review, shunt-related complications occurred in 45% of cases. Complications include shunt blockage (25%), shunt migration (20%), preterm labour and miscarriage (5–15%), amniorrhexis (2–5%), chorio-amniotis and iatrogenic gastroschisis.[61]

Fetal cystoscopy

As discussed previously, cystoscopy has been used to help in the diagnosis of obstructive uropathy by Quintero et al.[3] They then developed the technique further and in 1995 reported intra-uterine endoscopic ablation of posterior urethral valves.[62] The group then went on to use cystoscopy to position urethral vesico-amniotic shunts.[3] The same treatment was also reported by a European centre in 2003 by Welsh et al.,[29] who successfully treated 6/10 fetuses by hydro-ablation or guide-wire passage; five of these fetuses survived.

More recently, the group looked at fetal hydrolaparoscopy and endoscopic cystotomy in two cases of complicated lower urinary tract obstruction; this was successful in one case and in the second resulted in fetal death following premature rupture of the membranes. The authors concluded that this technique should only be used in complicated cases where conventional shunting is not possible.[58] While technically more complicated, it is felt that cystoscopy may have advantages over shunting in that it may allow restoration of normal fetal bladder dynamics as opposed to the situation of chronic bladder decompression seen with shunting.[63] This technique needs further development and research; with improvements in technology. it may be more widely adopted.

Systematic review of the medical literature and meta-analysis of prenatal bladder drainage (until 2003)

Numerous small studies on the effect of fetal urinary shunting have been reported, each using different criteria for fetal selection, different surgical techniques, and different outcome measures. In 2003, our group[78] published a systematic review and meta-analysis of the literature on prenatal therapy for bladder outflow obstruction. The review identified 16 observational studies (Fig. 3), including nine uncontrolled case series (n = 146 fetuses) and seven controlled case series (n = 195 fetuses).

The review demonstrated a lack of high-quality evidence to inform clinical practice reliably on prenatal bladder drainage in fetuses with ultrasound evidence of lower urinary tract obstruction. One part of the problem is related to patient selection and reporting bias, in that the treated fetuses comprised a heterogeneous mix of underlying aetiologies that were perhaps selectively included in publications due to favourable outcome. Another part of the problem is related to imprecision, in that many studies were small as regards number of patients with wide confidence intervals and uncertainty around the estimates of effect (Fig. 3).

Clarke et al.[78] generated pooled odds ratios (OR) as a summary measure of effect and the results were stratified according to predicted prognosis (based on

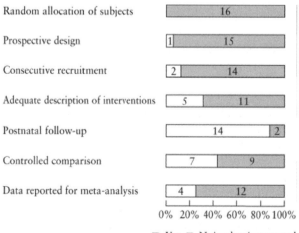

Fig. 3 Quality of evidence on prenatal bladder drainage in fetuses with ultrasound evidence of lower urinary tract obstruction (search, selection and quality assessment of studies). *Reprinted from* Kilby MD, Somerset DA, Khan KS[79] © International Society of Ultrasound in Obstetrics and Gynecology 2004

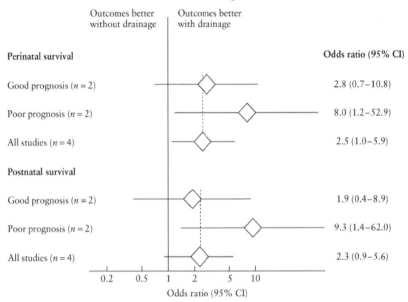

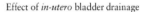

Fig. 4 Summary of effects of prenatal bladder drainage on perinatal and postnatal survival in fetuses with ultrasound evidence of lower urinary tract obstruction (analysis corrected for voluntary pregnancy terminations) (*Reprinted with the permission from* Clark TJ, Martin WL, Divakaran TG *et al.*[78] © WB Saunders 2003)

combination of ultrasound appearance and fetal urinary analytes). Within the controlled studies, vesico-amniotic drainage *in utero* (either open, fetoscopic or percutaneous procedures) appeared to improve overall perinatal survival as compared to the non-drainage group (OR 2.5; 95% CI 1.0–5.9; $P < 0.03$). However, subgroup analysis indicated that this improved survival was predominantly noted in fetuses with a defined 'poor prognosis' where there appeared to be marked improvement (OR 8.0; 95% CI, 1.2–52.9; $P < 0.03$; Fig. 4).

The review was unable to comment upon the indication or timing of the vesico-amniotic shunting because the studies included were relatively small.

Outcome
There has been concern raised about the effectiveness of *in utero* intervention, Holmes *et al.*[64] looked at the long-term outcome of 36 patients, with favourable fetal electrolytes and oligohydramnios treated at the University of California over an 18-year period. Fourteen of the patients had PUV (39%), only eight (57%) survived. Of these survivors, 63% had chronic renal impairment and underwent urinary diversion/reconstruction procedures. Their long-term outcomes indicate that intervention may help in getting the fetus to term but that the long-term sequelae of PUV, such as renal impairment, may not be preventable.[64]

These figures are supported by the case series of Freedman *et al.*[65] who followed 34 patients to a mean age of 54.3 months. Five (36%) had renal failure and successful transplantation, six (43%) had renal insufficiency and six (43%) had normal renal function. They also found that height was below the 25th percentile in 12 (86%) with seven (50%) below the 5th percentile. Of the children, 14% were incontinent with 50% acceptable continent; the remaining 36% had not yet commenced toilet training.[65]

It is thus important when counselling parents that they are aware that there is still a considerable uncertainty as to the development chance of renal failure but that these children are expected to have normal cognitive abilities and achieve acceptable continence with medical and surgical care.[65]

One study, by Holmdahl et al.,[66] has looked at long-term follow-up of 19 boys with PUV to 44 years of age and found that 32% were uremic, 21% had moderate renal failure and 48% had not been checked since adolescence. There were signs of bladder dysfunction in 40%, all with symptoms of detrusor weakness; all, however, were continent. The ability to father children was dependent on whether or not the man was uremic.[66] It is important to realise that these boys received no antenatal intervention only postnatal treatment and that many advances have been made in this area since the period that these boys were treated (1956–1970). This paper does, however, point out the importance of extended long-term follow-up for these patients.

THE FUTURE

As already discussed, there is much on-going research into new ways to diagnose congenital urinary tract abnormalities such as MRI, new markers for fetal renal impairment and new treatment modalities (e.g. fetal cystoscopy).

The results of the systematic review by Clark et al.[78] revealed a lack of high-quality evidence to answer the question as to whether prenatal intervention was effective. They suggested a multicentre, randomised, controlled trial to assess the short- and long-term effects of prenatal bladder drainage. This has been shown to be feasible via the Eurofetus twin–twin transfusion study.

PLUTO

The University of Birmingham will soon be commencing recruitment to the PLUTO study, a randomised, controlled trial to investigate the role of fetal vesico-amniotic shunting in moderate/severe LUTO funded by *Wellbeing for Women*. This will commence as a multicentre trial within the UK and hopefully be extended later to Europe. It is hoped that over a 2-year period, 200 women will be recruited; criteria being singleton, viable intra-uterine gestation with diagnosis of isolated bladder outflow obstruction at < 28 weeks (hydronephrosis, megacystis, oligo-hydramnios < 5th centile and no other structural or chromosomal abnormalities). Eligible women that consent will be randomised to either vesico-amniotic shunting or conservative observation. Where possible, fetal urine will be sampled and analysed for calcium, sodium and urinary β_2-microglobulin. Follow-up will initially be over a 12-month period with primary outcome measures being perinatal mortality and serum creatinine. Secondary outcome measures will be degree of reflux on micturating cysto-urethrography, bladder wall thickness and renal pelvic dilatation on postnatal ultrasound. Serious adverse events such as miscarriage, premature rupture of membranes, preterm labour and shunt complications will also be collected.

Further information can be obtained at <www.bctu.bham.ac.uk/fetalbladder> (Fig. 5).

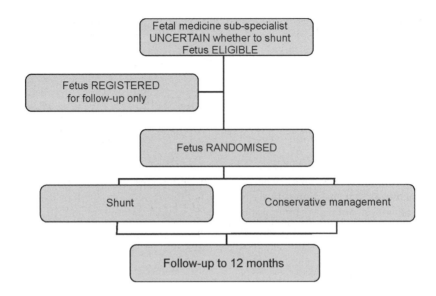

Fig. 5 Algorithm of PLUTO study.

CONCLUSIONS

Lower urinary tract obstruction is a heterogeneous condition with a natural history that is associated with high morbidity and mortality. Technical advances have allowed the introduction of tests to determine renal function and options for *in utero* treatment. Despite this, the evidence can still not identify an acceptable method to predict long-term renal function nor can we be certain that prenatal intervention is successful. Further research into these important areas is required.

References

1 Steinhardt G, Hogan W, Wood E, Weber T, Lynch R. Long-term survival in an infant with urethral atresia. J Urol 1990; 143: 336–337
2 Brand JR, Kaminopetros P, Cave C, Irving HC, Lilford RJ. Specificity of antenatal ultrasound in the Yorkshire Region: a prospective study of 2261 ultrasound detected anomalies. Br J Obstet Gynaecol 1994; 101: 392–397
3 Quintero RA, Johnson MP, Romero R et al. *In-utero* percutaneous cystoscopy in the management of fetal lower obstructive uropathy. Lancet 1995; 346: 537–540
4 Merrill DC, Weiner CP. Urinary tract obstruction. In: Fisk NM, Moise Jr KJ. (eds) Fetal Therapy: Invasive and Transplacental. Cambridge: Cambridge University Press, 1997; 273–286
5 Freedman AL, Johnson MP, Gonzalez R. Fetal therapy for obstructive uropathy: past, present, future? Pediatr Nephrol 2000; 14: 167–176
6 Parkhouse HF, Barratt TM, Dillon MJ et al. Long term outcome of boys with posterior urethral valves. Br J Urol 1988; 62: 59–62
7 Parkhouse HF, Woodhouse CR. Long-term status of patients with posterior urethral valves. Urol Clin North Am 1990; 17: 373–378
8 Anumba DO, Scott JE, Plant ND, Robson SC. Diagnosis and outcome of fetal lower urinary tract obstruction in the northern region of England. Prenat Diagn 2005; 25: 7–13
9 Vergani P, Ghidini A, Locatelli A et al. Risk factors for pulmonary hypoplasia in second-trimester premature rupture of membranes. Am J Obstet Gynecol 1994; 170: 1359–1364

10 Harrison MR, Ross NA, Noall RA. Correction of congenital hydronephrosis *in utero*. I: The model: fetal urethral obstruction produces hydronephrosis and pulmonary hypoplasia in fetal lambs. J Pediatr Surg 1983; 18: 247

11 Harrison MR, Nakayama DK, Noall RA *et al*. Correction of congenital hydronephrosis *in utero*. II: Decompression reverses the effects of obstruction on the fetal lung and urinary tract. J Pediatr Surg 1982; 17: 965

12 Nakayama DK, Glick PL, Villa RL *et al*. Experimental pulmonary hypoplasia due to oligo-hydramnios and its reversal by relieving thoracic compression. J Pediatr Surg 1983; 18: 347

13 Glick PL, Harrison MR, Noall RA *et al*. Correction of congenital hydronephrosis *in utero*. III: Early mid-trimester ureteral obstruction produces renal dysplasia. J Pediatr Surg 1983; 18: 681

14 Glick PL, Harrison MR, Adzick NS. Correction of congenital hydronephrosis *in utero*. IV: *In utero* decompression prevents renal dysplasia. J Pediatr Surg 1984; 19: 649–657

15 Berman DJ, Maizels M. The role of urinary obstruction in the genesis of renal dysplasia. A model in the chick embryo. J Urol 1982; 128: 1091–1096

16 Robyr R, Benachi A, Ikha-Dahmane F, Martinovich J, Dumez Y, Ville Y. Correlation between ultrasound and anatomical findings in fetuses with lower urinary tract obstruction in the first half of pregnancy. Ultrasound Obstet Gynecol 2005; 25: 478–482

17 Kaefer M, Peters CA, Retik AB, Benacerraf BB. Increased renal echogenicity: a sonographic sign for differentiating between obstructive and nonobstructive etiologies of in utero bladder distension. J Urol 1997; 158: 1026–1029

18 Arger PH, Coleman BG, Mintz MC *et al*. Routine fetal genitourinary tract screening. Radiology 1985; 156: 485–489

19 Abbott JF, Levine D, Wapner R. Posterior urethral valves: inaccuracy of prenatal diagnosis. Fetal Diagn Ther 1998; 13: 179–183

20 Hutton KA, Thomas DF, Arthur RJ, Irving HC, Smith SE. Prenatally detected posterior urethral valves: is gestational age at detection a predictor of outcome? J Urol 1994; 152: 698–701

21 Dinneen MD, Dhillon HK, Ward HC, Duffy PG, Ransley PG. Antenatal diagnosis of posterior urethral valves.[see comment]. Br J Urol 1993; 72: 364–369

22 McHugo J, Whittle M. Enlarged fetal bladders: aetiology, management and outcome. Prenat Diagn 2001; 21: 958–963

23 Oliveira EA, Diniz JS, Cabral AC *et al*. Predictive factors of fetal urethral obstruction: a multivariate analysis. Fetal Diagn Ther 2000; 15: 180–186

24 Xu W, Gelber S, Orr-Urteger A *et al*. Megacystis, mydriasis and ion channel defect in mice lacking the alpha3 neuronal nicotinic acetylcholine receptor. Proc Natl Acad Sci USA 1999; 96: 5746–5751

25 Xu W, Orr-Urteger A, Nigro F *et al*. Multiple autonomic dysfunction in mice lacking the beta2 and beta4 subunits of neuronal nicotinic acetylcholine receptors. J Neurosci 1999; 19: 9298–9305

26 Richardson C, Morgan J, Jasani B *et al*. Megacystis-microcolon-intestinal hypoperistalsis syndrome and the absence of the alpha3 nicotinic acetylcholine receptor subunit. Gastroenterology 2001; 121: 350–357

27 Lev-Lehman E, Bercovich D, Xu W, Stockton DW, Beaudet AL. Characterization of the human beta4 nAChR gene and polymorphisms in CHRNA3 and CHRNB4. J Hum Genet 2001; 46: 362–366

28 Cassart M, Massez A, Metens T *et al*. Complementary role of MRI after sonography in assessing bilateral urinary tract anomalies in the fetus. AJR Am J Roentgenol 2004; 182: 689–695

29 Welsh A, Agarwal S, Kumar S, Smith RP, Fisk NM. Fetal cystoscopy in the management of fetal obstructive uropathy: experience in a single European centre.[see comment]. Prenat Diagn 2003; 23: 1033–1041

30 Glick PL, Harrison MR, Golbus MS *et al*. Management of the fetus with congenital hydronephrosis II: Prognostic criteria and selection for treatment. J Pediatr Surg 1985; 20: 376–387

31 Crombleholme TM, Harrison MR, Golbus MS *et al*. Fetal intervention in obstructive uropathy: prognostic indicators and efficacy of intervention. Am J Obstet Gynecol 1990; 162: 1239–1244

32 Lipitz S, Ryan G, Samuell C *et al*. Fetal urine analysis for the assessment of renal function in obstructive uropathy. Am J Obstet Gynecol 1993; 168: 174–179

33 Johnson MP, Bukowski TP, Reitleman C, Isada NB, Pryde PG, Evans MI. *In utero* surgical treatment of fetal obstructive uropathy: a new comprehensive approach to identify appropriate candidates for vesicoamniotic shunt therapy. Am J Obstet Gynecol 1994; 170: 1770–1776

34 Dommergues M, Muller F, Ngo S *et al*. Fetal serum beta2-microglobulin predicts postnatal renal function in bilateral uropathies. Kidney Int 2000; 58: 312–316

35 Nicolini U, Tannirandorn Y, Vaughan J, Fisk NM, Nicolaidis P, Rodeck CH. Further predictors of renal dysplasia in fetal obstructive uropathy: bladder pressure and biochemistry of 'fresh' urine. Prenat Diagn 1991; 11: 159–166

36 Johnson MP, Corsi P, Bradfield W *et al*. Sequential urinalysis improves evaluation of fetal renal function in obstructive uropathy.[see comment]. Am J Obstet Gynecol 1995; 173: 59–65

37 Muller F, Bernard M-A, Benkirane A *et al*. Fetal urine cystatin C as a predictor of postnatal renal function in bilateral uropathies [2]. Clin Chem 1999; 45(12)

38 Bussieres L, Laborde K, Souberbielle JC, Muller F, Dommergues M, Sachs C. Fetal urinary insulin-like growth factor I and binding protein 3 in bilateral obstructive uropathies. Prenat Diagn 1995; 15: 1047–1055

39 Eugene M, Muller F, Dommergues M, Le ML, Dumez Y. Evaluation of postnatal renal function in fetuses with bilateral obstructive uropathies by proton nuclear magnetic resonance spectroscopy. Am J Obstet Gynecol 1994; 170: 595–602

40 Foxall PJ, Bewley S, Neild GH, Rodeck CH, Nicholson JK. Analysis of fetal and neonatal urine using proton nuclear magnetic resonance spectroscopy. Arch Dis Child 1995; 73: F153–F157

41 Daikha-Dahmane F, Dommergues M, Muller F *et al*. Development of human fetal kidney in obstructive uropathy: correlations with ultrasonography and urine biochemistry. Kidney Int 1997; 52: 21–32

42 Nolte S, Mueller B, Pringsheim W. Serum alpha1-microglobulin and beta2-microglobulin for the estimation of fetal glomerular renal function. Pediatr Nephrol 1991; 5: 573–577.

43 Berry SM, Lecolier B, Smith RS *et al*. Predictive value of fetal serum beta2-microglobulin for neonatal renal function. Lancet 1995; 345: 1277–1278

44 Ciardelli V, Rizzo N, Farina A, Vitarelli M, Boni P, Bovicelli L. Prenatal evaluation of fetal renal function based on serum beta(2)-microglobulin assessment. Prenat Diagn 2001; 21: 586–588

45 Tassis B, Trespidi L, Tirelli AS, Pace E, Boschetto C, Nicolini U. Serum B2-microglobulin in fetuses with urinary tract anomalies. Am J Obstet Gynecol 1997; 176: 54–57

46 Nolte S. Estimation of fetal renal function by microprotein determination (alpha1- and beta2-microglobulin) in fetal blood. Z Geburtshilfe Perinatol 1991; 195: 153–158

47 Cagdas A, Aydinli K, Irez T, Temizyurek K, Apak MY. Evaluation of the fetal kidney maturation by assessment of amniotic fluid alpha-1 microglobulin levels. Eur J Obstet Gynecol Reprod Biol 2000; 90: 55–61.

48 Cobet G, Gummelt T, Bollmann R, Tennstedt C, Brux B. Assessment of serum levels of alpha-1-microglobulin, beta-2-microglobulin, and retinol binding protein in the fetal blood. A method for prenatal evaluation of renal function. Prenat Diagn 1996; 16: 299–305

49 Greco P, Loverro G, Caruso G, Clemente R, Selvaggi L. The diagnostic potential of fetal renal biopsy. Prenat Diagn 1993; 13: 551–556

50 Bunduki V, Saldanha LB, Sadek L, Miguelez J, Miyadahira S, Zugaib M. Fetal renal biopsies in obstructive uropathy: feasibility and clinical correlations – preliminary results. Prenat Diagn 1998; 18: 101–109

51 Chevalier RL. Biomarkers of congenital obstructive nephropathy: Past, present and future. J Urol 2004; 172: 852–857

52 Farmer DL. Fetal surgery: a brief review. Pediatr Radiol 1998; 28: 409–413

53 Harrison MR, Golbus MS, Filly RA *et al*. Fetal surgery for congenital hydronephrosis. N Engl J Med 1982; 306: 591–593

54 Harrison MR, Golbus MS, Filly RA *et al*. Fetal hydronephrosis: selection and surgical repair. J Pediatr Surg 1987; 22: 556–558

55 Crombleholme TM, Harrison MR, Langer JC *et al*. Early experience with open fetal surgery for congenital hydronephrosis. J Pediatr Surg 1988; 23: 1114–1121

56 Wilson RD, Johnson MP, Flake AW *et al*. Reproductive outcomes after pregnancy complicated by maternal-fetal surgery. Am J Obstet Gynecol 2004; 191: 1430–1436

57 Bealer JF, Raisanen J, Skarsgard ED *et al*. The incidence and spectrum of neurological injury after open fetal surgery. J Pediatr Surg 1995; 30: 1150–1154

58 Quintero RA, Morales WJ, Allen MH, Bornick PW, Johnson P. Fetal hydrolaparoscopy and endoscopic cystotomy in complicated cases of lower urinary tract obstruction. Am J Obstet Gynecol 2000; 183: 324–330

59 Manning FA, Harrison MR, Rodeck C. Catheter shunts for fetal hydronephrosis and hydrocephalus. Report of the International Fetal Surgery Registry. N Engl J Med 1986; 315: 336–340

60 Coplen DE. Prenatal intervention for hydronephrosis. J Urol 1997; 157: 2270–2277

61 Rodeck CH, Nicolaides KH. Ultrasound guided invasive procedures in obstetrics. Clin Obstet Gynaecol 1983; 10: 515–539

62 Quintero RA, Hume R, Smith C et al. Percutaneous fetal cystoscopy and endoscopic fulguration of posterior urethral valves [see comment]. Am J Obstet Gynecol 1995; 172: 206–209

63 Agarwal SK, Fisk NM. In utero therapy for lower urinary tract obstruction. Prenat Diagn 2001; 21: 970–976

64 Holmes N, Harrison MR, Baskin LS. Fetal surgery for posterior urethral valves: long-term postnatal outcomes. Pediatrics 2001; 108: E7

65 Freedman AL, Johnson MP, Smith CA, Gonzalez R, Evans MI. Long-term outcome in children after antenatal intervention for obstructive uropathies [see comment]. Lancet 1999; 354: 374–377

66 Holmdahl G, Sillen U. Boys with posterior urethral valves: outcome concerning renal function, bladder function and paternity at ages 31 to 44 years. J Urol 2005; 174: 1031–1034

67 Thomas DF, Irving HC, Arthur RJ. Pre-natal diagnosis: how useful is it? Br J Urol 1985; 57: 784–787

68 Mahoney BS, Callen PW, Filly RA. Fetal urethral obstruction: US evaluation. Radiology 1985; 157: 221–224

69 Nakayama DK, Harrison MR, de Lomimier AA. Prognosis of posterior urethral valves presenting at birth. J Pediatr Surg 1986; 21: 43–45

70 Hayden SA, Russ PD, Pretorius DH, Manco-Johnson ML, Clewell WH. Posterior urethral obstruction: prenatal sonographic findings and clinical outcome in 14 cases. J Ultrasound Med 1988; 7: 371

71 Reuss A, Wladimiroff JW, Stewart PA, Scholtmeijer RJ. Non-invasive management of fetal obstructive uropathy. Lancet 1988; ii: 949–951

72 Harrison MR, Golbus MS, Filly RA (eds). The Unborn Patient: Prenatal diagnosis and treatment, 2nd edn. Philadelphia, PA: WB Saunders, 1990

73 Muller F, Dommergues M, Mandelbrot L, Aubry MC, Nihoul-Fekete C, Dumez Y. Fetal urinary biochemistry predicts postnatal renal function in children with bilateral obstructive uropathies. Obstet Gynecol 1993; 82: 813–820

74 Bokenkamp A, Dieterich C, Dressler F et al. Fetal serum concentrations of cystatin C and beta$_2$-microglobulin as predictors of postnatal kidney function. Am J Obstet Gynecol 2001; 185: 468–475

75 Nicolini U, Fisk NM, Rodeck CH, Beacham J. Fetal urine biochemistry: an index of renal maturation and dysfunction. Br J Obstet Gynaecol 1992; 99: 46–50

76 Muller F, Dommergues M, Bussieres L et al. Development of human renal function: reference intervals for 10 biochemical markers in fetal urine. Clin Chem 1996; 42: 1855–1860

77 Nicolini U, Spelzini F. Invasive assessment of fetal renal abnormalities: urinalysis, fetal blood sampling and biopsy. Prenat Diagn 2001; 21: 964–969

78 Clark TJ, Martin WL, Divakaran TG, Whittle MJ, Kilby MD, Khan KS. Prenatal bladder drainage in the management of fetal lower urinary tract obstruction: a systematic review and meta-analysis. Obstet Gynecol 2003; 102: 367–382

79 Kilby MD, Somerset DA, Khan KS. [Editorial] Potential for correction of fetal obstructive uropathy: time for a randomized controlled trial? Ultrasound Obstet Gynecol 2004; 23: 527–530

Anna Marie O'Neill   Irina D. Burd
Juan Carlos Sabogal   Jolene Seibel-Seamon
Stuart Weiner

Doppler ultrasound in obstetrics: current advances

Doppler ultrasonography has been the subject of numerous randomized controlled trials since its introduction to obstetrics in the 1970s. It is a non-invasive tool that has proven useful in the evaluation of maternal and fetal hemodynamics. As normal pregnancy progresses there are many changes occurring in maternal, fetal, and placental vasculature to accommodate the metabolic needs of the fetus. Abnormalities in one or more of these vascular systems occur prior to the clinical and laboratory appearance of, or as a result of, many pathological conditions of pregnancy. The ability to obtain information on the velocity and impedance of blood flow through maternal and fetal vessels using Doppler velocimetry has become an important tool in the evaluation and management of high-risk pregnancies. Essentially, every

Anna Marie O'Neill MD
Instructor, Department of Obstetrics and Gynecology, Jefferson Medical College of Thomas Jefferson University, Division of Maternal-Fetal Medicine, 834 Chestnut Street, Suite 400, Philadelphia, PA 19107, USA

Irina D. Burd MD PhD
Department of Obstetrics and Gynecology, Jefferson Medical College of Thomas Jefferson University, Division of Maternal-Fetal Medicine, 834 Chestnut Street, Suite 400, Philadelphia, PA 19107, USA

Juan Carlos Sabogal MD
Department of Obstetrics and Gynecology, Jefferson Medical College of Thomas Jefferson University, Division of Maternal-Fetal Medicine, 834 Chestnut Street, Suite 400, Philadelphia, PA 19107, USA

Jolene Seibel-Seamon MD
Department of Obstetrics and Gynecology, Jefferson Medical College of Thomas Jefferson University, Division of Maternal-Fetal Medicine, 834 Chestnut Street, Suite 400, Philadelphia, PA 19107, USA

Stuart Weiner MD (for correspondence)
Associate Professor of Obstetrics and Gynecology, Division of Maternal-Fetal Medicine, and Director, Division of Reproductive Imaging and Genetics, Jefferson Medical College of Thomas Jefferson University, 834 Chestnut Street, Suite 400, Philadelphia, PA 19107, USA
E-mail: lynn.stierle@jefferson.edu

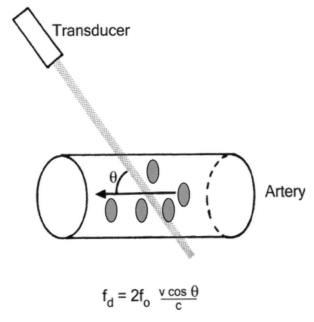

Fig. 1 Doppler effect (adapted from Copel *et al.*[1]) where: f_d = reflected frequency; f_0 = frequency of emitted sound wave; v = velocity of red blood cells; c = speed of sound waves traveling in tissues; and θ = angle between sound wave and path of blood cells.

$$f_d = 2f_0 \, \frac{v \cos \theta}{c}$$

fetal vessel has been interrogated in the research setting in an effort to improve our understanding of the pathophysiology of such conditions as intra-uterine growth restriction (IUGR), pre-eclampsia, fetal anemia, and fetal hypoxia. Information obtained from Doppler interrogation, in many cases, is also being used in the management of these conditions.

The physical phenomenon known as the Doppler effect was described by Christian Doppler in 1842. The Doppler effect is the shift in frequency of waves of energy which results from a source moving with respect to the observer. In Doppler ultrasonography, the source is the stationary transducer emitting sound waves at a constant frequency. The sound wave strikes a moving medium – the red blood cells – and is reflected back to the transducer. The frequency of the returning sound waves is determined by the velocity of the red blood cells. Because velocity is a vector, it has a magnitude (termed speed) and a direction. The angle at which the sound wave strikes the red blood cell has an effect on the reflected signal as described in the Doppler equation (Fig. 1).[1]

Calculations of flow or velocity are dependent on the angle between sound waves emitted from the transducer and flow within the vessel, or angle of insonation. As the angle of insonation increases, so does the error in these calculations. To minimize this effect, angle independent ratios are used to describe flow. The indices most commonly used are the S/D ratio, pulsatility index PI (S–D/A), and the resistance index RI (S–D/S) and are derived from the following: peak-systolic velocity (S) which is a result of cardiac contraction; end-diastolic velocity (D), which depends on vessel wall compliance, peak flow, heart rate and vascular impedance; and average velocity over the cardiac cycle (A). The PI and RI are useful when diastolic flow is absent, and the PI contains information about the shape of the waveform.

Several different types of Doppler technology are currently used in obstetrics. **Continuous wave Doppler** has two separate crystals within the transducer – one that transmits a continuous sound wave, and the other that receives the reflected sound wave. It is non-selective in that it recognizes all signals along its path, and cannot be used to visualize blood vessels. Portable Doptone and fetal heart rate monitoring equipment utilize this technology. **Pulsed wave Doppler** has a single crystal within the transducer that emits a brief sound wave, and must wait until the reflected sound wave is received before emitting the subsequent signal. It allows precise targeting and visualization of the specific vessel of interest and can be used to obtain information about the characteristics of blood flow within the vessel. **Color Doppler imaging** is used to identify the specific vessel of interest that is then interrogated with pulsed Doppler. Color Doppler displays the presence and direction of blood flow, and can highlight gross anomalies in vasculature or blood flow. It is used extensively in fetal echocardiography. **Power Doppler** has the greatest sensitivity and is used to detect low flow and low intensity signals such as those characteristic of venous circulation. However, it is not capable of determining direction of flow. **High definition Doppler** is the newest addition to Doppler technology in obstetrics. It combines the sensitivity of power Doppler with the ability to demonstrate direction of flow of color Doppler and is useful in interrogation of the fetal venous circulation.

In this chapter, we shall briefly review the application of Doppler to three areas of current interest in clinical obstetrics: (i) uterine artery studies; (ii) evaluation of fetal anemia; and (iii) fetal well-being and hypoxia.

UTERINE ARTERY DOPPLER

The majority of blood flow to the uterus is supplied by the uterine arteries. Throughout gestation, uterine blood flow increases 10–12-fold as a result of a combination of the physiological modification and trophoblastic invasion of the spiral arteries within the myometrium and decidua, and the 50% increase in maternal blood volume. The shape of the uterine artery Doppler waveform is unique and changes as gestation advances. In early pregnancy, the uterine circulation is characterized by high vascular impedance and low flow, giving a waveform with persistent end-diastolic velocity and continuous forward blood flow throughout diastole. As the trophoblastic invasion and spiral artery modification proceed, placental perfusion increases and uteroplacental circulation becomes a high-flow, low-resistance system giving a waveform with greater end-diastolic flow.

When the normal trophoblastic invasion and modification of spiral arteries is interrupted, there is increased impedance to flow within the uterine arteries and decreased placental perfusion. These pathological processes are key features common to the development of pre-eclampsia and IUGR, and are suspected when the RI fails to decrease in the second trimester, or with the appearance of diastolic notching in the umbilical artery waveform (Fig. 2).[2]

A prospective trial by Zimmermann et al.[3] evaluated the utility of uterine artery Doppler interrogation performed between 21 and 24 weeks in the

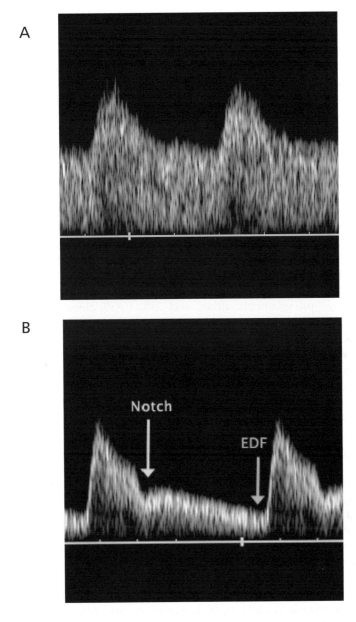

Fig. 2 Uterine artery waveforms at 24 weeks' gestation (from Nicolaides *et al.*[2]). (A) Normal uterine artery waveform. Forward flow present throughout diastole. (B) Abnormal uterine artery waveform demonstrating notching in early diastole (EDF = end-diastolic flow).

prediction of subsequent development of pre-eclampsia and IUGR. They identified 175 women at high risk for developing hypertensive disorders of pregnancy or IUGR, and 172 low-risk pregnancies. Persistent notching or elevated RI in the uterine arteries or an elevated RI in the uteroplacental arteries were defined as pathological Doppler signs. A positive medical history alone was associated with a 3-fold greater risk of developing pre-eclampsia and/or IUGR. In the high-risk group, a single pathological Doppler sign accounted for an additional 3–4-fold increased risk, and the combination of all three pathological signs, a 7-fold additional increase in risk for developing disease later in pregnancy. In this group, pre-eclampsia and/or IUGR were found in 58.3%, compared to 8.3% if Doppler results were normal. Doppler was less informative in the low-risk population. Here, pre-eclampsia and/or IUGR were seen in 6.1–6.4% in the group with abnormal Doppler findings compared to 5.2% in pregnancies with normal findings.[3]

Papageorghiou *et al.*[4] conducted a multicenter cohort study of approximately 8000 unselected singleton pregnancies to determine the utility of transvaginal color Doppler assessment of the uterine arteries in the prediction of subsequent development of pre-eclampsia and/or IUGR. Bilateral notching or an elevated PI were considered abnormal findings. The sensitivity, specificity, and positive and negative predictive values of an abnormal finding for identifying pregnancies at risk for developing both pre-eclampsia and IUGR were 83.3%, 88.5%, 3.8%, and 99.9%, respectively, with a likelihood ratio of 7.3 (95% CI 6.0–8.2). However, the sensitivities in predicting only one of these pathological outcomes independent of the other were much lower (41% for pre-eclampsia alone, and 24% IUGR alone). The authors concluded that uterine artery Doppler screening at 23 weeks is most informative in identifying the more severely affected fetuses and may have a role in routine pregnancy care.[4]

Christina *et al.*[5] conducted a multicenter prospective screening trial of 30,784 unselected low-risk singleton pregnancies that incorporated mid-trimester uterine artery Doppler interrogation and evaluation of patient-specific risk based on maternal demographic and anthropometric data in the development of an integrated risk assessment model. They determined that a combined assessment will identify about 70% of women who subsequently develop pre-eclampsia, compared to a 45% detection rate based on screening alone.[5]

Based on the currently available data, there is insufficient evidence to recommend uterine artery Doppler as a general screening modality for all pregnancies. When performed in a high-risk population, it does have some value in identifying pregnancies that may warrant more frequent blood pressure assessment. Patients with abnormal uterine Doppler parameters should be counseled on performing fetal kick counts, and on reporting symptoms of pre-eclampsia at each prenatal visit. There is no proven prophylaxis for pre-eclampsia, but recent and on-going clinical trials are evaluating the role of aspirin, vasodilators, and antioxidants.

EVALUATION OF FETAL ANEMIA

In the US, the most common causes of fetal anemia are maternal allo-immunization, infection with parvovirus B19 and fetomaternal hemorrhage. Maternal trauma and abuse may also be significant contributors. Maternal allo-immunization to red-cell antigens is the most common of the three, and has been estimated to occur in 35 per 10,000 live births.[6] To detect the fetuses at risk for hydrops before 34 weeks of gestation (10% of the entire population at risk),[7] either serial percutaneous umbilical blood sampling (PUBS) or amniocentesis were historically performed.

Amniocentesis is less invasive than PUBS and has been used since 1961 to diagnose fetal anemia indirectly by assessing the amniotic fluid optical density deviation at a wavelength of 450 nm[8] as a marker for the presence of bilirubin from breakdown of hemoglobin. Prior to 27 weeks of gestation, this method lacks accuracy[9] in predicting the severity of anemia,[10] and correlates poorly with the severity of fetal anemia in cases in of sensitization to Kell antigens where erythropoiesis may be suppressed.[11]

Although PUBS allows direct measurement of fetal hemoglobin, this is an invasive procedure associated with risk of infection, fetal bradycardia, premature rupture of membranes, bleeding from the cord puncture site, worsening of fetal allo-immunization and fetal demise of 1%.[8,12,13] It is estimated that if each fetus at risk for anemia were to undergo one PUBS procedure, there would be at least 140 fetal losses every year.[14]

The most reliable non-invasive test for predicting fetal anemia is Doppler study of blood flow velocity in the fetal middle cerebral artery (MCA). Studies that have evaluated the efficacy of non-invasive measurements such as the PI and the RI, which are independent of blood velocity in detecting fetal anemia, have failed to find a good correlation between ultrasound findings and the presence of fetal anemia.[15–18]

Peak systolic velocity (PSV) in the fetal middle cerebral artery (MCA)

Cerebral arteries respond quickly to hypoxemia, owing to the strong dependence of brain tissue on oxygenation. The velocity of blood flow in several circulatory beds, including the brain, is increased in a fetus with anemia because of an increased cardiac output and a decrease in blood viscosity.[19–21] MCA is one of the cerebral vessels that is easily visualized with an angle of insonation close to zero degrees, and this measurement has a low intra-observer and interobserver variability.[10] The PSV should be measured at the highest point of the Doppler waveform and the measurement should be repeated multiple times during periods of fetal apnea (Fig. 3).

Vyas et al.,[22] in a study of 24 previously untransfused, non-hydropic fetuses from red cell iso-immunized pregnancies at 18–35 weeks of gestation, were the first to propose a significant correlation between an increase in mean velocity in the middle cerebral artery and the degree of fetal anemia measured in samples obtained by cordocentesis.

Later, Mari et al.[23] found a significant association between MCA PSV and fetal hematocrit at PUBS. In this prospective study of 16 fetuses from iso-immunized pregnancies, all of the anemic fetuses had PSV above the normal mean for gestation, whereas none of the fetuses with PSV below the normal mean were anemic.[23] On the basis of these results, they suggested that, in the management of isoimmunized pregnancies, the indication for PUBS should be a peak systolic velocity above the normal mean for gestation. These results were used as preliminary data for a multicenter, prospective study involving 111 fetuses from iso-immunized pregnancies.[14] In this study, measurements of MCA PSV were found to predict the presence of moderate or severe anemia in fetuses with a sensitivity of 100% and a false positive rate of 12%. The data were obtained by many operators in different medical centers using different ultrasound equipment; this consistency suggests that others should be able to

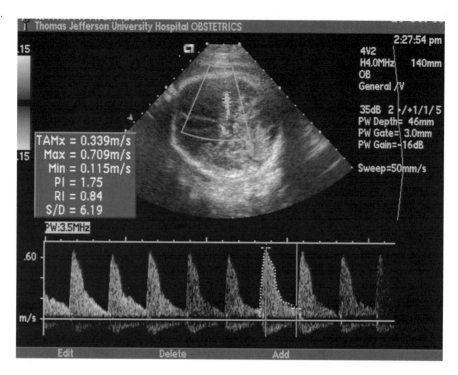

Fig. 3 MCA Doppler waveform assessment.

obtain similar results. In a large prospective intent-to-treat trial of 125 cases of red cell allo-immunization, previous findings were confirmed, and the detection of moderate-to-severe anemia with MCA PSV over 1.5 multiples of the median (MOM) showed a sensitivity of 88% and specificity of 87%.[24]

In studies comparing conventional management with amniocentesis determination of the ΔOD 450 to that with MCA PSV, MCA PSV has a better predictive value for moderate-to-severe anemia in red cell allo-immunization, eliminated the need for amniocentesis, and decreased the number of PUBS performed on non-anemic fetuses.[25,26] A management algorithm utilizing MCA PSV is presented in Figure 4.[27]

In addition to studies of red cell allo-immunization, evaluation of MCA PSV in cases of parvoviral infection showed that fetal anemia could be detected with a sensitivity of 94–100% and specificity of 93–100%.[28,29]

EVALUATION OF FETAL WELL-BEING

Doppler in intra-uterine growth restriction

The use of Doppler ultrasound has allowed the identification of abnormal patterns of resistance to blood flow in specific fetal vessels including the umbilical artery (UA), MCA, and ductus venosus (DV). In recent years, the characterization of such patterns and surveillance of fetuses demonstrating these abnormal patterns has contributed significantly to a decrease in perinatal morbidity and mortality. Furthermore, color flow analysis of different flow

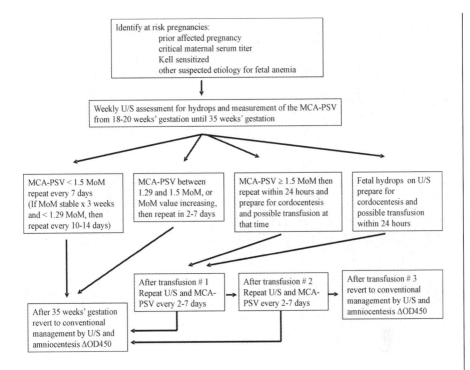

Fig. 4 Management algorithm for RBC iso-immunized pregnancies. MCA, middle cerebral artery; PSV, peak systolic velocity; U/S, ultrasound; MoM, multiples of the median. *With permission from* Pereira L.[48]

patterns within the fetal heart has enabled the clinician to identify the presence of congestive heart failure and predict fetal demise.

Alfirevic *et al.*[30] published a systematic review with meta-analysis addressing the usefulness of Doppler in the surveillance of high-risk pregnancies. Two groups of high-risk pregnant patients were identified and allocated to either a standard fetal assessment protocol or to standard fetal assessment plus Doppler ultrasound testing. Their results showed a decrease in perinatal mortality in the second group. The use of Doppler reduced the odds for perinatal death by as much as 38% (95% CI 15–55%).[30] However, it has also been shown that the use of Doppler in a low-risk population confers no benefit to patients over standard fetal surveillance.[31]

In fetuses demonstrating IUGR, a characteristic adaptive vascular mechanism is the cornerstone for fetal survival; this change in the normal vascular physiology and distribution of blood flow is now very well characterized. The identification of a pattern demonstrating fetal adaptation to impaired uteroplacental blood flow constitutes one of the most useful criteria in the diagnosis and surveillance of fetuses affected by IUGR.[32] Abnormal UA Doppler findings have proven useful in distinguishing the constitutionally small and healthy fetus from the fetus with IUGR.

The umbilical artery (UA) was the first vessel to be studied by Doppler ultrasonography. By about 15 weeks of gestation, diastolic flow can be identified in the UA. With advancing gestational age, the end-diastolic velocity

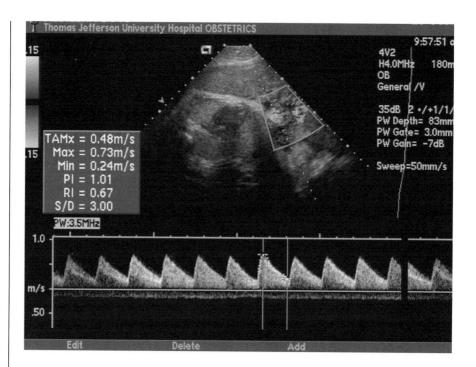

Fig. 5 Normal umbilical artery waveform. Forward flow is present throughout the cardiac cycle.

increases secondary to the decrease in placental resistance. This is reflected in a decrease in the S/D or PI. The interrogation of the UA produces a waveform with both systolic and diastolic flow in the normal fetus, suggesting continuous placental perfusion (Fig. 5). As the chorionic vascular bed undergoes an atherosclerotic-like process with local ischemia and necrosis in a pregnancy affected by IUGR, the UA shows increasing impedance that initially blunts forward flow during diastole, and ultimately reverses it at a later stage.[33] These findings have been associated with adverse perinatal outcome, and demand a closer follow-up of fetal condition.[34] Once reversal of diastolic flow is identified, administration of steroids for fetal lung maturity in the premature fetus and delivery must be considered.

MCA is another vessel well-characterized by Doppler interrogation and has been shown to be affected by IUGR as well. MCA, typically a vessel of higher impedance when compared with the UA (see Fig. 3), normally exhibits a low amplitude of diastolic flow which increases in the presence of fetal hypoxia as a marker of adaptive cerebral vasodilation, resulting in a decreased PI value. Although this may be an isolated finding in fetuses affected by IUGR, it more commonly represents a later stage in the hypoxic process and typically occurs after changes in the UA. The sequence of abnormal events that herald adverse perinatal outcome begins with an absence of UA end diastolic flow which is seen in more than 50% of affected fetuses about 15 days prior to acute deterioration requiring urgent delivery. Later findings include abnormal Doppler pulsatility of the MCA (with decreased PI) and ductus venosus (DV;

with absent or reversed flow during atrial contraction), and reversed flow in UA, are seen within 4–5 days of delivery.[35] Late changes are significantly associated with perinatal death.

Monitoring effects of fetal exposure to NSAIDs

The use of non-steroidal anti-inflammatory drugs (NSAIDs) has become more frequent in the management of the pregnant patient with preterm labor or polyhydramnios. A known effect of these medications is the premature closure of the ductus arteriosus (DA) *in utero* that may lead to fetal heart failure. The use of systolic peak velocity through the DA by means of Doppler assessment has been used to monitor on this side effect of NSAIDs, offering evidence to either continue or stop the medication.[36]

Doppler in fetal hypoxia

Fetal oxygenation requires oxygen transport across the placenta, oxygen association onto fetal hemoglobin, and fetal consumption after delivery at the cellular level. All four steps are essential for fetal growth and metabolism. Hypoxemia is defined as a decrease in oxygen content in fetal blood, while hypoxia is a decrease in oxygenation at the cellular level. Prolonged hypoxia results in metabolic acidosis. Asphyxia is defined as hypoxia with metabolic acidosis.

When fetal oxygenation is compromised, the fetus has a host of adaptive responses prior to decompensation. Initially, the fetus decreases its oxygen demands by conserving energy which manifests as decreased fetal movement. There is also redistribution of blood flow to the most critical organs – the brain, heart, coronaries, and adrenals – as evidenced by vasodilation of vascular beds supplying these organs. Dilation of cerebral vasculature results in decreased impedance demonstrated by cephalization of flow and a decreased PI. With prolonged hypoxemia, however, there is a loss of cephalization as cerebral impedance increases, reflected in an increasing PI. Cerebral edema may play a role in this loss of cephalization. The uteroplacental bed responds with rising umbilical artery impedance demonstrated by an increased S/D or PI, and absent or reversed end diastolic flow. Studies evaluating high-risk pregnancies with PUBS to determine fetal oxygenation and acid/base status have shown a significant association between abnormal UA Doppler waveforms and fetal acid–base abnormalities. Fetal hypoxia was present in 67–80% of fetuses with absent end-diastolic flow in the UA, and 45% were acidotic.[37] The time course from onset of abnormal arterial Doppler indices to onset of late decelerations in the fetal heart rate pattern, indicating acute fetal decompensation, is somewhat inversely related to gestational age with the less mature fetus showing a greater lag time. Late decelerations will develop about 2 weeks from the onset of abnormal Doppler indices in the immature fetus,[38] and sooner in the fetus near term.

Fetal venous Doppler interrogation is also used in monitoring the fetus at risk of hypoxia or acidemia. Most commonly, the umbilical vein, the inferior vena cava, and the ductus venosus are studied in assessing fetal well-being. In a healthy pregnancy, the umbilical vein demonstrates a non-pulsatile constant forward flow from about 12 weeks of gestation onward. The rest of the venous system demonstrates a complex triphasic waveform representing systole (S-wave), diastole (D-wave), and atrial systole (a-wave). With advancing gestation, venous flow velocities increase as placental resistance and afterload decrease. The DV maintains the highest forward velocity throughout gestation. Venous Doppler velocimetry reflects cardiac function, and abnormal waveforms indicate reduced cardiac contractility.[39–42]

In response to hypoxia, umbilical venous blood flow is redistributed through the DV to maintain oxygenation of brain and heart and bypasses the hepatic circulation. With progressive hypoxia, there is an increase in right ventricular afterload causing a reversal of flow in the inferior vena cava during atrial contraction. With further deterioration, the DV and umbilical vein will develop end-diastolic pulsations indicating a loss of forward flow during atrial contraction. These end-diastolic venous pulsations generally coincide with the onset of acidemia and late decelerations on the fetal heart tracing.[42–44]

Several recent studies have looked at the Doppler assessment of fetal hypoxia in the intrapartum period. A study of 92 full-term intrapartum gravidas by Siristatidis et al.[45] observed an alteration in UA Doppler velocimetry indices during labor indicated fetal hypoxia demonstrated by pulse oximetry. With pulse oximetry readings of < 40%, both RI and PI were increased. If pulse oximetry readings of < 30% were sustained for more than 2 min, there was an even greater increase in both of these indices. They noted a strong correlation between fetal pulse oximetry, Doppler velocimetry of the MCA and UA, and fetal morbidity.[45] In a more recent study, these investigators made similar observations in an additional 60 term fetuses and concluded that UA velocimetry correlated with perinatal outcome.[46]

In a study by Arbeille et al.,[47] a combination of the intensity and duration of the fetal flow redistribution (hypoxia) in the antenatal period were used to design a Doppler Hypoxic Index which correlated with the occurrence of abnormal fetal heart tracing during delivery.

Management of the fetus demonstrating abnormal Doppler indices is gestational-age dependent. In the mature fetus, there is little to be gained by continuing pregnancy, and the time course to decompensation is generally shorter in these fetuses; therefore, delivery is recommended. Induction of labor would be reasonable in those with a re-assuring fetal heart tracing. In the immature fetus, close surveillance is indicated. Once absent end-diastolic flow in the UA is demonstrated, twice weekly biophysical profile (BPP) testing and repeat of Doppler indices, daily fetal kick counts, and growth scans every 2–3 weeks should be initiated. With reversal of end-diastolic flow in the UA or cephalization in the MCA, hospitalization with continuous oxygen therapy, bed rest, daily BPP, and daily Doppler studies are indicated. Steroids for fetal lung maturity should be administered as these fetuses are likely to decompensate within hours to days. A pulsatile pattern in the DV Doppler is highly suggestive of fetal acidemia and is an indication to deliver. A fetus with either reversed end diastolic flow in the UA and/or a pulsatile DV pattern has little reserve and will not likely tolerate labor.

CURRENT AREAS OF DOPPLER INVESTIGATION IN OBSTETRICS

1. Randomized trials are currently in progress to characterize better the gestational age dependence on the timing of fetal adaptation and ultimate decompensation in relation to abnormalities in arterial and venous Doppler indices. The effects of intervention at various gestational ages is also being evaluated.

2. Management of pregnancy that continues beyond 40 weeks is an area of current Doppler investigation. Elective induction of pregnancy for this indication may carry an increased risk of cesarean section with its associated increased maternal morbidity and implications for future pregnancies. This risk is weighed against the risk to the fetus for increased morbidity and mortality with prolonged gestation. The PI of both the UA and MCA as well as their ratio, UA PI/MCA PI referred to as the cerebroplacental ratio, have been studied and reference ranges have been reported. Further investigation may demonstrate a role for these Doppler indices in fetal surveillance of prolonged pregnancies.

3. 3-D power Doppler is particularly sensitive for detecting low velocity flow which is then rendered to give a detailed image of fine vascular structures. It has been used investigationally to characterize complex fetal vascular anomalies and to evaluate placental development. Since tertiary stem villi can be visualized, there is a potential for earlier detection of abnormal placentation to detect pregnancies at high risk for pre-eclampsia or IUGR, or evaluation of a suspected placenta abruption or accreta. Other applications include demonstration of vascular anastamoses in monochorionic or conjoined twin pregnancies, better characterization of mass lesions by identifying feeding vessels, and evaluation of lung development in suspected pulmonary hypoplasia.

KEY POINTS FOR CLINICAL PRACTICE

- There is currently insufficient evidence to implement uterine artery Doppler as a screening modality in women at low risk for developing pre-eclampsia and/or IUGR.

- The addition of uterine artery Doppler to maternal history significantly increases the sensitivity for predicting pre-eclampsia in a high-risk population; however, there are currently no proven prophylactic therapies to offer those patients identified as high risk.

- Measurement of the fetal MCA PSV is a reliable indicator of severe fetal anemia and has become standard of care in the management of pregnancies at risk of fetal anemia, regardless of etiology.

- Doppler velocimetry is a useful tool in distinguishing the healthy, constitutionally small fetus from the IUGR fetus.

(continued on next page)

KEY POINTS FOR CLINICAL PRACTICE *(continued)*

• Both the IUGR fetus and the hypoxic fetus demonstrate similar patterns of abnormal Doppler indices in the progression from adaptation to acute decompensation. Absence of end diastolic flow in the UA is followed by a decrease in the MCA PI. Without intervention, reversal of flow in the UA ensues. Pulsatile flow in the DV and umbilical vein are late findings and predict the proximate onset of late decelerations in the fetal heart tracing.

• Management of the fetus demonstrating Doppler signs of IUGR or hypoxia are gestational-age dependent, but in many cases iatrogenic preterm birth is indicated.

References

1 Copel JA, Grannum PA, Hobbins JC *et al*. Doppler ultrasound in obstetrics. Williams Obstetrics, 17th edn (Suppl 16). Norwalk, CT: Appleton and Lange, 1988

2 Nicolaides KH, Rizzo G, Hecker K, Ximenes R. Diploma in Fetal Medicine Series. ISUOG Educational Series, 2002

3 Zimmermann P, Eirio V, Koskinen J *et al*. Doppler assessment of the uterine and uteroplacental circulation in the second trimester in pregnancies at high risk for pre-eclampsia and/or intrauterine growth retardation: comparison between different Doppler parameters. Ultrasound Obstet Gynecol 1997; 9: 330–338

4 Papageorghiou AT, Yu CKH, Bindra R *et al*. Multicenter screening for pre-eclampsia and fetal growth restriction by transvaginal uterine artery Doppler at 23 weeks of gestation. Ultrasound Obstet Gynecol 2001; 18: 441–449

5 Yu CKH, Smith GCS, Papageorghiou AT *et al*. An integrated model for the prediction of preeclampsia using maternal factors and uterine artery Doppler velocimetry in unselected low-risk women. Am J Obstet Gynecol 2005; 193: 429–436

6 Public Health Service. Centers for Disease Control and Prevention congenital malformation surveillance. Teratology 1993; 48: 545–709

7 Bowman JM. Hemolytic disease (erythroblastosis fetalis). In: Creasy RK, Resnik R. (eds) Maternal–Fetal Medicine, 4th edn. Philadelphia, PA: W.B. Saunders, 1999; 736–767

8 Daffos F, Capella-Pavlovsky M, Forestier F. Fetal blood sampling during pregnancy with use of a needle guided by ultrasound: a study of 606 consecutive cases. Am J Obstet Gynecol 1985; 153: 655–660

9 American College of Obstetricians and Gynecologists. Management of isoimmunization in pregnancy. ACOG educational bulletin. No. 227. Washington, DC: ACOG, 1996

10 Mari G, Andrignolo A, Abuhamad AZ *et al*. Diagnosis of fetal anemia with Doppler ultrasound in the pregnancy complicated by maternal blood group immunization. Ultrasound Obstet Gynecol 1995; 5: 400–405

11 Caine ME, Mueller-Heubach E. Kell sensitization in pregnancy. Am J Obstet Gynecol 1986; 154: 85–90

12 Royston P. Constructing time-specific reference ranges. Stat Med 1991; 10: 675–690

13 Ghidini A, Sepulveda W, Lockwood CJ, Romero R. Complication of fetal blood sampling. Am J Obstet Gynecol 1993; 168: 1339–1344

14 Mari G. Noninvasive diagnosis by Doppler ultrasonography of fetal anemia due to maternal red-cell alloimmunization. N Engl J Med 2000; 342: 9–14

15 Nicolaides KH, Fontanarosa M, Gabbe SG, Rodeck CH. Failure of ultrasonographic parameters to predict the severity of fetal anemia in rhesus isoimmunization. Am J Obstet Gynecol 1988; 158: 920–926

16 Copel JA, Grannum PA, Green JJ, Belanger K, Hobbins JC. Pulsed Doppler flow-velocity waveforms in the prediction of fetal hematocrit of the severely isoimmunized pregnancy. Am J Obstet Gynecol 1989; 161: 341–344

17 Hecher K, Snijders R, Campbell S, Nicolaides K. Fetal venous, arterial, and intracardiac blood flows in red blood cell isoimmunization. Obstet Gynecol 1995; 85: 122–128

18 Bahado-Singh R, Oz U, Mari G, Jones D, Paidas M, Onderoglu L. Fetal splenic size in anemia due to Rh-alloimmunization. Obstet Gynecol 1998; 92: 828–832

19 Fan FC, Chen RY, Schuessler GB, Chien S. Effects of hematocrit variations on regional hemodynamics and oxygen transport in the dog. Am J Physiol 1980; 238: H545–H552

20 Rosenkrantz TS, Oh W. Cerebral blood flow velocity in infants with polycythemia and hyperviscosity: effects of partial exchange transfusion with Plasmanate. J Pediatr 1982; 101: 94–98

21 Moise Jr KJ, Mari G, Fisher DJ, Huhta JC, Cano LE, Carpenter Jr RJ. Acute fetal hemodynamic alterations after intrauterine transfusion for treatment of severe red blood cell alloimmunization. Am J Obstet Gynecol 1990; 163: 776–784

22 Vyas S, Nicolaides KH, Campbell S. Doppler examination of the middle cerebral artery in anemic fetuses. Am J Obstet Gynecol 1990; 162: 1066–1068

23 Mari G, Adrignolo A, Abuhamad AZ et al. Diagnosis of fetal anemia with Doppler ultrasound in the pregnancy complicated by maternal blood group immunization. Ultrasound Obstet Gynecol 1995; 5: 400–405

24 Zimmermann R, Durig P, Carpenter Jr RJ, Mari G. Longitudinal measurement of peak systolic velocity in the fetal middle cerebral artery for monitoring pregnancies complicated by red cell alloimmunisation: a prospective multicentre trial with intention-to-treat. Br J Obstet Gynaecol 2002; 109: 746–752

25 Nishie EN, Brizot ML, Liao AW, Carvalho MHB, Toma O, Zugaib M. A comparison between middle cerebral artery peak systolic velocity and amniotic fluid optical density at 450 nm in the prediction of fetal anemia. Am J Obstet Gynecol 2003; 188: 214–219

26 Pereira L, Jenkins T, Berghella V. Conventional management of fetal alloimmunization compared to management by middle cerebral artery peak systolic velocity. Am J Obstet Gynecol 2003; 189: 1002–1006

27 Chervenak FA, Kurjak A. Textbook of Perinatal Medicine. London: Taylor & Francis, 2006; in press

28 Delle Chiaie L, Buck G, Grab D, Terinde R. Prediction of fetal anemia with Doppler measurements of the middle cerebral artery peak systolic velocity in pregnancies complicated by maternal blood group alloimmunization or parvovirus B19 infection. Ultrasound Obstet Gynecol 2001; 18: 232–236

29 Cosmi E, Mari G, Delle Chiaie L et al. Noninvasive diagnosis by Doppler ultrasonography of fetal anemia resulting from parvovirus infection. Am J Obstet Gynecol 2002; 187: 1290–1293

30 Alfirevic Z, Neilson JP. Doppler ultrasonography in high risk pregnancies: Systematic review with meta-analysis. Am J Obstet Gynecol 1995; 172: 1379–1387

31 Bricker L. Routine Doppler ultrasound in pregnancy. Cochrane database systematic review. Jan 2000

32 Fleisher AC, Romero R, Manning FA, Jeanty P, James AE. The principles and practice of Ultrasonography in Obstetrics and Gynecology, 5th edn. Prentice Hall, 1996

33 Callen PW. Ultrasonography in obstetrics and gynecology, 4th edn. Philadelphia, PA: W.B. Saunders, 2000

34 Bashat AA, Gembruch U, Reiss I et al. Relationship between arterial and venous Doppler and perinatal outcome in fetal growth restriction. Ultrasound Obstet Gynecol 2000; 16: 407–413

35 Ferrazzi E, Bozzo M, Rigano S et al. Temporal sequence of abnormal Doppler changes in the peripheral and central circulatory systems of the severely growth-restricted fetus. Ultrasound Obstet Gynecol 2002; 19: 140–146

36 Kiserud T. The ductus venosus. Semin Perinatol 2001; 25: 11–20

37 Nicolaides KH, Bilardo CM, Soothill PW, Campbell S. Absence of end diastolic frequencies in the umbilical artery: a sign of fetal hypoxia and acidosis. BMJ 1988; 297: 1026–1027

38 Bekedam DJ, Visser GHA, van der Zee AGJ, Snijders RJM, Poelmann-Weesjes G.

Abnormal velocity waveforms of the umbilical artery in growth-retarded fetuses: relationship to antepartum late heart rate decelerations and outcome. Early Hum Dev 1990; 24: 79–89

39 Gudmundusson S, Tulzer G, Huhta JC, Marsal K. Venous Doppler in the fetus with absent end diastolic flow in umbilical artery. Ultrasound Obstet Gynecol 1996; 7: 262–267

40 Rizzo G, Capponi A, Soregaroli M, Arduini D, Romanini C. Umbilical vein pulsations and acid base status at cordocentesis in growth retarded fetuses with absent end diastolic velocity in umbilical artery. Biol Neonate 1995; 68: 163–168

41 Arduini D, Rizzo G, Romanini C. Changes of pulsatility index from fetal vessels preceding the onset of late decelerations in growth-restricted fetuses. Obstet Gynecol 1992; 79: 605

42 Hecher K, Campbell S. Characteristics of fetal venous blood flow under normal circumstances and during fetal disease. Ultrasound Obstet Gynecol 1996; 7: 68

43 Hecher K, Campbell S, Doyle P, Harrington K, Nicolaides K. Assessment of fetal compromise by Doppler ultrasound investigation of the fetal circulation. Arterial, intracardiac, and venous blood flow velocity studies. Circulation 1995; 91: 129

44 Arduini D, Rizzo G, Romanini C. Changes in pulsatility index from fetal vessels preceding the onset of late decelerations in growth-retarded fetus. Obstet Gynecol 1997; 79: 605

45 Siristatidis C, Salamalekis E, Kassanos D, Loghis C, Creatsas G. Evaluation of fetal intrapartum hypoxia by middle cerebral and umbilical artery Doppler velocimetry with simultaneous cardiotocography and pulse oximetry. Arch Gynecol Obstet 2004; 270: 265–270

46 Siristatidis C, Salamalekis E, Kassanos D, Creatsas G. Alterations in Doppler velocimetry indices of the umbilical artery during fetal hypoxia in labor, in relation to cardiotocography and fetal pulse oximetry findings. Arch Gynecol Obstet 2005; 272: 191–196

47 Arbeille P, Perrotin F, Salihagic A, Sthale H, Lansac J, Platt LD. Fetal Doppler Hypoxic Index for the prediction of abnormal fetal heart rate at delivery in chronic fetal distress. Eur J Obstet Gynecol Reprod Biol 2005; 121: 171–177

48 Pereria L. Doppler in fetal anemia. In: Chervenak FA, Kurjak A. (eds) Textbook of Perinatal Medicine. London: Taylor and Frances, 2006: in press.

Chloe Vera   Ruth C. Fretts

8

Pregnancy and advanced maternal age

As women increasingly delay childbearing, questions surrounding the counseling and management of older mothers have become central to the practice of obstetrics. Advanced maternal age, generally held to signify age after 35 years at the time of delivery, is a term that implies decreased fertility and increased risk. This chapter will review the effects of age on fertility, pregnancy and delivery.

INCIDENCE AND EPIDEMIOLOGY

The global total fertility rate fell from 5 children per woman-lifetime in 1950–1955 to 2.7 children in 2000–2005.[1] Within the US, as well as in other industrialised countries, the crude birth rate (the number of live births per 1000 population) has dropped with women having fewer children. In the US, the crude birth rate dropped from 24.1 in 1950 to 14.9 in 2002. Similarly, the overall fertility rate (the number of live births per 1000 women aged 15–44 years) has dropped from 106.2/1000 to 64.8/1000.[2] The implication, that women are having fewer children than they were 50 years ago, seems obvious. One would expect that the effect would be that fewer older women are having children; however, although overall birth rates for older women have decreased, there is evidence that women are merely delaying childbearing. At age 40–44 years, the number of women who had not had at least one birth was 15.8/1000 in 2002, compared with 15.1/1000 in 1960. However, at every other age group, the number of women who had not yet had a live birth was significantly higher in

Chloe Vera MD
Department of Obstetrics and Gynecology, Brigham and Women's Hospital, Boston, Massachusetts, USA
E-mail: Cvera@Partners.org

Ruth C. Fretts MD MPH (for correspondence)
Assistant Professor, Harvard Medical School, Harvard Vanguard Medical Associates, Boston, Massachusetts, USA
E-mail: Rfretts@vmed.org

2002 than in 1960. For example, 66.5% of women aged 20–24 years had not had a child yet in 2002, versus 47.5% in 1960. Similarly, at age 25–29 years, 41.3% in 2002 versus 20% in 1960 had not yet given birth, suggesting that women were simply having children later rather than opting not to have children at all.[2]

The reasons for this shift toward later childbearing are multiple. Women are attaining higher educational levels than in previous decades; within non-industrialised countries, the age of first birth and the interval between births increases as women's status increases. Factors in particular that are related to this phenomenon are related to the free choice of a partner, women's education and the wealth of the family.[3] Within the US in 2002, 25.9% of women with live births had > 16 years of education, compared with 8.6% in 1970.[4] Level of education correlates with knowledge and use of contraception, age at first birth and total number of children. The changing role of women in the workplace, with more career opportunities available, has undoubtedly affected childbearing. Control of fertility with increased contraceptive options plays a part. Likewise, the availability of assisted reproductive technologies to older women has allowed many to achieve pregnancy and childbearing. A retrospective study of all deliveries in the US from 1997–1999 identified 539 deliveries to women over age 50 years, for a rate of four per 100,000.[5] These women are more likely to conceive with assisted reproductive technologies. The oldest woman to conceive a pregnancy naturally was 57 years old; births to women as old as 66 years have been reported using assisted reproductive technology.

PRECONCEPTIONAL ISSUES

Fertility declines with advancing maternal age. In 2002, fertility rates for women aged 35–39 years were 41.4/1000, for women aged 40–44 years 8.3/1000, and for women aged 45–54 0.5/1000 as compared to 103.6/1000 for women aged 20–24 years and 113.6/1000 for women aged 25–29 years.[2]

There are multiple factors, both physiological and acquired, that contribute to this diminished fertility with increasing age. Acquired pathology contributing to infertility, particularly tubal disease, accumulates over time. The role of structural lesions that increase with advancing age, such as uterine fibroids and endometrial polyps, is unclear but may also play a role in decreased fertility. Ovarian oocyte reserve declines with increasing number of ovulatory cycles. This decreased ability of the ovary to ovulate is illustrated by data from assisted reproductive technology clinics. In 2002, 19.9% of *in vitro* fertilization (IVF) cycles in women aged 41–42 years were cancelled as opposed to only 9.2% in women under aged 35 years.[6] Finally, oocyte quality diminishes over time as well.

The risk of aneuploidy rises significantly with advancing maternal age (Table 1).[7,8] Normal physiology predicts higher rates of aneuploidy with aging; as oocytes reach metaphase I during the fetal period and remain aligned on the metaphase plate until the oocyte is stimulated to divide, just prior to ovulation. Errors accumulated over time seem to increase the risk of non-disjunction, leading to unequal chromosome products at completion of division. Aneuploidy reduces implantation rates and results in abnormal development in implanted embryos. Estimates of the rates of aneuploidy have become more

Table 1 Age-specific risk for chromosomal abnormalities in live-born infants

Maternal age at delivery (years)	Risk of trisomy 21	Risk of any chromosomal abnormality
20	1/1667	1/526
22	1/1429	1/500
24	1/1250	1/476
26	1/1176	1/476
27	1/1111	1/455
28	1/1053	1/435
29	1/1000	1/417
30	1/952	1/385
31	1/909	1/385
32	1/769	1/322
33	1/602	1/286
34	1/485	1/238
35	1/378	1/192
36	1/289	1/156
37	1/224	1/127
38	1/173	1/102
39	1/136	1/83
40	1/106	1/66
41	1/82	1/53
42	1/63	1/42
43	1/49	1/33
44	1/38	1/36
45	1/30	1/21
46	1/23	1/16
47	1/18	1/13
48	1/14	1/10
49	1/11	1/8

Data modified from maternal age-specific rates by Hook EB, Cross PK, Schreinemacher DM. JAMA 1983: 249 and Hook EB. Obstet Gynecol 1981:58; 282.

precise recently with the advent of pre-implantation genetic diagnosis (PGD). In a recent, randomized, controlled trial involving PGD for women of advanced maternal age (defined as age ≥ 37 years), aneuploidy was observed in 43.2% of the tested embryos.[9] A prospective cohort study of women with recurrent miscarriage in which PGD and IVF was performed showed an aneuploidy rate of 43.9% for patients younger than age 37 years and 67.0% in patients older than 37 years. The on-going pregnancy rate per cycle was 25.7% in the younger versus 2.9% in the older patients.[10] Although this study represents an overestimate of aneuploidy risk in older women (as those with recurrent miscarriages likely have a higher baseline aneuploidy rate) the effects of age on aneuploidy rates are clear.

The options for treatment of infertility are somewhat dependent on the cause, but as women age, they increasingly must turn to assisted reproductive technologies (ARTs), including ovulation induction with intra-uterine insemination (IUI) and IVF. IUI and IVF for age-related infertility can accelerate the time to conception, but oocyte quality can still affect outcomes. Although these treatment options improve the likelihood of achieving pregnancy when compared to expectant management, ARTs cannot compensate for the entire natural decline of fertility with advancing age.[11]

Advanced maternal age affects the success of ovulation induction with IUI. This may, at least partially, be due to diminished ovarian reserve. One study examining the effects of diminished ovarian reserve found that only about 5% of women with the diagnosis will achieve pregnancy, even with ovulation induction; the overall poor pregnancy prognosis for these women was heightened by increasing maternal age.[12] A single-center review of pregnancy outcomes in 168 consecutive women aged ≥ 40 years who underwent ovulation induction with IUI (total of 469 cycles) showed decreasing fertility rates with increasing age.[13] For women aged 40, 41, and 42 years, per cycle fecundity rates were 9.6, 5.2, and 2.4, respectively, with no viable pregnancies occurring in women aged ≥ 43 years. This stands in contrast to the per cycle live birth rate in women under 35 years of age (17–22%) and women aged 35–40 years (8–10%).[6]

As maternal age increases, the success of IVF using fresh, non-donor eggs decreases. A woman's chance of progressing from the beginning of ART to pregnancy and live birth (using her own eggs) decreases at every stage of ART as her age increases: the likelihood of a successful response to ovarian stimulation and progression to egg retrieval decreases, cycles that have progressed to egg retrieval are slightly less likely to reach transfer, the percentage of cycles that progress from transfer to pregnancy decreases, and cycles that have progressed to pregnancy are less likely to result in a live birth because the risk for miscarriage is greater. In 2002, 42.5% of cycles in women aged less than 35 years resulted in pregnancies, while only 17.3% of cycles in women aged 41–42 years resulted in pregnancies. Live birth rates are lower, with only 10.7% of cycles in women aged 41–42 years resulting in live births Fig. 1).[6]

For older women without ovarian reserve, egg donation represents the only option likely to succeed. The success of egg donation does not significantly

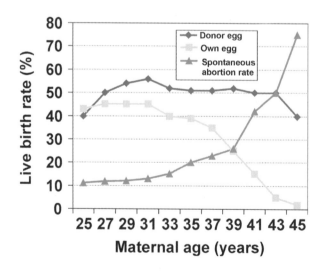

Fig. 1 Live birth rates using fresh and donor eggs and the spontaneous abortion rate.

Table 2 Demographic characteristics and medical history by parity and maternal age

	Nulliparous			Multiparous		
	20–29 yr	40+ yr	P	20–29 yr	40+ yr	P
History of infertility	3.6%	20.3%	< 0.01	1.3%	6.8%	< 0.01
History of IVF use	0.3%	8.7%	< 0.01	0.2%	2.3%	< 0.01
History of SAB	11.8%	34.4%	< 0.01	19.5%	41.1%	< 0.01
Hypertension	0.5%	0.9%	NS	0.6%	2.1%	< 0.01
Diabetes	0.3%	0.5%	NS	0.5%	0.8%	NS
Cardiac	2.2%	3.9%	< 0.01	1.9%	4.1%	< 0.01
Leimyomas	1.1%	10.1%	< 0.01	1.1%	4.6%	< 0.01

SAB, spontaneous abortion. yr = years old.

Hypertension and diabetes as pre-existing conditions.

Adapted from Bianco et al.[27]

vary according to the recipient's age up to age 50 years, after which there may be a small decline due to lower rates of implantation. In the largest study of delivery outcomes in recipients of donated eggs, implantation rates (number of fetal heart beats/number of embryos transferred) with fresh egg donation in women aged 49 years and under (n = 13,000 egg donations) and aged 50–54 years (n = 300 egg donations) were 22% and 16%, respectively, and the delivery rates (live birth/retrieval) were 40% and 32%, respectively.[14] The risk of aneuploidy are related to the age of the egg donor; however, risks of third trimester complications such as gestational diabetes and hypertension are elevated with maternal age (Table 2).

The data regarding successful pregnancy outcomes after pre-implantation genetic diagnosis for aneuploidy screening in older women are limited. Several retrospective or comparative studies have suggested no improvement in pregnancy rates. The one prospective, randomized, clinical trial comparing PGD for aneuploidy screening with traditional blastocyst transfer in couples with advanced maternal age showed similar positive pregnancy test rates and implantation rates (defined as presence of fetal heart beat), although significantly fewer embryos were available for transfer in the PGD group.[9]

FIRST TRIMESTER COMPLICATIONS

Although it is difficult to quantify the number of spontaneous abortions accurately, it is well established that older women are at increased risk (Table 3). Data from the FASTER (First and Second Trimester Evaluation of Risk) trial, in which approximately 30,000 women at 10–14 weeks' gestational age were enrolled in a prospective multicenter investigation of singleton pregnancies, revealed increasing rates of both threatened abortion and miscarriage with advancing maternal age. Although the rates found in this study likely underestimate true incidence (as women with losses prior to 10–14 weeks were never enrolled), adjusted odds ratios for miscarriage were 2.0 (95% CI 1.5–2.6) for women aged 35–39 years and 2.4 (95% CI 1.6–3.6) for women aged ≥ 40 years when compared with women under age 35 years.[15]

Table 3 Percentage loss by maternal age at conception

Maternal age (years)	Spontaneous abortions (%)	Ectopic pregnancies(%)	Stillbirth rate/1000
12–19	13.3	2.0	5.0
20–24	11.1	1.5	4.2
25–29	11.9	1.6	4.0
30–34	15.0	2.8	4.4
35–39	24.6	4.0	5.0
40–44	51.0	5.8	6.7
≥ 45	93.4	7.0	8.2

Adapted from Figures 2, 4, 5 in Nyobo Andersen et al.[16] This estimates the total spontaneous abortion rate under the assumption that only 80% of women with abortions in recognized pregnancies were hospitalized.

The leading cause of death in early pregnancy, ectopic gestation, remains one of the most significant obstetric complications. There is evidence associating advancing maternal age with increased risk of ectopic pregnancy. Older data suggested up to an 8-fold increased risk of ectopic pregnancy in women > 35 years compared to younger women.[16,17] This trend was supported by a recent study examining the ectopic pregnancy rate in a large managed care organization, with the rate of ectopic pregnancy in women aged 40–49 years (42.52/1000 pregnancies, 95% CI 36.39–48.75) roughly 4 times that of women aged 15–19 years (12.55/1000, 95% CI 10.42–14.68).[18]

Cardiac malformations, clubfoot, and diaphragmatic hernia appear to be more common in offspring of older women. As these abnormalities are structural and usually unrelated to aneuploidy, they are generally diagnosed in the second trimester by ultrasound. The increased risk of congenital anomalies in offspring of older women has been demonstrated by several large series. One series including over 100,000 abortions, stillbirths, and live births reported that cardiac defects were 4 times more common in infants of women 40 years of age compared to those aged 20–24 years. In addition, women > 35 years of age had a significantly higher risk of offspring with clubfoot or diaphragmatic hernias. However, the overall increase from age-related risk for women aged > 35 years was only 1%.[19] Another study looked at over one million singleton infants born at 20 weeks of gestation in Atlanta from 1968 to 2000 who did not have a chromosomal abnormality. Advanced maternal age (35–40 years) was associated with a small increased incidence in several congenital anomalies including all heart defects, tricuspid atresia, right outflow tract defects, hypospadias second degree or higher, other male genital defects and craniosynostosis.[20] The FASTER trial, which again included over 30,000 singleton pregnancies, reported congenital anomaly rates for women < 35, 35–39, and 40 years of age of 1.7%, 2.8%, and 2.9%, respectively.[15]

FIRST VERSUS SECOND TRIMESTER SCREENING FOR ANEUPLOIDY

The current American College of Obstetricians and Gynecologists (ACOG) recommendation regarding screening for fetal aneuploidy is that women with

Table 4 Antepartum complications by maternal age and parity

	Nulliparous			Multiparous		
	20–29 yr	40+ yr	P	20–29 yr	40+ yr	P
Gestational diabetes	1.7%	7.0%	< 0.01	1.6%	7.8%	< 0.01
Pre-eclampsia	3.4%	5.4%	< 0.01	1.0%	2.7%	< 0.01
Placenta previa	0.03%	0.25%	< 0.01	0.13%	0.05%	< 0.01
Prematurity	9.1%	14.1%	< 0.01	10.3%	13.7%	< 0.01

Adapted from Gilbert et al.[26]

singleton pregnancies who will be age 35 years or older at delivery and women with twin pregnancies aged 33 years or older at delivery should be offered prenatal diagnosis, and that all women should be offered screening.[21] This recommendation is based on age-related risk of Down syndrome and represents a consensus opinion.

In the first trimester, chorionic villus sampling is recommended for diagnosis of aneuploidy. Amniocentesis is not recommended during the first trimester because of higher rates of pregnancy loss following the procedure compared with traditional (15–17 weeks) timing.[21]

LATE PREGNANCY ISSUES

As women age, they have a greater opportunity to acquire conditions that can influence their health and the health of the fetus. Because of this, women aged 35 years or older can expect to have twice the rates of antepartum hospitalization than their younger counterparts.[15,22–28] The two most common medical problems complicating pregnancy (Table 4) are hypertension (pre-existing and pregnancy related) and diabetes (pregestational and gestational).

Hypertension

Hypertension is the most frequent medical problem encountered in pregnancy with older women having a 2-fold higher risk of being diagnosed with this problem. Similarly, the incidence of pre-eclampsia in the general obstetric population is 3–4%; this increases to 5–10% in women over age 40 years and is as high as 35% in women over age 50 years.[29] With careful monitoring and appropriately timed intervention, maternal and fetal morbidity and mortality can be reduced, but this is associated with an increase in preterm birth, small for gestational age infants, and cesarean delivery.[26,30,31]

Diabetes mellitus

The prevalence of diabetes increases with maternal age; the rates of both pre-existing diabetes mellitus and gestational diabetes increase 3–6-fold in women 40 years of age or older compared to women aged 20–29 years.[15,26,29]

Pre-existing diabetes is associated with an increased risk of congenital anomalies, perinatal mortality, and perinatal morbidity, while the most common complication from gestational diabetes is macrosomia.[32]

Abnormal placentation

Placental abruption and placental previa do occur more commonly in older women, with a large portion of this risk associated with increasing parity. Gilbert et al.,[26] however, did find a 10-fold increased risk of placenta previa in nulliparous women 40 years of age or older when compared to women aged 20–29 years, although the absolute risk of this was small (0.25% versus 0.03%).

Perinatal morbidity

Advanced maternal age is responsible for a substantial proportion of the recent increase in rate of low birthweight (LBW) and preterm (PTD) delivery observed in the past several years.[5,31,33,34] Cnattingius et al.,[35] in a large Swedish cohort study, found that nulliparous women aged 35–40 years with singleton gestations had a near 2-fold increased risk of preterm delivery, and a 1.7-fold increased risk of delivering a small for gestational age baby compared to women aged 20–24 years.

A US population-based study found a linear increase in the risk of delivering a low birth weight, such that women 40 years of age or older had a 2.3-fold increased risk of delivering a low birth weight infant when compared to women aged 20–24 years (95% CI 1.6–3.4). Smoking has been associated with an increased perinatal morbidity in all age groups, but the risk is particularly high in smokers aged 30–39 years.[36]

Perinatal mortality

Historically, a significant proportion of perinatal deaths seen in older women were related to an increase in lethal congenital and chromosomal anomalies. Currently, in industrialised countries, the increased perinatal mortality experienced by older women is largely due to non-anomalous fetal deaths and perinatal losses associated with multiple gestations. Large studies clearly show an increased risk of unexplained fetal death among older gravida, even after controlling for risk factors such as hypertension, diabetes, antepartum bleeding, and multiple gestation.[38-41]

In our population-based analysis of obstetrical outcome at the Royal Victoria Hospital in Montreal, we found that older women were at higher risk of fetal death compared to younger women (for women 35–39 years of age as compared with women < 30 years of age, OR 1.9, 95% CI 1.3–2.7; for those ≥ 40 years, OR 2.4, 95% CI 1.3–4.5) even after controlling for potential confounders such as hypertension diabetes, abruption placenta, placenta previa, previous abortion and multiple gestation.[38]

Jacobsson et al.,[39] in a large population-based study from Sweden, reported higher rates of fetal/neonatal death in older mothers after adjusting for confounders such as parity, congenital malformations, smoking, and maternal disease. The rates of fetal death for women 20–29, 40–44, and ≥ 45 years of age were 3.2, 6.4, and 11.6 per 1000, respectively.[39]

Dysfunctional labor and cesarean delivery

Women 35 years of age or older are more likely to be delivered by cesarean section. The cesarean delivery rate in the general obstetric population of the US is almost 30%, compared to almost 50% in women aged 40–45 years[26,40] and almost 80% in women aged 50–63 years.[26] The reasons for this are multifactorial; while there appears to be a linear relationship between dysfunction labor and maternal age, other factors likely come into play, such as the increased risk of medical complications, inductions of labor, and malpositions seen in older gravida. Physicians and patients alike probably have a lower threshold to perform a cesarean delivery in older women and we are seeing a growing acceptance of primary elective cesarean deliveries.

Maternal mortality

While advancing maternal age is associated with an increased risk of maternal mortality, in industrialised countries this is still a rare event. Within some areas of the US, the leading causes of maternal mortality are non-obstetric, such as death from trauma. The obstetrically related deaths in the US from 1991 to 1997, for women aged 26–29 years was 9/100,000 live births, the risk for women aged 35–39 years was 21/100,000 live births, and for women 40 years of age or older, the rate was 46/100,000.[41,42] The most common causes of death were related to hypertension, hemorrhage, and thrombo-embolism.[43,44]

In non-industrialised nations where maternal mortality is many fold higher, the lack of adequate care contributes substantially to these maternal losses, and plays a much larger role than maternal characteristics.[45]

KEY POINTS FOR CLINICAL PRACTICE

- Women must often balance the biological advantages of having a child at a younger age against economic and social advantages of obtaining an education and establishing a career.

- At intervals, young women should be educated about the risks of delaying childbearing. Unfortunately, high-profile pregnancies in older women have given women the impression that late pregnancies are easy to achieve and have good outcomes.

- The most significant hurdle for older women is their age-related risk of infertility, including changes in uterine or hormonal function and oocyte quality

- Evaluation of ovarian reserve using a day 3 FSH and estradiol assay or clomiphene citrate challenge test is reasonable but women should not be falsely re-assured that, if they have adequate testing, a pregnancy is guaranteed.[46]

(Continued on next page)

KEY POINTS FOR CLINICAL PRACTICE (continued)

- If conception has not occurred after 6 months of actively attempting pregnancy, the couple should be referred to a clinician who can initiate an infertility evaluation and help formulate a plan to optimize the establishment of pregnancy.

- Women should be counseled on the age-related risk of fetal aneuploidy and offered prenatal screening and prenatal diagnosis. A detailed second trimester ultrasound examination provides the opportunity to detect anomalies related or unrelated to aneuploidy that occur more often in older women.

- Women should be counseled that they have an increased risk of both early and late complications of pregnancy which includes spontaneous abortion, chromosomal abnormalities, ectopic pregnancy, some congenital anomalies, placenta previa, gestational diabetes, pre-eclampsia, and caesarean delivery. Such complications may, in turn, result in preterm birth.

- Because the risk of unexplained stillbirth appears to increase late in pregnancy, older women without medical or pregnancy complications may benefit from liberal use of antepartum testing, although this has not been proven. Quantifying these risks may be helpful for women. In a decision analysis model, Fretts et al.[47] showed that weekly antepartum testing and labor induction predicted a significant reduction the number of otherwise unexplained fetal deaths. In this model, weekly testing starting at 37 weeks of gestation would drop the risk of fetal death from 5.2 to 1.3 per 1000 pregnancies. A strategy of antepartum testing in older women does increase the chance that a women having an induced delivery. It was estimated that 14 additional caesareans would need to be performed to avert one unexplained fetal death.[47]

References

1 Cohen JE. Human population: the next half century. Science 2003; 302: 1172–1175
2 National Center for Health Statistics. Birth rate for women aged 15–44. <http://www.cdc.gov/nchs/pressroom/04facts/birthrates.htm> (Accessed 3/7/05)
3 Larsen U, Hollos M. Women's empowerment and fertility decline among the Pare of Kilimanjaro region, Northern Tanzania. Soc Sci Med 2003; 57: 1099–1115
4 Mathews TJ, Ventura SJ. National Vital Statistics Report. Birth and Fertility Rates by Educational Attainment: United States, 1994–1997; 45: 1
5. Salihu HM, Shumpert MN, Slay M, Kirby RS, Alexander GR. Childbearing beyond maternal age 50 and fetal outcomes in the United States. Obstet Gynecol 2003; 102: 1006–1014
6 Centers for Disease Control. Assisted Reproductive Technology (ART) Report: 2002 National Summary (Accessed 5/5/05)
7 Hook EB. Rates of chromosome abnormalities at different maternal ages. Obstet Gynecol 1981; 58: 282.

8 Hassold T, Chiu D. Maternal age-specific rates of numerical chromosome abnormalities with special reference to trisomy. Hum Genet 1985; 70: 11

9 Staessen C, Paltteau P, Van Assche E et al. Comparison of blastocyst transfer with or without preimplantation genetic diagnosis for aneuploidy screening in couples with advanced maternal age: a prospective randomized controlled trial. Hum Reprod 2004; 19: 2849–2858

10 Platteau P, Staessen C, Michiels A et al. Preimplantation genetic diagnosis for aneuploidy screening in patients with unexplained recurrent miscarriages. Fertil Steril 2005; 83: 393–397

11 Leridon H. Can assisted reproduction technology compensate for the natural decline in fertility with age? A model assessment. Hum Reprod 2004; 19: 1548–1553. Epub 2004 Jun 17

12 Scott RT, Opsahl MS, Leonardi MR, Neall GS, Illions EH, Navot D. Life table analysis of pregnancy rates in a general infertility population relative to ovarian reserve and patient age. Hum Reprod 1995; 10: 1706–1710

13 Corsan G, Trias A, Trout S, Kemmann E. Ovulation induction combined with intrauterine insemination in women 40 years of age and older: is it worthwhile? Hum Reprod 1996; 11: 1109–1112

14 Toner JP, Grainger DA, Frazier LM. Clinical outcomes among recipients of donated eggs: an analysis of the U.S. national experience, 1996–1998. Fertil Steril 2002; 78: 1038–1045.

15 Cleary-Goldman J, Malone FD, Vidaver J et al. Impact of maternal age on obstetric outcome. Obstet Gynecol 2005; 105: 983–990

16 Nyobo Andersen A, Wohlfahrt J, Christens P, Olsen J, Malbye M. Maternal age and fetal loss: population based register linkage study. BMJ 2000; 320: 1708

17 Storeide O, Velhomen M, Eide M et al. The incidence of ectopic pregnancy in Hordaland county, Norway 1976–1993. Acta Obstet Gynecol Scand 1997; 76: 345

18 van den Eeden, SK, Shan J, Bruce C, Glasser M. Ectopic pregnancy rate and treatment utilization in a large managed care organization. Obstet Gynecol 2005 ;105: 1052–1057

19 Hollier LM, Leveno KJ, Kelly MA, McIntire DD, Cunningham FG. Maternal age and malformations in singleton births. Obstet Gynecol 2000; 96: 701–706

20 Reefhuis J, Honein MA. Maternal age and non-chromosomal birth defects, Atlanta 1968–2000: teenager or thirty-something, who is at risk? Birth Defects Res A Clin Mol Teratol 2004; 70: 572–579

21 American College of Obstetricians and Gynecologists. Prenatal diagnosis of fetal chromosomal abnormalities. Practice Bulletin #27., Washington, DC: ACOG, 2001

22 Newcomb WW, Rodriguez M, Johnson JW. Reproduction in the older gravida. A literature review. J Reprod Med 1991; 36: 839

23 Hollander D, Breen JL. Pregnancy in the older gravida: how old is old? Obstet Gynecol Surv 1990; 45: 106

24 Prysak M, Lorenz RP, Kisly A. Pregnancy outcome in nulliparous women 35 years and older. Obstet Gynecol 1995; 85: 65

25 Edge V, Laros Jr RK. Pregnancy outcome in nulliparous women aged 35 or older. Am J Obstet Gynecol 1993; 168: 1881

26 Gilbert WM, Nesbitt TS, Danielsen B. Childbearing beyond age 40: pregnancy outcome in 24,032 cases. Obstet Gynecol 1999; 93: 9

27 Bianco A, Stone J, Lynch L et al. Pregnancy outcome at age 40 and older. Obstet Gynecol 1996; 87: 917-922

28 Seoud MA, Nassar AH, Usta IM et al. Impact of advanced maternal age on pregnancy outcome. Am J Perinatol 2002; 19: 1

29 Paulson RJ, Boostanfar R, Saadat P et al. Pregnancy in the sixth decade of life. Obstetric outcomes in women of advanced reproductive age. JAMA 2002; 288: 2320

30 Barton JR, Bergauer NK, Jacques DI, Coleman SK. Does advanced maternal age affect pregnancy outcome in women with mild hypertension remote from term? Am J Obstet Gynecol 1997; 176: 1236

31 Zeitlin JA, Ancel PY, Saurel-Cubizolles MJ, Papiernik E. Are risk factors the same for small for gestational age versus other preterm births? Am J Obstet Gynecol 2001; 185: 208

32 Casey BM, Lucas MJ, McIntire DD, Leveno KJ. Pregnancy outcomes in women with gestational diabetes compared with the general obstetric population. Obstet Gynecol 1997; 90: 869

33 Tough SC, Newburn-Cook C, Johnston DW, Svenson LW. Delayed childbearing and its impact on population rate changes in lower birth weight, multiple birth, and preterm delivery. Pediatrics 2002; 109: 399

34 Aldous MB, Edmonson MB. Maternal age at first childbirth and risk of low birth weight and preterm delivery in Washington State. JAMA 1993; 270: 2574

35 Cnattingius S, Forman MR, Berendes HW, Isotalo L. Delayed childbearing and risk of adverse perinatal outcome. A population-based study. JAMA 1992; 268: 886

36 Salihu HM, Shumpert MN, Aliyu MH et al. Smoking-associated fetal morbidity among older gravidas: a population study. Acta Obstet Gynecol Scand 2005; 84: 329

37 Fretts RC, Usher RH. Fetal death in women in the older reproductive age group. Contemp Rev Obstet Gynecol 1997; Sept; 173–179

38 Fretts RC, Schmittdiel J, McLean FH, Usher RH, Goldman MB. Increased maternal age and the risk for fetal death. N Engl J Med 1995; 333: 953

39 Fretts RC, Usher RH. Causes of fetal death in women of advanced maternal age. Obstet Gynecol 1997; 89: 40

40 Huang DY, Usher RH, Kramer MS, Yang H. Determinants of unexplained antepartum fetal deaths. Obstet Gynecol 2000; 95: 215

41 Froen JF, Arnestad M, Frey K et al. Risk factors for sudden intrauterine unexplained death: Epidemiological characteristics of singleton cases in Oslo, Norway, 1986–1995. Am J Obstet Gynecol 2001; 184: 694

42 Jacobsson B, Ladfors L, Milsom I. Advanced maternal age and adverse perinatal outcome. Obstet Gynecol 2004; 104: 727

43 Callaway LK, Lust K, McIntyre HD. Pregnancy outcomes in women of very advanced maternal age. Aust NZ J Obstet Gynaecol 2005; 45: 12

44 Callaghan WM, Berg CJ. Pregnancy-related mortality among women aged 35 years and older, United States, 1991–1997. Obstet Gynecol 2003; 102: 1015

45 Ghosh MK. Maternal mortality. A global perspective. J Reprod Med 2001; 46: 427

46 American Society of Reproductive Medicine. Aging and infertility in women: a committee opinion. Fertil Steril 2002; 78: 215

47 Fretts RC, Elkin EB, Myers ER, Heffner LJ. Should older women have antepartum testing to prevent unexplained stillbirth?. Obstet Gynecol 2004; 104: 56

Louise Ashelby   Cathy Winter   Robert Fox

Fluid balance in pre-eclampsia: what we know and what we don't

Pre-eclampsia is a multisystem disorder of vascular function, specific to pregnancy, which is typically characterised by hypertension, proteinuria, oedema, and fetal compromise. It arises in the placenta, probably as a result of ischaemia, and propagates throughout the maternal vascular tree such that all organ systems can be affected. It has consistently been one of the top causes of maternal mortality in the UK since the start of the Confidential Enquiry into Maternal Mortality in 1952 and it is now the commonest obstetric association of perinatal death.

Renal dysfunction is an almost ubiquitous feature, as revealed by high rates of proteinuria. In contrast, renal failure is uncommon. Despite its relative rarity and the fact that recovery rates in the short-to-medium term are very high and nearly always with no residual impairment, knowledge of the risk of renal failure gave rise to renal rescue strategies incorporating fluid challenge and/or forced diuresis. Unfortunately, this development appeared to be followed by a rise in the number of deaths from pulmonary oedema as a result of overzealous fluid administration.[1] In the UK, deaths from respiratory complications rose to outnumber those from intracranial haemorrhage that had previously accounted for about 75% of cases (Table 1).[2] By the 1991–1993 triennium, the situation had reversed and pulmonary complications outstripped deaths from intracranial haemorrhage three to one. The realisation that deaths from pulmonary complications had risen resulted in a swing to

Louise Ashelby MB ChB
Specialist Obstetric Registrar, Maternity Unit, Taunton & Somerset NHS Trust, Taunton TA1 5DA, UK

Cathy Winter RCM
Specialist Midwife, Maternity Unit, Taunton & Somerset NHS Trust, Taunton TA1 5DA, UK

Robert Fox MD MRCPI MRCOG (for correspondence)
Consultant Obstetrician, Maternity Unit, Taunton & Somerset NHS Trust, Taunton TA1 5DA, UK
E-mail: robert.fox@tst.nhs.uk

Table 1 Trends in maternal deaths from intracranial haemorrhage and pulmonary complications of pre-eclampsia[2]

| | Number of deaths | |
Triennium	Intracranial haemorrhage*	Pulmonary#
1982–1984	13	3
1985–1987	11	10
1988–1990	12	10
1991–1993	5	11
1994–1996	4	8
1997–1999	7	2
2000–2002	9	1

*Intracerebral and subarachnoid; #ARDS and pulmonary oedema.

fluid restriction, and in turn that was associated with a fall in the number of deaths from respiratory complications.

Both schools of thought continue to have advocates even though their mantras of force diuresis and keep dry represent diametrically opposing philosophies.[3] If renal rescue is to be employed, a crucial question is, can effective action be taken to protect the kidney and yet safely avoid pulmonary oedema? The purpose of this review is to see what evidence, if any, exists to support one or other line of management.

Medline was searched for the following terms singly and in combination: pre-eclampsia, eclampsia, fluid management, fluid balance, crystalloid, colloid, diuresis, diuretics, pulmonary oedema, renal dysfunction, renal failure, furosemide and dopamine. The citation lists of articles and standard textbooks were reviewed for other publications. Cochrane and SIGN databases were also searched. We found fewer than 20 original articles directly concerned with fluid management in pre-eclampsia and only three randomised-controlled trials of the management of a condition that complicates about 5% of pregnancies. This compares with more than 300 articles on biochemical screening for trisomy 21 which has an incidence of less than 1 in 500 maternities.

PHYSIOLOGICAL ADAPTATION IN NORMAL PREGNANCY

Fluid balance

A woman normally comprises of 60% water (about 42 l), of which 14 l are extracellular and 28 l are intracellular. The extracellular fluid subdivides into 10.5 l of interstitial fluid and 3.5 l of blood plasma. Fluid transport between blood plasma and the interstitial fluid is governed by forces described in the Starling hypothesis; arteriolar blood pressure, venous pressure at the end of the capillary, protein content of the plasma (colloid osmotic pressure of plasma, COPp), interstitial fluid pressure (colloid osmotic pressure of interstitial fluid, COPi), capillary permeability, and lymphatic drainage. Anything that disturbs one or more of these factors can result in the shift of fluid from one compartment to another.

Haemodynamics

In the normal pregnant woman there is an early increase in cardiac output associated with a fall in peripheral vascular resistance that causes a reduction in systemic blood pressure. This is thought to be mediated by the differential relationships of thromboxane A, endothelin, nitric oxide and prostacyclin. Along with the rise in cardiac output there is a rise in renal artery blood flow and glomerular filtration. Total body fluid is increased partly as a result of a rise in blood volume but there is also a rise in interstitial fluid in normal pregnancy (seen as mild oedema). Oncotic protein serum concentrations fall in normal pregnancy, often dramatically so, and this might account for the change in interstitial fluid (oedema) but the precise mechanism is not known.

PATHOPHYSIOLOGY OF PRE-ECLAMPSIA

Aetiology

The origin of pre-eclampsia is not the focus of this review and will only be covered briefly. It is still only partly understood but what seems likely is that placental microfragmentation results from ischaemia of which there are several proposed causes including abnormal trophoblast invasion, diabetic vascular disease, thrombophilia, acute hypovolaemia and placenta oedema (mirror syndrome). Debris enters the circulation and one or more chemical agents promote a micro-angiopathy with wide-spread damage to the maternal vascular endothelium and small infarcts. There is also an increased sensitivity to native pressor agents such as angiotensin II, catecholamines and arginine vasopressin (AVP formerly called anti-diuretic hormone). The two primary consequences are vasoconstriction (with hypertension) and increased capillary permeability (with oedema and proteinuria). The loss of protein through the kidney and of fluid into the interstitial space reduces the circulation blood volume which probably increases the placental ischaemia. The loss of plasma protein and fluid also promote sodium retention. As well as eclampsia, secondary events include vessel rupture (resulting from the effect of hypertension on injured vessel walls in intracranial haemorrhage), and liver dysfunction with intravascular coagulation (HELLP syndrome) (Fig. 1).

Fluid imbalance in pre-eclampsia

The patient with pre-eclampsia is often in positive fluid balance on calculation of total body fluid, and the excess fluid is mainly in the interstitial space due to salt retention, low oncotic pressure, and increased capillary permeability. In marked contrast, the plasma volume is usually reduced and there is haemoconcentration (as evidenced by high haemoglobin concentrations). The COPp is reduced due to hypoproteinaemia. Oedema is usually prevented from forming due to reduction in COPi, but this buffering mechanism does not apply in severe pre-eclampsia.[4] As the fluid leaks out of the capillaries into the interstitial fluid, oedema forms, usually manifesting clinically as simple peripheral oedema but in severe disease there can be oedema of the brain, lungs and larynx.

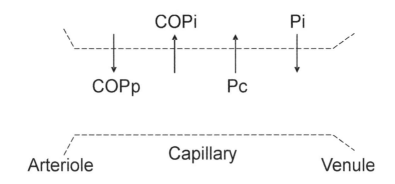

Fig. 1 Transcapillary fluid dynamics. COPp, plasma colloid osmotic pressure; COPi, interstitial colloid osmotic pressure; Pc, capillary hydrostatic pressure; and Pi, interstitial hydrostatic pressure.

Circulatory dynamics in pre-eclampsia

As a consequence of arterial vasospasm, the mean arterial pressure and SVR are usually high. In contrast, pulmonary vascular resistance is usually normal and pulmonary artery pressures (PAPs) may be low, particularly in the presence of severe vascular depletion. In general, women with pre-eclampsia have a normal heart rate and cardiac output for pregnancy. The ventricular function is usually hyperdynamic but a minority have depressed left ventricular function which is nearly always associated with severely elevated systemic vascular resistance (SVR). The central venous pressure (CVP) is usually normal in pre-eclampsia and, therefore, is not a reliable measurement of blood volume. In addition, it does not correlate well with pulmonary capillary wedge pressure, thought to be the result of differential responses of pulmonary and systemic vascular systems. The pulmonary capillary wedge pressures (PCWPs) may be low, normal or high, but is usually low-normal reflecting intravascular volume depletion. PCWP is a poor guide to cardiac output, therefore.

Renal pathology in pre-eclampsia

Renal problems are a common feature of pre-eclampsia. There appear to be several components to the renal dysfunction; reduced renal blood flow secondary to reduced circulating volume (pre-renal component), afferent arteriolar vasoconstriction and glomerular damage secondary to deposition of fibrinogen degradation products in the capillary bed (intrinsic renal components). There may also be a small effect from ureteric compression in late labour (post-renal component). In women who suffer placental abruption and severe hypovolaemia, acute tubular necrosis may also develop (intrinsic renal component).

The alteration in renal function affects both water homeostasis (oliguria/anuria) and the ability to excrete metabolites (decreased creatinine clearance). These two often run hand-in-hand but it is common to have a degree of dissociation; oliguria with no alteration in intrinsic renal function (creatinine clearance). The reverse can also be true with a good fluid output being maintained despite a marked increase in serum creatinine levels. This is an important observation with reference to fluid management; if urinary output can be maintained despite a declining glomerular filtration rate, it is simpler to regulate blood volume and so haemofiltration might be avoided (see below).

It is also crucial to understand that oliguria does not necessarily indicate severe volume depletion, particularly around the time of delivery. It may be a reflection of severe glomerular damage (see above), the progress of which will not be modulated by fluid challenge, but more often it is simply the response to physiological stress (mediated through arginine vasopressin release from posterior pituitary). An unpublished study of hourly urine production rates after caesarean section in normal woman undertaken in Bristol found a high rate of oliguria. It should also be borne in mind that urine flow is also reduced at night (again AVP-mediated nocturnal oliguria). Against this, it must be recognised that acute renal failure is extremely rare in the absence of HELLP syndrome and placental abruption.[6]

Polyuria and placental vasopressinase

Although one tends to think of oliguria in pre-eclampsia, curiously it may rarely present with severe polyuria. This may be due to a transient (gestational) form of diabetes insipidus. It is related to excessive placental vasopressinase activity causing degradation of maternal AVP. Gestational diabetes insipidus, although rare, is often associated with pre-eclampsia or HELLP syndrome, presumably because of volume depletion causing placental ischaemia and triggering the fragmentation cascade. In these patients, fluid restriction should be avoided as it may lead to dehydration and severe haemoconcentration both of which may worsen placental ischaemia.[5] It is usually responsive to treatment with synthetic dDAVP, which is not broken down by placental vasopressinase. If this approach is taken, supervision by a specialist endocrinologist is needed to avoid severe water retention.

Pulmonary oedema

Pulmonary oedema is a complication of pre-eclampsia which can lead to hypoxia-acidosis, hypercapnia and death from respiratory failure. The postpartum period is a particularly risky time for developing pulmonary oedema due to the physiological changes associated with delivery; 70% of cases present between 16–72 h following delivery.[7,8] The mortality is less than 10%.

The rate of transfer of fluid across the pulmonary capillary bed is a function of PCWP, plasma colloid osmotic pressure (COPp) and capillary permeability. PCWP is usually normal in pre-eclampsia and the threshold at which pulmonary oedema develops appears to be lower in pregnancy than in non-pregnant adults.[9] Bhatia and colleagues[10] studying plasma COPp and fibronectin levels showed that increased capillary permeability resulting from vessel injury was a key factor in the development of oedema. The altered capillary permeability associated with pre-eclampsia causes a non-cardiogenic form of pulmonary oedema, similar to adult respiratory distress syndrome

(ARDS). Pulmonary oedema is more likely to develop postpartum because of the decrease in plasma oncotic pressure associated with intravenous infusion of clear fluids around the time of delivery, and an increase in PCWP caused by autotransfusion as the uterus contracts. It should not be forgotten that, occasionally, an increase in the PCWP can occur in pre-eclampsia because of left ventricular failure (cardiogenic component), as a result of increased afterload (severe hypertension).

Pulmonary oedema can arise spontaneously in pre-eclampsia (without the infusion of fluids) but analysis of cases by Lehmann and co-researchers[11] in the 1980s indicates that it is highly probable that the chance of pulmonary oedema is increased by excessive intravenous fluid infusion. It may also be made more likely by pre-existing cardiac disease and certain medications such as β-mimetic tocolytics. There were also concerns that labetalol therapy increased the risk of pulmonary oedema but recent studies concluded that it is the severity of the disease process rather than the use of labetalol *per se*.[12]

MANAGEMENT OF FLUID BALANCE IN PRE-ECLAMPSIA

There is a lack of evidence from randomised, controlled trials to support current practice in many aspects of fluid management in pre-eclampsia. The paucity of good quality research data has been shown to create uncertainty amongst clinicians.[13] There are many local protocols for the active management of oliguria but none have been conclusively shown to have a beneficial effect on the incidence of acute renal failure and pulmonary oedema.[14] Nevertheless, there are some facts which can be used to guide safe practice.

Preventing problems

Before problems arise there are certain steps that can be taken to prevent renal dysfunction, fluid imbalance and pulmonary oedema (summarised in Table 2). A prerequisite for excellent care is a multiprofessional team approach from specialist midwives, obstetricians and anaesthetists. Nevertheless, it is important for one person to take overall responsibility for fluid management so that inadvertent over prescription by the different doctors involved in the patient's care can be avoided.[2]

Perhaps the most important intervention is timely delivery, both in terms of decision making and decision-to-delivery interval. One study has shown that expectant antepartum management for preterm disease improves neonatal outcomes but increases the chance of maternal complications.[15] Careful vigilance is needed to prevent the disease progressing unchecked but the difficulty with this advice is that the ability to predict events in pre-eclampsia is limited; too often, the first sign of a problem arising is the problem itself.

Even though it seems obvious advice, it is nonetheless important to mention that strict input/output monitoring is needed to avoid inadvertent fluid overload. Accurate charting of all administered fluids is essential including drug infusions which should be given in concentrated solutions using syringe drivers. With this in mind, anaesthetists should be aware of the risks of excess fluid administration when pre-loading prior to epidural anaesthesia. Some practitioners prefer to use ephedrine instead of fluid preload to prevent

- Timely delivery
- Strict fluid balance including hourly urometry
- Avoid sharp falls in blood pressure (sublingual nifedipine and bolus i.v. oxytocin)
- Avoid simultaneous pharmacological interventions*
- Avoid β-mimetic tocolysis
- Avoid ergometrine#
- Replace sudden blood losses promptly but carefully
- Avoid non-steroidal anti-inflammatory agents

*Includes combining epidural anaesthesia and anti-hypertensive agents.
#Widely known for hypertensive effect – also increases PCWP by 35%.[45]

hypotension,[16] but we could find no specific research comparing the different regimens.

Non-steroidal anti-inflammatory agents such as diclofenac should be avoided as these can induce sudden anuria in susceptible patients.[17] Sudden large losses of blood should be replaced promptly and acute hypovolaemia avoided. Women with pre-eclampsia who lack the normal hypervolaemia of pregnancy are much less tolerant of blood loss at delivery.[18] Acute tubular necrosis may be precipitated by acute hypovolaemia on the background of intravascular depletion, renal artery vasospasm and micro-angiopathy. It is hard to define what constitutes a significant obstetric haemorrhage in this context but a loss of greater than 500 ml and/or that which causes tachycardia should be taken seriously.

Although prompt treatment of severe hypertension is thought to be essential to reduce the chance of intracerebral haemorrhage, overly rapid or vigorous treatment of hypertension, particularly with vasodilators, can lead to collapse requiring fluid resuscitation. This fluid can be later displaced into interstitial tissues as vasodilatation reverses and blood pressure rises. Sublingual nifedipine and bolus doses of hydralazine, in particular, are known to provoke sharp falls in blood pressure.[19] This also applies to intravenous bolus doses of oxytocin (10 IU or more) which promote vasodilatation;[20] oxytocin infusions are preferred if large doses are needed.[2] Tocolysis with β-adrenergic agents is also contra-indicated because of the risk of precipitating non-cardiogenic pulmonary oedema.[21]

Clinical monitoring

Standard peripartum observations

Pre-eclampsia is an unpredictable condition, particularly postpartum, and high dependency care is advised for all women regardless of (apparent) severity. The intensity and location of care depends partly on the presence or absence of complications. The minimum should be regular review of symptoms together with frequent cardiovascular and respiratory measurements (pulse, blood pressure, and respiratory rate as well as temperature and oxygen saturation using a digital transcutaneous oximetry). A urinary catheter should be inserted and hourly urine output should be recorded. The purpose of urinary output monitoring is not that oliguria can be managed aggressively; but rather that it used as an indicator of worsening disease and, particularly in the case of anuria, as a sign that fluid overload might occur. Normal urine output should be greater than 0.5–1 ml/kg body weight/h. This is usually between 25–100 ml/h. Oliguria can be more simply defined as hourly urine flow of fewer than 25 ml/h for 2 h, and severe oliguria as below 10 ml/h for 2 h. Blood haematology and biochemistry should be undertaken at least daily and often more frequently than this.

Invasive monitoring

It has been advised that indications for invasive monitoring in pre-eclampsia may include refractory hypertension, refractory pulmonary oedema, refractory severe oliguria in presence of HELLP syndrome, severe haemorrhage, and multi-organ failure.[3,22]

The central venous pressure (CVP) is a measurement of the preload to the right side of the heart and is a (rough) guide to circulating blood volume; underfill and overfill. CVP monitoring is often used to guide fluid management and monitor fluid administration, during haemorrhage for example. Internal jugular and subclavian routes have no advantage over peripheral long lines which are probably safer and should be favoured.

CVP readings outside of pregnancy should normally be 10–15 mmHg but in pre-eclampsia lower readings should be expected and a lower criterion is needed to define when the vascular compartment is full (0–5 mmHg); pulmonary oedema can develop at lower pressures because of increased capillary permeability.[23] The CVP response to fluid infusion is probably of more value than the absolute level of a single reading (Fig. 2). Even so, the interpretation is fraught with difficulties – use by relatively inexperienced staff including general obstetricians and non-specialist midwives not being the least of these. The flat line trace, for instance, might simply reflect a poorly sited catheter tip. At all times, it is important to treat the patient and not simply the CVP reading.

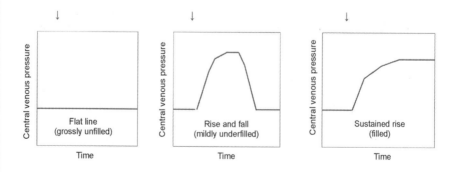

Fig. 2 CVP response to fluid infusion (commencement of fluid infusion indicated by vertical arrow).

An alternative to CVP measurement is the pulmonary artery or Swan-Ganz catheter (SGC). This is a triple lumen polyvinylchloride catheter with a balloon tip that is floated into the pulmonary artery. SGCs are used to measure CVP, pulmonary artery pressure (PAP), and pulmonary capillary wedge pressure (PCWP) simultaneously. In many critical care situations, left ventricular end-diastolic pressure can be derived from the PCWP to aid assessment of cardiac function.[24] Theoretically, these clinical data might be used to predict development of pulmonary oedema and help distinguish between cardiac and non-cardiac causes. Indeed, some have argued that the SGC is a better means of monitoring aggressive fluid replacement and vasoactive drug therapy than isolated CVP measurement because it gives a direct measure of the pulmonary vascular dynamics in pre-eclampsia.[25] It is true that in severe pre-eclampsia there is more discrepancy between CVP and pulmonary artery pressure.[25] However, just as CVP is a less reliable guide to circulating volume in pre-eclampsia, PCWP is a less reliable guide to cardiac function. In addition, although the Swan-Ganz catheter does provide more information on haemodynamics, it is associated with a high rate of serious complications – reported in 3–24% of cases.[22] These adverse events include fatal cardiac arrhythmias, thrombo-embolism, pulmonary infarction, sepsis and pneumothorax. Gilbert and colleagues[27] described it as being 'useful subjectively' in pre-eclampsia but stressed that this is impression is not borne out by scientific analysis. Moreover, a recently published trial of SGC use in a general ITU showed no evidence of benefit.[28] As there are no studies that demonstrate any benefit from SGC monitoring in pre-eclampsia, their use is not advised as a routine for severe oliguria, if at all. If they are employed, we recommend that SGCs are inserted only by experienced operators and that their use should be limited to an ITU setting.

Intravenous fluid therapy

Crystalloid or colloid?
Because serum oncotic protein levels are low, many advocate the use of colloid infusions (synthetic products or human albumin solutions). These do initially increase the colloid osmotic pressure. In contrast, crystalloid solutions dilute the oncotic proteins and reduce COPp. It is thought that the rise in COPp after colloid infusion will draw fluid back into the circulation and some have argued that colloid infusion may contribute to fluid overload particularly in the postpartum period.[29,30] In contrast, crystalloid will move more quickly across the endothelium into the interstitial space.[23] A recent study found that the elimination and distribution of crystalloid fluids is faster in women with pre-eclampsia than with matched controls.[31] Although this hypothesis probably holds true in the short term, colloid will also move across the capillary membrane into the interstitium causing a rise in COPi and drawing more fluid into the interstitial tissues. The initial improvement in haemodynamics with colloid might later reverse, therefore, and lead to increased oedema.[18] Moreover, if oedema does develop, one has to ask what is easier to shift out of the interstitium – colloid or crystalloid? There is no evidence to suggest that use of colloid fluid improves clinical outcome in pre-eclampsia so crystalloids remain the most commonly used fluid in practice.[23] A randomised, controlled

trial of colloid and crystalloid infusion in critically ill patients (non-gestational cases) used all-cause mortality rates to compare outcome. No benefit was found. The collaborators concluded that colloid therapy cannot be supported for volume replacement in critically ill patients.[32] Use of albumin for fluid resuscitation in critically ill patients has been debated. The recent SAFE trial comparing use of human albumin versus saline solutions in intensive care found that there were similar outcomes in both groups.[34] A systematic Cochrane review went further and stated that mortality was increased with use of albumin in critical care situations.[35] A recent Cochrane review of use of plasma volume expansion with colloid for the antenatal treatment of pre-eclampsia concluded that there was insufficient evidence to determine the effects.[33] The value of albumin in the peripartum management of pre-eclampsia has not been tested. In the absence of any proven benefit, with reason to believe it might be harmful, and because its cost is much greater, we advise that colloid should be avoided in favour of crystalloid solutions.

Hartmann's solution or normal saline?

Reid and colleagues[36] compared the effects of a 1-h infusion of 2 l normal (0.9%) saline with 2 l Hartmann's solution in healthy, non-pregnant subjects. They found that plasma volume expansion is greater and more sustained with normal saline than with Hartmann's solution. However, those subjects infused with Hartmann's solution developed their diuresis more quickly and to a greater degree (1000 m over 6 h compared with 450 ml). These data suggest that Hartmann's solution might be more suitable for women with pre-eclampsia but specific research would be necessary to confirm this.

Sliding scale insulin infusion

In women with diabetes mellitus who are on a sliding scale insulin regimen, care should be taken with infusion of dextrose solutions as these become simple water after metabolism of the glucose. Consideration should be given to use of 10% solutions at half rate so as to limit the water load which will distribute to all tissues.

Standard fluid volume regimen

The crux of this debate is the balance between the wish to avoid renal failure and the desire to prevent pulmonary oedema. With the evidence that aggressive volume expansion was associated with an unacceptably high rate of pulmonary oedema,[1] others have experimented with more moderate fluid replacement regimens. At present, there are no comparative trial data to determine which practice is best. However, Cunningham and Pritchard[37] have reported that conservative fluid management of a series of 245 women with eclampsia (not pre-eclampsia) resulted in no cases of renal failure. Cunningham later confirmed this result on 400 patients and wrote: 'For these reasons, until it is understood how to contain more fluid within the intravascular compartment and, at the same time, less fluid outside the intravascular compartment, we remain convinced that, in the absence of marked fluid loss, fluids can be administered safely only in moderation'. This information strongly supports restricted fluid replacement for those with oliguria in the absence of HELLP syndrome.[18]

Diagnosis – full clinical and biochemical review
    Check urinary catheter
    Look for evidence of sepsis and haemorrhage (and correct)
    Test for HELLP syndrome

Treatment of moderate oliguria in absence of HELLP syndrome
    Reduce magnesium sulphate infusion (to avoid toxicity)
    Maintain close observation
    Continue to infuse crystalloid fluid slowly (1 ml/kg/h of Hartmann's solution)
    Monitor for pulmonary oedema

Treatment of severe oliguria in presence of HELLP syndrome*
    Either   Continue with expectant management

    Or   Measure central venous pressure
           Underfilled – consider fluid infusion ± furosemide infusion
           Filled or overfilled – consider low-dose dopamine infusion

*Insufficient data to determine best practice.

The precise nature of a conservative fluid regimen varies from unit to unit. Some employ a simple formula such as a maximum of 2.5 l in 24 h or 1 ml/kg/h,[4] whereas others prefer to calculate the rate as previous hour's urinary output plus 40 ml, or 1 ml/kg/h. Once a patient is able to tolerate oral intake, it is sensible to allow free oral fluids and decrease intravenous fluids steadily in line with this.

Management of oliguria (Table 3)

Diagnosis
The first consideration is the cause of the reduced output. It should not be assumed automatically that it is exclusively the result of the pre-eclamptic process. Often it is simply physiological oliguria and, in the case of sudden-onset anuria, it may be nothing more than blockage of the urinary catheter. More rarely, it might reflect occult haemorrhage or sepsis and these require specific therapy. In some cases, it will be a sign of worsening pre-eclampsia and the patient should be completely reviewed including a repeat blood screen to test for HELLP syndrome.

Magnesium sulphate
Because magnesium is cleared almost exclusively by renal clearance, infusions of magnesium should be reduced by half if oliguria develops to avoid toxic accumulation in blood.[18] The effects of magnesium on fluid dynamics also deserves special consideration. It has been shown to promote a naturesis in pregnant women with essential hypertension,[38] but in the context of tocolysis, magnesium therapy was found to be associated with a risk of pulmonary oedema.[39] Sibai[40] reviewed four large trials of magnesium sulphate prophylaxis in pre-eclampsia. He concluded that the available evidence to date

confirms the efficacy of magnesium sulphate in reduction of seizures in women with eclampsia and severe pre-eclampsia but that this benefit does not influence maternal mortality and morbidity overall.[40] Magnesium toxicity should be considered if oxygen saturation falls.

Management of low-risk cases

Given that renal failure is very rare in the absence of HELLP, sepsis or haemorrhage, there is much to be said for an expectant approach for those with moderate oliguria; most women will improve spontaneously and the risk of fluid overload is small.[41] It is possible that a very small proportion of such women will require dialysis but it is likely to be very much less than 1% of cases and that might be small price to pay for avoiding pulmonary oedema. How long to maintain a conservative approach is another important question. Some advocate action after 6 h or so, but others choose not to act unless a complication or severe oliguria intervenes. In the absence of evidence of benefit and with the knowledge of risk of pulmonary oedema, we advise that expectant management is continued for moderate oliguria.

Management of high-risk cases

For those women who develop severe oliguria/anuria in the presence of HELLP, sepsis or haemorrhage, the risk of renal failure is much greater. Although it seems logical to conclude that improved outcome from an interventionist approach with HELLP syndrome is more likely, the balance between benefit and harm has not been demonstrated clinically. Controlled studies have shown that treatment with either continuous furosemide or renal-dose dopamine infusion will promote a diuresis,[14,42–44] but all-cause morbidity and mortality rates have not been reported as yet. All things considered, we favour an expectant approach but each physician must make his or her own judgement. If intervention is contemplated, the first step is to measure CVP and decide action according to the degree of vascular filling (see below).

CVP indicates grossly underfilled vascular compartment

A pre-renal effect is then the most likely component, and more fluid should be given alone in the first instance (250 ml of Hartmann's solution over 30 min – see Fig. 2). This will be followed by a diuresis in about 25% of women but it is not clear whether this is cause or co-incidence. Next, a furosemide infusion (5 mg/h) can be used if there is no response. Most will respond to this. If the response is great (> 200 ml/h), it is important to replace the fluid to avoid volume depletion.

CVP indicates filled vascular compartment

If the vascular compartment is filled, then an intrinsic renal component is more likely (afferent arteriolar spasm or glomerular capillary damage). Dopamine administration (3 µg/kg/min) with fluid restriction is then a more logical approach as this will treat any arteriolar vasoconstriction (but not glomerular capillary damage).[14] Mantel and colleagues were able to triple the urine output to > 50 ml/h without any deterioration in pulse or blood pressure. All of this should be undertaken in an intensive care setting and in conjunction with advice from a specialist in intensive medicine or a renal physician.

Diagnosis

If oxygen saturation values decrease or supplemental oxygen is needed to maintain them, pulmonary oedema should be considered a possibility but not assumed. Rarely, aspiration of gastric contents occurs during eclampsia and other causes such as magnesium toxicity, atelectasis, pneumonia, pulmonary embolism and occult Eisenmenger's syndrome may need to be considered. If pulmonary oedema is diagnosed, it is important to distinguish between ARDS-type respiratory problems from cardiogenic forms (silent myocardial infarct, gestational cardiomyopathy, *etc.*) particularly in elderly or diabetic women.[45] A full respiratory and cardiovascular examination should be performed for pulse, blood pressure, oxygen saturation, respiratory rate, presence of cardiac murmurs, and added respiratory sounds. Plain chest radiology is one of the most sensitive detectors of early pulmonary oedema but its interpretation is made difficult by the knowledge that some radiological evidence of pulmonary oedema is present in up to a third of pre-eclamptic patients in the 6 days following delivery.[13] Other investigations could include arterial blood gases, ECG and cardiac enzymes. If there is doubt about ventricular function (cardiogenic pulmonary oedema), echocardiography should be undertaken. Monitoring should continue with cardiovascular/respiratory observations and continuous pulse oximetry,

Treatment

The patient should be sat upright and given oxygen by face mask. Furosemide should be given intravenously where there is evidence of fluid overload but care must be taken to monitor for cardiovascular collapse if the intravascular compartment is depleted. The action of furosemide is complex and includes reduction of pulmonary artery pressure as well as diuresis. In severe cases, continuous positive airway pressure (CPAP) ventilation may be beneficial as found in other causes of pulmonary oedema.[46] The involvement of obstetric anaesthetists, respiratory physicians, and intensive care units may be necessary depending on the clinical scenario.

CONCLUSIONS

The most certain finding of this review is the paucity of information about fluid management in pre-eclampsia; further research is undoubtedly necessary to improve our knowledge and management of this important area of obstetric medicine. What is evident is that anuric ARF is very rare, despite a period of moderate oliguria being very common, and that it recovers quickly in nearly all women with no residual impairment.[47] When it does occur, renal failure is usually associated with haemorrhage, sepsis or HELLP. The rarity and reversibility of ARF has to be contrasted with the potentially fatal course of pulmonary oedema in 10% of affected women.

Although there is a lack of random-allocation studies, observational data strongly suggest that for the vast majority women with moderate oliguria and otherwise uncomplicated pre-eclampsia, a conservative hands-off approach with non-invasive monitoring and simple fluid replacement using crystalloids is all that is required. This cautious approach should help prevent fluid overload and limit the risk of pulmonary oedema for the large majority of women who do not have HELLP syndrome, sepsis or acute blood loss. That is not to say that moderate oliguria should be ignored entirely. It is essential to consider the underlying cause which might include occult haemorrhage or sepsis. Furthermore, reductions in urine output might also be the only outward sign of worsening pre-eclampsia and the development of HELLP syndrome in particular; a full clinical review including blood haematology and biochemistry is important.

Although this information implies that aggressive management of moderately oliguric women with uncomplicated pre-eclampsia is unjustified because it is unnecessary and unsafe, is it wrong for all patients? The chance of renal failure is much higher for those with HELLP syndrome, sepsis or haemorrhage and so the balance of risk and benefit might be different. Clearly, sepsis and haemorrhage demand specific treatment. For those women with HELLP combined with severe oliguria, intervention might be justified but there are no comparative data with which to guide clinical management. It is known that intravenous furosemide and low-dose dopamine will have a positive effect on urine production but there is no evidence that this halts the damage to glomerular capillary bed from fibrinogen deposition; creatinine levels may continue to rise inexorably. One theoretical advantage of maintaining a fluid output is that haemofiltration, which requires full anticoagulation, might be delayed or avoided altogether, but this must be weighed against the risks of pulmonary oedema (from fluid overload) or acute tubular necrosis (from hypovolaemia through diuresis – pre-renal crisis). The stark fact is that evidence of true benefit, or even safety, of such interventions is lacking.

If active management of severe oliguria is chosen, CVP monitoring might allow clinicians to elicit the underlying pathophysiology (renal or pre-renal) and so avoid both volume depletion and fluid overload but it must be borne in mind that CVP is probably less reliable in pre-eclampsia than for other clinical situations. There is no evidence to support frequent use of Swan-Ganz catheters in severe pre-eclampsia and as they have a high rate of complication and it could be argued that their risks are likely to outweigh their theoretical benefit.

There is evidently a great need for better quality information through research into clinical outcomes according to treatment modality. Thus far, too often, management has been based on what seems plausible or that which (falsely) re-assures the clinician, and not enough on robust scientific evidence. In addition, too much research has been of an epidemiological nature or has concentrated on surrogate markers of improvement – none of which have been properly validated. There is an important need to determine the most appropriate volume and type of fluid replacement (crystalloid, synthetic colloid or human albumin) for different clinical situations, and for a direct comparison of expectant and active management for severely oliguric women at higher risk of renal failure.

References

1 Lopez-Llera M. Complicated eclampsia: fifteen years' experience in a referral medical center. Am J Obstet Gynecol 1982; 142: 28–35

2 Department of Health, Scottish Executive Health Department, and Department of Health, Social Services and Public Safety, Northern Ireland. Why Mothers Die. Fifth Report on Confidential Enquiries into Maternal Deaths in the United Kingdom, 1997–1999. London: RCOG Press, 2001

3 Young PF, Leighton NA, Jones PW, Anthony J, Johanson RB. Fluid management in severe preeclampsia (VESPA): survey of members of ISSHP. Hypertens Pregnancy 2000; 19: 249–259

4 O'Donnel E, Grady K, Cox C. Eclampsia, pre-eclampsia, HELLP, fatty liver and hepatic rupture. In: Johnson RB. (ed) Managing Obstetric Emergencies. Oxford: Bios, 1999; 66–72

5 Oian P, Maltau JM, Noddeland H, Fadnes HO. Transcapillary fluid balance in pre-eclampsia. Br J Obstet Gynaecol 1986; 93: 235–239

6 Gul A, Aslan H, Cebeci A, Polat I, Ulusoy S, Ceylan Y. Maternal and fetal outcomes in HELLP syndrome complicated with acute renal failure. Ren Fail 2004; 26: 557–562

7 Krege J, Katz VL, Bowes Jr WA. Transient diabetes insipidus of pregnancy. Obstet Gynecol Surv 1989; 44: 789–795

8 Benedetti TJ, Kates R, Williams V. Hemodynamic observations in severe preeclampsia complicated by pulmonary oedema. Am J Obstet Gynecol 1985; 152: 330–334

9 Cotton DB, Gonik B. Cardiovascular alterations in severe pregnancy induced hypertension: relationship of CVP to pulmonary capillary wedge pressure. Am J Obstet Gynecol 1985; 151: 762–764

10 Bhatia RK, Bottoms SF. Mechanisms for reduced colloid osmotic pressure in preeclampsia. Am J Obstet Gynecol 1987; 157: 106–108

11 Lehmann DK, Mabie WC, Miller Jr JM, Pernoll ML. The epidemiology and pathology of maternal mortality: Charity Hospital of Louisiana in New Orleans, 1965–1984. Obstet Gynecol 1987; 69: 833–840

12 Gilson GJ, Kramer RL, Barada C, Izquierdo LA, Curet LB. Does labetalol predispose to pulmonary edema in severe pregnancy-induced hypertensive disease? J Matern Fetal Med 1998; 7: 142–147

13 Engelhardt T, MacLennan FM. Fluid management in pre-eclampsia. Int J Obstet Anaesth 1999; 8: 253–259

14 Kirshon B, Lee W, Mauer M. Effects of therapy in the oliguric patient with pre-eclampsia. Am J Obstet Gynecol 1988; 159: 604–607

15 Sibai BM, Taslimi M, Abdella TN, Brooks TF, Spinnato JA, Anderson GD. Maternal and perinatal outcome of conservative management of severe pre-eclampsia in midtrimester. Am J Obstet Gynecol 1985; 152: 32–37

16 Shearer VE, Ramin SM, Wallace DH, Dax JS, Gilstrap 3rd LC. Fetal effects of prophylactic ephedrine and maternal hypotension during regional anesthesia for cesarean section. J Matern Fetal Med 1996; 5: 79–84

17 Tomaszewski M, Zukowska-Szcsechowska E, Zywiec J, Grzeszczak W. Anuria in a patient with chronic renal failure and liver affection after a single dose of diclofenac. Nephron 2001; 88: 287–288

18 Hypertensive disorders in pregnancy. In: Cunningham FG. (ed) Williams Obstetrics, 21st edn. New York: McGraw Hill, 2003; 567–618

19 Hata T, Manabe A, Hata K, Kitao M. Changes in blood velocities of fetal circulation in association with fetal heart rate abnormalities: effect of sublingual administration of nifedipine. Am J Perinatol 1995; 12: 80–81

20 Weis Jr FR, Markello R, Mo B, Bochiechio P. Cardiovascular effects of oxytocin. Obstet Gynecol 1975; 46: 211–214

21 Bader AM, Boudier E, Martinez C et al. Etiology and prevention of pulmonary complications following beta-mimetic mediated tocolysis. Eur J Obstet Gynecol Reprod Biol 1998; 80: 133–137

22 Fox DB, Troiano NH, Graves CR. Use of pulmonary artery catheter in severe pre-eclampsia: a review. Obstet Gynecol Surv 1996; 51: 684–695

23 Brown MA, Zamit VC, Lowe SA. Capillary permeability and extracellular fluid volumes in pregnancy induced hypertension. Clin Sci 1989; 77: 599–604

24 Cotton DB, Benedetti TJ. Use of the Swan-Ganz catheter in obstetrics and gynaecology. Obstet Gynecol 1980; 56: 641–645

25 Benedetti TJ, Cotton DB, Read JA. Hemodynamic observations in severe pre-eclampsia with a flow directed pulmonary artery catheter. Am J Obstet Gynecol 1980; 136: 465–469

26 Clark SL, Cotton DB. Clinical indications for pulmonary artery catheterization in the patient with severe pre-eclampsia. Am J Obstet Gynecol 1988; 158: 453–458

27 Gilbert WM, Towner DR, Field NT, Anthony J. The safety and utility of pulmonary artery catheterization in severe preeclampsia and eclampsia. Am J Obstet Gynecol 2000; 182: 1397–1403

28 Harvey S, Harrison DA, Singer M et al. and PAC-Man Study Collaboration. Assessment of the clinical effectiveness of pulmonary artery catheters in management of patients in intensive care (PAC-Man): a randomised controlled trial. Lancet 2005; 366: 472–477

29 Moise Jr KJ, Cotton DB. The use of colloid osmotic pressure in pregnancy. Clin Perinatol 1986; 13: 827–842

30 Wasserstrum N. Issues in fluid management during labour: maternal plasma volume status and volume loading. Clin Obstet Gynecol 1992; 35: 514–526

31 Drobin D, Hahn RG. Distribution and elimination of crystalloid fluid in pre-eclampsia. Clin Sci 2004; 106: 307–313

32 Schierhout G, Roberts I. Fluid resuscitation with colloid or crystalloid in critically ill patients: a systematic review of randomised trials. BMJ 1998; 316: 961–964

33 Duley L, Williams J, Henderson-Smart DJ. Plasma volume expansion for treatment of pre-eclampsia. The Cochrane Database of Systematic Reviews 1999, Issue 4. Art No: CD001805. DOI: 10.1002/14651858. CD001805

34 The Safe Study Investigators. A comparison of albumin and saline for fluid resuscitation in the intensive care unit. N Engl J Med 2004; 350: 2247–2256

35 Cochrane Injuries Group. Human albumin administration in critically ill patients: systematic review of randomised controlled trials. BMJ 1998; 317: 235–240

36 Reid F, Lobo DN, Williams RN, Rowlands BJ, Allison SP. (Ab)normal saline and physiological Hartmann's solution: a randomized double-blind crossover study. Clin Sci (Lond) 2003; 104: 25–26

37 Pritchard JA, Cunningham FG, Pritchard SA. The Parkland Memorial Hospital protocol for treatment of eclampsia: Evaluation of 245 cases. Am J Obstet Gynecol 1984; 148: 951–962

38 Samol JM, Lambers DS. Magnesium sulfate tocolysis and pulmonary edema. Am J Obstet Gynecol 2005; 192: 1430–1432

39 Ohtomo T, Kikuchi K, Komura H et al. The effects of intravenous infused magnesium on hemodynamics and renal water-sodium metabolism. Nippon Jinzo Gakkai Shi 1989; 31: 977–984

40 Sibai BM. Magnesium sulfate prophylaxis in pre-eclampsia: lessons from randomized trials. Am J Obstet Gynecol 2004; 105: 402–410

41 Ventura JE, Villa M. Acute Renal Failure in pregnancy. Ren Fail 1997; 19: 217-220.

42. Keiseb J, Moodley J, Connolly CA. Comparison of the efficacy of continuous furosemide and low dose infusion in pre-eclampsia/eclampsia-related oliguria in the immediate postpartum period. Hypertens Pregnancy 2002; 21: 225–234

43 Mantel GD, Makin JD. Low dose dopamine in post partum pre-eclamptic women with oliguria: a double blind, placebo controlled, randomised trial. Br J Obstet Gynaecol 1997; 104: 1180–1183

44 Katz VL, Dotters DJ, Droegemueller W. Low dose dopamine in the treatment of persistent oliguria in pre-eclampsia. Int J Gynecol Obstet 1990; 31: 57–59

45 Sciscione AC, Ivester T, Largoza M, Manley J, Shlossman P, Colmorgen GH. Acute pulmonary edema in pregnancy. Obstet Gynecol 2003; 101: 511–515

46 Pang D, Keenan SP, Cook DJ, Sibbald WJ. The effect of positive pressure airway support on mortality and the need for intubation in cardiogenic pulmonary edema: a systematic review. Chest 1998; 114: 1185–1192

47 Mjahed K, Alaoui SY, Barrou L. Acute renal failure during eclampsia: incidence risks factors and outcome in intensive care unit. Ren Fail 2004; 26: 215–221

48 Secher NJ, Arnsbo P, Wallin L. Haemodynamic effects of oxytocin (syntocinon) and methyl ergometrine (methergin) on the systemic and pulmonary circulations of pregnant anaesthetized women. Acta Obstet Gynecol Scand 1978; 57: 97–103

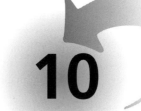

Jai B. Sharma   Suneeta Mittal

Prevention of pre-eclampsia

Pre-eclampsia, as defined by the Working Group of the National High Blood Pressure Education Program, is hypertension (blood pressure > 140/90 mmHg using Korotkoff V sound for diastolic blood pressure) associated with proteinuria (300 mg or more in 24-h urine).[1] Pre-eclampsia community guideline (PRECOG) takes only diastolic blood pressure of ≥ 90 mmHg to define hypertension.[2] It is a major cause of maternal and perinatal mortality and morbidity world-wide causing 15% of all direct maternal deaths in the UK and 24% of all maternal deaths in India.[3–5] There is a 5-fold increase in perinatal mortality in pre-eclampsia with iatrogenic prematurity being the main culprit.[6] Eclampsia is a more significant cause of perinatal mortality and morbidity in non-industrialised countries (up to 40% perinatal deaths).[7] We observed an overall perinatal mortality rate of 106/1000 births (59, 90 and 400/1000 births in mild, severe pre-eclampsia and eclampsia, respectively). These data of 271 consecutive cases of pre-eclampsia and eclampsia were collected from three hospitals in Delhi (Sharma JB, Zutshi V, Bhatia P, Bhasin S, Mittal S. 2004, unpublished data). Fortunately, especially in western countries, there have been falling trends in the cause of late fetal deaths in the last decade in relation to pre-eclampsia from 3.5/10,000 total births (1982–1990) to 2.1/10,000 total births (1991–2000), but it is still a significant cause of perinatal mortality.[8] Different management would reasonably have expected to alter the outcome for 46% of maternal deaths and 65% of fetal deaths due to pre-eclampsia reported through confidential enquiries into maternal deaths and stillbirths

Jai B. Sharma MD DNB MRCOG MFFP MAMS FICOG (for correspondence)
Assistant Professor, Department of Obstetrics and Gynaecology, All India Institute of Medical Sciences, New Delhi – 110 029, India
E-mail: jbsharma@eth.net

Suneeta Mittal MD FAMS FICOG FIMSA FICMCH, FRCOG(Hon)
Professor and Head, Department of Obstetrics and Gynaecology, All India Institute of Medical Sciences, New Delhi – 110 029, India
E-mail: smittal@aiims.ac.in

and deaths in infancy as there has been a failure to identify and respond to signs and symptoms of pre-eclampsia from 20 weeks' gestation.[2]

The various risk factors for development of gestational hypertension and pre-eclampsia are shown in Table 1.[9] Various factors like primigravidity, extremes of age, multiple pregnancy, obesity, history of hypertension or pre-eclampsia,

Table 1   Risk factors for pre-eclampsia[9,10]

	Relative risk (RR)	95% CI
Genetic factors		
Genetic pre-disposition		
Race and ethnicity: more common in Blacks and Asians		
Family history of pre-eclampsia	2.90	1.70–4.93
Pregnancy by ovum donation		
Age and parity		
Teenage pregnancy		
Age more than 40 years	1.96	1.34–2.87
Long interval between pregnancies		
Nulliparity	2.91	1.28–6.61
Partner-related factors		
Change of partner		
Partner who fathered a pre-eclamptic pregnancy in another woman		
Limited sperm exposure		
Pregnancy due to donor insemination		
Presence of underlying disorders		
Chronic hypertension		
Diabetes mellitus	3.56	2.54–4.99
Renal disease		
Obesity (body mass index > 35 kg/m^2)		
(i) Before pregnancy	2.47	1.66–3.67
(ii) At booking	1.55	1.28–1.88
Maternal low birth weight		
Polycystic ovarian syndrome		
Migraine		
Collagen vascular disorders		
Uncontrolled hyperthyroidism		
Factor V Leiden deficiency, activated protein-C deficiency and thrombophilia		
Sickle cell disease or trait and other haemoglobinopathies		
Anti-phospholipid antibodies	9.72	4.34–21.75
Protein-S deficiency and hyperhomocysteinaemia		
Women with excessive snoring		
Previous pre-term birth		
Pregnancy-related risk factors		
Multiple pregnancy	2.93	2.04–4.21
Hydatidiform mole		
Hydrops fetalis		
Congenital and chromosomal fetal anomalies (trisomy 13, triploidy)		
Urinary tract infection		
Miscellaneous factors		
Smoking (reduced risk)		
Psychological strain and stress at working place		
Previous history of pre-eclampsia	7.19	5.85–8.83
Raised blood pressure (diastolic > 80 mmHg) at booking	1.38	1.01–1.87
CI = Confidence interval		

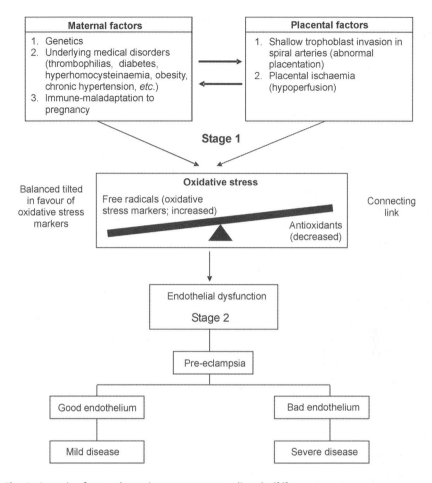

Fig. 1 Genesis of pre-eclampsia as a two-stage disorder[12,13]

history of medical problems like renal disease, diabetes and neurofibromatosis are more common in pre-eclamptic women.[9,10] Duckitt and Harrington[9] systematically reviewed controlled studies published from 1966–2002 and calculated unadjusted relative risks for various risk factors for pre-eclampsia (Table 1).

Aetiopathogenesis of pre-eclampsia needs to be fully understood before scientific foundations of preventive modalities can be laid. The precise aetiology of pre-eclampsia remains unknown. However, four hypotheses – placental ischaemia theory, very low-density lipoproteins (VLDL) versus toxicity preventing activity, immune maladaptation theory and genetic imprinting – have been extensively investigated, which are not mutually exclusive, but are probably interactive.[11] Dekker and Sibai[11] tried to unify the hypotheses on genesis of pre-eclampsia by proposing that in genetically susceptible individuals immune maladaptation, cytokine-mediated oxidative stress markers cause endothelial cell dysfunction with placental ischaemia and increased syncytiotrophoblast deportation.

Roberts et al.[12] proposed that maternal endothelial cell dysfunction is the key event resulting in diverse clinical manifestations of pre-eclampsia and considered pre-eclampsia as a 2-stage disorder.[13] The initiation of pre-eclampsia seems to be related to decreased placental perfusion (stage 1) which then results in the maternal syndrome of pre-eclampsia (stage 2). The linkage of the two stages is an important target area for prevention of pre-eclampsia (Fig. 1).

Oxidative stress is the presence of active oxygen species in excess of the available antioxidant buffering capacity. These products can damage DNA, proteins and lipids and can alter the structure and function of the cells of the body. Oxidative stress has been implicated in many human diseases like atherosclerosis, cancers and in pre-eclampsia.[14] Oxidative stress markers have been observed to be raised and anti-oxidants have been found to be lower in maternal sera, decidua and placenta.[14,15] We observed significantly raised levels of oxidative stress markers (malondialdehyde, glutathione peroxidase and superoxide dismutase) and significantly reduced levels of anti-oxidants lycopene and vitamins C in 50 women with varying grades of pre-eclampsia in contrast to 50 normal pregnant women and the alterations were higher in more severe disease (Sharma JB, Mittal S, Sharma A, Bahadur A. 2004 unpublished data).

PREVENTION OF PRE-ECLAMPSIA

Prevention of pre-eclampsia, if possible, would be a great step forward in prenatal care. The prevention of any condition has three aspects. Primary prevention means avoiding occurrence of a disease; secondary prevention for pre-eclampsia would mean breaking off the disease process before emergence of obvious clinical disease.[16] Tertiary prevention implies prevention of complications caused by the disease process and is almost equivalent to the treatment and is beyond the scope of this chapter.

Primary prevention

Although primary prevention is the best prevention for any disease, it would only be feasible if the aetiology is well understood and if it is possible to avoid or modify the causes. The primary event for the development of pre-eclampsia appears to be a failure of the second wave of trophoblast invasion from 16–20 weeks' gestation with failure to destroy the muscularis layer of the spiral arterioles. This causes shallow endovascular cytotrophoblast invasion with enhanced inflammatory response and endothelial cell dysfunction as key features in the pathogenesis of pre-eclampsia. The mechanisms for these are not yet clearly understood.[11] Primary prevention may be possible to some extent by modification of some of the risk factors of pre-eclampsia listed in Table 1. As the disease occurs more often in nulliparous women or in multiparous women with change of partners, there appears to be a protective effect of long-term sperm exposure on the frequency of the disease. Hence, it is recommended to have pregnancies with low-risk men, to stay with the same partner and to have children at an age when the endothelium is still able to cope with the inflammatory stress associated with the pregnant state. Similarly, avoidance of other high-risk factors presented in Table 1 may help in primary prevention of the disease in some cases. Thus, prevention or effective treatment of obesity or both could result in a significant reduction in the frequency of pre-eclampsia and should be encouraged.[16] Similarly, women with diabetes, chronic hypertension, renal and other medical disorders should have their primary condition under control before venturing into conception.

Although cigarette smoking is associated with a 30–40% reduction in the risk of pre-eclampsia, possibly mediated by nicotine through inhibition of interleukin-2 and tumour necrosis factor production by mononuclear cells, it cannot be recommended due to substantial harmful effects of smoking on maternal general health, increased frequency of fetal growth restriction and risk of placental abruption.[16] Hence, although it is recommended to modify the risk factors for pre-eclampsia, it would be possible only in the minority of cases. However, using the relative risk of pre-eclampsia in high-risk situations as suggested by Duckitt and Harrington,[9] early diagnosis of pre-eclampsia with timely referral for consultant care using PRECOG guidelines[2] can help in their timely management and can prevent them from going into severe pre-eclampsia.

Secondary prevention

Secondary prevention is the most important modality for pre-eclampsia and is almost synonymous with its prevention. Secondary prevention of any disease is feasible if the following three basic requirements for prevention are fulfilled and available:[16] (i) accurate knowledge of pathogenesis and genetics (pathophysiological mechanisms); (ii) availability of methods for early detection (effective screening methods); and (iii) means of intervention and modification of the pathophysiology.

Unfortunately, in spite of extensive research world-wide, none of the three criteria are available for pre-eclampsia to make a strong case for successful secondary prevention. The screening methods that have been tested by various researchers include history taking, examination and laboratory diagnosis. In spite of the availability of many modalities for screening, none is sensitive and specific enough to be used as a screening method, especially in low-risk women.[6] Presence of dichotic notch showing abnormal wave forms in uterine/uteroplacental Doppler flow studies has been used by many researchers, but is a very poor predictor of pre-eclampsia. Blood pressure measurement remains the cornerstone of early diagnosis although it has limitations including measurement errors associated with sphygmomanometry and the effect of maternal posture on blood pressure in pregnant women.[6] Middle trimester mean arterial pressure (MAP; [2 x diastolic blood pressure] + systolic blood pressure)/3) has been recommended as a better screening method.[6] Though some tests are useful to detect patients at risk, there is no one test which is truly predictive of pre-eclampsia. The multifactorial origin of the disease suggests that it is highly unlikely that there will be a single predictive test available in future to predict pre-eclampsia.

Non-pharmacological interventions

Bed rest
It was recommended initially for women at high risk of developing pre-eclampsia by many obstetricians and midwives in the hope that it reduces oedema and lowers blood pressure by increasing urinary output. However,

bed rest (either in hospital or at home) was not found to be effective to prevent the occurrence of pre-eclampsia, modify the course of the disease, decrease the incidence of preterm delivery, low birth weight or the perinatal mortality.[17] In fact, bed rest can be harmful to pregnant women and should not be routinely recommended.

Life-style changes
Regular antenatal care is mandatory for the prevention and early detection of pre-eclampsia. Job stress including lack of control over work pace, timing and frequency of breaks may be related to various adverse events including pre-eclampsia. In a preliminary study, pregnant women who were exposed to high job stress were found to be at greater risk of developing pre-eclampsia and gestational hypertension than were women exposed to low job stress.[18] In this study, evaluation was based on scores assessing the psychological demand of the job and decision-making attitude. So reducing job stress may be beneficial in the prevention of pre-eclampsia.[18]

Regular physical activity
Physical conditioning and pre-eclampsia have opposite effects on critical physiological functions. Regular prenatal exercise may prevent or oppose the progression of the disease as suggested by epidemiological studies.[19] The protective effect results from one or more of the following mechanisms: (i) stimulation of placental growth and vascularity; (ii) reduction of oxidative stress; and (iii) exercise induced reversal of maternal endothelial dysfunction.

However, there is not enough evidence yet for their efficacy in prevention of pre-eclampsia. There is a need for controlled, randomised, clinical trials examining the effects of prenatal exercise on biochemical markers for endothelial dysfunction, placental dysfunction and oxidative stress, which, if proven efficacious, would provide a low-cost intervention that could improve prenatal care for women at risk of this disease. Similarly, there is a need to evaluate the role of relaxation exercises, meditation and Yoga which have been used in the management of hypertension in non-pregnant state but there is no data available on their role in pregnancy.

Nutritional interventions

Dietary sodium restriction
Although sodium and water retention are universal in pregnancy, there are no differences in total body water or serum sodium concentrations between women with mild or severe pre-eclampsia as compared to gestationally age-matched pregnant women without hypertension. Dietary sodium restriction has been found to be useful in long-term management of chronic hypertension in men; however, there is no convincing evidence of its efficacy in prevention or treatment of hypertension during pregnancy.[20] The physiological volume expansion of uncomplicated pregnancy and the association of chronic hypertension, pre-eclampsia and intra-uterine growth restriction with plasma volumes lower than those measured in normal pregnancy are the common reasons cited for why sodium restriction generally is not recommended to treat hypertension during pregnancy. In chronic hypertensive women who are

determined to be salt-sensitive and who have responded to such therapy before pregnancy, sodium restriction and even diuretic therapy may be considered. There is, however, no data supporting salt restriction to prevent pre-eclampsia or to influence perinatal outcome.[20]

Dietary protein and energy intake
Several nutritional interventions have been suggested to prevent pre-eclampsia including increasing protein and energy intake generally or restricting protein or energy intake for obese women. However, a recent overview of randomised trials of nutritional interventions during pregnancy reported no benefit of such measures in the prevention of pre-eclampsia.[21]

Control of obesity
Although obesity is a known risk factor for superimposed pre-eclampsia, there is no evidence that limiting weight gain during pregnancy reduces its occurrence. Hence weight reduction is not recommended during pregnancy even in obese women.[21]

Change in dietary habits
There is some suggestion that nutrients in dietary form may have effects that are different from those observed with supplements including calcium supplementation. Thus, a study by the Dietary Approaches to Stop Hypertension (DASH) Collaborative Group demonstrated that dietary manipulation could significantly lower both systolic and diastolic blood pressure.[22] However, the results have not been confirmed by other studies.

Fish oils
Some studies showed the protective effect of n-3 fatty acids (omega-3 fatty acids) in prevention of pre-eclampsia. When they are included in the diet, eicosapentaenoic acid and docasahexaenoic acid compete with arachidonic acid. They inhibit synthesis of arachidonic acid from linoleic acid, and compete with arachidonic acid for the 2-position in membrane phospholipids, thereby lowering plasma and cellular concentrations of arachidonic acid. In addition, eicosapentaenoic acid competes with arachidonic acid as the substrate for cyclo-oxygenase, inhibiting the production of thromboxane-A_2 by platelets and producing low amounts of physiologically inactive thromboxane-A_3. The production of prostaglandin-I_2 in endothelial cells is not inhibited significantly. Many trials have been performed including the large European Multicentre Fish Oil Supplementation trial (FOTIP trial).[23] In six multicentre trials, women with high-risk pregnancies were randomly assigned to receive fish oil or olive oil from around 20 weeks' gestation. Although fish oil reduced the risk of preterm delivery from 33% to 21% (RR 0.54; 95% CI 0.30–0.98), none of the other parameters like prevalence of pre-eclampsia or intra-uterine growth restriction were affected. Hence, fish oils are unlikely to be beneficial in prevention of pre-eclampsia.

Alcohol intake
In non-pregnant patients, high alcohol intake is related to hypertension, but in pregnancy it is not associated with an increased risk of gestational

hypertension, pre-eclampsia or eclampsia. There is no definite evidence that consumption of less than 120 g of alcohol per week causes any adverse effects on pregnancy outcome including fetal growth, though, there are some suggestions that excessive consumption of alcohol can cause or aggravate maternal hypertension.[24]

Arginine supplementation
Dietary supplementation with L-arginine has been found to be useful in the prevention of pre-eclampsia.[25] However, it was an isolated study and no other study has confirmed its findings.

Japanese herbal medicine
Takei et al.[26] performed an experimental study on pregnant rats by creating a pre-eclampsia like syndrome including hypertension and intra-uterine growth retardation by N-omega-nitro-L-arginine methyl ester (L-NAME). They then tested a traditional herbal medicine Toki-shakuyaku-san (TS) for beneficial effects in this model. They observed inhibition of L-NAME-induced hypertension with the herbal medicine which was nitric oxide independent and concluded that the herbal medicine TS may be beneficial for the treatment and prevention of pre-eclampsia.

Pharmacological interventions

Role of antihypertensive drugs
It is generally agreed that women with pre-existing chronic hypertension are at significantly higher risk of developing pre-eclampsia than their normotensive counterparts. The various antihypertensive medications like methyldopa, labetolol and atenolol have been evaluated in various randomised trials for their efficacy in prevention of superimposed pre-eclampsia. Critical analysis of all these trials failed to find any reduction in the incidence of pre-eclampsia.[27]

Role of diuretics
Diuretics have been tried in pregnancy to reduce the incidence of pre-eclampsia. A meta-analysis of 9 randomised trials using diuretics (mainly hydrochloro-thiazide) in pregnancy involving more than 7000 women revealed no reduction in the incidence of pre-eclampsia or perinatal mortality, although the incidence of oedema and hypertension was reduced.[28] In the light of current evidence, diuretics cannot be recommended in clinical practice to prevent pre-eclampsia as they are not effective and may have deleterious effects such as reduced renal and placental perfusion. Thiazide diuretics should be avoided because of the risk of serious sodium and potassium depletion, haemorrhagic pancreatitis and severe thrombocytopenia in some newborns.

Zinc supplementation
Zinc concentrations are reduced among women with hypertensive disorders of pregnancy, including pre-eclampsia suggesting that pre-eclampsia results from zinc deficiency and that it may be prevented by dietary zinc supplementation. However, recent randomised clinical trials have failed to demonstrate the efficacy of zinc supplementation for the prevention of pre-eclampsia.[29]

Magnesium

Given the proven benefit of magnesium for the prevention and treatment of severe pre-eclampsia and eclampsia, the implication of dietary magnesium deficiency during pregnancy in the pathogenesis of pre-eclampsia, and a report of decreased intracellular magnesium concentration in women with pre-eclampsia, dietary supplementation with magnesium has been investigated as a potential preventive measure. A Cochrane review of two trials could detect no apparent effect of magnesium supplementation on the prevention of pre-eclampsia (mean supplement dose 365 mg and 500 mg).[30] The methodological quality of these trials was poor especially in relation to concealment of treatment and supplements were oral with poor absorption. Hence, routine magnesium supplementation to prevent pre-eclampsia cannot be recommended in the general population. However, this conclusion is unrelated to, and differs from, that of the effectiveness of parenteral magnesium sulphate for the treatment of severe pre-eclampsia and eclampsia, where it is considered to be the best and gold standard treatment.

Role of folic acid and other B-vitamins

Women with pre-eclampsia have been shown to have elevated blood levels of homocysteine which occur prior to the onset of the disease. Elevated levels of homocysteine may damage the lining of blood vessels leading to signs and symptoms of pre-eclampsia including rise in blood pressure, proteinuria and oedema. The total plasma homocysteine concentration is increased in pre-eclampsia and is significantly correlated with cellular fibronectin concentration suggesting that homocysteine plays a role in promoting endothelial dysfunction in pre-eclampsia.[31] Homocysteine concentrations have also been weakly and negatively correlated with plasma folate concentration., In fact, Leeda et al.[31] studied women with hyperhomocysteinemia and history of pre-eclampsia or fetal growth restriction with an abnormal methionine loading test and supplemented them with 5 mg folic acid and 250 mg of vitamin B_6 for at least 10 weeks in pregnancy. Vitamin B_6 and folic acid corrected the methionine-loading test in patients with hyperhomocysteinemia with a favourable perinatal outcome. In another trial studying the effect of vitamin B_6 on incidence of pre-eclampsia, supplementation of vitamin B_6 twice a day significantly reduced the incidence of pre-eclampsia.[16] Although the metabolic correction of hyperhomocysteinemia occurs, it is unknown currently whether or not metabolic correction translates into improved perinatal and maternal outcome.[16] Women who are deficient in vitamin B_2 (riboflavin) are more likely to develop pre-eclampsia than women with normal vitamin B_2 levels.[32] However, the results were observed in a non-industrialised country where deficiencies are more common than in the West. Although insufficient vitamin B_2 may cause biochemical changes simulating abnormalities underlying the disease process of pre-eclampsia, there is no definite scientific evidence that any of B vitamins can prevent pre-eclampsia.[32]

Low-dose aspirin

As pre-eclampsia is associated with vasospasm, endothelial cell dysfunction and activation of coagulation–haemostasis systems and as the biochemical studies suggested that these abnormalities are probably caused by an

Table 2 Results of larger multicentre trials of aspirin to prevent pre-eclampsia

Reference and country	Drug used (dose)	Patients chosen	Events/total (%) Study	Events/total (%) Control	RR	CI	Usefulness	Comments
Sibai et al. (1993)[34] USA	Aspirin 60 mg vs placebo	Nulliparous	69/1485 (4%)	94/1500 (6.3%) (P = 0.09)	0.74	0.55–1.00	Not useful	Increased rate of perinatal deaths due to abruptio placentae
Parazini et al. (1993)[35] Italy	Aspirin 50 mg or no treatment	Obstetric history	12/497 (2.12%)	9/423 (1.88%)	1.13	0.48–2.67	Not useful	–
Redman et al. (1994)[36] CLASP multi-national	Aspirin 60 mg vs placebo	Obstetric history	267/3992 (6.7%)	302/3982 (7.6%) (NS)	0.88	0.75–1.03	Not useful	Decrease in pre-eclampsia, preterm labour (NS;) increase in abruption (NS)
Atallah et al. (1996)[37] ECPPA Brazil	Aspirin 60 mg vs placebo	Obstetric history	32/476 (6.7%)	30/494 (6.1%) (NS)	1.11	0.68–1.79	Not useful	
Golding et al. (1998)[38] Jamaica	Aspirin 60 mg vs placebo	Nulliparous	215/3023 (7.1%)	189/3026 (6.3%) (NS)	1.14	0.94–1.38	Not useful	Increase in abruption (NS)
Rotchell et al. (1998)[39] Barbados	Aspirin 75 mg vs placebo	All pregnant women	40/1819 (2.2%)	46/1822 (2.5%) (NS)	0.87	0.57–1.32	Not useful	
Caritis et al. (1998)[40] USA	Aspirin 60 mg vs placebo	High-risk women	231/1254 (18.4%)	254/1249 (20.3%) (NS)	0.91	0.77–1.06	Not useful	

PE, pre-eclampsia; NS, not significant.

imbalance in the production of prostaglandins, prostacyclin (vasodilator and inhibitor of platelet aggregation) and thromboxane-A_2 (vasoconstrictor and platelet aggregator) with balance tilted in favour of thromboxane-A_2.[33] Low-dose aspirin (50–150 mg/day) therapy during pregnancy selectively inhibits platelet thromboxane-A_2 biosynthesis with minimal effects on prostacyclin production, thus altering the balance in favour of prostacyclin.[33]

The initial smaller studies on high-risk women showed favourable results with low-dose aspirin with significant (up to 70%) reduction in the incidence of pre-eclampsia.[33] Unfortunately, the initial encouraging results of aspirin to prevent pre-eclampsia could not be confirmed by larger multicentre trials (Table 2).[34–40] None of these studies observed any reduction in the incidence of pre-eclampsia in women given low-dose aspirin in comparison to placebo treatment. Another worrying point in the American study[34] was the incidence of perinatal death secondary to abruptio placentae, which was significantly higher in the aspirin-treated group (0.7% versus 0.1%) than in the placebo group. The largest trial to date was the CLASP study,[36] a multicentre trial recruiting 9364 pregnant women between 12–32 weeks' gestation from 213 centres across 16 countries between January 1988 and December 1992. This was a randomised, placebo-controlled trial co-ordinated by the Clinical Trials Unit in Oxford. The eligibility for entrance to this study were patients who in the opinion of the clinician were at significant risk of pre-eclampsia or intra-uterine growth restriction for pharmacological antiplatelet therapy with no significant contra-indications. Overall, the use of low-dose aspirin in pregnant women was associated with a 12% reduction in the incidence of pre-eclampsia (non-significant) and it reduced the incidence of preterm delivery in the high-risk group (19.7% in aspirin group versus 22.3% in placebo group). Although aspirin-treated women had a higher incidence of abruptio placentae, this did not reach statistical significance (1.8% versus 1.5%) compared to the placebo group.

Duley et al.[41] performed a systematic review of antiplatelet drugs for prevention of pre-eclampsia and its consequences by taking into consideration all the suitable trials from the literature. They included 39 randomised trials in their meta-analysis and divided their meta-analysis into moderate- and high-risk women. The included trials recruited 30,563 women with most studies comparing aspirin alone with placebo (28,802 women), while four studies used a combination of aspirin and dipyridamole compared with control, one used heparin with dipyridamole compared with control and another compared ozagrel hydrochloride with placebo. There was no overall difference in the risk of pregnancy-induced hypertension in the 27 trials.[41] However, there was 15% reduction in risk of pre-eclampsia associated with antiplatelet drugs (32 trials, 29,331 women; RR 0.85; 95% CI 0.78–0.92; number needed to treat was 100). There were no significant differences between the treatment and control groups in the risk of eclampsia, maternal deaths, caesarean section, induction of labour, antenatal admission or placental abruption. There was a small (8%) reduction in the risk of preterm delivery (RR 0.92; CI 0.88–0.97; number needed to treat, 72). There was also a 14% reduction in perinatal deaths in the antiplatelet group compared with the control group (RR 0.86; CI 0.75–0.98; number needed to treat, 250). However, there were no significant differences between treatment and control group in the risk of low birth weight babies, admission to special care baby unit, intraventricular haemorrhage, neonatal bleeding, child health and development at 12–18 months (one trial).

In an update, the authors[42] concluded that among women at moderate risk, low-dose aspirin was associated with a moderate reduction in pre-eclampsia (RR 0.85; CI 0.77–0.94). Overall, 89 women would have to be treated during most of their pregnancy to prevent one case of pre-eclampsia. In high-risk women, low-dose aspirin had a protective effect (RR 0.73; CI 0.64–0.83) with greater effect among women treated with higher doses than 75 mg/day of aspirin (RR 0.49; CI 0.38–0.63). The Cochrane reviewers concluded that despite the potential benefits overall, it was not possible to make clear recommendations.[42]

Although low-dose aspirin corrects the prostacyclin/thromboxane-A$_2$ imbalance, it does not prevent pre-eclampsia possibly because such an imbalance is not the only, and certainly not the major, pathogenic biochemical pathway.[16] Some investigators have suggested using higher doses of aspirin and to start it earlier. Low-dose aspirin has been studied in combination with other antiplatelet drugs. In a South African study, addition of ketanserin to aspirin was associated with a substantial decrease in the frequency of superimposed pre-eclampsia and an improvement in pregnancy outcome among patients with mild-to-moderate, mid-trimester hypertension.[43] Many advocates of aspirin argue that the benefits of low-dose aspirin in larger multicentre trials were not observed due to selecting low-risk women. But the large multicentre study by Caritis *et al.*[40] enrolled high-risk women (insulin-treated diabetes mellitus, chronic hypertension, multiple pregnancy or a history of pre-eclampsia) and even this study failed to demonstrate any benefits of low-dose aspirin to prevent pre-eclampsia even in high-risk women. Most studies found no increase in antepartum or postpartum haemorrhage but the Jamaican study[38] showed increased chance of haemorrhage. In summary, due to heterogenesis, the results of various studies on aspirin are not consistent with one another. The results of available trials do not support the wide-spread and routine prophylactic or therapeutic use of antiplatelet therapy among all women judged to be at risk of pre-eclampsia or intra-uterine growth restriction. The only group in whom the use of low-dose aspirin may be justified are those at especially high risk of early onset pre-eclampsia, as starting early aspirin has been found to have a favourable effect on prostanoids in these women. So, the hoped-for benefits from low-dose aspirin which was thought to be a wonder drug have not been realised.[33]

Role of heparin

Subcutaneous heparin alone or more often in combination with low-dose aspirin and/or dipyridamole has been used to prevent pre-eclampsia with significant reduction in its incidence. The incidence of pre-eclampsia was 2.3% with the combination regimen as compared to 26% with low-dose aspirin and 28% with no treatment.[44] Treatment with heparin and low-dose aspirin has also been associated with lower incidence of pre-eclampsia and improved perinatal survival in women with anti-phospholipid syndrome.[44] The scientific basis for using heparin to prevent pre-eclampsia is to modify the endothelial cell dysfunction and activation of the coagulation system, which are central in the pathophysiology of pre-eclampsia. There is, however, insufficient data available to recommend its use routinely in the prevention of pre-eclampsia except in cases of antiphospholipid syndrome. Moreover, its use during pregnancy can cause adverse reactions like increased chances of spontaneous abortion, abruptio placentae, postpartum haemorrhage and osteoporosis in the mother.

Calcium supplementation

Data from epidemiological and observational studies have shown that there is an inverse relationship between calcium intake and the frequency of pre-eclampsia and eclampsia. Observational data have also suggested that the higher the level of calcium intake the greater the protection against eclampsia. The results of most of the trials of calcium supplementation in prevention of pre-eclampsia are given in Table 3.[45–60] As is clear from the table, smaller initial studies showed better results. There have been three major studies by Lopez-Jaramillo et al.[48,49,56] done in Ecuador in a population with low calcium levels. All three trials demonstrated a significant reduction in the incidence of pre-eclampsia. However, the largest and the most definitive study was conducted by Levine et al.[57] from the US which was a randomised trial sponsored by the National Institute of Child Health and Human Development. In this trial, using double masking, 4589 healthy nulliparous women were randomly administered either 2 g/day of supplemental calcium (2295 women) or placebo (2294 women). Supplemental calcium did not prevent any of the hypertensive disorders due to pregnancy including gestational hypertension or pre-eclampsia. However, Cochrane Database[59,60] in their meta-analysis observed a modest reduction in pre-eclampsia and the effect was greatest in women at high risk of hypertension and those with low baseline calcium intake. Hence, calcium supplementation is only recommended in communities with lower calcium levels. The World Health Organization (WHO) is conducting a double-blind, randomised, controlled trial in 7 locations world-wide where calcium intake is below 600 mg/day. The pregnant women receive an extra 1.5 g of calcium carbonate or placebo per day with treatment commenced after gestational week 20. Its results should be available in the near future.

Role of nitric oxide donors

Nitric oxide (NO) is a major paracrine mediator and important regulatory agent in various female reproductive processes. It is released by endothelial cells, is a potent vasodilator and inhibits platelet aggregation and adhesion to vascular endothelial surfaces. Research indicates that pre-eclampsia is characterised by impaired NO synthesis with diminished production of second messenger, cyclic guanosine monophosphate (cGMP). In an experimental study, infusion of the NO synthase inhibitor, nitro-L-arginine-methyl ester (L-NAME), in pregnant rats produced proteinuric hypertension which has been used as an animal model for pre-eclampsia.[61] Small studies have shown the beneficial effects of nitric oxide donors in improving placental flow and uteroplacental perfusion in women with pre-eclampsia. Nakatsuka et al.[61] used transdermal isosorbide dinitrate for a mean duration of 11.1 ± 7.2 days in two women with pre-eclampsia associated with oligohydramnios and increased pulsatility index (PI) in uterine artery. Pulsed Doppler ultrasound showed that average PI was significantly decreased in uterine artery ($P < 0.003$) and umbilical artery ($P < 0.004$). The amniotic fluid pocket increased 4-fold. Similar findings were reported in another study in 17 patients of pre-eclampsia

Table 3 Efficacy of calcium supplementation in prevention of pre-eclampsia

Reference	Calcium salt (mg/day)	Control	Pre-eclampsia incidence Study (calcium) (%)	Control (Placebo) (%)	Statistical analysis (P-value or 95% CI)	Other parameters & outcome	Conclusion
Kawasaki et al. (1985)[45]	Calcium aspirate (600)	No control	1:22 (4.5)	15:72 (21.2)	P < 0.05	Nil	Reduction in PE
Marya et al. (1987)[46]	Calcium carbonate (375) with vitamin D_3	Placebo	11:188 (6)	16:182 (9)	P = 0.65 (95% CI 0.31–1.38)	No effect	No reduction in PE
Villar et al. (1987)[47]	OS-Cal tablets (1500)	Placebo	1:25 (4)	3:27 (11.1)	P = 0.37 (95% CI 0.05–2.83)	–	Reduction in PE
Lopez-Jaramillo et al. (1989)[48]	Calcium gluconate (2000)	Placebo	0:55 (0)	12:51 (24)	P = 0.10 (95% CI 0.03–0.32)	–	Reduction in PE (OR 0.15; 95% CI 0.04–0.61%)
Lopez-Jaramillo et al. (1990)[49]	Elemental calcium (2000)	Placebo	0:22 (0)	8:34 (23.5)	P = 0.15 (95% CI 0.03–0.69)	Decrease	Significant reduction in PE. (OR 0.28; 95% CI 0.02–0.30). No effect on preterm delivery
Mantanaro et al. (1990)[50]	Calcium carbonate (2000)	Placebo	2:86 (2.4)	9:86 (10.5)	P = 0.27 (95% CI 0.08–0.90)	–	Reduction in PE (OR 0.28; 95% CI 0.09–84)
Villar & Repke (1990)[51]	OS-Cal tablets (2000)	Placebo	0:90 (0)	3:88 (3.4)	P = 0.13 (95% CI 0.01–1.26)	–	No effect on PE. Reduction in preterm deliveries (OR 0.32; 95% CI 0.13–77)
Belizan et al. (1991)[52]	Calcium carbonate (2000)	Placebo	13:579 (2.6)	23:588 (3.9)	P = 0.66 (95% CI 0.34–1.26)	–	Reduction in PE (OR 0.63; 95% CI 0.44–0.90)
Cong et al. (1993)[53]	Shengu capsules-NA	Placebo	5:50 (10)	6:50 (12)	P = 0.19 (95% CI 0.009–4.10)	–	Reduction in PE (OR 0.22; 95% CI 0.05–0.96)
Sanchez-Ramos et al. (1994)[54]	Calcium carbonate (2000)	Placebo	4:29 (13.8)	15:34 (44)	P = 0.37 (95% CI 0.15–0.92)	–	Reduction in PE (OR 0.46; 95% CI 0.25–0.86)
Purvar et al. (1996)[55]	Elemental calcium (2000)	Placebo	2:96 (2.1)	11:93 (11.8)	P = 0.13 (95% CI 0.01–0.64)	–	Reduction in PE
Lopez-Jaramillo et al. (1997)[56]	Calcium carbonate (2000)	Placebo	4:125 (32)	21:135 (15.5)	P < 0.001	–	Decreased systolic blood pressure by 9.1 mmHg, diastolic by 6 mmHg
Levine et al. (1997)[57]	Calcium carbonate (2000)	Placebo	158:2295 (6.9)	163:2294 (7.3)	P = 0.94 (95% CI 0.76–1.16)	Non significant	No effect on caesarean delivery, preterm delivery, PE
Herrere et al. (1998)[58]	Elemental calcium	Placebo	4:43	16:43	P = 0.001; 0.25 (95% CI 0.09–0.69)	–	Reduction in diastolic blood pressure by 7 mmHg. Increase in gestation and birth weight
Hofmeyr et al. (2003)[59]	Elemental calcium	Placebo	0:68	–	RR 0.21 (95% CI 0.11–0.39)	–	Modest decrease in risk of PE. No effect on preterm delivery rate, still births or deaths
Atallah et al. (2005)[60]	Elemental calcium	Placebo	10 trials, 6634 women	–	RR 0.58 (95% CI 0.43–0.79)		Modest decrease in risk of PE

PE, pre-eclampsia; OR, odds ratio; CI, confidence interval.

who received transdermal glycerine trinitrate (GTN). There was a significant fall in mean pulsatility and resistance index of $18 \pm 4\%$ and $17 \pm 3\%$, respectively.[62] However, the data on the role of nitric oxide donors in preventing pre-eclampsia are limited and conflicting. A large, multicentre, randomised, double blind, placebo-controlled trial is currently under way in various hospitals in India by the Indian Council of Medical Research (An ICMR Task Force Study, personal communication) to see the impact of transdermal GTN patch 5 mg/day and aspirin 75 mg/day in the prevention of pre-eclampsia and its complications. Its results are likely to be available in 2 years.

Role of antioxidants

As discussed above, oxidative stress seems to play a major role in the aetio-pathogenesis of pre-eclampsia. Oxidative stress markers are significantly raised while antioxidants are concomitantly reduced in maternal tissues, decidua and placenta[14,15] in pre-eclamptic women compared to normotensive women. None-theless, the role of oxidative stress in pre-eclampsia is not without controversy as some studies have found no evidence of lipid peroxidation or deficiency of antioxidant activity.

The best test of whether oxidative stress causes pre-eclampsia is by its successful prevention by antioxidant therapy. In fact, many such trials have been completed with promising results.[63-69] Unfortunately, the first trial using 1000 mg vitamin C, 800 IU of vitamin E and 200 mg of allopurinol per day from 24–32 weeks' gestation for 14 days by Gulmezoglu et al.[63] on 56 patients with severe pre-eclampsia did not find any benefit with antioxidant therapy. This was probably due to the fact that disease was already too advanced for antioxidants to show any benefit. It is likely that by the time pre-eclampsia is clinically evident, irreversible changes are already present and thus therapy must be begun before this time.

Chappell et al.[64] tested the efficacy of antioxidant therapy before clinically evident disease. They identified some high-risk women by history (previous pre-eclampsia, pre-existing hypertension) but identified most by abnormal uterine artery Doppler studies at 20 and 24 weeks of gestation. The uterine artery Doppler study they used had a positive predictive value of 20%, when there is evidence of increased resistance at 20 and 24 weeks' gestation. On the basis of abnormal Doppler (diastolic notch in uterine artery), they randomised women at 20 weeks to receive either 1000 mg of vitamin C and 400 IU of vitamin E or placebo. The women whose waveforms became normal by 24 weeks were classified as being at low risk and were withdrawn from further treatment. It was an intent-to-treat trial and there was a significant reduction in markers of endothelial activation (plasminogen activator inhibitor [PAI-1]/PAI-2 ratio). Supplementation with vitamins C and E was associated with a 21% decrease in the PAI-1/PAI-2 ratio during gestation (95% CI 4–35; $P = 0.015$). In the intention-to-treat cohort, pre-eclampsia occurred in 24 (17%) of 142 women in the placebo group and 11 (8%) of 141 women in the vitamin group (adjusted odds ratio 0.39; 95% CI 0.17–0.90; $P = 0.02$). In the cohort who completed the study (81 placebo group, 79 vitamin group), the odds ratio for pre-eclampsia was 0.24 (95% CI 0.08–0.70; $P = 0.002$).

In a further analysis, Chappell et al.[65] studied 79 women who were at high risk taking vitamin supplements (vitamin C, 1000 mg; vitamin E, 400 IU/D), 81 high-risk women who were taking placebo and compared them with 32 women who were at low risk and who were not taking any supplements. They observed

Table 4 Study design of randomised controlled trials on antioxidants to prevent pre-eclampsia

Reference & country	Patients (n)	Patients' characteristics	Antioxidants and daily dosage	Start treatment (weeks' gestation)	Treatment duration (weeks)
Gulmezoglu et al. (1997)[63] South Africa	56	Severe PE	Vitamin C (1000 mg), vitamin E (800 IU), Allopurinol (200 mg)	24–32	2
Chappell et al. (1999)[64] UK	283	High-risk (h/o previous PE, chr HTN and abnormal uterine artery Doppler)	Vitamin C (1000 mg), vitamin E (400 IU)	16–20	20–24
Chappell et al. (2002)[65] UK	193	Low and high risk	Vitamin C (1000 mg), vitamin E (400 IU)	16–20	20–24
Pressman et al. (2003)[66] USA	20	Elective LS patients	Vitamin C (500 mg), vitamin E (400 IU)	35	2–4
Sharma et al. (2003)[67] India	251	Primigravidas	Lycopene (4 mg)	16–20	20–24
Han et al. (1993)[68] China	100	High risk	Selenium (100 µg)	32–34	6–8
Lumbanraja (2004; unpub. data) Indonesia	28	Mild PE	NAC (600 mg)	32–37	2
Wibowo et al. (2004; unpub. data) Indonesia	25	Severe PE	NAC (40 mg/kg), vitamin E (10 IU)	Not mentioned	5 days
Mose et al. (1999; unpub. data) Indonesia	50	High risk	Garlic (1050 mg)	26–32	2
Ziaei et al. (2001)[69] Iran	100	High risk	Garlic (800 mg)	28–32	8

PE, pre-eclampsia; NAC, chr HTN = chronic hypertension; N-acetylcysteine; Unpub. data = unpublished data.

abnormal indices of oxidative stress and placental function in the high-risk placebo group. Ascorbic acid, PAI–2 and placental growth factor concentrations were decreased, and 8-epi prostaglandin $F_2\alpha$, leptin and PAI-1/ PAI-2 ratio were increased in high risk placebo group as compared to women who were at low risk. In the group that received vitamin supplements, ascorbic acid, 8-epi-prostaglandin $F_2\alpha$, leptin and PAI-1/PAI-2 values were similar to women who were at low risk. They thus concluded that antioxidant supplementation in women who were at risk of pre-eclampsia was associated with improvement in biochemical indices of the disease.[65]

There have been many studies on the role of various antioxidants like vitamins C and E,[64,65] lycopene,[67] selenium,[68] N-acetylcysteine (Lumbanraja *et al.* 2004 unpublished data; Wibowo *et al.* 2004, unpublished data) and garlic (Ziaei et al.,[69] Mose *et al.*, 1999, unpublished data) in prevention of pre-eclampsia (Table 5). The study design and results of these studies are shown in Tables 4 and 5, respectively. Thus, most of the antioxidants have shown promising results when started early in pregnancy (16– 20 weeks), before the clinically evident disease, while the treatment was ineffective if started late or when the disease was clinically evident.[63] Most authors used combinations of vitamins C and E as antioxidants. Antioxidants are inhibitors of reactive oxygen species and the likely explanation of their beneficial effects is through this mechanism. Vitamin C (ascorbic acid) is a potent scavenger of superoxide radicals and may help to preserve nitric oxide. In addition, both vitamin E (α-tocopherol) and vitamin C decrease low-density lipoprotein (LDL) oxidation.[63,64] Ascorbic acid can also help to maintain intracellular glutathione concentration.

We have used the antioxidant lycopene (LycoRed™ containing Lyc-O-Mato®; Jagsonpal Pharmaceuticals Limited, Delhi, India) 2 mg twice daily in 116 primigravidas and similar-looking placebo tablets in another 135 primigravidas in a double-blind, randomised, controlled trial at 16–20 weeks' gestation and continued the treatment until delivery (total duration 20–24 weeks).[67] There was a significant reduction in pre-eclampsia in the lycopene group compared to the placebo group (8.6% versus 17.7%; 51.4% reduction; P = 0.043). Mean diastolic blood pressure was significantly lower in the lycopene group than in the placebo group (86.7 ± 3.8 mmHg versus. 92.2 ± 5.98 mmHg; P = 0.033). The mean fetal weight was also significantly higher in the lycopene group than in the placebo group (2751.17 ± 315.76 g versus 2657.26 ± 444.30 g; P = 0.0491). The incidence of intra-uterine growth retardation (IUGR) was also significantly lower in the lycopene group than the placebo group (12.1% versus 23.7%; P = 0.033). Lycopene is the dominant carotenoid in human serum and constitutes about 50% of all carotenoids found in the serum. It has been shown in experiments to have the highest oxygen quenching capacity (strongest antioxidant and is twice as powerful as β-carotene in neutralising free radicals). Lycopene is a natural extract, derived from tomatoes.[67] Its antioxidant property protects the cells from DNA damage and it also has a role in growth control and cell-to-cell communication. Levels of lycopene have been found to be reduced in pre-eclampsia (Sharma JB *et al.* 2004, unpublished data).

Antioxidant studies in progress

Encouraged by the initial promising results of antioxidants in prevention of pre-eclampsia, several large trials are currently in progress world-wide. There

Table 5 Results of studies of antioxidants in prevention of pre-eclampsia

Reference	Gulmezoglu *et al*. (1997)[63]
Results	1 eclampsia in each group (RR 0.74;95% CI 0.43–1.28)
Maternal outcome	Delivered within 2 weeks (RR 0.68; 95% CI 0.45–1.04)
Perinatal outcome	No significant difference. Still birth (RR 0.84; 95% CI 0.36–1.93); neonatal death (RR 5.0; 95% CI 0.64–39.06); perinatal death (RR 1.29; 95% CI 0.67–2.48)
Biochemical marker	No significant difference in lipid peroxidates, uric acid decreased, vitamin E increased
Comments	No improvement
Reference	Chappell *et al*. (1999)[64]
Results	Pre-eclampsia 8% versus 17% (OR 0.39; 95% CI 0.17–0.90; $P = 0.02$)
Maternal outcome	
Perinatal outcome	SGA infants – 32% in placebo, 23% in vitamin group
Biochemical marker	21% reduction in PAI-1/2 ratio (95% CI 4–35; $P = 0.015$)
Comments	Significant reduction in pre-eclampsia
Reference	Chappell *et al*. (2002)[65]
Results	Pre-eclampsia 8% in vitamin, 26% in placebo groups
Maternal outcome	
Perinatal outcome	SGA infants: 25% in vitamin group, 36% placebo in high-risk, 15% in low-risk groups
Biochemical marker	Decreased vitamin C, PAI 2, PGF and increase of 8-epi $PGF_2\alpha$, leptin, PAI 1/2 ratio in high-risk placebo versus low risk
Comments	Significant improvement in biochemical markers
Reference	Pressman *et al*. (2003)[66]
Results	
Maternal outcome	
Perinatal outcome	
Biochemical marker	Plasma levels of vitamin E increased. No change in vitamin C levels. Vitamins C and E correlate with amniotic fluid and chorioamnion levels, respectively
Comments	
Reference	Sharma *et al*. (2003)[67]
Results	Pre-eclampsia 17.7% in placebo and 8.6% in lycopene (54.1% decrease)
Maternal outcome	Mean diastolic blood pressure in lycopene group < placebo ($P = 0.012$)
Perinatal outcome	Mean fetal weight in lycopene > placebo ($P = 0.049$), IUGR 23.7% in placebo and 12% in lycopene (49.3% reduction)
Biochemical marker	
Comments	Significant reduction in pre-eclampsia
Reference	Han *et al*. (1993)[68]
Results	Decrease in incidence of PET, HTN and gestational oedema
Maternal outcome	NS in PPH
Perinatal outcome	NS in birth weight
Biochemical marker	Increased selenium in maternal and umbilical cord
Comments	Useful to prevent pre-eclampsia
Reference	Lumbanraja (2004) unpublished data
Results	33.3% in treatment and 76.9% in placebo groups developed severe PET ($P = 0.003$)
Maternal outcome	
Perinatal outcome	No asphyxia in treatment group, 23% in placebo group
Biochemical marker	
Comments	Useful
Reference	Wibowo *et al*. (2004) unpublished data
Results	Increased length of conservative treatment in NAC group
Maternal outcome	Systolic and diastolic blood pressure decreased after NAC treatment
Perinatal outcome	
Biochemical marker	NS in TNF, IL-6 and fibronectin
Comments	Useful

Table 5 *(continued)* Results of studies of antioxidants in prevention of pre-eclampsia

Reference	Mose *et al.* (1999) unpublished data
Results	78.1% in preventing pre-eclampsia
Maternal outcome	Decrease in systolic blood pressure 7.4%, decrease in diastolic blood pressure 15.1%
Perinatal outcome	Birth weight in garlic group > controls
Biochemical marker	
Comments	Limited use
Reference	Ziaei *et al.* (2001)[69]
Results	NS in preventing pre-eclampsia but prevents HT
Maternal outcome	
Perinatal outcome	Decreased total cholesterol after garlic treatment
Biochemical marker	
Comments	No decrease in pre-eclampsia

is a study on at-risk women in the UK, which also includes WHO network centres in non-industrialised countries.[13] In the UK, the Diabetes and Pre-eclampsia Intervention Trial (DAPIT) study group is performing a randomised, multicentre, double-blind, placebo-controlled trial that will recruit 756 pregnant women with type-1 diabetes from 20 metabolic antenatal clinics in the UK over 4 years.[70] Women will be randomised to receive daily vitamin C (1000 mg) and vitamin E (400 IU) or placebo at 8–22 weeks of gestation until delivery. Maternal venous blood will be obtained at randomisation, 26 and 34 weeks for markers of endothelial activation and oxidative stress and to assess glycaemic control. The primary outcome is pre-eclampsia. Secondary outcomes include endothelial activation (PAI 1/PAI 2) and birth-weight centile. This study is likely to be completed by 2008. It will increase our understanding of the pathogenesis of the complications associated with diabetic pregnancies. If the treatment is successful, it may have major cost and health implications with significant improvement in maternal and perinatal outcomes.[70]

There are on-going studies on low-risk women in Canada, Mexico and the US. The largest study is being conducted in the US by the National Institute of Child Health and Human Development Maternal Fetal Medicine Network for clinical trials with support from National Heart, Lung and Blood Institute (NICHD/NHLB) and is enrolling 10,000 women.[13] This trial is randomising women to treatment with 1000 mg of vitamin C and 400 IU of vitamin E at 8–16 weeks' gestation and is powered to see differences in maternal and fetal outcomes, rather than merely a reduction in the frequency of pre-eclampsia. The primary outcomes are gestational hypertension and markers of maternal morbidity (severe hypertension, eclampsia, hepatic or renal dysfunction or thrombocytopenia) or markers of perinatal outcome (still births, indicated preterm birth, or small for gestational age babies). There is also a pathophysiology/prediction component in which 2000 treated and 2000 placebo group (total 4000 women) will have biological samples obtained before randomisation and then intermittently throughout the pregnancy. The study may also determine if any subsets of women are more or less likely to benefit from antioxidant therapy as well as what components of the pathophysiology of pre-eclampsia are likely to be modified by the therapy. The results are likely to be available by 2007, which, if proven beneficial, will be a significant landmark in the prevention of pre-eclampsia. If the results of this largest trial turn out to be unfavourable, antioxidant therapy may have the same fate as low-dose aspirin therapy. Considering the aetiopathogenesis of this disease, theories and failure of various preventive modalities, emergence of an effective preventive measure is unlikely.[71]

ACKNOWLEDGEMENTS

We are grateful to the WHO, Geneva, Indian Council of Medical Research, New Delhi, National Institute of Health, Hyderabad, India and Dr Sangeeta Sharma, Paediatrician, L.R.S. Institute of Tuberculosis and Respiratory Diseases, New Delhi for their help in the preparation of this article.

KEY POINTS FOR CLINICAL PRACTICE

- Pre-eclampsia is a leading cause of severe obstetric morbidity for both mother and fetus throughout the world.

- Pre-eclampsia continues to be a disease of theories and no one theory can explain its aetiopathogenesis. Probably more than one theory works. The basic defect is placental ischaemia followed by release of oxidative stress markers in maternal tissues causing vasospasm and various lesions of pre-eclampsia in various target organs, leading to clinical syndrome of the disease.

- Although many screening methods are available, none are sensitive or specific enough to be used routinely in low-risk women.

- Primary prevention is identification of risk factors, quantify them as suggested by Duckitt and Harrington[9] and using the pre-eclampsia community guideline (PRECOG),[2] the women at risk should be identified and referred for early consultant care to manage the disease in its early stage to prevent its development into severe disease.

- Secondary prevention though the ideal type of prevention does not really exist. The various modalities such as physical activity, dietary modification, use of aspirin and calcium supplementation have been tried with promising initial results but are not convincingly effective for universal use. Role of antioxidants like vitamins C and E or lycopene have been found to be effective in initial smaller studies but results of larger trials are awaited. To date, no proven effective modality exists for prevention of pre-eclampsia.

- As the exact aetiology and aetiopathogenesis of pre-eclampsia is not known, prevention of pre-eclampsia is still a distant dream.

- Use of pre-eclampsia community guideline (PRECOG)[2] to screen for and detect onset of pre-eclampsia, improvement of antenatal care along with active management of the disease on its development will improve both maternal and perinatal outcome, as pre-eclampsia matters.[72]

1 Working Group Report on High Blood Pressure in Pregnancy. National Institute of Health, National Heart, Lung and Blood Institute, National High Blood Pressure Education Program, NIH Publication No. 00-3029, Revised July 2000

2 The pre-eclampsia community guideline (PRECOG): how to screen for and detect onset of pre-eclampsia in the community. BMJ 2005; 330: 576–580

3 WHO. WHO International Collaborative Study of Hypertensive Disorders of Pregnancy. Geographic variation in the incidence of hypertension in pregnancy. Am J Obstet Gynecol 1988; 158: 80–83

4 Confidential Enquiry into Maternal Deaths. Why mothers die 2000-2002. The sixth report of the confidential enquiries into maternal deaths in the united kingdom. London: Royal College of Obstetricians and Gynaecologists Press; 2004

5 Bedi N, Kamboj I, Dhillon BS, Saxena BN, Singh P. Maternal deaths in India – Preventable tragedies (An ICMR Task Force Study). J Obstet Gynaecol Ind 2001; 51: 86–92

6 Farag K, Hassan I, Ledger WL. Prediction of preeclampsia. Obstet Gynecol Surv 2004; 59: 464–482

7 Nanda S, Sharma JB, Gulati N. Perinatal mortality in eclampsia. J Obstet Gynaecol Ind 1989; 39: 792–795

8 Bell R, Parker L, MacPhail S, Wright C. Trends in the cause of late fetal deaths, 1982–2000. Br J Obstet Gynaecol 2004; 111: 1400–1407

9 Duckitt K, Harrington D. Risk factors for pre-eclampsia at antenatal booking: systematic review of controlled studies. BMJ 2005; 330: 565–577

10 Sharma JB, Gulati N, Malik S. Maternal and perinatal complications in neurofibromatosis during pregnancy. Int J Gynecol Obstet 1991; 34: 221–225

11 Dekker GA, Sibai BM. Etiology and pathogenesis of preeclampsia. Am J Obstet Gynecol 1998; 179: 1359–1375

12 Roberts JM, Taylor RN, Musci TJ, Rodgers GM, Hubel CA, McLaughlin MK. Preeclampsia: An endothelial cell disorder. Am J Obstet Gynecol 1989; 161: 1200–1204

13 Roberts JM, Speer P. Antioxidant therapy to prevent preeclampsia. Semin Nephrol 2004; 24: 557-564.

14. Hubel CA. Oxidative stress in the pathogenesis of pre-eclampsia. Proc Soc Exp Biol Med 1999; 222: 222–235

15 Sharma JB, Mittal S. Oxidative stress and preeclampsia. Obstet Gynaecol Today 2004; IX: 551–554

16 Dekker G, Sibai B. Primary, secondary and tertiary prevention of pre-eclampsia. Lancet 2001; 357: 209–215

17 Allen C, Glasziou P, Del Mar C. Bed rest: a potentially harmful treatment needing more care evaluation. Lancet 1999; 354: 1229–1233

18 Marcoux S, Berube S, Brisson C, Moudor M. Job strain and pregnancy induced hypertension. Epidemiology 1999; 10: 376–382

19 Weissgerber TL, Wolfe LA, Davies GA. The role of regular physical activity in preeclampsia prevention. Med Sci Sports Exer 2004; 36: 2024–2031

20 Steegers EA, Eskes TK, Jongsma HW, Hein PR. Dietary sodium restriction during pregnancy: a historical review. Eur J Obstet Gynecol Reprod Biol 1991; 40: 83–90

21 Kramer MS. Energy/protein restriction for high weight-for-height or weight gain during pregnancy. (Cochrane Review), in The Cochrane Library, Issue 1. Chichester, UK, John Wiley, 2004

22 Appel LJ, Moore TJ, Obarzanek E et al. A clinical trial of the effects of dietary patterns on blood pressure. N Engl J Med 1997; 336: 1117–1124

23 Olsen S, Secher NJ, Tabor A, Weber T, Walker JJ, Gluud C. Randomised clinical trials of fish oil supplementation in high risk pregnancies. Br J Obstet Gynaecol 2000; 107: 382–395

24 Royal College of Obstetricians and Gynaecologists: alcohol consumption in pregnancy. Guideline Report 9. London, Royal College of Obstetricians and Gynaecologists, 1996

25 Ekerhovd E. Dietary supplementation with L-arginine in women with preeclampsia. Acta Obstet Gynecol Scand 2004; 83: 871–872

26 Takei H, Nakai Y, Hattori N *et al*. The herbal medicine toki-shakuyaku-san improves the hypertension and intrauterine growth retardation in preeclampsia rats induced by N-omega-nitro-L-arginine methylester. Phytomediane 2004; 11: 43–50

27 Sibai BM, Treatment of hypertension in pregnant women. N Engl J Med 1996; 335: 257–265

28 Collins R, Yusuf S, Peto R. Overview of randomized trials of diuretics in pregnancy. BMJ 1985; 29: 17–23

29 Jonsson B, Hauge B, Larsen NF, Hald F. Zinc supplementation during pregnancy: a double blind randomized clinical trial. Acta Obstet Gynaecol Scand 1996; 75: 725–729

30 Makrides M, Crowther CA: Magnesium supplementation in pregnancy. (Cochrane Review), in The Cochrane Library, Issue 1, Chichester, UK, John Wiley, 2004

31 Leeda M, Riyazi N, de Vries JIP, Jokobs C, van Geijn HP, Dekker GA, Effects of folic acid and vitamin B6 on women with hyperhomocysteinemia and a history of pre-eclampsia or fetal growth restriction. Am J Obstet Gynecol 1998; 179: 135–139

32 Wacker J, Fruhauf J, Schulz M, Chiwora FM, Volz J, Becker K. Riboflavin deficiency and preeclampsia. Obstet Gynecol 2000; 96: 38–44

33 Sibai BM. Prevention of preeclampsia. A big disappointment. Am J Obstet Gynecol 1998; 179: 1275–1278

34 Sibai BM, Caritis SN, Thom E, Klebanoff M, McNellis D, Rocco L. Prevention of preeclampsia with low-dose aspirin in healthy, nulliparous, pregnant women. The National Institute of Child Health and Human Development Network of MFM Units. N Engl J Med 1993; 329: 1213–1218

35 Italian study of Aspirin in Pregnancy Group. Low-dose aspirin in prevention and treatment of intrauterine growth retardation and pregnancy-induced hypertension. Lancet 1993; 341: 396–400

36 CLASP (Collaborative Low-dose Aspirin Study in Pregnancy) Collaborative Group. A randomised trial of low-dose aspirin for the prevention and treatment of preeclampsia among 9,364 pregnant women. Lancet 1994; 343: 619–629

37 ECPPA (Estudo Collaborative Para Prevencao da Pre-eclampsia com Aspirina) Collaborative Group. Randomised trial of low-dose aspirin for the prevention of maternal and fetal complications in high risk pregnant women. Br J Obstet Gynaecol 1996; 103: 39–47

38 Golding J, on behalf of the Jamaica Low-Dose Aspirin Study group. A randomized trial of low-dose aspirin for primiparae in pregnancy. Br J Obstet Gynaecol 1998; 105: 293–299

39 Barbados Low-Dose Aspirin Study in Pregnancy (BLASP). A randomized trial for the prevention of pre-eclampsia and its complications. Br J Obstet Gynaecol 1998; 105: 286–292

40 Caritis SN, Sibai BM, Hauth J, Lindheimer MD, Klebanoff M, Thom E. Low-dose aspirin therapy for the prevention of preeclampsia in high-risk women. N Engl J Med 1998; 338: 701–705

41 Duley L, Smart DH, Knight M, King J. Antiplatelet drugs for prevention of pre-eclampsia and its consequences: systematic review. BMJ 2001; 322: 329–333

42 Knight M, Duley L, Henderson-Smart DJ, King JF. Antiplatelet agents for preventing and treating pre-eclampsia (Cochrane Review), in The Cochrane Library, Issue 1. Chichester, UK, John Wiley, 2004

43 Steyn DW, Odendaal HJ. Randomized controlled trial of Ketanserin and aspirin in prevention of pre-eclampsia. Lancet 1997; 350: 1267–1271

44 Kutteh WH. Antiphospholipid antibody associated recurrent pregnancy loss: treatment with heparin and low-dose aspirin is superior to low-dose aspirin alone. Am J Obstet Gynecol 1996; 174: 1584–1589

45 Kawasaki N, Matsui K, Masaharu I, Nakamura T, Yoshimura T, Hidetaka U. Effect of calcium supplementation on the vascular sensitivity to angiotensin II in pregnant women. Am J Obstet Gynecol 1985; 153: 576–582

46 Marya RK, Rathee S, Manrow M. Effect of calcium and vitamin D supplementation on toxemia of pregnancy. Gynaecol Obstet Invest 1987; 24: 38–42

47 Villar J, Repke JT, Belizan JM, Pareja G. Calcium supplementation reduces blood pressure during pregnancy: results of a randomized controlled clinical trial. Obstet Gynecol 1987; 70: 317–322

48 Lopez-Jaramillo P, Narvaez M, Weigel RM, Yepez R. Calcium supplementation reduces the risk of pregnancy-induced hypertension in an Andes population. Br J Obstet Gynaecol 1989; 96: 648–655

49 Lopez-Jaramillo P, Narvaez M, Felix C, Lopez A. Dietary calcium supplementation and prevention of pregnancy hypertension. Lancet 1990; 335: 293–295

50 Montanaro D, Boscutti G, Mioni G et al. Calcium supplementation decreases the incidence of pregnancy-induced hypertension (PIH) and preeclampsia. Presented at the Seventh World Congress of Hypertension in Pregnancy, 1990; Perugia, Italy. Abstract 91

51 Villar J, Repke JT. Calcium supplementation during pregnancy may reduce preterm delivery in high-risk populations. Am J Obstet Gynecol 1990; 163: 124–131

52 Belizan JM, Villar J, Gonzalez L, Campodonico L, Bergel E. Calcium supplementation to prevent hypertensive disorders of pregnancy. N Engl J Med 1991; 325: 1399–1405

53 Cong KJ, Chi SL, Liu CR. Calcium and pregnancy-induced hypertension. Am J Obstet Gynecol 1993; 28: 1–10

54 Sanchez-Ramos L, Briones DK, Kaunitz AM, Del Vale GO, Gandier FL, Walker DC. Prevention of pregnancy-induced hypertension by calcium supplementation in angiotensin II-sensitive patients. Obstet Gynecol 1994; 84: 349–353

55 Purwar M, Kulkarni H, Motghare V, Dhole S. Calcium supplementation and prevention of pregnancy-induced hypertension. J Obstet Gynaecol Res 1996; 22: 425–430

56 Lopez-Jaramillo P, Delgado F, Jacome P, Teran E, Ruano C, Rivera J. Calcium supplementation and the risk of preeclampsia in Ecuadorian pregnant teenagers. Obstet Gynecol 1997; 90: 162–167

57 Levine RJ, Hauth JC, Curt LB et al. Trial of calcium to prevent pre-eclampsia. N Engl J Med 1997; 337: 69–76

58 Herrera JA, Arevalo-Herrera M, Herrera S. Prevention of preeclampsia by linoleic and calcium supplementation: a randomized controlled trial. Obstet Gynecol 1998; 91: 585–590

59 Hofmeyr GJ, Roodt A, Atallah AN, Duleh L, Calcium supplementation to prevent preeclampsia-a systematic review. South Afr Med J 2003; 93: 224–228

60 Atallah AN, Hofmeyr GJ, Duley L. Calcium supplementation during pregnancy for preventing hypertensive disorders and related problems (Cochrane Review), in the Cochrane Library, Issue I, Chichester UK. John Willey, 2004

61 Nakatsuka M, Takata M, Tada K et al. Long term transdermal nitric oxide donors improves uteroplacentation in women with pre-eclampsia. J US Med 2002; 8: 831–836

62 Cacciatore B, Halmesmaki E, Kaaja R, Teramo K, Ylikorkala O. Effects of transdermal nitroglycerin on impedance to flow in the uterine, umbilical and fetal middle cerebral arteries in pregnancies complicated by pre-eclampsia and intrauterine growth retardation. Am J Obstet Gynecol 1998; 1: 140–145

63 Gulmezoglu AM, Hofmeyr GJ, Oosthuisen MMJ. Antioxidants in the treatment of severe pre-eclampsia: An explanatory randomized controlled trial. Br J Obstet Gynaecol 1997; 104: 689–696

64 Chappell LC, Seed PT, Briley AL et al. Effect of antioxidants on the occurrence of pre-eclampsia in women at increased risk: a randomized trial. Lancet 1999; 354: 810–816

65 Chappell LC, Seed PT, Kelly FJ et al. Vitamin C and E supplementation in women at risk of pre-eclampsia is associated with changes in indices of oxidative stress and placental function. Am J Obstet Gynecol 2002; 187: 777–784

66 Pressman EK, Cavanaught JL, Mingione M, Norkus EP, Woods JR. Effects of maternal antioxidant supplementation on maternal and fetal antioxidant levels: a randomized, double-blind study. Am J Obstet Gynecol 2003; 189: 1720–1725

67 Sharma JB, Kumar A, Kumar A et al. Effect of lycopene on pre-eclampsia and intra-uterine growth retardation in primigravidas. Int J Gynecol Obstet 2003; 81: 257–262

68 Han L, Zhou SM. Effects of selenium supplement on prevention of pregnancy-induced hypertension. Zhonghua Yi Xue Za Zhi 1993; 73: 647–648

69 Ziaei S, Hantoshzadeh S, Rezasoltani P, Lamyian M. The effect of garlic tablet on plasma lipids and platelet aggregation in nulliparous pregnants at high risk of preeclampsia. Eur J Obstet Gynecol Reprod Biol 2001; 99: 201–216

70 Holmes VA, Young IS, Maresh MJA, Pearson DWM, Walker JD, McCance DR. On behalf of the DAPIT Study Group. The Diabetes and Pre-eclampsia Intervention Trial. Int J Gynecol Obstet 2004; 87, 66–71

71 Sharma JB, Mittal S. Prevention of pre-eclampsia: Where do we stand? Int J Gynecol Obstet Ind 2006; In press

72 Greer IA. Pre-eclampsia matters. BMJ 2005; 330: 549–550

Charlotte L. Deans   Anselm Uebing   Philip J. Steer

Cardiac disease in pregnancy

The incidence of clinically significant cardiac disease in pregnancy is reported to be between 0.1–4%,[1,2] with an average in most studies of about 0.8%. Fifty years ago, when the first triennial maternal mortality report was published, 121 women died from cardiac causes; of these 85% had rheumatic heart disease and 25% died in labour. In the most recent report for 2000–2002, although mortality is now much lower overall, 44 women still died from heart disease related to pregnancy. It is now the second most common cause of death after psychiatric causes, more frequent even than those from the previous most common direct cause, thrombo-embolism (30 deaths).[3] In 1961–1963, deaths from congenital heart disease were reported for the first time and the mortality rate in this group has remained relatively constant over the years. Women with congenital lesions now account for 70–80% of patients with heart disease seen in pregnancy in the UK as the incidence of rheumatic heart disease has declined substantially in the industrialised world (although it is still a major scourge in non-industrialised countries). Moreover, as 0.8% of babies born have congenital heart defects and as surgical management is so much better than it was in the past, more women will be surviving into the reproductive age group over the next decade and beyond. Deaths from acquired heart disease appear to be increasing in parallel to the increasing rate of obesity and hypertension in the population, and advancing maternal age.

Charlotte L. Deans MBBS MRCOG (for correspondence)
Maternal Medicine Clinical Fellow, Chelsea and Westminster Hospital, 369 Fulham Road, London SW10 9NH, UK
E-mail: charlottedeans@hotmail.com

Anselm Uebing MD
Fellow in Adult Congenital Heart Disease, Royal Brompton Hospital, London, UK

Philip J. Steer BSc MB BS MD FRCOG
Professor of Obstetrics and Gynaecology, Chelsea and Westminster Hospital, 369 Fulham Road, London SW10 9NH, UK

This chapter aims to give an overview of both the general and lesion-specific principles of managing a patient with cardiac disease antenatally, on the labour ward and postnatally.

PHYSIOLOGICAL EFFECTS OF PREGNANCY ON THE CARDIOVASCULAR SYSTEM

Haemodynamic changes start early in pregnancy. By weeks 6–8, peripheral vasodilatation has lead to a fall in systemic vascular resistance and to compensate for this the cardiac output has increased by 20%. This is achieved mainly by an increase in stroke volume and, to a smaller extent, by an increase in heart rate. Cardiac output increases to about a maximum of 40% above non-pregnant values by 24–28 weeks and then plateaus, so it from this time onwards when the cardiac function will be maximally challenged. Patients with obstructive heart lesions such as aortic and mitral stenosis and co-arctation, will be less able to compensate for this extra work load and are, therefore, at particular risk of heart failure in pregnancy. Increased cardiac output also increases the risk of aortic root rupture in vulnerable patients (*e.g.* Marfan's syndrome, repaired co-arctation).

In labour, especially the second stage, there is additional stress to the cardiovascular system, when the sympathetic response to pain and uterine contractions produce a further increase in cardiac output, blood pressure and circulating volume. Hence, labour and delivery must be carefully planned and managed to avoid critical changes that could overwhelm the already compromised responses of patients with cardiac disease.

Postpartum, there are further changes to the circulating volume as immediate relief of inferior vena caval compression, and uterine contraction and retraction redistributes blood into the systemic circulation, and fluid is transferred from the extravascular spaces (oedema) back into the vascular compartment. Continued vigilance is required, especially with respect to fluid balance. Cardiac output returns to normal about 2 weeks after delivery.

RISKS TO THE MOTHER

Ideally, pre-pregnancy counselling should be available to all women with cardiac disease; this will include a thorough assessment of their non-pregnant cardiac status and a full and frank discussion of the potential risks of pregnancy. A woman's ability to cope with the additional strain of pregnancy will depend on the nature of the cardiac defect and presence or absence of risk factors, which include: (i) presence of cyanosis; (ii) pulmonary hypertension; (iii) left outflow tract obstructive lesions; (iv) previous peripartum cardiomyopathy; (v) impaired myocardial function; and (vi) poor functional class (New York Heart Association NYHA).

The risk of pregnancy-associated death needs to be addressed, and a statistical estimate of this outcome should be given to the woman and her family (together with an emphasis on the uncertainty of prediction – some women with a 50% risk will survive, and some women with a 1% risk will die). This discussion must be clearly documented in the notes. Therapeutic termination of pregnancy in women with a high risk of mortality (*e.g.*

Table 1 Approximate mortality rates associated with pregnancy

•	Entirely healthy woman	1 in 20,000
•	Average for population	1 in 10,000
•	Corrected Fallot's or similar	1 in 1000
•	Severe aortic stenosis	1 in 100
•	Pulmonary hypertension	1 in 3
•	Eisenmenger's complex	1 in 2

Adapted from Steer PJ. Pregnancy and contraception. In: Gatzoulis MA, Swan L, Therrien J, Pantely GA. (eds) Adult Congenital Heart Disease: a practical guide. Oxford: BMJ Publishing/Blackwell, 2005; 16–35.[4]

pulmonary hypertension either primary or Eisenmenger's syndrome, dilated cardiomyopathy, Marfan's syndrome with dilated aortic root and severe obstructive lesions) should also be offered (Table 1).

As well as the risk of death, pregnancy in women with cardiac disease is associated with significant morbidity including endocarditis, arrhythmias, paroxysmal embolic events, heart failure and pulmonary hypertension.

RISKS TO THE FETUS

Recurrence

In the general population, the incidence of structural cardiac defects is 0.8%. This is increased to 3–50% in babies of women with cardiac disease, depending on the defect.[5] Conditions such as Marfan's syndrome with autosomal dominant inheritance have a 50% risk of recurrence in the offspring, and left heart obstructive lesions have a higher recurrence rate than right-sided lesions. A nuchal translucency measurement taken at 11–13 weeks, in combination with maternal age and biochemistry, has an 85% sensitivity for detection of Downs' syndrome, with a false positive rate of 5%. In fetuses with a nuchal translucency > 95th centile, it is estimated that 2% will have a major cardiac defect.[6] In a recent study of over 8000 fetuses, those with a nuchal translucency of > 3.5 mm with normal chromosome analysis, 1 in 43 had a cardiac defect.[7] Cardiac anatomy is difficult to image reliably in the first trimester. However, moderate-to-severe lesions can be detected by fetal echocardiography at 14–16 weeks and 80% of major lesions will be detected at routine 20 week anomaly scanning. A particularly detailed fetal cardiac ultrasound is also recommended in women with congenital cardiac defects themselves, and this should be performed at 18–22 weeks by a specialist fetal cardiologist. Post-natally, babies should be examined carefully; repeat echocardiography or ultrasound is performed if there is any clinical suspicion of a defect.

There is a risk of intra-uterine growth restriction especially in women with cyanosis, left outflow obstruction, hyper- or hypotension and for those taking β-blockers. This may, in turn, lead to iatrogenic premature delivery and associated neonatal morbidity. Serial ultrasound growth measurements are necessary in such pregnancies. In lower risk patients, clinical assessment of the

Table 2 Cardiac drugs to be avoided

DRUGS TO BE AVOIDED	FETAL ADVERSE EFFECT
ACE inhibitors	Neonatal renal failure, IUGR, decreased skull ossification
Warfarin	Skeletal and CNS abnormalities. Intracranial haemorrhage
Amiodarone	Hypothyroidism, possible brain damage
Phenytoin	Cardiac and orofacial defects, IUGR
Spironolactone	Anomalies of external genitalia

DRUGS CONSIDERED RELATIVELY SAFE

Adenosine
Amiloride
β-Blockers
Calcium channel blockers
Digoxin
Flecainide
Heparin
Lidocaine

fundal height taken at each visit is probably sufficient, with ultrasound requested if growth restriction is suspected.

Fetal abnormalities

Fetal abnormalities are associated with certain medications likely to be used in this group of patients, for example anticoagulants (warfarin), ACE inhibitors, and certain anti-arrhythmic drugs (*e.g.* amiodarone). Table 2 lists commonly used drugs and their safety profile.

Antenatal management

A joint clinic with a multidisciplinary team consisting of an obstetrician, cardiologist, anaesthetist and specialist midwives is essential. Of the cardiac deaths reported to the Confidential Enquiry between 2000–2002, 40% were noted to have received substandard care. An appropriate model of care was recognised as crucial even in 1952 when the first Confidential Enquiry into Maternal Death report published the statement that 'all patients known or suspected to be suffering from heart disease should be referred for their care in pregnancy and confinement to a hospital where they can receive the necessary supervision'. This advice remains as pertinent today.

In a combined clinic setting, a comprehensive, detailed plan for antenatal and intrapartum care is discussed and documented. The level of risk and need for surveillance should be determined on an individual basis. Since most general obstetricians will only see a small number of patients with cardiac disease, referral to a specialist clinic for assessment of risk is advisable. Women with low-risk lesions such as mild or moderate regurgitation or isolated small septal defects, can be reviewed in these clinics either preconceptually or early in the pregnancy and a plan formulated for their care. Clear recommendations regarding her management are given to the woman, her family and all the care providers at the local hospital and primary care team where on-going antenatal surveillance and delivery may be appropriate. This assessment is also an opportunity to re-iterate general advice about dental hygiene and endocarditis prophylaxis, as, following discharge from paediatric services, some women with congenital defects may not have had any further specialist follow-up. Ideally, a preconception counselling service should be developed to bridge that gap. Antenatally, on-going communication with the specialist clinic should be available in case of any change or deterioration in the maternal or fetal condition.

Women seen by their GP or midwife at booking with a possible cardiac history or previously undiagnosed heart murmur can also be reviewed in this clinic and then referred for further investigations, or re-assured and discharged, as appropriate. Between 15–52% of cardiac abnormalities are first diagnosed during pregnancy[8] as this is often when women, especially from immigrant populations, first have contact with the healthcare system. It is, therefore, important that the careful examination of the heart and lungs in all pregnant women at booking is not overlooked. Benign soft ejection systolic flow murmurs are present in a about 80% of pregnant women and those of a low grade (for example no more than 1/6) are unlikely to be of any clinical significance. Referral for echocardiography would be indicated in women with a history of cardiac symptoms or surgery or when the past medical history is not known, as in women recently arrived in the UK. Women who have been brought up in the UK, who have had routine medicals without any abnormality being detected, who played normal games at school, who are asymptomatic, and have no more than a grade 1/6 mid-systolic murmur are unlikely to have a significant cardiac lesion.

Table 3 Classification of cardiac defects

LOW RISK
- Small ASD or VSDs
- Repaired defects with no cardiac dysfunction
- Mitral valve prolapse with no significant regurgitation
- Repaired co-arctation
- Repaired tetralogy of Fallot

MODERATE RISK
- Mitral stenosis
- Aortic stenosis
- Systemic right ventricle
- Mechanical prosthetic valves
- Large left to right shunt
- History of previous peripartum cardiomyopathy with no residual ventricular dysfunction
- Fontan type circulation

HIGH RISK
- Marfan's syndrome with aortic root dilatation or major valvular involvement
- Severe aortic stenosis
- Eisenmenger's syndrome and other pulmonary hypertension

Adapted from Siu S, Colman J. Heart disease and pregnancy. Heart 2001; 85: 710–715.

Women with moderate-to-severe lesions[9] should be cared for in a tertiary unit with a multidisciplinary team available 24 hours a day. Table 3 lists a classification system for severity of cardiac lesions and conditions.

Initial assessment of all women should include a thorough history, including all previous investigations and surgical procedures. Relevant information needed is:

- *age at diagnosis of defect*
- *previous surgery*
- *results of previous investigations, e.g. echo and ECG (copies for later comparison are useful)*
- *history of previous cardiac events (arrhythmias/ischaemic events, etc.)*
- *medication (previous/current)*
- *exercise tolerance (and prepregnancy comparison)*
- *history of palpitations/chest pain/syncope/oedema*
- *previous pregnancies and obstetric complications*
- *previous concurrent medical history, e.g. diabetes/hypercholesterolaemia*
- *smoking and alcohol consumption*
- *any family history of cardiac conditions.*

A full cardiovascular examination must be performed including pulse rate and rhythm, blood pressure (to the nearest 2 mmHg – see <http://www.bhsoc.org/Guidelines_how_to_measure_blood_pressure.htm>) heart sounds and grade of any murmur heard, and auscultation of lung bases.

These observations are the baseline for reference throughout the pregnancy where a change in murmur intensity, for example, can be the first sign of developing endocarditis.

A recent echocardiogram, ECG and arterial oxygen saturation (when indicated) are useful. Important features from an echo report and their implications are documented in Table 4. A chest X-ray with lead apron covering the maternal abdomen will expose the patient to < 0.001 rad (which is equivalent to 20 h air travel) and should be performed if necessary. Magnetic resonance imaging is also safe in pregnancy.

Subsequent visit frequency is individualised to each woman, but, in all, increased surveillance will be necessary. At each visit, direct questioning about symptoms such as breathlessness, palpitations and chest pain will alert the clinician to any deterioration. The pulse, blood pressure, heart sounds and chest examination are recorded at each visit. At Chelsea and Westminster Hospital, a specifically designed antenatal record sheet (Appendix 1) is inserted in the notes which highlights all these key aspects of care and acts as an aide memoir for the clinician.

Women need to be monitored especially carefully for any signs of pregnancy-induced hypertension and/or pre-eclampsia, as these conditions have a particularly adverse effect in women with structural cardiac lesions (for example, the vasoconstriction and coagulopathies associated with pre-eclampsia are particularly problematic). Women with ischaemic heart disease and pre-existing hypertension, with or without renal impairment, are at particularly increased risk. Anaemia and hyperthyroidism need to be

Table 4 Interpretation of echocardiography results

Measurement	Normal values	Measurement of special importance in:
DIMENSIONS		
Left ventricular end diastolic (LVEDD; cm)	4.0–5.2	• Left heart obstructive lesions (aortic diameter stenosis, HOCM)
Left ventricular end systolic diameter (LVESD; cm)	2.3–3.5	• Left heart regurgitant lesions (aortic regurgitation, mitral regurgitation)
		• Left ventricular dysfunction (cardiomyopathy)
Left ventricular shortening fraction (LVSF) %*	28–44	
Aortic valve annulus (cm)	1.6–2.6	• Marfan's syndrome
Sinus of valsalva (cm) #	2.2–3.6	• Tetralogy of Fallot and pulmonary atresia with ventricular septal defect
Sinotubular junction (cm)	2.8–2.6	• Bicuspid aortic valve with ascending aortopathy
Right ventricular outflow tract dimension from parasternal long-axis M-mode cm†	1.9–3.8	• Right heart regurgitant lesions (pulmonary regurgitation, tetralogy of Fallot after repair, tricuspid regurgitation, Ebstein's anomaly of the tricuspid valve)
		• Atrial septal defect
Left atrial diameter (cm)	2.7–4.0	• Mitral valve disease (stenosis and regurgitation)
		• Left ventricular dysfunction
Right atrial diameter (cm)	3.1–4.5	• Tricuspid valve disease (stenosis and regurgitation)
		• Pulmonary valve disease (pulmonary stenosis and regurgitation, tetralogy of Fallot)
Aortic valve are (cm²)*	> 1.5	Aortic valve stenosis
Mitral valve area (cm²)*	> 2	Mitral stenosis/rheumatic heart disease
PEAK FLOW VELOCITIES		
Right ventricular inflow (cm/s)	30–70	Tricuspid valve stenosis
Main pulmonary artery (cm/s)	60–90	• Pulmonary stenosis
		• Double chambered right ventricle
Left ventricular inflow (cm/s)	60–130	• Mitral valve stenosis
Left ventricular outflow/ ascending aorta (cm/s) (mmHg)*	100–170 (4–12)	• Aortic valve stenosis
		• HOCM

† As a result of the complex geometry of the right ventricle, reliable judgement of size and function of this heart chamber is difficult. In patients where right ventricular function is crucial (*e.g.* transposition of the great arteries after atrial switch operation, congenitally corrected transposition of the great arteries, tetralogy of Fallot, pulmonary hypertension) repeated echocardiography should alwaysbe performed by a single experienced investigator. The judgement of right ventricular size and function results from multi-view 2-dimensional echocardiography. The same applies for ventricular function of patients with complex congenital heart disease (*e.g.* functionally univentricular hearts etc.)

*left heart obstruction (mitral valve area <2 cm², aortic valve area <1.5 cm², left ventricular outflow tract peak Doppler gradient >30 mmHg prior to pregnancy) and ventricular dysfunction are established generic risk factors for adverse cardiac events (symptomatic arrhythmia, stroke, pulmonary oedema, overt heart failure or death) in pregnant women with heart disease.

#Pregancy is considered to carry a high risk for aortic dissection in women with Marfan's syndrome and an aortic diameter at sinus level >4 cm.

Normal values from: Feigenbaum H. Echocardiography, 4th edn. Philadelphia:Lea & Febiger, 1986; Chambers J. Echocardiography in primary care. New York:The Pantheon, 1996; and Walsh C and Wilde P. Practical Echocardiography. London:Greenwich Medical Media, 1999 recognised and treated promptly as they can precipitate or aggravate arrhythmias. Infections such as urinary tract infections need to be treated promptly and effectively if endocarditis is to be avoided.

In the event of preterm labour, β_2-agonists, such as ritodrine and salbutamol, are strictly contra-indicated because of their sympathomimetic side effects such as tachycardia, palpitations and hypotension. Atosiban, an oxytocin receptor antagonist, has fewer side effects and can be used with appropriate monitoring. Steroid administration for fetal lung maturity can also be used as a single course.

Intrapartum management

A plan for delivery needs to be agreed upon antenatally in the joint clinic and documented clearly in the notes. Obstetric risk factors are noted, the cardiologist makes an assessment of cardiac function and reserve, and analgesia is discussed with the anaesthetic consultant. A plan is formulated and, in our unit, a proforma is filled out and secured in the labour page of the patient's hand-held notes (Appendix 2).

Historically, delivery has often been recommended to be by caesarean section. However, the key objective is to avoid stressing the mother's cardiovascular system. Our experience suggests that this is most effectively done by allowing spontaneous labour, providing the best possible analgesia using regional blockade, and avoiding maternal bearing down by performing an instrumental delivery. Caesarean section is associated with a higher risk of haemorrhage, infection and deep vein thrombosis. However, emergency caesareans do pose a higher risk than elective caesareans, and every effort should be made to reduce their impact, either by performing an elective section when vaginal birth is in any way contra-indicated, or by intervening early in cases of slow progress or fetal compromise. With careful monitoring and adherence to suggested guidelines, vaginal delivery poses fewer risks to the woman. Appropriate levels of monitoring are decided antenatally and most women with even mild heart disease should be monitored throughout labour using ECG and oxygen saturation monitors. Blood pressure monitoring with automated external devices can be unreliable in pregnancy, and, moreover, cease to give a reading when maternal cardiac output falls to a low level. Thus, we prefer to use an intra-arterial line which is relatively simple and quick to set up and produces an accurate measure of blood pressure under all conditions. In more severe cases, invasive blood pressure and central venous pressure monitoring can also be useful if substantial blood loss is anticipated. Continuous electronic fetal monitoring is recommended: assessment of fetal condition is not only vital in itself, but can also be an important indicator of uterine perfusion and, therefore, indirectly of maternal cardiac status. Particular attention should be paid to the fetal heart rate patterns of those babies identified antenatally as growth restricted.

Regional block is nowadays almost always performed using a slow, incremental, low-dose, epidural blockade. This minimises changes in peripheral resistance and blood pressure and allows the woman's cardiac output to keep up with the relatively slow rate of change in demand. Considerable caution should be used when employing a spinal blockade, as hypotension can be quite acute, resulting in destabilisation of the maternal condition. Some have advocated the use of ephedrine epidural which has minimal cardiovascular effects and, therefore, can be used safely to avoid hypotension, but there are some conditions (notably the arrhythmogenic right ventricle) in which ephedrine is contra-indicated because of its effect to increase myocardial excitability.

Induction of labour is considered for the usual obstetric indications. If Syntocinon is needed to augment labour, we recommend that the concentration of Syntocinon infused be doubled compared with the standard dilutions used (that is, 10 U of Syntocinon in a litre of Hartmann's solution rather than 5 U) and the infusion rate halved, to reduce the volume of fluids given. A long, protracted labour should be avoided and, therefore, a close eye should be kept on the partogram and signs of obstructed labour identified early. In patients with limited cardiac reserve, a time limit for bearing down in the second stage should be set antenatally. In severe disease (*e.g.* aortic or pulmonary stenosis), an elective lift-out forceps with no maternal effort performed in theatre is recommended. In mild-to-moderate cases, a shortened and bearing down period of 20–30 min may be appropriate before an assisted delivery is undertaken.

Antibiotic prophylaxis for endocarditis is not considered necessary if the woman has a spontaneous vaginal delivery, unless she has artificial heart valves or has had endocarditis previously. However, it is recommended for all women with a structural defect requiring an instrumental or operative delivery, and also if an extensive or third degree tear occurs, or if the placenta requires manual removal. Current recommendations for prophylaxis are 1 g of amoxicillin and 120 mg of gentamicin intravenously immediately after the delivery (in theatre) followed by an oral 5-day course of ampicillin. Vancomycin or teicoplanin can be used in patients allergic to penicillin.

Careful management of the third stage is also very important. It is easy to breathe a sigh of relief after the successful delivery of a healthy baby and then underestimate the implications of the haemodynamic changes that occur afterwards. An increase in circulating volume as the uterus retracts and blood redistributes from the placental bed back into the main circulation predisposes the patient to overload. Syntocinon has unpredictable effects on blood pressure; and both hyper- and hypotensive changes can occur. For example, a 50% reduction in blood pressure has been reported following the bolus injection of 10 U of Syntocinon. Moreover, because of its antidiuretic properties, in large doses it is associated with fluid retention and pulmonary oedema. In our unit, Syntocinon is administered as a slow infusion (8–12 mU/min over a minimum of 4 h) rather than as a bolus. At caesarean section, removal of the placenta by controlled cord traction is recommended. It is also not advisable to remove the placenta rapidly, as this can cause major changes in blood pressure either from circulatory overload following accelerated contraction and retraction of the uterus, or from sudden blood loss leading to under filling of the circulation. Haemorrhage secondary to atony can be dealt with using β-lynch uterine compression sutures at caesarean or insertion of a Cook's balloon catheter after vaginal delivery. This avoids the use and possible side effects of oxytocics. Prostaglandins also have adverse cardiovascular effects. Hemabate (prostaglandin F2α) can cause systemic and pulmonary hypertension and should be avoided. Misoprostol 1 mg per rectum is useful to control haemorrhage but can also cause hypotension and, rarely, hyperpyrexia. Clearly, a massive obstetric haemorrhage can be life-threatening; therefore, all measures should be used appropriately according to the benefit and risk assessment made by the consultant obstetrician and anaesthetist at the time.

Specialist midwives attached to the joint clinic play an important role in the antenatal preparation of these women for labour and their intrapartum and postnatal high-dependency care. However, even if labour is progressing normally and a spontaneous vaginal delivery is expected, it must be remembered by the labour ward team that these women have a serious medical condition which can be labile and unpredictable. Very close surveillance must always be maintained. In an emergency situation such as maternal collapse, cardiac causes (*e.g.* arrhythmias) as well as the usual obstetric ones must be quickly considered.

Postpartum

The patient should be monitored in a high-dependency setting. Management in the immediate postpartum period aims to avoid significant changes in the blood volume and blood pressure.[5] It is important that a strict input/output chart is maintained and caution must be taken with fluid replacement, especially blood transfusion (which is liable to cause circulatory overload unless diuretics are also given). Vaginal and surgical drain loss should be watched closely and vigilance for secondary postpartum haemorrhage maintained. Return to the postnatal ward should be delayed for 48–72 h depending on the individual patient. Postnatal care in the high dependency unit and the length of stay should be discussed antenatally and documented clearly.

Thromboprophylaxis with low molecular weight heparin is recommended until the patient is fully mobile. Most cardiac medications are safe with breastfeeding, except for some β-blockers, such as sotalol or propanolol, which can cause fetal bradycardia.[4] Liaison with neonatologists is recommended, especially if the baby is premature or growth restricted. Women should be reviewed daily and discharged by a senior obstetrician. A follow-up postnatal appointment for the joint clinic should be made at 6–8 weeks.

Contraception

Contraceptive advice is needed from adolescence onwards, and the implications of an unplanned pregnancy in an unprepared cardiac patient should be discussed with all young adults with congenital heart disease. Barrier methods of contraception are unreliable and the combined contraceptive pill is contra-indicated in all conditions where thrombosis (*e.g.* atrial fibrillation, pulmonary hypertension and cyanotic heart disease) and paradoxical embolism (atrial septal defect) are a risk. Progesterone-only preparations have a better side-effect profile and long-acting, slow-release preparations, such as implanon and the Mirena intra-uterine system (IUS), have improved efficacy compared to oral preparations. Insertion of a Mirena coil should be performed in a hospital environment with full anaesthetic support as the vaso-vagal response to cervical dilatation is unpredictable. Pre-insertion screening for genito-urinary infection is recommended as is endocarditis prophylaxis to cover the insertion procedure. Sterilisation may be considered if the couple have decided that they never want children or that their family is complete. Laparoscopic clip sterilisation carries greater risks compared to a vasectomy; however, it is recognised that women with serious defects have a shortened life-expectancy and the partner may wish to preserve his fertility to have a family in the future.

INDIVIDUAL DEFECTS

Left-to-right shunt lesions

Atrial and ventricular septal defects and patent ductus arteriosus are the three most common cardiac lesions seen at birth and make up 50% of congenital heart defects.[12] These are usually well tolerated in pregnancy[9,10] as the volume overload associated with increased cardiac output is counteracted by the decrease in peripheral vascular resistance. If no pulmonary hypertension is present and ventricular function is good, then pregnancy and labour are well tolerated. Potential problems are development of arrhythmias, ventricular dysfunction and development of pulmonary hypertension which can occur in larger defects. In women with unoperated atrial septal defects, there is also a risk of thrombo-embolic events which can lead to systemic events if there is a transient reversal of flow due to systemic vasodilatation and/or elevation in pulmonary resistance. Some authors recommend low-dose aspirin in these patients.[11] Echocardiography should be performed to exclude regurgitant lesions and assess ventricular function.

Co-arctation of the aorta

Co-arctation is a stenosis in the aortic arch usually at or distal to the site of the ductus arteriosus. It accounts for 7% of congenital heart lesions and is common in Turner's syndrome (up to 25%).[12] An associated bicuspid aortic valve is present in up to 85% together with associated anomalies of the head and neck vessels and aneurysm formation. The risk of aortic dissection and rupture is small, probably no more than 1%.

Most women will have had surgical repair in childhood. Long-term sequelae of this condition include hypertension and accelerated atherosclerotic disease. Management in pregnancy aims to control the blood pressure but to be mindful of the fact that pressures will be lower distal to the co-arctation. This may compromise placental perfusion and so fetal growth should be monitored carefully. Endocarditis prophylaxis is necessary.

Tetralogy of Fallot

This is the most common form of cyanotic heart disease which is characterised by four features – a ventricular septal defect, subvalvular pulmonary stenosis, overriding aorta and secondary right ventricular hypertrophy. In uncorrected cyanotic heart disease such as tetralogy of Fallot, the physiological changes in pregnancy will increase the right-to-left shunt and, therefore, increase the degree of hypoxaemia. Fetal risks are proportional to the level of cyanosis and there is an associated increase in fetal loss, prematurity and low birth weight.[13] Maternal oxygen saturations less than 85% result in a live birth rate of 12% compared to saturations > 90% producing a 92% live birth rate.[14] Maternal complications associated with cyanosis and subsequent increased haemoglobin concentration are thrombosis (including paradoxical emboli) and impaired renal function. In women with corrected Fallots and underlying good cardiac function, the risk of pregnancy is low, but right heart failure and arrhythmias are still potential hazards. Endocarditis prophylaxis is required.

Of patients with tetralogy of Fallot, 15% have a microdeletion of chromosome 22q11 known as the diGeorge syndrome or catch 22 (cardiac defect, abnormal facies, thymic hypoplasia, cleft palate and hypocalcaemia). There is an autosomal dominant inheritance pattern and preconception counselling should involve genetic screening if the patient is suspected of this diagnosis.

Marfan's syndrome

Marfan's syndrome is an autosomal, dominant, genetic condition with variable penetrance. The underlying pathology is an abnormality of elastic tissue. Aortic root dilatation and valvular (commonly mitral valve) prolapse and regurgitation can occur. These complications are increased in pregnancy due to the additional haemodynamic stress. A study of 45 pregnancies showed no increase in obstetric complications in women with a normal aortic root diameter (< 3.7 cm for adults) and no significant changes in echocardiographic data. An aortic root diameter > 4.0 cm or previous aortic root surgery was associated with dissection[15] and these risk factors need to be identified and discussed preconceptually. β-Blockade is recommended antenatally, as well as serial echocardiographic assessments.[9]

Endocarditis prophylaxis is required if there is mitral valve prolapse with regurgitation, and after surgical repair.[19]

Transposition of the great arteries

In patients with complete transposition of the great arteries, the right atrium connects to the right ventricle but this gives rise to the aorta, and the left atrium connects to the left ventricle which gives rise to the pulmonary artery. This situation is potentially lethal, so nearly all patients will have undergone surgical correction. This can be performed by creating an atrial connection (Mustard or Senning procedure) to re-direct blood from the right to left atrium then via the mitral valve to the left ventricle and to the connecting pulmonary artery; in the opposite direction, oxygenated blood from the left atrium is re-directed through the tricuspid valve to the right ventricle and out of the aorta to the body. This means that the right ventricle has to support the systemic circulation. An alternative is to perform an arterial switch so the pulmonary artery and aorta are switched position to re-instate 'normal' anatomy. Congenitally corrected transposition is rare but also creates a systemic right ventricle. This ventricle is less able to cope with the demands of the increased work load in pregnancy and dysfunction and failure can occur. When surgery has been performed in the atrial region, the sino-atrial node can be affected resulting in arrhythmias and atrioventricular heart block.[16–18]

Valvular heart disease

Generally, regurgitant lesions are better tolerated in pregnancy than stenotic lesions. This is because resistance to flow in stenotic lesions increases geometrically as cardiac output rises, whereas the proportion of regurgitation in women with regurgitant lesions increases only proportionately as cardiac output goes up. Pregnancy in women with mitral and aortic valve stenosis are associated with an increase in maternal morbidity and adverse fetal outcomes.[17] Mitral valve stenosis is the commonest rheumatic valvar lesion. It is classified according to the valve area – mild stenosis is when the valve area is < 4 cm^2 but > 1.5 cm^2; moderate 1.5–1 cm^2 and severe < 1 cm^2 (normal is 4–6 cm^2). Pregnancy hyperdynamic circulatory changes cause: (i) an increase in left atrial pressure; (ii) increased risk of atrial fibrillation; and (iii) left heart failure with pulmonary oedema.[18] Aortic stenosis is most commonly due to a congenital bicuspid aortic valve and this restricts the woman's ability to increase cardiac output, leading to increased left ventricular pressures which can precipitate heart failure or ischaemia.[9] In severe symptomatic cases (gradient across the valve > 50 mmHg according to the American Heart Association classification), antenatal balloon valvuloplasty may be necessary. Bypass surgery should be avoided if possible as it carries a 30% risk of fetal death,[19,28] although this can be reduced to about 10% if hypothermia is not used. Women with severe lesions should be counselled preconceptually and should not plan to become pregnant until after surgical correction. Endocarditis prophylaxis is required.

Pulmonary stenosis, if severe, can also be associated with right heart failure and atrial dilatation leading to arrhythmias.

Mitral valve prolapse is present in 12–17% of women of childbearing age[20] and rarely gives rise to any cardiovascular complications. If it is found in isolation and is asymptomatic and mild, no particular precautions are necessary in pregnancy other than recommendations for endocarditis prophylaxis. Occasionally, prolapse may suddenly become much worse, in which case management as for mitral regurgitation becomes necessary.

Pregnancy with replacement heart valves

The likelihood of thrombosis increases 6-fold in pregnancy, and 11-fold in the puerperium. Thus, the risk of increased thrombo-embolic events in women with mechanical heart valves in pregnancy is dramatically increased. Bioprosthetic (pig or human cadaver) valves are, therefore, recommended for women of child-bearing age[21] to avoid the complications and fetal risks associated with the anticoagulant therapy needed for mechanical valves. The most effective anticoagulant from the cardiac point of view is warfarin, but warfarin crosses the placenta and can lead not only to embryopathy (facial and skeletal dysmorphism, cardiac defects, and intra-uterine growth restriction) but also to a high rate of fetal loss and placental haemorrhage. Selecting a safe and adequate anticoagulation regimen in pregnancy remains a challenge. Intravenous heparin is difficult to manage in pregnancy but the efficacy of subcutaneous low molecular weight heparin in preventing valve thrombosis still needs clarifying. A recent review of women given low molecular weight heparin found 8.6% had valve thrombosis.[29] It may be possible to reduce the level of risk by using doses even higher than those usually used to treat vein thrombosis, and such an approach requires monitoring of anti-factor Xa levels (level should be a minimum of 1.0 U/ml) to decrease the incidence of thrombo-embolic events. Fortunately, the use of warfarin in the puerperium is less problematic. Warfarin is safe in breastfeeding and can be recommenced immediately postpartum.

Rhythm disorders

Pregnancy can precipitate or exacerbate arrhythmias and the risk is relatively higher during labour and delivery. Management of arrhythmias is similar to that in the non-pregnant state. Conservative measures such as the avoidance of stimulants (for example, caffeine and alcohol) are recommended. Drug treatment is indicated when women are symptomatic and, fortunately, almost all commonly used anti-arrhythmic medications are safe. Exceptions are sotalol, which can be associated with fetal growth restriction (careful monitoring of fetal growth is necessary when this drug is used), and amiodarone which can cause neonatal hypothyroidism and should be avoided. Electrical cardioversion is generally safe in unstable patients in pregnancy,[22] although there is one case report in which the cardioversion appears to have caused the uterus to contract, with the resulting fetal bradycardia.

Eisenmenger's syndrome and pulmonary hypertension

Pulmonary hypertension is defined as any elevation of mean pulmonary artery pressure greater than 25 mmHg at rest or 30 mmHg with exercise. It can be primary (an idiopathic, rare condition) or secondary to a number of cardiac, respiratory and embolic causes. Both types are high risk in pregnancy. Pulmonary hypertension develops due to either increased pulmonary blood flow or damage to the pulmonary arterioles. In patients with cardiac defects, the most common causes are a large ventricular septal defect, as well as a patent ductus arteriosus and atrial septal defects. Eisenmenger's syndrome occurs when the increased pulmonary vascular blood flow produces a right-sided pressure greater than the left side and hence a reversal of the shunt; subsequently, cyanosis develops. This condition is associated with a 30–50% maternal mortality. Management involves anticoagulation, avoiding increases in pulmonary vascular resistance, and maintaining right ventricular preload and left and right ventricular contractility.[23] Therapy includes vasodilatation with calcium antagonists and reduction of pulmonary vascular resistance by nasally administered domiciliary oxygen. Intravenous prostacyclin and inhaled nitric oxide can are also used in more severe cases to dilate the pulmonary vasculature.

Cardiomyopathy

Cardiomyopathy is divided into two groups – conditions that predate pregnancy (hypertrophic, dilated and restrictive cardiomyopathy) and peripartum cardiomyopathy. Eight deaths attributable to cardiomyopathy were reported to in the 2000–2002 Confidential Enquiry. All were postpartum, and four were diagnosed as due to peripartum cardiomyopathy. The authors of the Confidential Enquiry concluded that peripartum cardiomyopathy is more common in older, obese multiparous women with hypertension. The diagnosis should be suspected when tachycardia, dyspnoea or pulmonary oedema develop in the context of these risks factors in the months following delivery. Management involves investigations for, and exclusion of, infectious, metabolic and toxic causes. Thrombo-embolic complications have been reported in as many as 50% of cases[23] and fatal arrhythmias and heart failure can also occur. Treatment with immunosuppressive therapy has been used, resulting in improved clinical features and ventricular function.[24] Mortality rates are high (25–50%). There is a high rate of recurrence of peripartum cardiomyopathy, and these women should probably be recommended to avoid pregnancy in future, although the risk may be lower if they appear to recover fully. However, women with long-standing cardiomyopathy who tolerated pregnancy well are probably likely to do equally well in another pregnancy. Detailed echocardiography is an important tool and assessment of left ventricular dysfunction at the time of diagnosis has prognostic value with regards to recovery of cardiac function.[25]

Ischaemic heart disease

Physiological changes in pregnancy increase the myocardial oxygen demand; although acute myocardial infarction is rare in pregnancy, it results in significant maternal and fetal morbidity and mortality when it does occur. Chronic hypertension with or without superimposed pre-eclampsia and diabetes are associated risk factors. The trend to delay child bearing until the thirties or even forties, advancing maternal age, compounded by increasing obesity and higher rates of smoking amongst young women are all factors that could lead to atherosclerotic complications being seen more commonly in pregnancy. Severe hypertensive disease in pregnancy confers an increased risk of development of ischaemic heart later in life, so dietary and life-style changes and on-going surveillance is recommended for these patients.[26] Coronary artery dissection is a rare complication but a major common cause of death if there is myocardial infarction in pregnancy.[3] Coronary artery spasm can be provoked by the use of prostaglandins and ritodrine, so these medications should be avoided in women with known ischaemic heart disease. It is also important not to underestimate the implications of a high systolic blood pressure even in the presence of a normal range diastolic value.

Treatment of acute myocardial infarction is the same as for the non-pregnant patient, and successful coronary angioplasty has been reported. Successful thrombolysis has also been reported[27] although there are risks of placental abruption and neonatal intracranial haemorrhage.[28]

SUMMARY

Cardiac disease in pregnancy kills more women than thrombo-embolism. Management of moderate-to-severe lesions needs to be in a combined clinic with an on-going multidisciplinary approach to care.

KEY POINTS FOR CLINICAL PRACTICE

- Thorough history and full cardiovascular examination of all women with previous cardiac symptoms, especially those recently arrived in the UK.

- Identification of risk factors and referral to specialist centre where appropriate.

- Full counselling concerning risks associated with pregnancy.

- Mortality is relatively rare but women are also at risk of morbidity from heart failure, arrhythmias and thrombo-embolic events.

- Fetal surveillance for recurrence of congenital heart disease, and growth restriction, is needed.

- Antibiotic prophylaxis for endocarditis should be used for all women at risk unless they have a normal uncomplicated vaginal delivery.

References

1 Siu SC, Sermer M, Colman JM *et al*. Prospective multicentre study of pregnancy outcomes in women with heart disease. Circulation 2001; 104: 515–521
2 McFaul PB, Dornan JC, Lamki H, Boyle D. Pregnancy complicated by maternal heart disease. A review of 519 women. Br J Obstet Gynaecol 1988; 95: 861–867
3 Lewis G, Drife JO. Why Mothers Die 2000–2002. The Sixth Report of Confidential Enquiries into Maternal and Child Health. London: RCOG Press, 2004
4 Steer PJ. Pregnancy and contraception. In: Gatzoulis MA, Swan L, Therrien J, Pantely GA. (eds) Adult Congenital Heart Disease: a practical guide. Oxford: BMJ Publishing/Blackwell, 2005; 16–35
5 Uebing A, Steer PJ, Yentis SM, Gatzoulis MA Pregnancy and congenital heart disease. BMJ 2006; 332(7538): 401–406
6 Hyett J, Perdu M, Sharland G *et al*. Using fetal nuchal translucency to screen for major congenital cardiac defects at 10–14 weeks gestation. BMJ 1999; 318: 81–85
7 Bahado-Singh RO, Wapner R, Thom E *et al*. Elevated first-trimester nuchal translucency increases the risk of congenital heart defects. Am J Obstet Gynecol 2005; 192: 1357–1361
8 Gei AF, Hankins GD. Cardiac disease and pregnancy. Obstet Gynecol Clin North Am 2001; 28: 465–512
9 Siu SC, Colman J. Congenital heart disease. Heart 2001; 85: 710–715
10 Shime J, Mocarski E, Hastings D *et al*. Congenital heart disease in pregnancy: short and long term implications. Am J Obstet Gynecol 1987; 156: 313–322
11 Klein LL, Galan HL. Cardiac disease in pregnancy. Obstet Gynecol Clin North Am 2004; 31: 429–459
12 Gatzoulis M, Swan L, Thierrien J, Pantley GA. Adult Congenital Heart Disease: a practical guide. Oxford:BMJ publishing/Blackwell, 2005
13 Whittemore R, Hobbins JC, Engle MA. Pregnancy and its outcome in women with and without surgical treatment of congenital heart disease. Am J Cardiol 1982; 50: 641–651
14 Presbiteo P, Somerville J, Stone S *et al*. Pregnancy in cyanotic congenital heart disease. Outcome of mother and fetus. Circulation 1994; 89: 2673–2676
15 Rossiter JP, Repke JT, Morales AJ *et al*. A prospective longitudinal evaluation of pregnancy in the Marfan syndrome. Am J Obstet Gynecol 1995; 173: 1599–1606
16 Thierrien J, Barnes I, Somerville J. Outcome of pregnancy in patients with congenitally corrected transposition of the great arteries. Am J Cardiol 1999; 84: 820–824
17 Malhotra M, Sharma JB, Tripathii R, Arora P, Arora R. Maternal and fetal outcome in valvular heart disease. Int J Gynaecol Obstet 2004; 84: 11–16
18 Desai DK, Adanlawo M, Naidoo DP *et al*. Mitral stenosis in pregnancy: a four year

experience at King Edward VIII Hospital, Durban, South Africa. Br J Obstet Gynaecol 2000; 107: 953–958

19 Chambers CE, Clark SL. Cardiac surgery during pregnancy. Clin Obstet Gynecol 1994; 37: 316–323

20 Savage DD, Garrison RJ, Devereux RB *et al.* Mitral valve prolapse in the general population. 1. Epidemiologic features : the Framingham Study. Am Heart J 1983; 106: 571–576

21 Mihaljevic T, Paul S, Leacche M, Rawn JD, Cohn LH, Byrne JG. Valve replacement in women of childbearing age : influences on mother, fetus and neonate. J Heart Valve Dis 2005; 14: 151–157

22 Gowda RM, Khan IA, Mehta NJ *et al.* Cardiac arrhythmias in pregnancy : clinical and therapeutic considerations. Int J Cardiol 2003; 88: 129–133

23 Van Mook WNKA, Peeters L. Severe cardiac disease in pregnancy, part II: impact of congenital and acquired cardiac diseases during pregnancy. Curr Opin Crit Care 2005; 11: 435–448

24 Midei MG, DeMent SH, Feldman AM *et al.* Peripartum myocarditis in peripartum cardiomyopathy. Circulation 1990; 81: 922–928

25 Chapa JB, Heiberger HB, Weinert L, Decara J, Lang RM, Hibbard JU. Prognostic value of echocardiography in peripartum cardiomyopathy. Obstet Gynecol 2005; 105: 1303–1308

26 Wikstrom AK, Haglund B, Olvosson M, Lindeberg SN. The risk of maternal ischaemic heart disease after gestational hypertensive disease. Br J Obstet Gynaecol 2005; 112: 1486–1491

27 Schumacher B, Belfort MA, Card RJ. Successful treatment of acute myocardial infarction during pregnancy with tissue plasminogen activator. Am J Obstet Gynecol 1997; 176: 716–719

28 Roth A, Elkayam U. Acute myocardial infarction associated with pregnancy. Ann Intern Med 1996; 125: 751–762

29 Oran B, Lee-Parritz A, Ansell J. Low molecular weight heparin for the prophylaxis of thromboembolism in women with prosthetic mechanical heart valves during pregnancy. Thromb Haemost 2004; 92: 747–751

Antenatal records for women with cardiac disease

Name: Cardiac lesion
S/B cardiologist   S/B Anaesthetist
Fetal cardiac scan   Fetal anomaly scan

EDD: Delivery plan:

Date						
Gestation						
SOB						
Palpitations						
Other symptoms						
BP						
Pulse rate						
Pulse rhythm						
Murmur						
Lung bases						
Oedema						
SFH						
Presentation						
5ths palp						
FH						
Urine						
Next appt						
Signature						

Abbreviations: S/B seen by; EDD, estimated date of delivery; SOB, short of breath; BP, blood pressure; SFH, symphysis-fundal height; appt, appointment.

APPENDIX 2

Joint Cardiac Obstetric Service (JCOS) management plan for delivery

Cardiac diagnosis...

Please circle agreed plan and tick box when actioned:

If admitted to labour ward, Please inform:

Obstetrician on call   Consultant/registrar

Anaesthetist on call   Consultant/registrar

Cardiac team   Y/N

Antenatal admission: From .... weeks

Mode of delivery: Elective lower caesarean section/trial of vaginal delivery

CAESAREAN SECTION:
    Anaesthetic technique: epidural/spinal/general/other
    Maternal monitoring: ECG/SaO$_2$/non-invasive BP/invasive BP/CVP
    3rd stage: Prophylactic compression suture/Syntocinon 5 U over 10–20 min
               /Syntocinon – low-dose infusion (8–12 mU/min)

Vaginal delivery 1st stage
    HDU chart/TEDS in labour/medication to be continued ....
    Prophylactic antibiotics: Elective/if operative delivery
    Epidural for analgesia: none/when requested/as soon as in established labour
    Comments re anaesthetic ....
    Maternal monitoring: ECG/SaO$_2$/non-invasive BP/invasive BP/CVP

Vaginal delivery 2nd stage
    Normal second stage/short second stage (then assist if not delivered within
    maximum min pushing)/elective assisted delivery only

Vaginal delivery 3rd stage
    Normal active management (oxytocin and CCT)/Syntocinon infusion 8–12 mU/min
    Continue Syntocinon infusion ...... h

Post delivery
    High Dependency Unit (min stay .... h)/LMW heparin (duration ......)
    Other drugs postpartum ....

Please inform the consultant obstetrician on call if there is departure from planned management or if new clinical situations develop.

Delivery management plan for women with cardiac disease. Courtesy of High Risk Obstetric Team, Chelsea & Westminster Hospital, London, UK. ECG, electrocardiogram; SaO$_2$, oxygen saturation; BP, blood pressure; CVP, central venous pressure; HDU, high dependency unit; TEDS, thrombo-embolic deterrent stockings; CCT, controlled cord traction; LMW, low molecular weight heparin.

Alok Ash

High-dependency care in obstetrics

High-dependency care may be required for the pregnant woman who becomes sick or for the sick woman who becomes pregnant.[1] Pregnancy and childbirth is a physiological process and, in the majority of the women, proceeds uneventfully. However, in a small proportion, it can pose major health risks, the most extreme of which is maternal mortality. Traditionally, maternal mortality has been used as a measure of the success of obstetric intervention, but is now too rare to reflect accurately the quality of obstetric care in the industrialised world, with only < 1% of about half a million maternal deaths occurring every year world-wide.[2] Death only represents the tip of a morbidity iceberg the size of which is unknown (Fig. 1). There are approximately 118 life-threatening events of 'near-miss mortality' or severe acute maternal morbidity (SAMM) for each maternal death.[3] According to a recent World Health Organization (WHO) systematic review, the global prevalence of SAMM (defined as severe life-threatening obstetric complication necessitating an urgent medical intervention in order to prevent likely death of the mother) varies from 0.01% to 8.23%, with an inverse trend with the development status of the country.[4] It is suggested that SAMM on its own[5] or as a ratio of SAMM:mortality[3] should be used as a quality indicator of maternity care. It is these 'near misses' or SAMMs that require high-dependency care.

WHAT IS HIGH-DEPENDENCY CARE?

A UK Department of Health (DH) document[6] defines high-dependency care as a level of care between that on a general ward and on an intensive care unit (ICU). Such care involves the monitoring and support of patients requiring

Alok Ash MBBS MD(Cal) FRCOG
Consultant Obstetrician, Guy's and St Thomas's Hospital NHS Foundation Trust, and Honorary Senior Lecturer, King's College London, Consultants' Office, 10th Floor, North Wing, St Thomas's Hospital, Lambeth Palace Road, London SE1 7EH, UK
E-mail: Alok.Ash@gstt.nhs.uk

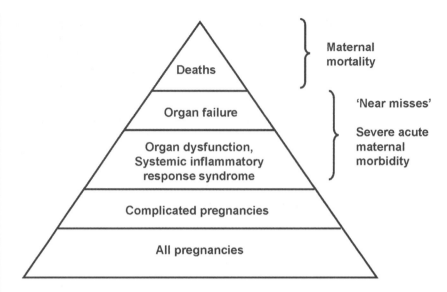

Fig. 1 Diagrammatic sequence of events from a normal healthy pregnancy through 'near misses' to death in a pregnant population (not in proportion). Adapted with the permission of the Royal College of Obstetricians and Gynaecologists and Professor RC Pattinson from Mantel *et al.* Severe acute maternal morbidity: a pilot study of a definition for a near-miss. *J Obstet Gynaecol* 1998; **105**: 985–990.

only basic respiratory support or the support of only one other organ system with acute or acute-on-chronic single organ failure, and 'step-up' or 'step-down' support between levels of care. However, procedures like intubation with mechanical ventilation for advanced respiratory support, invasive investigations and monitoring (beyond central venous and long arterial lines), or multiple organ support are usually not the remit of high-dependency care. Patients should be admitted to the ICU should these be necessary.

BACKGROUND

Obstetric ICUs and high-dependency units (HDUs) are a relatively recent phenomenon. In the UK, although *Confidential Enquiry into Maternal Deaths* (CEMD) dates back to 1952, it was not until the 1988–1990 report[7] that the need for a 'properly equipped, staffed and supervised high-dependency care area in every consultant obstetric unit' had been highlighted. The subsequent enquiries[8–10] report 35–53% of all direct and indirect maternal deaths involved (or needed) intensive care and emphasise the lack of, and a need for, on-site ICU facilities.

The principles behind the pathogenesis and treatment of critical care illness began to take shape in the 1980s. In the UK, joint training posts in critical care medicine were introduced in 1986.[11] In the US, in 1988, the Society for Critical Care Medicine promulgated the definitions and established the guidelines for the design and staffing of ICUs. The evolution of critical care in obstetrics has followed this development generally.[12–14] While critical care concept and need were being highlighted, spiralling medical costs prompted an evaluation of intensive care use in general. The concept of intermediate care was proposed for patients who did not require intensive care *per se*, but who needed more care than could be provided on a general ward.[15,16]

Since late 1980s and early 1990s, dedicated obstetric intensive care has become well established in some maternity units in the US,[12] South Africa,[17] and The Netherlands.[18] A UK national survey conducted in 1994 found that only 41% of maternity units had designated obstetric HDU beds and 19% did not have an ICU on site.[19] Until 2003, only about half a dozen centres in the US[20] have reported a fully operational, designated, obstetric ICU. In the UK, by January 2002, increasing numbers of the nationally available 1319 HDU beds were to be found in obstetric units.[11]

WHY A DEDICATED OBSTETRIC HDU?

Several policy documents[21-23] and successive CEMDs[8-10] recommend the provision of a specially designated obstetric HDU on-site. The availability of a dedicated HDU within an obstetric setting has a number of potential advantages:

1. Altered maternal physiology, the presence of a fetus and diseases specific to pregnancy pose various challenges in providing care to critically ill obstetric patients. Medical conditions might present risk to the pregnancy and pregnancy may modify the disease state. Drug therapy may be affected by altered pharmacokinetics, or have impact on the developing fetus. A dedicated obstetric HDU with the knowledge, familiarity, experience and expertise of an obstetrician and a specialist team would be the best place to monitor and treat the critically ill obstetric patients.[12,24]

2. High bed-occupancy rate in ICUs (often > 90% in the UK[11]) can reduce the availability of emergency beds. From a general ICU, it is difficult to identify the avoidable obstetric ICU admissions due to lack of antenatal data and a control obstetric population (*i.e.* who do not require ICU admission). A dedicated obstetric HDU, as a 'step-down' unit, can act as a gateway for initial assessment before triaging the more critically ill women to the ICUs. This can be economical in view of the spiralling medical cost of general ICU usage.

3. Early intervention and treatment in an HDU can prevent serious complications and reduce the need and avoid the hazards of transfer patients to the ICU at a separate location.[25,26] Emergency transport to an ICU raises concern about the standard of care for escorting critically ill patients[27] because of specific risks that differ from other adult transport. There are two (more, in multiple pregnancy) patients to consider and this is a group particularly at risk from improper positioning.[25]

4. Obstetric patients in ICU need continuing obstetric and midwifery input throughout their stay and this presents a significant challenge to shared care. On an obstetric HDU, improved continuity of antenatal, intrapartum and postnatal care can be provided by the same team. Delivery of the baby takes place in a more familiar and better-equipped environment with minimal disruption of mother-to-baby bonding.

5. Care in an obstetric HDU may avoid exposure of the critically ill pregnant mother with her altered cell-mediated immunity and high levels of circulating

corticosteroids to a potentially hazardous ICU environment with the risk of hospital-acquired infection.

6. An obstetric HDU would fulfil the need of most tertiary centres, as there will be more centralised care of the critically ill women. The academic centres attached to them will also benefit for the teaching and training of the trainee doctors, nurses and midwives, who can learn a great deal about HDU and rare medical complications of pregnancy.

7. High dependency care, as opposed to full intensive care has indeed been recognised as a valid option in terms of efficacy and cost benefit.[28]

However, many hospitals with smaller maternity units lack the volume to justify such units as they may not be able to fulfil the criteria and maintain the contemporaneous skills.[29] It would not be cost-effective either.

THE UNIT

It is important to note that obstetric care is not considered in the UK DH document[6] cited above and that the definition refers to the category of care, not to geographical areas within which care is provided (*i.e.* HDU is not a place but a service). Thus a high-dependency care may not be restricted to an HDU set-up.[1] In most cases, however, the obstetric HDU is a highly specialised and discrete area within the maternity ward, usually on the delivery suite/labour ward specially equipped for critical care (Table 1). The philosophy is: put the sickest patients in a room (HDU) with the best team trained to treat them.[12]

PLANNING AND DESIGNING AN OBSTETRIC HDU

Critically ill patients consume significant resources. Accordingly, healthcare managers are increasingly cost conscious and often demand evidence of cost effectiveness for an obstetric HDU in terms of workload, manpower perspective and expenses. Knowledge of the local obstetric population, prevalence of particular medical or obstetric disorders, obstetric admission rate, mean length of stay (bed occupancy rate) in the ICUs, *etc.* could help design a business plan for beds, facilities, staffing, funding, *etc.* for an obstetric HDU. One has to consider the cost of initial capital expenditure, purchase of new technology, recruitment of staff, rolling annual cost and other indirect costs (training, consumables, IT facility, *etc.*).

In Europe and the US, about 0.1–0.9% of women during pregnancy, labour and puerperium develop complications that will require intensive care.[12,17,30] Taking the upper limit, the index for which maternity services should make provision is up to 10 high-dependency cases per 1000 deliveries per year.[23] In the UK, there are approximately 670,000 maternities in each year;[10,11] so, on an average obstetric HDU/ICU admissions might be required in as many as 7000 cases yearly (20,000 cases in the US for approximately 4 million births per year[31]).

It is important that adequate space is allocated to optimise the care of the HDU, to provide space for equipment, facilitate all cleaning regimens and prevent infection. Current standards suggest a minimum of 20 m² floor area is

Facilities
- Adjustable electric beds suitable for vaginal delivery (obstetric beds)
- Adjustable lights
- Effective temperature control
- Emergency call bell
- Medical gases – oxygen, Entonox
- Suction apparatus (wall-mounted or free-hand)
- Motorised syringe pumps
- Cardiorespiratory monitoring equipment
- Pulse oxymeter
- ECG machine
- ICU broadsheet observation chart for documentation
- Fetal monitors (CTG machine)
- Cardiac arrest trolley
- Blood gas analyser
- Blood fridge with 'O'-negative blood readily available
- X-ray view box
- Work station with computer and telephone
- Drug cupboard (with a stock of emergency drugs)
- Ready access to a portable ultrasound machine

Interventions
- Peripheral line(s)
- Central venous line
- Arterial line
- Basic respiratory monitoring and support with oxygen via face mask, nebuliser, peak flow meter
- Pulse oxymetry
- Arterial blood gas analysis
- ECG
- Blood transfusion
- Management of sickle crisis
- Management of PTE and DVT
- Management of other medical disorders (asthma, diabetic keto-acidosis, thyroid storm, *etc.*)
- Intravenous magnesium sulphate
- Fetal monitoring (CTG)
- Physiotherapy

ECG, electrocardiography; PTE, pulmonary thrombo-embolism; DVT, deep vein thrombosis; CTG, cardiotocography.

required for each general bed, but this should be at least 32.5 m² for HDU cubicles.[32] In the author's unit with an annual delivery of 5500, there is a 3-bedded obstetric HDU. This is in keeping with an incidence of (equates to the need of) 0.55% of pregnant women requiring HDU care per year.

STAFFING: THE HDU TEAM

An obstetric HDU should be adequately staffed by appropriately trained personnel, who should work as a team. At Guy's & St Thomas's Hospital, London, the team consists of 7 obstetricians, 3 HDU-trained specialist midwives, 4 obstetric anaesthetists, 4 neonatologists, 1 obstetric physician (Head of Obstetrics), with the back-up support of haematologist, pharmacist, theatre personnel, imaging department and designated physiotherapist. It is essential that in a complicated pregnancy, in addition to professional competence, the team operates with effective communication, mutual respect and clear patterns of responsibility.[21] An average nurse:patient ratio of 1:2 is specified together with 'continuous availability' of medical staff.[6]

It is vital to have a team leader (usually a senior obstetrician or an obstetric anaesthetist) who must take the ownership of overall responsibility. The team leader should be overseen by the head or director of the maternity unit who would ensure quality, safety and appropriateness of care. The director also oversees the administrative aspects of the unit including current policies and future strategies, and education and training of staff. There should be regular meetings between the director and the HDU team, plus clinical case conferences at regular intervals. This team should also have the direct responsibility for the generation of the HDU guidelines.

The HDU care should be provided on a 24-h basis with at least one team member as part of the delivery suite's 'core' staff in each shift, others being available when needed during 'out of hours' according to a dedicated 'on-call' rota.

INDICATIONS FOR ADMISSION TO THE HDU

The two most common primary reasons for obstetric HDU admission are respiratory failure and haemodynamic instability. Pulmonary oedema which may be due to peri-operative fluid overload, congestive heart failure, complication of severe pre-eclampsia or tocolytic therapy with β-agonists, is the commonest cause of respiratory failure,[33] whereas haemodynamic instability arise mostly from obstetric haemorrhage and postoperative complications. Antenatal admissions are more common with medical complications and hypertensive disease of pregnancy, while post-partum patients are admitted more with haemodynamic instability. Post-partum admissions have also been shown to be associated with a high incidence of sepsis or systemic inflammatory response syndrome (SIRS).[31] Usually, two-thirds of the admissions are due to obstetric disorders and one-third due to medical disorders. The most common obstetric cause of admission is hypertensive disease of pregnancy with associated complications such as renal failure, placental abruption and coagulopathy. Haemorrhage is the second most common cause followed by sepsis, and medical complications of pregnancy. The major indications of HDU admission are shown in Table 2. Differences in local prevalence of the disease, availability of concurrent HDU/ICU facilities and ICU admission criteria may account for the differences in the reported relative frequencies of indications among studies.

THE CARE

The principles of obstetric HDU care rest on a good understanding of the pathophysiology of the specific conditions of pregnancy. Early and aggressive intervention is an important strategy in the care of these patients to ensure best possible outcome for both mother and baby.

All patients admitted to the HDU must be evaluated by the HDU multidisciplinary team. On a daily basis, there should be a consultant

Table 2 Main indications of admission to the HDU

Hypertensive disease of pregnancy
      Severe pre-eclampsia with or without HELLP syndrome
      Eclampsia
Major obstetric haemorrhage
      Antepartum haemorrhage – major placenta praevia, placental abruption
      Postpartum haemorrhage
      Peripartum hysterectomy
Sepsis
Acute fatty liver of pregnancy
Pulmonary thrombo-embolism and deep vein thrombosis
Complications of pre-existing medical disorders in pregnancy
      Severe asthma
      Epilepsy
      Renal disease
      Peripartum cardiomyopathy
      Decompensated valvular heart disease/prosthetic heart valve
      Sickle cell crisis
      Poorly controlled diabetes/diabetic keto-acidosis
      Other endocrine disease (*e.g.* Addison's)
Uterine rupture and other complicated genital tract trauma
Post-caesarean complications – bowel perforation, ileus
Complications of anaesthesia
Surgical conditions in pregnancy, *e.g.* appendicitis, cholecystitis, pancreatitis.

These indications are not mutually exclusive. In many cases, there may be more than one condition that necessitates HDU admission.

obstetrician in charge of the 'shop floor' for both HDU and the labour ward of a high-risk maternity unit. There should be a regular ward round at least twice a day by the HDU team and a formal handover between shifts. This assures a formal multidisciplinary review of each patient and forward planning of daily care, provides on-site teaching and training, improves communication between the members of the team, patient and relatives, and reduces the risk of duplication or omission of aspects of patient care. However, too big a team may not be appropriate by the bedside of the critically ill.

Patients are evaluated every 15–60 min depending on the severity of the case with basic observations and clinical monitoring of organ functions (pulse, blood pressure, temperature, respiratory rate, oxygen saturation, urine output, Glasgow Coma Scale). In parallel with appropriate investigations (full blood count, coagulation screen, blood glucose, C-reactive protein, arterial blood gases, renal function tests, liver function tests, cardiac enzymes, urine microbiology and blood culture, appropriate imaging as indicated), specific management of the primary condition should be instituted without delay. A broad ICU observation chart is useful.

Provision of oxygen is vital to the critically ill obstetric patients for the following reasons:

1. As the entire cardiac output passes through the pulmonary vasculature with each cardiac cycle, conditions like pulmonary oedema, acute

respiratory distress syndrome (ARDS) and SIRS would affect the exchange of gases across the alveolocapillary membrane due to endothelial injury and toxic inflammatory mediator release, and compromise patients with minimal reserve. Multiple fetuses can exaggerate these effects.

2. In pregnancy, there is an increase of metabolic rate of 15–20% above the baseline. Provision of oxygen is paramount to the hypermetabolic anaemic patient.

3. Pregnant patients hyperventilate leading to respiratory alkalosis. To compensate, the kidneys increase the excretion of bicarbonate, causing a compensatory metabolic acidosis. This leads to intolerance to hypoxia because the patient's buffering ability is significantly decreased. Maternal metabolic acidosis also causes uterine vasoconstriction compromising uteroplacental perfusion.

Maternal organ perfusion and oxygen supply can be improved by maximising oxygen delivery, correction of hypovolaemia and improving cardiac contractility. Fluid therapy in acutely ill obstetric patients, with severe pre-eclampsia or major obstetric haemorrhage for example, requires a cautious balance between intravascular volume expansion to prevent hypoperfusion injury to the kidney and cerebral ischaemia on the one hand, and iatrogenic pulmonary oedema on the other. This should be ideally guided by central venous pressure (CVP) measurement or more accurately pulmonary artery wedge pressure, in which case a transfer to the ICU would be indicated. The patient should be placed in a 15° left lateral tilt with oxygen administered via face mask. Caution is required for vomiting and aspiration during mask ventilation in pregnancy. Haemoglobin should be maintained between 8–10 g/dl to provide the optimum balance between oxygen carrying capacity and blood viscosity.[30] If cardiac output is still low despite adequate fluid resuscitation, inotropes may be required to increase cardiac contractility in the ICU. The usual adrenal and corticosteroid response to stress may be absent or deficient in the critically ill, hence intravenous corticosteroids should be considered.[30] Sepsis should be aggressively treated with broad-spectrum antibiotics with a cover for Gram-negative organisms as well as anaerobes. Septic shock is associated with multi-organ failure and requires a transfer to the ICU. In cardiopulmonary arrest, resuscitation should follow standard protocols with modification of positioning in 15° left lateral tilt to avoid aortocaval compression, which might reduce cardiac output by as much as 25%. During electrical cardioconversion and defibrillation, fetal monitoring leads must be removed to prevent arcing. Compliance to the local HDU protocol (see below) with dated and timed documentation of records is essential. Figure 2 shows an outline of management.

Approximately 4.5% of patients admitted to the obstetric HDU will require transfer to the ICU (see Table 3 for indications), which is about 2% of all general ICU admissions when an obstetric HDU is in operation[12] with a higher incidence (up to 10%) in non-industrialised countries.[34]

The fetus in HDU care

Generally, fetal morbidity and mortality reflect maternal condition closely, for example, with rates of 45–50% for premature deliveries in maternal

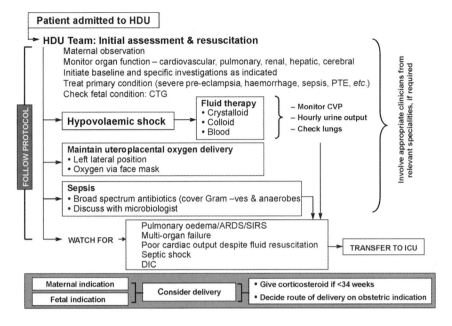

Fig. 2 Outline of management. PTE, pulmonary thrombo-embolism; DIC, disseminated intravascular coagulopathy.

pneumonia and 25% in ARDS.[30] Umbilical venous blood returning to the fetus has a low oxygen tension, but the fetus is usually well adapted to living in a hypoxic environment with a left shift of the oxygen dissociation curve of fetal haemoglobin, high cardiac output and a high fetal haemoglobin concentration.[30] However, as the uterine vasculature is maximally dilated in pregnancy, maternal illness tends to affect fetal oxygenation adversely. Adequate maternal oxygen saturation and maintenance of perfusion and oxygen delivery to the placenta is vital for fetal survival in the critically ill mother. Simple measures such as avoidance of supine hypotension by a 15° left

Table 3 Indications of transfer from obstetric HDU to ICU

Need for advanced respiratory support
Endotracheal intubation* and mechanical ventilation
Continuous positive airway pressure or non-invasive ventilation
Adult respiratory distress syndrome
Need for Swan-Ganz catheter
Vasoactive infusion/inotropic support
Disseminated intravascular coagulopathy
Multi-organ failure
Pulmonary thrombo-embolism requiring thrombolytic therapy
Any other condition(s) not considered suitable for HDU
*Consideration should be given to improved stabilisation and elective intubation prior to transfer.[11]

lateral tilt, and oxygen via face-mask can improve uteroplacental oxygen delivery. Fetal condition should be observed by continuous electronic fetal monitoring with a cardiotocograph (CTG) machine. There is, however, some concern that high maternal oxygen level may actually harm the baby by worsening the fetal acidosis.[30] Early delivery may be required for maternal or/and fetal indication, and should be considered with antenatal corticosteroids for fetuses < 34 weeks administered 24 h prior to delivery, if the situation permits. Route of delivery should be decided upon by obstetric indication and individual circumstances.

The nature of HDU obstetric patients demands an on-site presence of a specialised neonatal unit providing level-3 perinatal intensive care[35] and a neonatologist should be in attendance during delivery.

GUIDELINES AND PROTOCOLS

As HDU care involves management of critically ill obstetric patients, guidelines and protocols should be in place to encourage appropriate responses to these critical situations and justify actions that are sufficient and efficient, neither excessive nor deficient. The American College of Critical Care Medicine has published guidelines for general intensive and intermediate care.[36] Unfortunately, there are no specific guidelines from the speciality (obstetrics and gynaecology) organisations that describe a plan of care of critically ill pregnant women.[24] In the UK, the CEMD simply recommends access to care, but does not address the issue of guidelines for such a care.[1]

It is reasonable to apply the general ICU guidelines to obstetric HDU. Guidance may also be obtained and collated from management guidelines on the relevant maternal conditions (*e.g.* eclampsia, thrombo-embolic disease in pregnancy and puerperium, chicken pox in pregnancy, massive obstetric haemorrhage, *etc.*) from speciality organisations, for example, the clinical green-top guidelines of The Royal College of Obstetricians and Gynaecologists (RCOG). As far as practicable, these guidelines should be evidence-based, properly referenced, and modified in the light of local experience in agreement with the multidisciplinary team. Each unit should formulate specific protocols, update them regularly and make them available in paper and/or electronic versions in the HDU for ready reference. This should include strict criteria for admission, investigations, intervention (medical, surgical, anaesthetic, obstetric), ICU referral, discharge, aftercare and follow-up.

AFTERCARE AND FOLLOW-UP

In addition to the physical illness, the delivery of a baby to the mother in the HDU setting adds stress to both parents with substantial psychological morbidity. The mother would require: (i) information about the newborn; (ii) conditions allowing visit to the neonatal care unit; (iii) access to the partner for support; and (iv) their own time together. A clear policy of allowing the partner's presence and provision of regular information with appropriate briefing to the parents should be in place. There are reports of critically ill mothers subsequently developing post-traumatic stress syndrome.[37] Emotional support and post-partum counselling are important to help reduce the stress of the critical illness and improve 'family morbidity' before discharge from the hospital.[7] Help from a qualified stress or bereavement counsellor (in the event of a perinatal death), and support group is extremely useful. A discharge summary should be sent to the patient's general practitioner (GP) soon after discharge from the HDU.

Ideally, care should extend beyond the HDU site. Follow-up arrangements must be made (if required more than once) with the consultant obstetrician. The patient should be given the opportunity to revisit her illness, with proper and detailed explanation, and discuss on-going care, if any, required. Subsequent reproductive outcome may be compromised in some of the 'near misses' with a high rate of loss of fertility potential, with its attendant psychological morbidity.[38] Advice on future pregnancy should, therefore, be an integral part of such a follow-up. In addition to informing the GP, it is author's practice to give the patient a copy of her case summary containing advice for any subsequent pregnancy for her future reference.

OUTCOME

How does obstetric critical care mortality compare with general critical care mortality? In the ICU setting, to compensate for age and illness, comparison of standardised mortality ratios has been used based on the severity scoring systems, *e.g.* the Acute Physiology and Chronic Health Evaluation (APACHE II),[39] Acute Physiology, Age and Chronic Health Evaluation (APACHE III),[40] Simplified Acute Physiology Score (SAPS II),[41] Mortality Probability Model,[42] *etc.* Several investigators have applied these scoring tools derived from non-obstetric populations to obstetric populations with conflicting results: 0–36% for maternal mortality[13,14,43–45] and 6–14% for perinatal mortality.[26,33,43] It must be emphasised that, although most widely used, the original database of APACHE II was developed about 20 years ago on mixed ICU patient populations and very few obstetric patients were included. Many physiological changes during pregnancy, such as higher respiratory and heart rate, lower haematocrit and creatinine levels, development of a low resistance placental circulation, *etc.* can affect the variables of APACHE II and SAPS II. For example, a systolic blood pressure of 70–90 mmHg may be normal in pregnancy, but given a high score on SAPS II; a serum creatinine value of 75–125 mmol/l is normal in a non-obstetric patient but high in pregnancy assigning a lower score on APACHE II, causing false prediction for mortality rate.[33] Little is known regarding the ability to assess severity of illness and predict outcomes in obstetric patients as there are no current models that are designed specifically for use in obstetric patients. Data extrapolated from the general ICU statistics would, therefore, not accurately reflect the outcome of obstetric HDU/ICU patients. Any outcome measure of obstetric HDU care is thus difficult. Moreover, as mentioned earlier, the reduction in maternal mortality has weakened the value of this traditional quality-assurance indicator. SAMM would be a better indicator, but currently no data exist on the predictors of SAMM either.[3] It has been suggested, therefore, that a separate scoring system be developed for pregnant patients to devise a reliable model to predict outcomes on initial presentation.[46] Such a model would also allow proper mobilisation of resources (*e.g.* notifications of consultants, blood bank, transfer centre).

Maternal survival appears to be as good as or better than general ICU populations, possibly because of their young age, lack of co-morbidity and reversibility of many of the predisposing conditions. However, patients with failure of two or more organ systems for > 48 h usually do not survive.[47] The most common pathological cause of death in obstetric patients admitted to ICUs is ARDS secondary to major haemorrhage and sepsis.[30] The four most common direct obstetric causes of maternal death are: thrombosis and thrombo-embolism, haemorrhage, hypertensive disease of pregnancy and sepsis.[11] The actual HDU care aside, the survival of a pregnant woman is dependent on many inter-related factors, *e.g.* the severity of the disease at admission, her basic health, quality of antenatal care, the healthcare facilities and access to them. Other risk factors include maternal age > 34 years, social exclusion, non-white,[3] and differences in the risk profile of the population served. Lack of antenatal care and ICU facilities, plus delay in ICU referral are two important causes of poor maternal and perinatal outcome in non-industrialised countries.[48]

RECORD KEEPING, DATA COLLECTION AND AUDIT

Ideally, record keeping for HDU should be paperless via an efficient computerised database to which only designated staff should have authorised access. Harmer[49] stressed on the importance of monitoring obstetric admissions to ICUs and recommended that the sub-speciality societies explore the feasibility of such data collection. Scarpinato[50] identified a serious lack of knowledge of obstetric critical care and called for increased reporting of such data. The South West Thames database on ICU admissions encountered the problem of missing values of up to 28%.[45] These findings highlight a definite need for setting up a robust HDU database. The information technology (IT) department should be closely involved to design an appropriate tool for the local database with easy and universally accepted search/key words that would specifically 'flag' HDU admission. This will be extremely useful for future audit locally. With suitable interrogation and amalgamation, local data can be linked with a larger regional and national database (for example, the case mix programme of the Intensive Care National Audit and Research Centre [ICNARC]) providing a useful template for national and international comparisons of diseases, interventions and approaches of care between centres, allowing for regional, national and international variation. An additional advantage of such comparison would be to devise regional protocols of the management of the disorders requiring HDU care[51] and help research. The results of a UK national survey conducted in 2000 by the National Obstetric Anaesthetic Database (NAOD) are awaited (Holdcroft A. Personal communication).

Examples of auditable standards of practice comprise audit of referrals, morbidity-specific clinical management in compliance with the guidelines/ protocols, unplanned admission to the HDU/ICU, *etc.* Incorporation of near misses or SAMM into maternal death enquiries would strengthen these audits by allowing for more rapid reporting, more robust conclusions, comparisons to be made with maternal deaths, reinforcing lessons learnt, establishing requirements for intensive care and calculating comparative indices.[52] Unlike mortality, audit of SAMM would also allow interviews of patients, which helps improve service based on patients' feedback. This is, however, not an easy task due to the complexities in definition and case-identification of SAMM and general poor reporting quality of the studies,[4] thus limiting the comparability of the studies and utility of some data extracted. However, a recent Scottish population study[53] shows that categories of severe maternal morbidity can be identified, and it is feasible to establish a national reporting system of maternal morbidity as well as mortality. Some serious disorders of pregnancy are rare and difficult to study because routine information sources are inadequate; however, they are important causes of maternal or perinatal morbidity and/or mortality and would, therefore, warrant care in the HDU/ICU. A new UK Obstetric Surveillance System (UKOSS; a prospective monthly case-collection scheme) has recently been launched to investigate uncommon disorders of pregnancy.[54]

HOW TO REDUCE HDU AND ICU ADMISSION

Long-term measures

1. Continued improvement of socio-economic conditions should bring a concomitant increase in the standard of general health, nutrition, housing and education ensuring that women enter into their pregnancies more healthier. These issues are more sociopolitical than medical/obstetric and are important for non-industrialised countries on a global perspective.

2. Careful and critical review of all maternal and perinatal deaths and severe maternal morbidity is essential, no matter how small the hospital. This will pinpoint the avoidable organisational and human factors that may be preventable in the future.

3. Adequate training of personnel who look after high-risk pregnant women, along with continuing education and support.

Medium-term measures

High-quality antenatal care is the key to maintain a healthy pregnancy and reduce complications. Forward planning for careful selection, early identification and referral of high-risk pregnancies to the appropriate perinatal care team is important, particularly for those with pre-existing medical disorders. The setting of a 'one-stop shop' in high-risk antenatal clinics, as suggested by Steer and Yentis,[55] where women can see all the healthcare professionals of the perinatal care team, can offer a 'total' pregnancy care with proper planning of antenatal, intrapartum and postnatal management, including anaesthetic consideration and neonatal care.

Short-term measures

As pulmonary oedema, haemodynamic instability and sepsis comprise the main indications of obstetric HDU admission, clinicians should try to prevent the development of these conditions with judicious use of i.v. fluids, infection control measures, prevention and timely control of massive post-partum haemorrhage (PPH), *etc.*

POTENTIAL RISKS

Inappropriate referral and lack or delay in appropriate referral

Inappropriate HDU/ICU admission increases the anxiety level of the patients and their relatives. It also means improper utilisation of resources – highly trained staff, costly beds and facilities. One study in non-obstetric patients showed as many as 25% of all admissions to the ICU could be inappropriate, whereas 75% of the general ward admissions should have been cared in an HDU set-up.[56] Another study[26] showed 60% of the patients admitted to ICU could have been managed appropriately within the HDU setting. Failure to estimate the severity of illness correctly and refer to the HDU may represent a degree of substandard care. Using specific criteria for sub-optimal care, such as lack of knowledge, failure to seek advice, lack of experience, and unavailability of medical staff, McQuillan *et al.*[57] identified deficiencies in care contributing to more than half of all ICU admissions. There is no absolute method of distinguishing these cases, especially in early phase, but a high index of suspicion must be maintained by staff.[11]

Early referral and outreach

Transfer to the HDU/ICU from the community may be a problem. One of the key findings of *Comprehensive Critical Care*[58] is that there is a need to share critical care skills with staff in wards and the community. This report recommended the development of services such as Patient At Risk Team (PART) to identify critically ill patients in the community and arrange the transfer to the critical care beds. Although there is no specific reference to maternity services in the report, it is clearly an area that could benefit from such a scheme.

Inappropriate patient turnover

There should be agreed guidelines for transfer of the high-risk patients from the HDU to the general obstetric ward and the ICU, or there is risk of overstay and premature discharge (with the risk of re-admission).

HDU care error

Organisational and human factors can lead to errors contributing to adverse events, sometimes fatal. One observational study in the ICU showed an error rate of 1.7 per patient per day.[59] Root-cause analysis of these errors has shown that most adverse events usually occur as a result of the convergence of multiple system failures and about 30% are due to human errors.[60,61] Human errors can prolong ICU stay equivalent of 15% of ICU time.[62] It is reasonable to assume the same for the HDU.

Staff support

Working in the HDU can be very stressful. By its nature, HDU care is very challenging and demands a very high level of physical ability and mental alertness with the risk of fatigue and 'burn-out', and in some cases monotony, leading to drop-out. A good management should have systems in place for monitoring staff stress level. It is vital that the rota system takes this into account. It is crucial to have a 'core' HDU personnel, but equally important is 'recycling' of staff in both HDU and low-risk maternity areas with suitable spread of seniority and experience to safeguard against exhaustion and ensure skill mix. Undesirable and disastrous outcome can take a heavy toll on staff moral. There should be adequate staff support system and counselling facilities in traumatic circumstances.

RISK MANAGEMENT AND CLINICAL GOVERNANCE

HDU practice must be maintained at the highest possible standard. Teamwork dynamics, operational schedules and management protocols must be strictly adhered to. Any deviation from the protocol should be intensively scrutinised via critical incident reporting according to the risk management strategy of the unit, and audits should be regularly carried out. The whole exercise should be made an integral part of clinical governance scheme. Many aspects of HDU care could be an essential requirement for the Clinical Negligence Scheme for the Trust (CNST)[63] as well.

EVALUATION

The impact of an HDU should be evaluated from organisational, staffing and consumer perspectives. Ideally, such evaluation should be carried out before and after the development of the HDU and compared. One such evaluation study in Australia[64] in non-obstetric patients recorded a higher satisfaction level in patients, relatives and nurses after the change, *i.e.* establishment of an HDU.

The importance of adequate staffing and regular ward rounds cannot be over-emphasised. A literature review has shown that, in the absence of a daily ICU physician ward round, in-hospital and ICU mortality increases 3-fold, and the risk of developing complications (acute renal failure, septicaemia or cardiac arrest, the need for platelet transfusion or re-intubation) by a factor of 2 or 3 times, as well as increased length of stay and higher cost of care.[60] The ideal midwife (nurse):patient ratio is 1:1 to 1:2 depending on the case load.[12,20] ICU length-of-stay is higher when ICU nurses had to care for more than two patients.[60]

However, the impact of obstetric HDU on reducing admissions to ICU is not so easy to assess. Data from Dublin[25] show a sizeable, although not significant, reduction of 50% (from 0.08% to 0.04%)) in obstetric admissions to ICU following the setting-up of an obstetric HDU. The figure is 24% in a London teaching hospital.[1]

A quality assurance review should be carried out with detailed records of HDU patients collected regularly and analysed. This should be aimed at meeting the objectives of the HDU (Table 4). For a comparison of prevailing practices, similar units in other large tertiary centres should be surveyed.

TRAINING

Each member of the HDU team is required to have adequate knowledge and training on multi-organ pathophysiology in pregnancy including a clear

Table 4 Objectives of the HDU

- Provide best possible care for the critically ill obstetric patient on a designated site with the specialised facilities, knowledge and expertise
- Maximise resource utilisation between HDU and ICU
- Reduce maternal morbidity and mortality
- Improve perinatal outcome
- Ensure appropriate staffing with balanced skill mix
- Direct consultant input in the HDU care with a clearly defined care pathway
- Educate and train the multidisciplinary team
- Maintain effective team-work including communication between HDU staff and other healthcare professionals
- Perform internal audit and promote clinical research to further the knowledge of SAMM
- Educate patients in preventative aspects of obstetrics and improve their level of awareness about the disease process that might affect pregnancy outcome

understanding of fluid, electrolyte and acid–base balance, 12-lead ECG, defibrillation, basic adult and neonatal resuscitation. Lack of proper training and experience can lead to inappropriate management resulting in poor maternal and perinatal outcomes and potential for litigation.

Critical care in obstetrics should be given emphasis in specialist training in obstetrics and gynaecology.[65] The RCOG's core specialist training in obstetrics and gynaecology includes medical complications of pregnancy, and special-skill module training in maternal medicine and obstetric leadership on the labour ward requires management of medical disorders in pregnancy with two sessions on ITU and high-dependency care on labour ward, respectively, under the auspices of the British Maternal & Fetal Medicine Society (Special Skills Training in Obstetrics and Gynaecology <www.rcog.org.uk and www.bmfms.org.uk>). Senior clinicians should regularly update their knowledge and skill as a part of their continuing professional development (CPD) by attending relevant courses, *e.g.* advanced life support in obstetrics (ALSO),[66] management of obstetric emergency and trauma (MOET)[67] and visiting other units of excellence. Training programmes in acute obstetric emergencies have been recently systematically reviewed by Black and Brockenhurst.[68]

The role of the midwife in the HDU care was not specifically mentioned in any policy documents until the 1997 CEMD in the UK.[9] It states that: 'as members of the multidisciplinary team, midwives have an equal responsibility in ensuring high standards of care and positive outcome of pregnancy'. This has been echoed in other documents also:[21] '…as far as midwifery cover of high dependency care units is concerned, it will be necessary to develop a cadre of midwives who have particular experience and expertise in the management of critically ill women'. Currently in the UK, there are many established Nursing and Midwifery Council (NMC)-approved obstetric HDU courses for midwives run by various local education providers, universities and nursing/midwifery schools. Midwifery training should be regularly refreshed by attending compulsory study days. Hospitals can arrange exchange programmes of duty and training between ICU nurses and HDU midwives.

All team members must also attend regular in-house 'drills and skills' of common, as well as rare, obstetric emergencies.

In addition to the clinical skill courses, each member of the HDU team should have suitable training in communication and counselling skill of how to brief the patient and the anxious family members with balanced information, and help them to adapt to the HDU environment. It is important for the team to have the right attitude and behaviour.

The HDU director and the supervisor of midwives together should ensure round-the-year rolling training of the team to achieve and maintain competence.

FUTURE RESEARCH

The evidence base for many interventions and treatment in critical care in obstetrics is not robust. Although there have been many important randomised controlled trials (RCTs) in ICUs, few areas of obstetric critical care have been subjected to RCT analysis.[1] As a result, the risk:benefit balance of many interventions (*e.g.* invasive monitoring) in the acutely ill obstetric population is less certain than in their non-pregnant counterparts.[69]

Severe obstetric morbidity constitutes a serious maternal-fetal and public health problem world-wide.[11] There is a need for future studies to identify the predictive factors of SAMM. This would not only contribute to the assessment of quality of patient care in the HDU, but also enhance risk stratification of pregnant women in the evaluation of new therapies. Structured observational research would be good at identifying these problems,[70] as ethically and practically it would be difficult to conduct RCTs in critical obstetric illness. There is also a need for critical review with relevant research of strategies employed and the commitment and support from health policy makers.

CONCLUSIONS

The critically ill obstetric patient poses a unique challenge to the healthcare professionals, and requires the expertise of several sub-specialities. There are many potential benefits of a dedicated obstetric HDU to provide specialised care, intermediary between a general obstetric ward and an ICU. More and more obstetric units in the UK are having on-site HDUs.

A round-the-clock service must be provided by a trained multidisciplinary team following strict guidelines and protocols. Maternal management should focus on maintaining oxygen delivery, fluid balance, controlling sepsis and treating specific conditions of pregnancy. Fetal management aims to maintain placental perfusion and delivery at an appropriate time for fetal and/or maternal indication. Debriefing and aftercare with appropriate follow-up must be arranged including emotional support and advice on future pregnancy.

A quality assurance review of HDU care should be regularly carried out by high-quality record keeping, computerised data collection, well-designed audit, a robust risk management exercise, and regular training and education of the staff.

Different prognostic systems have been developed to predict the outcome of critically ill ICU patients, but currently there is no such model for critically ill obstetric patients. Moreover, ICU outcome measures are inappropriate, because maternal mortality is very rare in the industrialised world. SAMM can be a better quality indicator of maternity care, but no data exist on the predictors of SAMM. There is a need for future studies to identify the predictive factors of SAMM in order to improve maternal and perinatal outcome in these patients. The evidence base for many interventions and treatment in critical care in obstetrics is not robust, as few areas of obstetric critical care have been subjected to RCTs. Structured observational research may be considered as RCTs are ethically and practically difficult to carry out.

ACKNOWLEDGEMENT

I am grateful to Dr Diana Hamilton-Fairly, Consultant Obstetrician and Gynaecologist, Guy's & St Thomas's Hospital NHS Foundation Trust, London for her helpful comments on the manuscript.

References

1 Yentis SM. Intensive care. In: MacLean AB, Neilson J. (eds) Maternal morbidity and mortality. London: RCOG Press, 2002; 381–389
2 Bulletin of the World Health Organization. <http://www.who.int/reproductive-health/publications/maternal_mortality_2000/executive_summary.html> (Accessed 25 September 2005)
3 Waterstone M, Bewley S, Wolfe C. Incidence and predictors of severe obstetric morbidity: case-control study. BMJ 2001; 322: 1089–1093
4 Say L, Pattison RC, Gülmezoglu AM. WHO systematic review of maternal morbidity and mortality: the prevalence of severe acute maternal morbidity (near miss). Reprod Health 2004; 1: 3 <http://www.reproductive-health-journal.com/content/1/1/3>
5 Fitzpatrick C, Halligan A, McKenna P, Coughlan BM, Darling MRN, Phelan D. Near miss maternal mortality. Ir Med J 1992; 85: 37
6 Department of Health/NHS Executive. Guidelines on admission to and discharge from Intensive Care and High Dependency Units. London: DoH, 1996
7 Report on Confidential Enquiries into Maternal Death in the United Kingdom, 1988–90. Department of Health, Welsh Office, Scottish Home and Health Department, Department of Health and Social Services, Northern Ireland. London: HMSO, 1994
8 Report on Confidential Enquiries into Maternal Death in the United Kingdom 1991–1993. London: HMSO, 1994
9 Report on Confidential Enquiries into Maternal Death in the United Kingdom 1994–1996. London: HMSO, 1997
10 Why mothers die: Report on Confidential Enquiries into Maternal Death in the United Kingdom 1997–1999. London: HMSO, 2001
11 Why mothers die: Report on Confidential Enquiries into Maternal Death in the United Kingdom 2000–2002. London: RCOG Press, 2004
12 Mabie WC, Sibai BM. Treatment in an obstetric intensive care unit. Am J Obstet Gynecol 1990; 162: 1–4
13 Kilpatrick SJ, Matthay MA. Obstetric patients requiring critical care: a five-year review. Chest 1992; 101: 1407–1412
14 Mahutte NG, Murphy-Kaulbeck L, Le Q et al. Obstetric admission to the intensive care unit. Obstet Gynecol 1999; 94: 263–266
15 Teres D, Steingrub J. Can intermediate care substitute for intensive care? [Editorial]. Crit Care Med 1987; 15: 280
16 Popovitch J. Intermediate care units: graded care options. Chest 1991; 99: 4–5

17 Johanson RB, Anthony J, Dommisse J. Obstetric intensive care at Groote Schuur Hospital, Cape Town. J Obstet Gynaecol 1995; 15: 174–177

18 Visser W, Wallenburg HCS. Maternal and perinatal outcome of temporizing management in 254 consecutive patients with severe preeclampsia remote from term. Eur J Obstet Gynaecol Reprod Biol 1995; 63: 147–154

19 Cordingley JJ, Rubin AP. A survey of facilities for high risk women in consultant obstetric units. Int J Obstet Anesth 1997; 6: 156–160

20 Zeeman GG, Wendel GD, Cunningham EG. A blueprint for obstetric critical care. Am J Obstet Gynecol 2003; 188: 532–536

21 Changing Childbirth: Report of the expert maternity group (Cumberlage Report) 1993

22 First Class Delivery: improving maternity services in England and Wales. Audit Commission. London: HMSO, 1997

23 Towards safer childbirth. Minimum standards for the organisation of labour wards: Report of a joint working party, Royal College of Midwives and Royal College of Obstetricians and Gynaecologists. London: RCOG Press, 1999.

24 Kirshon B, Hinkley CM, Cotton DB et al. Maternal mortality in a maternal-fetal medicine intensive care unit. J Reprod Med 1990; 35: 25–28

25 Ryan M, Hamilton V, Bowen M, McKenna P. The role of high-dependency unit in a regional obstetric hospital. Anaesthesia 200; 55: 1155–1158

26 Wheatley E, Farkas A, Watson D. Obstetric admission to an intensive therapy unit. Int J Obstet Anesth 1996; 5: 221–224

27 Oakley PA. The need for standards for inter-hospital transfer. Anaesthesia 1994; 49: 565–566

28 Kilpatrick A, Ridley S, Plenderleith L. A changing role for intensive therapy: is there a case for high dependency care? Anaesthesia 1994; 49: 666–670

29 McCormack DM. Care of the obstetrical patient in the traditional intensive care unit. Crit Care Nurs Q 1998; 21: 1–11

30 Male D, Stockwell M, Jankowski S. Management of the critically obstetric patient. Curr Obstet Gynaecol 2002; 12: 322–327

31 Gilbert TT, Smulian JC, Martin AA, Ananth CV, Scorza W, Scardella AT. Obstetric admissions to the intensive care unit: outcomes and severity of illness. Obstet Gynecol 2003; 102: 897–903

32 Humphreys H, Moriarty J .Upgrading Intensive Care Units - Getting the Design Right Prevents Infection. Ir Med J Online Paper. Accessed 25 September 2005

33 Afessa B, Green B, Delke I, Koch K. Systemic inflammatory response syndrome, organ failure, and outcome in critically ill obstetric patients treated in the ICU. Chest 2001; 120: 1271–1277

34 Parikh CR, Karnad DR. Quality, cost and outcome of intensive care in a public hospital in Bombay, India. Crit Care Med 1999; 27: 1754–1759

35 British Association of Perinatal Medicine. Obstetric standard for the provision of perinatal care, November 1998

36 American College of Critical Care Medicine and the Society of Critical Care Medicine. Guidelines on admission and discharge for adult intermediate care units: Guidelines/Practice parameters Committee of the American College of Critical Care Medicine and the Society of Critical Care Medicine. Crit Care Med 1998; 26: 607–610

37 Umo-Etuk J, Lumley J, Holdcroft A. Critically ill parturient women and admission to intensive care: a 5-year review. Int J Obstet Anaesth 1996; 5: 79–84

38 Murphy DJ, Charlett P. Cohort study of near-miss maternal mortality and subsequent reproductive outcomes. Eur J Obstet Gynecol Reprod Biol 2002; 102: 173–178

39 Knaus WA, Draper EA, Wagner DP et al. APACHE II: A severity of illness classification system. Crit Care Med 1985; 13: 818–829

40 Knaus WA, Wagner DP, Draper EA et al. The APACHE III prognostic system: Risk prediction of hospital mortality for critically ill hospitalised adults. Chest 1991; 100: 1619–1639

41 Le Gall JR, Lemeshow S, Saulnier F. A new simplified acute physiology score (SAPS II) based on a European/North American multicenter study. JAMA 1993; 270: 2957–2963

42 Lemeshow S, Teres D, Klar J et al. Mortality probability models (MPM II) based on international cohort of intensive care unit patients. JAMA 1993; 270: 2478–2486.

43 El-Solh A, Grant B. A comparison of severity of illness scoring system for critically ill obstetric patients. Chest 1996; 110: 1299–1304

44 Lapinsky SE, Kruezynski K, Seawrad GR *et al*. Critical care management of the obstetric patients. Can J Anaesth 1997; 44: 325–329

45 Hazelgrove LF, Price C, Pappachan VJ, Smith GB. Multicentre study of obstetric admissions to 14 intensive care units in southern England. Crit Care Med 2001; 29: 770–775

46 Bhagwanjee S, Paruk F, Moodley J, Muckart DJ. Intensive care unit morbidity and mortality from eclampsia: an evaluation of the Acute Physiology And Chronic Health Evaluation II score and the Glasgow coma scale score. Crit Care Med 2000; 28: 120–124

47 Campbell L, Klocke RA. Update in non-pulmonary critical care: Implications for the pregnant patient. Am J Respir Crit Care Med 2001; 163: 1051–1054

48 Karnad DR, Lapsia V, Krishnan A, Salvi V. Prognostic factors in obstetric patients admitted to an Indian intensive care unit. Crit Care Med 2004; 32: 1294–1299

49 Harmer M. Maternal mortality – is it still relevant? Anaesthesia 1997; 52: 99–100

50 Scarpinato L. Obstetric critical care. Crit Care Med 1998; 26: 433

51 Waterstone M, Bewley S, Wolfe C. Preliminary results from a one-year prospective study of the incidence of severe obstetric morbidity. Br J Obstet Gynaecol 1998; 105 (Suppl 17): 35

52 Pattinson RC, Hall M. Near misses: a useful adjunct to maternal death enquiries. Br Med Bull 2003; 67: 231–243

53 Brace V, Penney G, Hall M. Quantifying severe maternal morbidity: a Scottish population study. Br J Obstet Gynaecol 2004; 111: 481–484

54 Knight M, Kurinczuk JJ, Tuffnell D, Brockenhurst P. The UK Obstetric Surveillance System for rare disorders of pregnancy. Br J Obstet Gynaecol 2005; 112: 263–265.

55 Steer P, Yentis S. ABC of Labour Care: Letters. BMJ 1999; 319: 1270

56 Loughrey JP, Fitzpatrick G, Connolly J, Donnelly M. High dependency care: impact of facilities for high-risk surgical patients. Ir J Med Sci 2002; 171: 211–215

57 McQuillan P, Pilkington S, Allan A *et al*. Confidential enquiry into quality of care before admission to intensive care. BMJ 1998; 316: 1853–1858

58 Comprehensive Critical Care: a Review of Adult Critical Care, Department of Health. London: HMSO, 1999

59 Coiera EW, Jayasuriya RA, Hardy J *et al*. Communication loads on clinical staff in the emergency department. Med J Aust 2002; 176: 415–418

60 Gatt S. Pregnancy, delivery and the intensive care unit: need, outcome and management. Curr Opinion Anaesth 2003; 16: 263–267

61 Joint Commission on Accreditation of Healthcare Organizations. Preventing Infant Death During Delivery. Oakbrook Terrace, Ill: Joint Commission on Accreditation of Healthcare Organizations; 2004. Sentinel Event Alert No. 30

62 Bracco D, Favre JB, Bissonnette B *et al*. Human errors in a multidisciplinary intensive care unit: a 1-year prospective study. Intensive Care Med 2001; 27: 137–145

63 Clinical Negligence Scheme for Trusts. Clinical Risk Management Standards for Maternity Services, 2002

64 Armstrong K, Young J, Hayburn A, Irish B, Nikoletti S. Evaluating the impact of a new high dependency unit. Int J Nurs Pract 2003; 9: 285–293

65 Bergström S. Obstetric ectoscopy: an eye-opener for hospital-based clinicians. Acta Obstet Gynecol Scand 2005; 84: 105

66 ALSO Instruction Manual. American Academy of Family Physicians. University of Wisconsin. 1996

67 Johanson RB, Cox C, O'Donnel E, Grady K, Howell CJ, Jones PW. Managing obstetric emergencies and trauma (MOET). Structured skills training using models and reality-based scenarios. Obstet Gynecol 1999; 1: 46–52

68 Black RS, Brockenhurst P. A systematic review of training in acute obstetric emergencies. Br J Obstet Gynaecol 2003; 110: 838–841.

69 Nolan TE, Wakefield ML, Devoe LD. Invasive haemodynamic monitoring in obstetrics. A critical review of its indication, benefits, complications and alternatives. Chest 1992; 101: 1429–1433

70 Carthey J. The role of structured observational research in health care. Qual Safety Health Care 2003; 12: ii13

Richard N. Brown

Antepartum haemorrhage: bleeding of placental and fetal origin

The criteria for the diagnosis of antepartum haemorrhage are varied but the most generally accepted definition describes antepartum haemorrhage as bleeding that occurs beyond the 20th week of gestation but prior to the onset of labour. Although the precise incidence cannot be defined as some episodes may not be recognised at all and in those cases where an episode of bleeding is appreciated by the mother not all are reported, it is clear that this is one of the commonest complications of pregnancy affecting up to 5% of all pregnancies.

The potential causes are very varied with these in the broadest terms being attributable either to a feto-placental site of origin or to a maternal site of

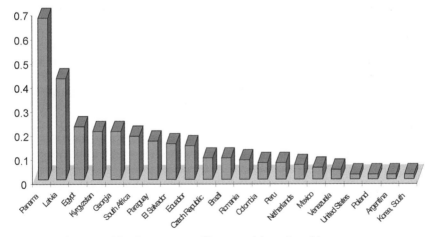

Fig. 1 Mortality rates (deaths per one million people) attributable to antepartum haemorrhage (World Health Organization Statistical Information Service).

Richard N. Brown MBBS MRCOG
Assistant Professor of Obstetrics and Gynecology, McGill University, Women's Pavilion, Royal Victoria Hospital, 687 Pine Avenue West, Montreal, Quebec H3A 1A1, Canada
E-mail: richard.brown@muhc.mcgill.ca

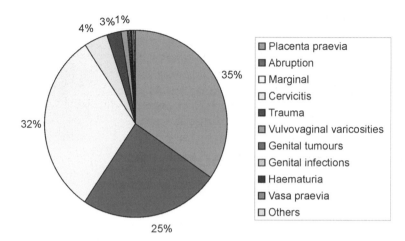

Fig. 2 The spectrum of causes of antepartum haemorrhage.

origin. The majority of episodes are 'minor' and these may not even be recognised if the bleeding is concealed and of insufficient quantity to result in signs or symptoms; however, there is always the possibility that the haemorrhage might be clinically significant at its presentation or become so later and that this may have detrimental consequences to either the mother, the fetus or both. In the non-industrialised world, maternal mortality consequent to antepartum haemorrhage remains a significant contributor to the high death rates still observed in association with childbirth (Fig. 1).

The broad and diverse spectrum of causes of antepartum haemorrhage is indicated in Figure 2. The two most important causes from an obstetric standpoint are placenta praevia and placental abruption. Together, these account for around 50% of the cases of antepartum haemorrhage. A significant proportion of antepartum bleeds, however, have no clear cause evident and are considered unexplained or unclassified,[1] although often these are speculatively classified as marginal bleeds or bleeds arising from the placental edge. In addition, bleeding may arise from any site within the lower genital tract and may indeed be unrelated to the pregnancy itself.

PLACENTA PRAEVIA

The term placenta praevia describes a placenta that is inserted, at least in part, in the lower uterine segment. Typically, four grades are used to describe this condition as summarised in Table 1.

The incidence is around 0.5% of pregnancies although this might have increased somewhat in recent years with the incidence being greater in black women and those from other minority groups as compared to white women (odds ratio [OR] 1.3). In addition, the incidence is greatest in those women aged 35 years or greater and in those aged 20 years or less (OR 4.7).[2,3]

Although some cases of placenta praevia are suspected on the basis of a history of antepartum haemorrhage, it is more common in current practice for this to be suspected as a consequence of routine antenatal second trimester

Table 1 Four grades of placenta praevia

Grade	
I	The placenta is sited within the lower uterine segment but the leading edge does not encroach on the internal cervical os
II	The leading placental edge reaches but does not cover the internal cervical os
III	The placenta partially or asymmetrically covers the internal cervical os
IV	The placenta wholly covers the internal cervical os

fetal sonography. Although first trimester trans-vaginal evaluation may allow exclusion of some cases of placenta praevia,[4] the value of this intervention is debatable given that routine second trimester sonography is ubiquitous in those healthcare systems capable of offering first trimester trans-vaginal sonography. If the findings of trans-abdominal sonography are uncertain or equivocal, then trans-vaginal sonography, which is safe to undertake in such circumstances, having no association with an increased risk of bleeding,[5,6] remains the gold standard for the diagnosis of placenta praevia. Should there be reasons to preclude a trans-vaginal approach than a perineal or trans-labial technique may be adopted with similar results.[7,8]

Amongst the neonatal complications associated with placenta praevia there have been observed increases in the incidence of major congenital anomalies (OR 2.48), in the risk of respiratory distress syndrome (OR 4.94) which is principally due to the increased frequency of preterm birth (almost 50%), and in the incidence of anaemia (OR 2.65). The perinatal mortality rate associated with placenta praevia is, as would be expected from these observations, increased (by a factor of between 2.9–4.25 as compared to control populations).[9–11] Although it has previously been suggested that there may be a relationship between the presence of placenta praevia and the rate of intra-uterine fetal growth restriction, more recent data have not supported such an association overall;[9] although it is perhaps more likely to observe a reduction in the fetal growth velocity in those cases that have been complicated by recurrent antepartum haemorrhages.

From the maternal perspective, the complications are mostly related to bleeding and its consequences. The relative risk of there being an observed episode of antepartum bleeding is increased by a factor of almost 10, although in up to 30% of cases there may be no bleeding. The incidences of intrapartum and postpartum bleeding are increased by factors of 2.5 and up to 1.9, respectively. Women with placenta praevia are also at greater risk of retroplacental haemorrhage with an increased likelihood ratio of placental abruption of 13.8.[3]

It has been speculated that women with placenta praevia may broadly be divided into two groups, those who have no bleeding and those who have recurrent episodes of bleeding with the prognosis from both a maternal and fetal point of view being worse in the latter.[12,13] Overall, however, the risk of the need for blood transfusion is increased by around 10-fold and the rate of peripartum hysterectomy is increased by a factor of 33.[14] Postpartum bleeding is exacerbated in these cases by the fact that the lower uterine segment has poor contractility as compared to the rest of the uterine body and upon placental separation there is a greater risk that this will result in bleeding from insufficiently occluded venous sinuses. This may also contribute to the small risk of air embolism associated with placenta praevia, as air may enter the systemic circulation through these low pressure venous sinuses. Although this would usually present immediately following the delivery there may be a delay of some hours before signs of the air embolism become evident. Despite these increased risks to the mother, the maternal mortality rate from placenta praevia in the industrialised world has fallen markedly to around 0.03–0.5%.

The precise reasons why some pregnancies are complicated by the implantation of the placenta into the lower uterine segment are unclear; although this may simply be a chance occurrence, there are a number of well-recognised associations. The risk of placenta praevia has been positively linked with maternal age, parity and previous cesarean section delivery.[15] With a single previous cesarean section, the relative risk is increased by a factor of 1.2 and after two previous cesarean sections by a factor of 2.1. A correlation of the risk with the number of previous cesarean sections has been observed with an incidence for placenta praevia approaching 10% having been reported in women who have had four prior cesarean section deliveries.[16,17] Furthermore, the incidence of an anteriorly sited placenta praevia has been reported to be increased in association with prior cesarean section as might be expected if there were a simple mechanical contribution due to the presence of a uterine scar influencing the site of placental implantation.[18] Seemingly, less dramatic uterine surgery, such as uterine curettage or surgical abortion, has also been linked with placenta praevia, with an increased incidence of both placenta praevia and of morbidly adherent placentation; a previous surgical abortion increases the risk by a factor of 1.8.[19,20]

Some reports have also indicated an increased incidence in association with multiple gestations,[10] though this has not been consistently evident.[15] There is, however, a well-established association between cigarette smoking and the incidence of placenta praevia with the risk being increased between 3–6-fold[21–23] and similarly with the use of cocaine the risk of placenta praevia is increased by a factor of 2.4.[24]

For those women who have had a placenta praevia in a previous pregnancy, the recurrence risk is increased by a factor of 8–10-fold.[25] Furthermore, although the aetiologies behind placenta praevia and placental abruption are not necessarily similar, the risk of a placenta praevia is also increased if the preceding pregnancy was complicated by abruption.[26]

Generally, the management of women with placenta praevia aims to allow the pregnancy to progress to as close to term as possible at which point delivery by cesarean section is undertaken for all cases except those cases of grade one placenta praevia where, although the placenta enters the lower segment, the distance between the leading placental edge and the cervix is deemed sufficient to allow vaginal delivery. Available data suggest that this should be a distance of at least 20 mm.[27]

Achieving an adequate gestation in cases of placenta praevia where complications such as episodes of bleeding have occurred may be supported by the adoption of an interventional rather than a conservative approach. Examples of this more 'aggressive' approach to treatment include the use of blood transfusion to manage significant episodes of bleeding which in themselves have not resulted in maternal or fetal compromise of a degree requiring immediate delivery. In addition, the use of tocolysis in threatened preterm labour associated with antepartum haemorrhage has been used successfully to achieve further prolongation of pregnancy.[28–30] As would be expected, improvements in birth weight have been observed with this strategy. Although a trend suggesting an increased frequency of bleeding episodes has been observed in pregnancies managed this way, this did not reach significance nor has there been evidence to suggest that this approach in itself results in an increased requirement for blood transfusion. Re-assuringly, therefore, and contrary to commonly voiced opinion, there does not appear to be any significant detrimental effect on the bleeding pattern as a consequence of the use of tocolytic therapy in patients with placenta praevia who have experienced an antepartum haemorrhage.

A perhaps still more aggressive intervention that has been considered in order to attempt to delay delivery further in this situation has been elective cervical cerclage. The data as to the benefit of this remain uncertain; two reports suggest a benefit from cerclage in respect of prolongation of pregnancy, birth weight and possibly the number of bleeding episodes although a third study has shown no such benefit.[31,32] The number of cases that have been treated in this way remains relatively small and further data may clarify the value or otherwise of this procedure when used in this indication. Therefore, at present, this intervention should perhaps remain confined to clinical studies.

In North American practice, it is often the norm to base the timing of the delivery upon objective evidence of fetal lung maturity by assessing the amniotic fluid lecithin and sphingomyelin ratio although this is rarely undertaken in the UK. Despite taking an aggressive approach to the management there must always be the acceptance that if an episode of haemorrhage is deemed sufficient to be or to potentially be a cause of maternal or fetal compromise then delivery will be indicated.

At present, the body of opinion is broadly split as to whether the management of women whose pregnancies are complicated by placenta praevia should be conducted with the patient admitted to the hospital or as an out-patient at home. Frequently, a combination of in-patient and out-patient care is employed and in each case the decision on the pattern of care will be based on the history of antenatal haemorrhage during the pregnancy, the grade of the placenta praevia, the patient's social circumstances and her wishes as well as the obstetrician's preferred practice. There are at present no good data to indicate that either in-patient or out-patient care leads to a superior outcome. Re-assuringly, perhaps more so for those obstetricians who adopt an out-patient approach, there are no data indicating that either form of care is associated with an increased incidence of adverse outcomes.[33]

The incidence of cesarean delivery is very much increased in these patients as expected since this is generally advocated for all other than some cases of grade I placenta praevia. In this latter group, the decision is dependent upon the distance between the leading placental edge and the internal cervical os, which should be at least 20 mm,[27] and other more general obstetric or maternal factors. The risk of fetal malpresentation due to the placenta preventing stabilisation and engagement of the fetal head within the pelvis is also increased and this, in part, contributes to the increased risk of cesarean delivery even in those cases where vaginal delivery would not be considered unsafe.

The principal factor of interest to the obstetrician undertaking the cesarean section is whether the placenta is sited posteriorly, where the method of the delivery follows an entirely normal pattern, or whether it is anteriorly sited as these latter cases are associated with a greater risk of intra-operative haemorrhage. When the placenta is anteriorly sited, it is often beneficial to perform a scan immediately prior to the cesarean section to localise the placenta precisely and determine whether there is an area of the lower uterine segment where the amniotic sac can be approached without having to incise through the body of the placenta. Even if this can be achieved, the intra-operative blood loss may still be greater than that of an uncomplicated cesarean delivery as the vascularity of the anterior uterine wall is much increased in these cases. However, when there is no such 'placenta-free window' of entry, then the choices lie between gaining access to the fetus using a transplacental approach, with the consequent haemorrhage from the placenta that must be anticipated, or adopting an upper segment ('classical') approach with the consequences that this may have in terms of the management of subsequent pregnancies. Most often, a lower segment approach is used in such cases but, if it is suspected that the placenta is not only low lying but may also be morbidly adherent, an upper segment cesarean section with the placental body being left intact and then if indicated being left *in situ* after the delivery may prove to be a preferred alternative to a lower segment delivery after which the risk of hysterectomy would be very high in such circumstances.

A commonly held view is that a delivery by cesarean section in cases of placenta praevia should be performed under general anaesthesia rather than using regional anaesthetic techniques principally because of the fears of haemorrhage and consequent hypotension. However, there is a growing body of data indicating the safety of regional techniques in such situations. Indeed, there are data indicating that the risk of haemorrhage may in fact be increased in women undergoing cesarean delivery under general anaesthesia and the use of regional techniques is now considered a safe alternative to general anaesthesia in both elective and emergency cesarean delivery in cases of placenta praevia.[2,34,35]

Cases where a placenta praevia is associated with a previous cesarean section or uterine scar are associated with a much greater risk of the placenta being morbidly adherent (placenta accreta, increta or percreta) than are cases of 'isolated' placenta praevia (18% versus 4.5%).[36] This, given the increased incidence of placenta praevia *per se* following prior cesarean delivery, must be acknowledged as a real concern by obstetricians given the rising cesarean section delivery rates that we have been experiencing over the last few decades, especially as the incidence of hysterectomy in such cases is very high (in excess of 90%) and that there is a notable increase in maternal morbidity and mortality.[37]

There are data reporting a positive predictive value for the detection of placenta accreta by ultrasound using colour Doppler imaging of 87.5%.[38]

Magnetic resonance imaging has also been employed with some success in identifying morbidly adherent placentation.[39] Although the maternal mortality rate for this condition is low, the frequency of major surgical intervention is very high with conventional management resulting in around 90% of women requiring a postpartum hysterectomy.[37] By contrast, a conservative approach, which involves leaving the placenta *in situ* and then typically employing conservative surgery such as internal iliac artery ligation or uterine artery embolisation, or a medical approach with the administration of systemic methotrexate, has been shown to be successful in avoiding hysterectomy in a similar proportion of women.[40]

VASA PRAEVIA

If feto-placental blood vessels rather than the placenta itself are present over the internal cervical os then the term vasa praevia is used. With an incidence of around 0.03%, this is a very rare complication of pregnancy which, in part because of its rarity, is associated with a very high perinatal mortality.

The typically quoted associations of vasa praevia are placentas that have a succenturiate or multi-lobed composition and low-lying placentas. Vasa praevia has also been reported to be associated with velamentous cord insertion which, in turn, has been identified as being increasingly common in pregnancies resulting from *in vitro* fertilisation perhaps due to the abnormal or disturbed orientation of the blastocyst on implantation and hence an increased incidence has been observed in pregnancies resulting from such assisted reproductive techniques.[41] Multiple pregnancies also carry an increased risk.

In cases where risk factors for the condition exist, then antenatal diagnosis based on the colour Doppler visualisation of these vessels by endocavitary ultrasound is well recognised.[42] However, often the diagnosis is first considered if vessels are felt during ante-natal or intra-partum vaginal examination or prior to amniotomy. A typical presentation is with unanticipated bleeding at amniotomy. A bedside test to determine whether blood encountered in such circumstances is of fetal origin relies on fetal haemoglobin's ability to withstand alkali denaturation. In most cases where haemorrhage is due to vasa praevia, the fetal haemorrhage would also present itself through cardio-tocographic evidence of fetal compromise with the diagnosis then being confirmed after delivery has been achieved, usually by immediate cesarean section.

PLACENTAL ABRUPTION

The premature separation of the placenta during the antenatal or intrapartum period of pregnancy is termed placental abruption. The incidence is up to 1.5% in pregnancies overall and 0.3% in pregnancies at term.[43,44] Histological examination of the placenta after delivery indicates that many cases are unrecognised with an incidence on histological examination of 4.5%.[45]

A broad distinction in the diagnosis of abruption is drawn between those where there is overt blood loss noted from the lower genital tract – revealed haemorrhage – and those where all bleeding is contained within the gravid uterus with no external bleeding being evident – concealed haemorrhage. The latter typically accounts for around one-third of cases. A more precise classification with four defined categories is also employed. Within this, grade 0 describes an asymptomatic and incidentally observed retro-placental clot. Grades 1–3 are all associated with symptoms although each of these may be either revealed or concealed. Grade 1 refers to haemorrhages where there is pain and uterine irritability but no maternal or fetal compromise. In grade 2 there is no maternal compromise but fetal compromise or distress is recognised. In grade 3 there is uterine tetany, maternal compromise and fetal demise.[46] Most often, the diagnosis of abruption will be based on the clinical history and examination findings. Ultrasonography is often used in those cases where immediate delivery is not indicated, but the sensitivity of ultrasound for the presence of an abruption is poor (24%).[47]

Amongst the factors that are associated with the development of abruption, cigarette smoking features highly with an increase in the risk of up to 90% and with a positive correlation between this risk and the amount smoked.[48] Hypertensive disorders, both pre-existing and of onset during the pregnancy, are also linked with abruption,[49] although hypertension may also develop *de novo* following an abruption. The combination of chronic hypertension and smoking has an additive effect on increasing the risk.

Direct abdominal trauma may also lead to placental haemorrhage and abruption; hence, pregnant women sustaining an abdominal injury such as a road traffic accident should also have an obstetric review after the event.[50] Within the context of direct abdominal trauma, the possibility of physical abuse by a partner or other individual should not be forgotten.[51] The prevalence of physical violence of domestic origin in pregnancy generally exceeds 1 in 100 and the risk of abruption in these cases is increased almost 4 times. Therefore, it is essential and should be routine that during the obstetric assessment an opportunity is made where, in an environment free of possible intimidation, the pregnant woman is able to express any concerns regarding issues such as abuse to which she might have been exposed. As this is a common problem, which all too often passes unrecognised or unreported, positive exclusion of physical abuse should perhaps be considered part of routine antenatal care.

Additional contributory factors include sudden uterine decompression (for example following membrane rupture in cases of polyhydramnios or following amnio-drainage procedures where there is over enthusiastic or overly rapid removal of fluid) and the manipulation associated with external cephalic version. Preterm, prelabour membrane rupture has also been demonstrated to carry an increased risk of abruption, most typically being observed in that group of women in whom the membrane rupture is preceded by bleeding.[52]

Over recent years, an increasing number of acquired and inherited thrombophilias have been identified and it has become apparent that these are associated with a variety of poor outcomes in obstetrics including abruption. Amongst the commoner factors so implicated are the factor V Leiden mutation, the prothrombin gene (G20210A) mutation, the antiphospholipid syndrome, anti-thrombin III (ATIII) deficiency, methylenetetrahydrofolate reductase polymorphisms, hyperhomocysteinaemia, protein C deficiency and protein S deficiency.[53,54] Women who carry these factors and who have previously experienced complications such as venous thrombosis undoubtedly benefit from thromboprophylaxis during pregnancy – in the case of defects such as ATIII deficiency this is indicated even in the absence of a past history as the risk of complications is very high. Thromboprophylaxis in these women will normally consist of mechanical measures (compression stockings, *etc.*) together with pharmacological agents, most typically the low-molecular weight heparins. The role of low-dose aspirin in this indication remains to be clarified.

It has been suggested that women whose pregnancies have been complicated by an abruption for which no other clear explanation is evident should be screened for thrombophilia. However, not all the available data have demonstrated significant differences in the rates of thrombophilias in such groups when compared to controls. Furthermore, there are no data available, at the present time, to indicate whether women with a thrombophilia who have not had a prior thrombotic complication and in whom thrombo-prophylaxis is, therefore, not unequivocally indicated, might benefit from thromboprophylaxis in order to reduce the risk of obstetric complications including abruption. As the value of therapeutic interventions in this group of women is yet to be determined, the value of screening women with abruption for thrombophilia has also yet to be proven. It has also been speculated that there may be an association between abruption and abnormal placentation or trophoblastic invasion as is the case with pre-eclampsia and that prophylactic low-dose aspirin might, therefore, reduce the incidence but this has not been supported by the results of trials using this treatment.[55]

Additionally, associations with diabetes, parity and maternal age have been reported although these have not been consistent findings. As previously noted, there is also an increased incidence of abruption associated with placenta praevia and as with placenta praevia it has also been reported that there is an increased risk in women who have previously been delivered by cesarean section.[56] Despite these various associations, in the majority of cases of placental abruption the aetiology remains uncertain. Abruption in a prior pregnancy is associated with a recurrence rate in excess of 10%. Although previously it has been felt that the likelihood of a poor outcome in a subsequent pregnancy is increased even in the absence of recurrent abruption, more recent data do not support this view.[49,57]

Principally in light of the link with hypertensive disorders and on the basis that abruption may be associated with early maldevelopment of the placental circulation, there have been a number of reports evaluating the use of both first and second trimester uterine artery Doppler ultrasonography in the screening of pregnancies with regard to adverse outcomes. The outcomes evaluated in such studies have generally included hypertensive complications and abruption and many studies report that abnormalities of uterine artery blood flow (an elevated resistance index, an elevated pulsatility index or the presence of a 'notch') identify a group of women at increased risk of these complications, including abruption. However data reviewing all cases of abruption have concluded that Doppler screening only identifies a small proportion of those women whose pregnancies are complicated by abruption and, therefore, does not allow useful prenatal prediction to be made.[58] Given the broad and diverse nature of contributory factors that has been referred to above, this is only to be expected. Another non-specific marker of poor obstetric outcome is an elevation in the maternal serum alpha-fetoprotein (AFP) level and this too has been noted to demonstrate an association with abruption, with the incidence of abruption in pregnancies complicated by an unexplained elevation in AFP (*i.e.* where a fetal neural tube defect, intra-uterine haemorrhage or multiple pregnancy has been excluded) being greater than that in controls at around 5%. However, at the present time, there are no tools that are sufficiently specific or sensitive that can be used as a means of identifying a population at risk of this complication nor has any antenatal intervention been shown to reduce the risk.

As alluded to by the classification mentioned above, placental abruption carries potential consequences to both mother and fetus. Maternal death may occur most usually as a consequence of massive haemorrhage or of various associated pathologies including disseminated intravascular coagulopathy (DIC), adult respiratory distress and renal failure which may all be interlinked. The mortality rate attributable to abruption in the western world is typically less than 1% but in non-industrialised areas where access to rapid cesarean delivery, blood transfusion and intensive care is limited much higher rates are observed. The latter, together with the availability of specialised neonatal care, also contributes to the higher perinatal mortality in these areas which may exceed 50%. Even in industrialised countries, perinatal mortality rates vary widely from almost 12% in the US in the mid-1990s to just under 2% in Norway in the early part of the same decade.[59,60]

With regard to the fetus there are increases in the reported incidences of fetal congenital malformation and growth restriction (IUGR) noted in association with abruption.[61] The link between abruption and IUGR may be either concurrent or consequential with growth restriction occurring both in association with abnormalities of placentation, where the risk of abruption might itself be increased, as well as in those cases where an abruption occurs that does not require immediate delivery but where the resulting loss of a proportion of functional placenta affects future fetal growth.

The management of abruption is guided by the grade at presentation according to the above classification, the presence of concomitant pathologies and the fetal gestation. In cases where there is any maternal or fetal compromise and fetal viability has been achieved, then early delivery is the norm. In most cases, this will be by cesarean section unless labour is already established and advanced as there is a risk of the uterine contractions resulting in expansion of the abruption and, therefore, a deterioration of both the maternal and fetal conditions. If the fetus is already dead, then vaginal delivery is the preferred method of delivery provided that the maternal condition permits this. If there are maternal complications such as DIC already established, although early delivery might be desirable the risks of surgery are very much increased and, therefore, pursuit of a vaginal delivery, whilst administering agents to correct the coaguloapthy, is often the better course to follow. If operative delivery is indicated then normalisation of the maternal condition and clotting systems with the use of blood products – red cells, platelets, fresh frozen plasma and cryoprecipitate – as advised by a haematologist is essential before surgery is undertaken.

In cases where there is asymptomatic evidence of abruption (grade 0) or where there is no maternal or fetal compromise and fetal viability has not yet been achieved, then conservative approaches may be adopted. As these have been successful there has been a move to extend this conservative approach to cases in the third trimester where optimum fetal lung maturation has not yet been achieved; in this approach, even tocolysis, which traditionally has been viewed as a contra-indicated intervention in cases of placental abruption, has been used. There are data to support the use of tocolytic therapies in such cases provided that this is undertaken in an environment where close maternal and fetal monitoring is undertaken and where the facilities for rapid cesarean section delivery are available.[62]

UNCLASSIFIED VAGINAL BLEEDING

A significant proportion of episodes of antepartum haemorrhage cannot clearly be attributed either to an abruption or a low-lying placenta. If a lower genital tract pathology such as a cervical ectropion is also excluded, then these bleeds are considered unclassified but are often termed marginal bleeds indicating a bleed from the placental margin rather than a bleed into the retro-placental space. This is essentially a diagnosis of exclusion. The principal concern of unclassified bleeds is their association with an increased risk of preterm delivery and also a small increase in the risk of fetal congenital abnormality.[1] In some centres, there has been a tendency for women who have experienced unclassified bleeds to be induced once they reach term but, as the principal morbidity in such cases is in fact related to preterm delivery there are no data to justify this course of action. As with other causes of APH, the management of these cases will depend on the perceived quantity of blood lost and the presence of any adverse consequences of this to the mother or fetus.

UMBILICAL CORD HAEMORRHAGE

A rare site of antepartum haemorrhage is the umbilical cord. Most haemorrhages within the cord or from the cord are iatrogenic as a consequence of fetal cord blood sampling; however, spontaneous cord haemorrhages have been reported and most often these have been associated with a poor perinatal outcome. Such haemorrhages may be spontaneous, for example umbilical vein rupture, or associated with pathologies of the umbilical cord such as a cord cyst. Demise may arise as a consequence of tamponade of the cord vessels within an intact cord or from fetal exsanguination.[63,64] An iatrogenic bleed may be managed conservatively if the bleed appears to be self-limiting with no evidence of compromise to the umbilical circulation or by delivery, if the thresholds for fetal viability or fetal lung maturity have been reached and concerns about the impact of the haemorrhage on the fetus or evidence of a continuing bleed are manifest.

KEY POINTS FOR CLINICAL PRACTICE

- Antepartum haemorrhage affects around 5% of pregnancies.

- Placenta praevia and placental abruption together account for around half of antepartum bleeds with a significant proportion of all bleeds being unclassified, *i.e.* of uncertain cause, although most of these are attributed to marginal placental haemorrhage.

- Placenta praevia complicates 0.5% of pregnancies.

- The rate of placenta praevia increases almost 2-fold after uterine curettage or abortion and 2-fold after two cesarean section deliveries. These latter factors also increase the rate of morbidly adherent placentation.

- Aggressive conservative management allows safe prolongation of pregnancy, reducing the perinatal morbidity and mortality.

- Placental abruption affects up to 1.5% of pregnancies although many more cases are unrecognised.

- The sensitivity for sonographic diagnosis of an abruption is poor (24%) nor is Doppler screening in early pregnancy able to predict the majority of cases.

References

1 Chan CC, To WW. Antepartum hemorrhage of unknown origin – what is its clinical significance? Acta Obstet Gynecol Scand 1999; 78: 186–190

2 Frederiksen MC, Glassenberg R, Stika CS. Placenta previa: a 22-year analysis. Am J Obstet Gynecol 1999; 180: 1432–1437

3 Iyasu S, Saftlas AK, Rowley DL, Koonin LM, Lawson HW, Atrash HK. The epidemiology of placenta previa in the United States, 1979 through 1987. Am J Obstet Gynecol 1993; 168: 1424–1429

4 Hill LM, DiNofrio DM, Chenevey P. Transvaginal sonographic evaluation of first-trimester placenta previa. Ultrasound Obstet Gynecol 1995; 5: 301–303

5 Farine D, Fox HE, Jakobson S, Timor-Tritsch IE. Vaginal ultrasound for diagnosis of placenta previa. Am J Obstet Gynecol 1988; 159: 566–569

6 Timor-Tritsch IE, Yunis RA. Confirming the safety of transvaginal sonography in patients suspected of placenta previa. Obstet Gynecol 1993; 81: 742–744

7 Hertzberg BS, Bowie JD, Carroll BA, Kliewer MA, Weber TM. Diagnosis of placenta previa during the third trimester: role of transperineal sonography. AJR Am J Roentgenol 1992; 159: 83–87

8 Jeanty P, d'Alton M, Romero R, Hobbins JC. Perineal scanning. Am J Perinatol 1986; 3: 289–295

9 Crane JM, Van den Hof MC, Dodds L, Armson BA, Liston R. Neonatal outcomes with placenta previa. Obstet Gynecol 1999; 93: 541–544

10 Ananth CV, Demissie K, Smulian JC, Vintzileos AM. Placenta previa in singleton and twin births in the United States, 1989 through 1998: a comparison of risk factor profiles and associated conditions. Am J Obstet Gynecol 2003; 188: 275–281

11 Ananth CV, Smulian JC, Vintzileos AM. The effect of placenta previa on neonatal mortality: a population-based study in the United States, 1989 through 1997. Am J Obstet Gynecol 2003; 188: 1299–1304

12 Gorodeski IG, Neri A, Bahary CM. Placenta previa – the identification of low- and high-risk subgroups. Eur J Obstet Gynecol Reprod Biol 1985; 20: 133–143

13 Lam CM, Wong SF, Chow KM, Ho LC. Women with placenta praevia and antepartum haemorrhage have a worse outcome than those who do not bleed before delivery. J Obstet Gynaecol 2000; 20: 27–31

14 Crane JM, Van den Hof MC, Dodds L, Armson BA, Liston R. Maternal complications with placenta previa. Am J Perinatol 2000; 17: 101–105

15 Parazzini F, Dindelli M, Luchini L *et al*. Risk factors for placenta praevia. Placenta 1994; 15: 321–326

16 Clark SL, Koonings PP, Phelan JP. Placenta previa/accreta and prior cesarean section. Obstet Gynecol 1985; 66: 89–92

17 Hershkowitz R, Fraser D, Mazor M, Leiberman JR. One or multiple previous cesarean sections are associated with similar increased frequency of placenta previa. Eur J Obstet Gynecol Reprod Biol 1995; 62: 185–188

18 To WW, Leung WC. Placenta previa and previous cesarean section. Int J Gynaecol Obstet 1995; 51: 25–31

19 Johnson LG, Mueller BA, Daling JR. The relationship of placenta previa and history of induced abortion. Int J Gynaecol Obstet 2003; 81: 191–198

20 Ota Y, Watanabe H, Fukasawa I *et al*. Placenta accreta/increta. Review of 10 cases and a case report. Arch Gynecol Obstet 1999; 263: 69–72

21 Castles A, Adams EK, Melvin CL, Kelsch C, Boulton ML. Effects of smoking during pregnancy. Five meta-analyses. Am J Prevent Med 1999; 16: 208–215

22 Handler AS, Mason ED, Rosenberg DL, Davis FG. The relationship between exposure during pregnancy to cigarette smoking and cocaine use and placenta previa. Am J Obstet Gynecol 1994; 170: 884–889

23 Williams MA, Mittendorf R, Lieberman E, Monson RR, Schoenbaum SC, Genest DR. Cigarette smoking during pregnancy in relation to placenta previa. Am J Obstet Gynecol 1991; 165: 28–32

24 Kistin N, Handler A, Davis F, Ferre C. Cocaine and cigarettes: a comparison of risks. Paediatr Perinat Epidemiol 1996; 10: 269–278

25 Monica G, Lilja C. Placenta previa, maternal smoking and recurrence risk. Acta Obstet Gynecol Scand 1995; 74: 341–345

26 Rasmussen S, Albrechtsen S, Dalaker K. Obstetric history and the risk of placenta previa. Acta Obstet Gynecol Scand 2000; 79: 502–507

27 Bhide A, Prefumo F, Moore J, Hollis B, Thilaganathan B. Placental edge to internal os distance in the late third trimester and mode of delivery in placenta praevia. Br J Obstet Gynaecol 2003; 110: 860–864

28 Cotton DB, Read JA, Paul RH, Quilligan EJ. The conservative aggressive management of placenta previa. Am J Obstet Gynecol 1980; 137: 687–695

29 Besinger RE, Moniak CW, Paskiewicz LS, Fisher SG, Tomich PG. The effect of tocolytic use in the management of symptomatic placenta previa. Am J Obstet Gynecol 1995; 172: 1770–1775

30 Silver R, Depp R, Sabbagha RE, Dooley SL, Socol ML, Tamura RK. Placenta previa: aggressive expectant management. Am J Obstet Gynecol 1984; 150: 15–22

31 Tessarolo M, Bellino R, Arduino S, Leo L, Wierdis T, Lanza A. Cervical cerclage for the treatment of patients with placenta previa. Clin Exp Obstet Gynecol 1996; 23: 184–187

32 Cobo E, Conde-Agudelo A, Delgado J, Canaval H, Congote A. Cervical cerclage: an alternative for the management of placenta previa? Am J Obstet Gynecol 1998; 179: 122–125

33 Mouer JR. Placenta previa: antepartum conservative management, inpatient versus outpatient. Am J Obstet Gynecol 1994; 170: 1683–1685

34 Bonner SM, Haynes SR, Ryall D. The anaesthetic management of Caesarean section for placenta praevia: a questionnaire survey. Anaesthesia 1995; 50: 992–994

35 Parekh N, Husaini SW, Russell IF. Caesarean section for placenta praevia: a retrospective study of anaesthetic management. Br J Anaesth 2000; 84: 725–730

36 Chattopadhyay SK, Kharif H, Sherbeeni MM. Placenta praevia and accreta after previous caesarean section. Eur J Obstet Gynecol Reprod Biol 1993; 52: 151–156

37 Armstrong CA, Harding S, Matthews T, Dickinson JE. Is placenta accreta catching up with us? Aust NZ J Obstet Gynaecol 2004; 44: 210–213

38 Chou MM, Ho ES, Lee YH. Prenatal diagnosis of placenta previa accreta by transabdominal color Doppler ultrasound. Ultrasound Obstet Gynecol 2000; 15: 28–35

39 Ha TP, Li KC. Placenta accreta: MRI antenatal diagnosis and surgical correlation. J Magn Reson Imaging 1998; 8: 748–750

40 Courbiere B, Bretelle F, Porcu G, Gamerre M, Blanc B. [Conservative treatment of placenta accreta]. J Gynecol Obstet Biol Reprod (Paris) 2003; 32: 549–554

41 Englert Y, Imbert MC, Van Rosendael E *et al*. Morphological anomalies in the placentae of IVF pregnancies: preliminary report of a multicentric study. Hum Reprod 1987; 2: 155–157

42 Catanzarite V, Maida C, Thomas W, Mendoza A, Stanco L, Piacquadio KM. Prenatal sonographic diagnosis of vasa previa: ultrasound findings and obstetric outcome in ten cases. Ultrasound Obstet Gynecol 2001; 18: 109–115

43 Saftlas AF, Olson DR, Atrash HK, Rochat R, Rowley D. National trends in the incidence of abruptio placentae, 1979-1987. Obstet Gynecol 1991; 78: 1081–1086

44 Sheiner E, Shoham-Vardi I, Hallak M *et al*. Placental abruption in term pregnancies: clinical significance and obstetric risk factors. J Matern Fetal Neonatal Med 2003; 13: 45–49

45 Fox H. Pathology of the Placenta. London: WB Saunders, 1978

46 Knuppel AR, Drukker JE. Bleeding in late pregnancy: antepartum bleeding. In: Hayashi RH, Castillo MS. (eds) High Risk Pregnancy: A Team Approach. Philadelphia, PA: WB Saunders, 1986

47 Glantz C, Purnell L. Clinical utility of sonography in the diagnosis and treatment of placental abruption. J Ultrasound Med 2002; 21: 837–840

48 Ananth CV, Smulian JC, Vintzileos AM. Incidence of placental abruption in relation to cigarette smoking and hypertensive disorders during pregnancy: a meta-analysis of observational studies. Obstet Gynecol 1999; 93: 622–628

49 Ananth CV, Savitz DA, Williams MA. Placental abruption and its association with hypertension and prolonged rupture of membranes: a methodologic review and meta-analysis. Obstet Gynecol 1996; 88: 309–318

50 Grossman NB. Blunt trauma in pregnancy. Am Fam Physician 2004; 70: 1303–1310

51 Janssen PA, Holt VL, Sugg NK, Emanuel I, Critchlow CM, Henderson AD. Intimate partner violence and adverse pregnancy outcomes: a population-based study. Am J Obstet Gynecol 2003; 188: 1341–1347

52 Major CA, de Veciana M, Lewis DF, Morgan MA. Preterm premature rupture of membranes and abruptio placentae: is there an association between these pregnancy complications? Am J Obstet Gynecol 1995; 172: 672–676

53 de Vries JI, Dekker GA, Huijgens PC, Jakobs C, Blomberg BM, van Geijn HP. Hyperhomocysteinaemia and protein S deficiency in complicated pregnancies. Br J Obstet Gynaecol 1997; 104: 1248–1254

54 Lockwood CJ. Inherited thrombophilias in pregnant patients: detection and treatment paradigm. Obstet Gynecol 2002; 99: 333–341

55 Subtil D, Goeusse P, Puech F *et al*. Aspirin (100 mg) used for prevention of pre-eclampsia in nulliparous women: the Essai Regional Aspirine Mere-Enfant study (Part 1). Br J Obstet Gynaecol 2003; 110: 475–484

56 Hemminki E, Merilainen J. Long-term effects of cesarean sections: ectopic pregnancies and placental problems. Am J Obstet Gynecol 1996; 174: 1569–1574

57 Toivonen S, Heinonen S, Anttila M, Kosma VM, Saarikoski S. Obstetric prognosis after placental abruption. Fetal Diagn Ther 2004; 19: 336–341

58 Toivonen S, Heinonen S, Anttila M, Kosma VM, Saarikoski S. Reproductive risk factors, Doppler findings, and outcome of affected births in placental abruption: a population-based analysis. Am J Perinatol 2002; 19: 451–460

59 Ananth CV, Wilcox AJ. Placental abruption and perinatal mortality in the United States. Am J Epidemiol 2001; 153: 332–337

60 Rasmussen S, Irgens LM, Bergsjo P, Dalaker K. Perinatal mortality and case fatality after placental abruption in Norway 1967–1991. Acta Obstet Gynecol Scand 1996; 75: 229–234

61 Raymond EG, Mills JL. Placental abruption. Maternal risk factors and associated fetal conditions. Acta Obstet Gynecol Scand 1993; 72: 633–639

62 Towers CV, Pircon RA, Heppard M. Is tocolysis safe in the management of third-trimester bleeding? Am J Obstet Gynecol 1999; 180: 1572–1578

63 Brown RN, Nicolaides KH. Umbilical cord haematoma associated with an umbilical cord cyst and fetal death at 28 weeks of gestation. J Ultrasound Med 2000; 19: 223–225

64 Romero R, Chevernak F, Cousta D. Antenatal sonographic diagnosis of umbilical cord hematoma. Am J Obstet Gynecol 1982; 143: 719

Kavita Goswami   Steven Thornton

The prevention and treatment of preterm labour

Preterm birth occurs in 7–12% of all deliveries, but accounts for over 85% of perinatal morbidity and mortality.[1] Although the death rate has decreased over the past few decades, this can be attributed to improvements in neonatal management rather than a reduction in preterm births.[2]

The mortality, morbidity and costs of preterm delivery are higher at lower gestational ages, for example, mortality rates are 90% at 23 weeks dropping to 2% at 34 weeks. Even in babies that survive, there is a high risk of short- and long-term morbidity.[3] Some associated conditions are acute and amenable to treatment but others such as cerebral palsy, neurodevelopmental, and pulmonary disorders can result in long-term, severe disability.

The immediate neonatal costs of caring for preterm infants are enormous but small in comparison to the long-term care of survivors who often require special needs education, mobility aids, and additional healthcare. It has been calculated that prematurity is responsible for 35% of all healthcare spending.[4] There are also major implications in terms of the psychological and social impact of disability on the individuals and their carers.

The devastating consequences of prematurity have led to attempts to improve outcome by predicting, preventing and treating preterm labour. These are discussed in this chapter.

Kavita Goswami BSc MBBS MRCOG MMedSci Dip Obs & Gynae USS
Consultant Obstetrician and Gynaecologist, University Hospitals of Coventry and Warwickshire, Clifford Bridge Road, Coventry CV2 2DX, UK
E-mail: kavita.goswami@uhcw.nhs.uk

Steven Thornton DM FRCOG (for correspondence)
Professor of Obstetrics and Associate Dean (Research), Warwick Medical School, The University of Warwick, Clifford Bridge Road, Coventry CV4 7AL, UK
E-mail: s.thornton@warwick.ac.uk

SCREENING AND PREDICTION

Many different approaches have been suggested for the screening and prediction of preterm labour such as salivary oestriol, home uterine-activity monitoring and measurement of plasma metabolites. Although these have not been demonstrated to be effective in routine clinical practice, some methods such as maternal risk scoring, fetal fibronectin (FFN) and cervical ultrasonography require further discussion.

Risk scoring

Scoring systems are based on factors which increase the risk of preterm delivery. The risk is highest with a previous preterm delivery but bleeding in pregnancy, urinary tract infection, higher order pregnancies, body mass index (BMI) < 20 kg/m^2, previous low birth weight babies and stress (particularly family illness, mortality, disruption, violence, or financial) are associated with preterm delivery.[5] Unfortunately, risk scores do not identify the majority of women who deliver preterm even when weighting is given to those with the highest predictive value. For this reason, they are of limited clinical use.

Fetal fibronectin (FFN) testing

The appearance of FFN in cervicovaginal secretions in the late second and early third trimester represents disruption of the chorio–decidual interface which can be caused by preterm labour, infection, stress or haemorrhage. Given the effect of preterm labour on FFN, testing has been used to determine the risk of preterm delivery in asymptomatic and symptomatic women.[6,7] Although quantification has not been helpful in routine clinical practice, a positive fibronectin test (based on an arbitrary cut-off) increases the risk of preterm delivery.

In asymptomatic women, the likelihood ratio for a positive result is 4.01 (95% CI 2.93–5.49) for predicting birth before 34 weeks' gestation, with a corresponding ratio for a negative result of 0.78 (95% CI 0.72–0.84). Among symptomatic women, the likelihood ratio for a positive results is 5.42 (95% CI 4.36–6.74) for predicting birth within 7–10 days of testing and the ratio for a negative result is 0.25 (95% CI 0.20–0.31).[8]

The result of FFN testing may help decision making regarding in-patient admission, *in-utero* transfer and administration of steroids. Although FFN is predictive, alterations in the subsequent management of a positive test need to be demonstrated to improve outcome. Nevertheless, the high negative predictive value can be used to influence management.

Other biochemical markers (interleukin-6, tumour necrosis factor, C-reactive protein, collagenase, granulocyte elastase, matrix metalloproteinases, human chorionic gonadotrophin, corticotrophin releasing hormone, estradiol, estriol-17B, relaxin, granulocyte colony-stimulating factor and progesterone) have been linked to subsequent preterm delivery but, at present, do not have the specificity to be useful in clinical practice.

Cervical sonographic assessment

Endovaginal ultrasonographic examination of the uterine cervix is more accurate than digital examination of the cervix in the assessment of the risk for preterm delivery in patients with symptoms of preterm labour and intact membranes.[9,10] It has a high sensitivity and positive predictive value, particularly in symptomatic women at high risk for preterm delivery (*i.e.* contractions, premature rupture of membranes, and history of preterm delivery).[11]

Measurement of cervical length provides accurate prediction of risk for early preterm delivery.[12] Routine measurement of cervical length at 22–24 weeks can, therefore, be used to identify a group at high risk of early preterm birth. There is a significant inverse association between cervical length and rate of spontaneous delivery before 33 weeks. When cervical length is 1.5 cm or less, 26% deliver before 34 weeks, compared with the UK national average of 1.5%.[13] At present, the management of women with a short cervix is controversial. Interventions have not been demonstrated to reduce the risk of preterm delivery, hence the rationale for undertaking a routine scan for cervical length has been questioned. The investigation may be helpful for women where cerclage is indicated from the clinical history but who decline the procedure (see below). However, there is only a reason to undertake the scan if cerclage would be undertaken if the cervix was subsequently demonstrated to be short. Cervical scanning may also be useful for research studies where a high-risk population needs to be identified. Although routine ultrasound screening is not currently indicated, future demonstration of interventions which improve outcome in women with a short cervix could lead to its wide-spread use. Furthermore, it may be helpful in threatened preterm labour to guide tocolytic or steroid administration. The combination with other tests such as maternal α-fetoprotein, alkaline phosphatase, and granulocyte colony-stimulating factor may enhance the ability to predict spontaneous preterm birth and so the future development of multiple-marker tests for spontaneous preterm birth is feasible.[14]

PREVENTION

Preventing the onset of preterm labour is generally unrewarding but behavioural and life-style modifications coupled with optimal management can reduce the incidence of delivery.

Smoking,[15] substance and physical abuse, malnutrition, and heavy physical activity[16] during pregnancy are risk factors. Smoking cessation decreases preterm births and increases birth weight.[17] Although trials have not demonstrated an improvement in outcome with all behavioural modifications, appropriate life-style changes such as adequate nutrition and avoidance of illicit drugs are likely to be beneficial.

In contrast, studies of social support and home visiting in pregnancy do not seem to be effective in preventing preterm birth.[18] Efforts to monitor high-risk women and to institute tocolytics and bed rest at the first signs of labour have not been effective. For women with uncomplicated twin pregnancy, such a policy may even be harmful since the risk of very preterm birth seems to be increased.[19]

There are a number of maternal and fetal conditions associated with preterm labour. Fetal abnormality, multiple pregnancy, genito-urinary infection and systemic maternal medical conditions are associated risks. Adhering to strict policies in reproductive medicine to prevent multiple pregnancy, detection and treatment of genito-urinary infections and optimal management of maternal or fetal conditions will reduce prematurity, albeit in only a small number of individuals.

Insertion of a vaginal pessary may be a cost-effective preventive treatment in patients at risk for spontaneous preterm birth but prospective controlled trials are needed.[20] Recent Cochrane reviews of multiple strategies for premature labour prevention have shown that most are unsuccessful. However, certain specific interventions such as cervical cerclage, administration of progesterone, detection and treatment of vaginal and intra-uterine infection may be of benefit. These require further evaluation.

Cervical cerclage

Cervical cerclage involves placing a stitch around the cervix. The rationale is that an intrinsically weak cervix could be held closed throughout pregnancy. Although this relatively simplistic view may be correct, it has recently been suggested that cerclage could prevent ascending infection by lengthening the cervical canal thereby preventing labour. The procedure is usually based on the techniques described by McDonald or Shirodkar. Since there are no controlled comparative clinical trials to support the use of the technically more demanding Shirodkar procedure, it seems reasonable, at present, to undertake McDonald cerclage unless there are specific indications.

The indications for cerclage are vague and there is a wide variation in obstetric practice. Frequently, past obstetric history has been taken as the major indication, in particular, a history of painless cervical dilatation, mid trimester rupture of the membranes, history of cervical damage, uterine developmental abnormalities or exposure to diethylstilboestrol *in utero*.

It has recently been suggested that a short cervix diagnosed by ultrasound scan in asymptomatic women may be an indication for cerclage. The results of trials and reviews have been inconsistent possibly due to differing inclusion criteria. Although some studies[12] suggest that ultrasound-directed cerclage may be helpful, this has not been confirmed in others.[22] The largest study has recently been reported by To *et al.*[13] who reported a multinational study where around 47,000 normal singleton pregnancies were screened for cervical length. In those where the cervix was 1.5 cm or less, women were randomly allocated to have a stitch inserted or conservative management. Overall, 1% of women had a short cervix and were eligible for randomisation. Those who had a stitch inserted, had the procedure done with mersilene tape, under spinal block with erythromycin cover. All women received steroids in the form of two doses of 12 mg of dexamethasone at 27 weeks, but they were not given tocolytics, antibiotics or bed rest. The vast majority (74% and 78%) of both groups delivered after 33 completed weeks. Cerclage did not improve the outcome in terms of preterm delivery, perinatal mortality or morbidity. Thus routine determination of cervical length in low-risk women followed by cerclage in those with a shortened cervix cannot be advocated.

Although cerclage may not be helpful in low-risk women identified to have a short cervix on ultrasound, the procedure may be helpful in individuals who are at risk based on their history. Meta-analyses[23,24] have suggested that prophylactic cerclage does not prevent preterm delivery in women at lower risk. However, a systematic review by Bachman *et al.*[25] demonstrated that cervical cerclage, in women at higher risk of preterm birth, reduces the incidence before 34 weeks' and 37 weeks' gestation with OR of 0.72 (95% CI 0.53–0.97) and 0.80 (95% CI 0.63–1.02), respectively. The reported number to be treated to prevent one additional preterm birth before 34 weeks was 24 women (95% CI 10–61). Similar conclusions were shown by the systematic review by Odibo *et al.*[26] who calculated that 20 cervical cerclages are required to prevent one delivery less than 34 weeks.

Although the meta-analyses are encouraging, the trials entered into the analyses require further discussion. The largest trial was that undertaken by the MRC/RCOG.[27] This recruited only those women whose obstetrician was uncertain whether or not to undertake cerclage. Therefore, those who were most likely to benefit were excluded. Even so, the trial demonstrated that cerclage was associated with a lower risk of delivery below 33 weeks. Therefore, although there is no definitive data to support cerclage, since the largest study demonstrated a benefit in some women, it would seem reasonable to use cerclage in appropriate cases.

Progesterone

Progesterone has many cellular functions which maintain pregnancy; in numerous species, withdrawal is a prerequisite for labour. Although its precise involvement in human labour is controversial, there is overwhelming evidence that it has a fundamental role in pregnancy. The administration of progesterone to prevent or treat preterm labour is not new. In the 1980s, meta-analyses suggested that progestational agents were not helpful for prevention or treatment of preterm labour in high-risk women but a meta-analysis of prophylactic treatment with one particular drug (17α-hydroxyprogesterone caproate, a metabolite of progesterone), showed a reduction in preterm delivery. The odds ratio for preterm birth in women who received this progesterone was 0.50 (95% CI 0.30–0.85), and for low birth weight (< 2500 g) 0.50 (95% CI 0.27-0.80) but administration did not influence perinatal mortality or morbidity.[28] This meta-analysis by Kierse[28] was largely ignored until interest was rekindled with the recent publication of a double blind randomised study of 17α-hydroxyprogesterone caproate compared to placebo for the prevention of preterm delivery in high-risk women.[29,30] This study demonstrated that weekly administration to women with a previous preterm delivery reduced the risk of delivery at less than 37 weeks from 54.9% to 36.3% (RR 0.66; 95% CI 0.54–0.81); $P < 0.001$). Delivery at less than 35 weeks of gestation reduced from 30.7% to 20.6% (RR 0.67; 95% CI 0.48–0.93) and delivery at less than 32 weeks of gestation reduced from 19.6% to 11.4% (RR 0.58; 95% CI 0.37–0.91). Based on these data, five or six women with a previous spontaneous preterm birth would need to be treated to prevent one birth less than 37 weeks' gestation and 12 women to prevent one birth less than 32 weeks' gestation. Perhaps the most encouraging outcome of this trial, and in contrast to almost all others, was that infants of women treated with 17α-hydroxyprogesterone caproate had significantly lower rates of the secondary outcomes of necrotising enterocolitis, intraventricular haemorrhage, and need for supplemental oxygen.

Although the results suggest that progesterone administration to high-risk women (defined as previous preterm delivery) is beneficial, caution is required for the following reasons: (i) there was an unusually high incidence of preterm delivery in the control group (55%); (ii) it is not known whether the results can be extrapolated to other high risk groups (such as multiple pregnancy); (iii) 17α-hydroxyprogesterone caproate is not readily available; (iv) there is a high risk of preterm delivery (36%) even in those women treated with the active agent; and (v) administration requires weekly intramuscular injections.

It is interesting that a smaller study[31] demonstrated that administration of vaginal progesterone was also associated with a reduced risk of preterm delivery. This not only provides supporting evidence from a second independent study for prophylactic progesterone, but also suggests that systemic administration is not mandatory since the effect may not be specific for 17α-hydroxyprogesterone caproate.

Although the safety of 17α-hydroxyprogesterone remains to be documented, so far there has been no reported increase in congenital anomalies or adverse effects.[32,33] Thus, in conclusion, although progesterone (possibly 17α-hydroxyprogesterone caproate) may be beneficial for the prevention of preterm delivery, its wide-spread administration cannot be advocated until safety is confirmed and improved outcome documented.

Role of infection

There is overwhelming evidence to implicate infection as a possible cause for preterm labour.[34-36] This may be in the form of abnormal vaginal flora (bacterial vaginosis such as anaerobes, *Gardenerella vaginalis* or *Mycoplasma hominis*), intra-uterine or genital tract infection (*Trichomonas vaginalis* or *Chlamydia trachomatis*).

Bacterial vaginosis

Around 50% of women with bacterial vaginosis are asymptomatic. If symptoms do occur, the most common is a thin, watery, malodorous, non-itchy discharge. The criteria used to diagnose bacterial vaginosis are vaginal pH > 4.5, presence of thin watery discharge, fishy odour (with 10% KOH), clue cells on a saline wet mount, and/or Gram stain.

A number of studies have confirmed that women with bacterial vaginosis during pregnancy have a significantly increased risk of delivering preterm compared to those with normal vaginal flora.[37-40] Bacterial vaginosis is associated with a higher incidence of late miscarriage or preterm birth (OR 5.5; 95% CI 2.3–13.3). The earlier the abnormal genital colonisation is detected, the greater is the risk of an adverse outcome. Abnormal genital tract flora at 26–32 weeks' gestation is associated with an odds ratio for preterm delivery of 1.4–2 whereas at 7–16 weeks the ratio is 5–7.5.[37]

Despite this association, the effects of treatment in low-risk women have been contradictory. In a large study by Carey *et al.*,[41] asymptomatic women were screened at 16–24 weeks and treated with metronidazole or placebo. A repeat vaginal smear and pH were done at 24–30 weeks and treatment repeated if indicated. There was no difference in low or very low birth weight babies before 32, 35 or 37 weeks. In this study, however, women with symptomatic bacterial vaginosis were excluded, treatment was given after 16 weeks, there were high number of exclusions for unexplained reasons, a high placebo response rate and the diagnosis (made by Gram stain) changed in many women before treatment.

In contrast, The study of Ugwundu et al.[42] demonstrated a reduction in the rate of miscarriage or spontaneous preterm delivery (95% CI 5.0–15.8) in asymptomatic women with bacterial vaginosis at 12–22 weeks' gestation who received clindamycin. In another study by Lamont and colleagues,[43] women with bacterial vaginosis were randomised to receive clindamycin or placebo. The placebo group had a lower gestational age at delivery and a higher rate of neonatal intensive care unit admission. Subgroup analysis demonstrated the greatest effect in women with florid abnormal genital tract flora. These two studies[42,43] in contrast to that of Carey et al.,[41] therefore, support the identification and treatment of bacterial vaginosis in low-risk women in early pregnancy.

In contrast to the contradictory results in low-risk women, detection and treatment of bacterial vaginosis in high-risk women is generally advocated. Hauth et al.[44] randomised 624 women at high risk of preterm birth to receive oral metronidazole and erythromycin or placebo (between 22–24 weeks). Repeat antibiotics were given if indicated by swabs taken after 2–4 weeks. The rate of preterm births in women receiving antibiotics was 31% compared to 49% for those given placebo ($P = 0.006$). There was no difference in the rate of preterm birth in women receiving antibiotics who did not have a diagnosis of bacterial vaginosis. A Cochrane Systematic Review[45] failed to provide a definitive answer perhaps although it was published before some of the double-blind, placebo-controlled trials were published.[42]

In conclusion, it seems reasonable to screen and treat bacterial vaginosis in high-risk women as early as possible in pregnancy. In those at low risk, treatment seems appropriate if abnormal genital flora are diagnosed fortuitously or symptoms are present.[46] In future, it may be appropriate to screen low-risk women if trials demonstrate a benefit of early treatment in these women.

The choice of treatment is controversial. Recent evidence[47] suggests that metronidazole may increase preterm delivery in women selected by history and positive FFN. In view of this, treatment with clindamycin seems prudent.

Genital tract infection

There is evidence that T. vaginalis in adolescent women is associated with preterm delivery and low birth weight.[48,49] An association between C. trachomatis and subsequent preterm birth has also been reported. Despite these associations, results of studies to evaluate treatment have been contradictory. Those conducted by the Maternal-Fetal Medicine Units (MFMU) network have shown an association between infection and preterm birth, but have not shown a beneficial effect of treatment of asymptomatic women. Indeed, treatment of T. vaginalis with metronidazole may be deleterious.[50] Further work is required to confirm or refute these observations.

TREATMENT

The current contentious areas are whether tocolysis should be used in uncomplicated preterm labour and, if so, which drug should be administered.

It is naive to believe that outcome will be improved in all pregnancies by delaying delivery. There are individuals in whom a delay in delivery will adversely affect outcome, such as those with preterm delivery precipitated by placental failure or abruption. It is, therefore, mandatory that, if tocolysis is administered, it is restricted to those who will benefit. Even with this proviso, there are arguments for not using tocolysis. These are: (i) a delay in delivery could prolong the fetal exposure to an adverse environment, for example that caused by unrecognised infection; (ii) cross-sectional outcome data which demonstrate improved outcome with gestational age may not be applicable to an individual in threatened preterm labour; and (iii) clinical trials and meta-analyses[51] have failed to demonstrate improved neonatal outcome in women treated with tocolytics.

There are good reasons, however, why clinical trials may not have demonstrated improved outcome. First, the delay in delivery may not have been used to undertake measures likely to benefit the fetus such as *in utero* transfer or administration of steroids. Second, there were flaws in many of the trials such as: (i) patients were recruited at a gestational age where a delay in delivery was unlikely to improve outcome; (ii) they were underpowered; (iii) patients were not in true preterm labour; (iv) an ineffective tocolytic was used; or (v) inappropriate outcomes were determined.

It is perhaps not surprising, therefore, that there is currently no consensus opinion on whether tocolysis should be used in uncomplicated preterm labour and a definitive trial is urgently needed. Current guidelines in the UK[52] support (but do not recommend) tocolysis if the time gained by delaying delivery is used to improve neonatal outcome. This essentially means transfer to a unit with appropriate neonatal facilities or administration of steroids. Maintenance tocolysis is not recommended for routine practice.[52]

Maternal administration of steroids

Administration of maternal steroids causes many effects in the fetus leading to increased maturation. There are major effects on the fetal lung (surfactant production and structural), gastrointestinal and central nervous systems. Maternal administration causes a reduction in neonatal death, respiratory distress syndrome, necrotising enterocolitis and intraventricular haemorrhage in babies born preterm.[53]

Betamethasone crosses the placenta. A randomised placebo trial of betamethasone demonstrated a significant reduction in respiratory distress in babies born before 32 weeks' gestation and improvement in other neonatal outcomes. Baud *et al.*[54] compared the neonatal outcome in a retrospective analysis of women who received betamethasone, dexamethasone or no steroids. Cystic periventricular leukomalacia occurred in 4.4% of infants whose mothers had received betamethasone, 11.4% of those who received dexamethasone and 8.4% without glucocorticoids. This suggests that betamethasone should be the steroid of choice for this indication.

The maximal beneficial effect of steroids is between 24 h and 7 days after administration. The data are consistent with an effect prior to and following this but the benefits are more difficult to document in clinical trials. Steroids are recommended between 24–36 weeks of gestation, for single or multiple pregnancies. This should include those with preterm prelabour ruptured membranes and mothers with diabetes (in whom careful control of blood glucose is required). Although definitive evidence of benefit in all these groups is lacking, the advantages conferred by administration outweigh the risks.[55,56]

The optimal gestational age at which steroids should be given has not been determined. Meta-analysis confirms that administration prior to 30 weeks confers a benefit although the lower limit of the gestational age is not known. The upper limit of the gestation age which confirms a benefit is also not known. The data show a non-significant improvement in outcome for babies delivered to mothers who receive steroids at gestational ages above 34 weeks. It is likely that the lack of significance is a consequence of the small improvement in outcome which can be achieved at higher gestational ages. However, given that steroids are not without adverse effects, the risk/benefit should be considered for each patient in whom steroids are contemplated at 34 weeks and above.

Perhaps more controversial is whether steroids should be given to all women in threatened preterm labour. Since the diagnosis is difficult and many women who present with preterm uterine activity ultimately deliver at term, administration to all women with symptoms will mean that many receive the drug unnecessarily. A case can, therefore, be made to administer steroids if additional investigations such as FFN suggest that delivery is likely. A description of the number needed to treat with positive or negative FFN at 31 weeks is provided in the systematic review by Honest et al.[8] Although further work is required to determine the precise risks and benefits, caution should be exercised in administration of steroids to women with very low risks of preterm delivery whilst ensuring that those who are reasonably likely to deliver receive a safe and effective drug.

The theoretical risk of maternal fetal infection following steroids has not been confirmed in trials. Nevertheless, steroids should be avoided in patients with chorio-amnionitis. Although the benefits of maternal steroids are numerous, there are concerns regarding adverse effects such as intra-uterine growth restriction. The adverse effects are likely to be increased by repeated courses and so only a single course is currently recommended. For this reason, since tocolysis is usually indicated in order to administer steroids (see above), tocolytics are not usually required on more than one occasion. It should be stressed, however, that clinical follow-up studies have been undertaken for up to 20 years in offspring whose mothers received steroids. These demonstrate that a single course is not associated with clinical adverse effects.[54]

Which tocolytic?

Guidelines from the UK Royal College of Obstetricians and Gynaecologists (RCOG) suggest that if tocolytics are administered, the first choice should be an oxytocin antagonist (atosiban) or a calcium channel blocker (nifedipine). Other drugs suggested to have tocolytic activity are either ineffective or have more worrying adverse effects.

Oxytocin antagonists
Atosiban is an oxytocin antagonist which also has activity at the vasopressin receptor. Since oxytocin has a fundamental role in the onset of parturition, inhibition is logical and represents a relatively specific method for delaying delivery.[57]

Large, double-blind, clinical trials have been undertaken to compare atosiban with placebo[58] or with β-sympathomimetics[59] in threatened preterm labour. Unfortunately, it was considered that these trials could not be done without rescue tocolysis. This means that any woman who did not respond to the original tocolytic could receive another drug. It is, therefore, impossible with this study design to determine the drug effect on neonatal outcome. The placebo controlled trials did not demonstrate a significant improvement in the primary end-point which was time between the beginning of treatment and delivery or therapeutic failure. Atosiban was, however, associated with a marked and significant reduction in women who remained undelivered and did not receive alternative tocolytics at 1, 2 and 7 days.

The comparator trials which pool results for all β-sympathomimetics, demonstrate that the proportion of women who delivered after 48 h or 7 days are similar in those who receive atosiban or β-sympathomimetics.[59] Since β-sympathomimetics effectively delay delivery, the implication is that atosiban is as effective, with the major advantage that side effects are markedly reduced. The long-term safety of atosiban has been determined by follow-up of babies for 2 years. To date there have been no major or consistent adverse effects reported in these children. Thus, based on the evidence available, atosiban seems a logical and rational treatment for preterm labour, albeit that the authors conclusions differ from those in a recent meta-analysis.[64]

Calcium channel blockers

Nifedine is the most commonly used calcium channel blocker for tocolysis. In contrast to the large studies for atosiban, many of the nifedipine trials are relatively small.[60] There are no good-quality, placebo-controlled, blinded trials. A meta-analysis of unblinded comparator trials[61] demonstrated that nifedipine was associated with a reduction in risk of birth within 1 week, reduction in neonatal respiratory distress syndrome, intraventricular haemorrhage and necrotising enterocolitis. These results should, however, be interpreted cautiously since rescue tocolysis was used in some of the studies (see above), different doses of nifedipine were used, very high infusion rates of ritodrine were administered in some studies and patients may not have been analysed on an intention-to-treat basis. There are no reports of long-term follow-up from these studies although initial concerns about fetal compromise[62] due to redistribution of uterine blood flow have not been confirmed in clinical studies.

The maternal side effects for calcium channel blockers are predominantly headache, dizziness, flushing, reflex tachycardia due to systemic hypotension and reduced atrioventricular conduction. Calcium channel blockers may predispose to pulmonary oedema. Co-administration of calcium channel blockers with magnesium sulphate can cause hypotension.

The decision regarding which drug should be used as the first-line tocolytic is, therefore, difficult and atosiban, although licensed, is more expensive than nifedipine. There are no direct comparative studies and indirect studies[63] are unlikely to be helpful given the quality of included trials and lack of quality outcome data.

Given that there are large double-blind studies of atosiban suggesting that it is efficacious, in the absence of such data for nifedipine, the authors favour an oxytocin antagonist as the first-line treatment of uncomplicated preterm labour.

KEY POINTS FOR CLINICAL PRACTICE

- Maternal risk scoring is of limited use.

- Studies of social support and home visiting in pregnancy do not suggest a beneficial effect in preventing preterm birth.

- Fetal fibronectin testing may be predictive for risk of preterm delivery in asymptomatic and symptomatic women. Although predictive, the subsequent management of a positive test needs to be demonstrated to improve outcome.

- There is a significant inverse association between cervical length and rate of spontaneous delivery before 33 weeks.

- It may be reasonable to restrict tocolysis and steroids to women with a positive fibronectin or a short cervix.

- Systematic reviews suggest that prophylactic cervical cerclage is effective in reducing the incidence of preterm birth before 34 weeks in appropriate women.

- Although progesterone (in particular 17α-hydroxyprogesterone caproate) may prevent preterm delivery, its wide-spread administration cannot be advocated until safety is confirmed and improved neonatal outcome confirmed.

- It seems reasonable to screen and treat bacterial vaginosis in high-risk women as early as possible in pregnancy. In those at low risk, treatment seems appropriate if abnormal genital flora are diagnosed fortuitously or symptoms are present.

- Current guidelines in the UK support (but do not recommend) tocolysis if the time gained by delaying delivery is used to improve neonatal outcome.

- Maternal administration of steroids causes a reduction in neonatal death, respiratory distress syndrome, necrotising enterocolitis and intraventricular haemorrhage in babies born preterm before 34 weeks. Betamethasone is the steroid of choice.

- UK Royal College of Obstetricians and Gynaecologists' guidelines suggest that if tocolytics are administered, the first choice should be an oxytocin antagonist (atosiban) or a calcium channel blocker (nifedipine).

References

1 Guyer B, Freedman MA, Strobino DM *et al.* Annual summary of vital statistics – 1998. Pediatrics 1999; 104: 1229–1246
2 Scheider H. Pharmacological intervention in preterm labour. Res Clin Forums 1994; 16: 59–83
3 Hack M, Flannery DJ, Schluchter M, Cartar L, Borawski E, Klein N. Outcomes in young adulthood of very low birth weight infants. N Engl J Med 2002; 346: 149–157

4 Lewit E, Baker L, Corman H, Shiono PH. The direct cost of low birth weight. Future Child 1995; 5: 35–56

5 Moutquin JM. Socio-economic and psychosocial factors in the management and prevention of preterm labour. Br J Obstet Gynaecol 2003; 110 (Suppl 20): 56–60

6 Goldenberg RL, Klebanoff M, Carey JC *et al.* Vaginal fibronectin measurements from 8 to 22 weeks gestation and subsequent spontaneous preterm birth. Am J Obstet Gynecol 2000; 183: 469–475

7 Leitich H, Kaider A. Fetal fibronectin – how useful is it in the prediction of preterm birth? Br J Obstet Gynaecol 2003; 110 (Suppl 20): 66–70

8 Honest H, Bachmann LM, Gupta JK, Kleijnen J, Khan K. Accuracy of cervical fetal fibronectin test in predicting risk of spontaneous preterm birth: systematic review. BMJ 2002; 325: 301–311

9 Gomez R, Galasso M, Romero R *et al.* Ultrasonographic examination of the uterine cervix is better than cervical digital examination as a predictor of the likelihood of premature delivery in patients with preterm labour and intact membranes. Am J Obstet Gynecol 1994; 171: 956–964

10 Berghella V, Tolosa JE, Kuhlmann K, Weiner S, Bolognese RJ, Wapner RJ. Cervical ultrasonography compared with manual examination as a predictor of preterm delivery. Am J Obstet Gynecol 1997; 177: 723–730

11 Hoesli I, Tercanli S, Hozgreve W. Cervical length assessment by ultrasound as a predictor of preterm labour – is there a role for screening? Br J Obstet Gynaecol 2003; 110 (Suppl 20): 61–65

12 Heath VC, Southall TR, Souka AP, Elisseou A, Nicolaides KH. Cervical length at 23 weeks of gestation: prediction of spontaneous preterm delivery. Ultrasound Obstet Gynecol 1998; 12: 301–303

13 To MS, Alfirevic Z, Heath VC *et al.* Fetal Medicine Foundation Second Trimester Screening Group. Cervical cerclage for prevention of preterm delivery in women with short cervix: randomised controlled trial. Lancet 2004; 363: 1849–1853

14 Goldenberg RL, Iams JD, Mercer BM *et al.* National Institute of Child Health and Human Development Maternal-Fetal Medicine Units Network. What we have learned about the predictors of preterm birth. Semin Perinatol 2003; 27: 185–193

15 Burguet A, Kaminski M, Abraham-Lerat L *et al.* Epipage Study Group. The complex relationship between smoking in pregnancy and very preterm delivery. Results of the Epipage study. Br J Obstet Gynaecol 2004; 111: 258–265

16 Papiernik E, J Bouyer, Collin D. Prevention of preterm births: a perinatal study in Haguenau, France. Pediatrics 1985; 76: 154

17 Lumley J, Oliver S, Waters E. Interventions for promoting smoking cessation during pregnancy. Cochrane database Syst Rev 2000; (2): CD 001055

18 Hodnett ED. Support during pregnancy for women at increased risk of low birth weight babies. Cochrane database Syst Rev 2003; (3): CD 000198

19 Crowther CA. Hospitalisation and bed rest for multiple pregnancy. Cochrane database Syst Rev 2001; (1): CD 000110

20 Arabin B, Halbesman JR, Vork F, Hubener M, van Eyck J. Is treatment with vaginal pessaries an option in patients with a sonographically detected short cervix. J Perinat Med 2003; 31: 122–133

21 Althuisius S, Dekker G, Hummel P, Bekedam D, Kuik D, van Geijn H. Cervical Incompetence Prevention Randomized Cerclage Trial (CIPRACT): effect of therapeutic cerclage with bed rest vs. bed rest only on cervical length. Ultrasound Obstet Gynecol 2002; 20: 163–167

22 Rust OA, Atlas RO, Reed J, van Gaalen J, Balducci J. Revisiting the short cervix detected by transvaginal ultrasound in the second trimester: why cerclage therapy may not help. Am J Obstet Gynecol 2001; 185: 1098–1105

23 Drakeley AJ, Roberts D, Alfirevic Z. Cervical cerclage for prevention of preterm delivery: meta-analysis of randomized trials. Obstet Gynecol 2003; 102: 621–627

24 Drakeley AJ, Roberts D, Alfirevic Z. Cervical stitch (cerclage) for preventing pregnancy loss in women. Cochrane Database Syst Rev. 2003; (1):CD003253

25 Bachmann LM, Coomarasamy A, Honest H, Khan K. Elective cervical cerclage for prevention of preterm birth: a systematic review. Acta Obstet Gynecol Scand 2003; 82: 398–404

26 Odibo AO, Elkousy M, Ural SH, Macones GA. Prevention of preterm birth by cervical cerclage compared with expectant management: a systematic review. Obstet Gynecol Surv 2003; 58: 130–136

27 MRC/RCOG Working Party on Cervical Cerclage. Final report of the Medical Research Council/Royal College of Obstetricians and Gynaecologists multicentre randomised trial of cervical cerclage. Br J Obstet Gynaecol 1993; 100: 516–523

28 Keirse MJNC. Progesterone administration in pregnancy may prevent pre-term delivery. Br J Obstet Gynaecol 1990; 97: 149–154

29 Meis PJ. National Institute of Child Health and Human Development Maternal-Fetal Medicine Units Network. 17 alpha-hydroxyprogesterone acetate to prevent recurrent preterm birth. Am J Obstet Gynecol 2002; 187: S54

30 Meis PJ, Klebanoff M, Thorn E et al. National Institute of Child Health and Human Development Maternal-Fetal Medicine Units Network. Prevention of recurrent preterm delivery by alpha-hydroxyprogesterone caproate. N Engl J Med 2003; 348: 2379–2385

31 Da Fonseca EB, Bittar RE, Carvalho MH, Zugaib M. Prophylactic administration of progesterone by vaginal suppository to reduce the incidence of spontaneous preterm birth in women at increased risk: a randomised placebo controlled double-blind study. Am J Obstet Gynecol 2003; 188: 419–424

32 Resseguie LJ, Hick JF, Bruen JA, Noller KL, O'Fallon WM, Kurland LT. Congenital malformations among offspring exposed in utero to progestins, Olmsted County, Minnesota, 1936–1974. Fertil Steril 1985; 43: 514–519

33 Spong CY. Recent developments in preventing recurrent preterm birth. Obstet Gynecol 2003; 101: 1153–1154

34 Lamont RF. The role of infection in preterm labour and birth. Hosp Med 2003; 64: 644–647

35 Lamont RF. Infection in preterm labour. Proceedings of the 40th Study group of the Royal College of Obstetricians and Gynaecologists. London: RCOG, 2001; 305–317

36 Lettieri L, Vintzileos AM, Rodis JM, Albini SM, Salafia CM. Does idiopathic preterm labour resulting in preterm birth exist? Am J Obstet Gynecol 1993; 168: 1480–1485

37 Hay PE, Lamont RF, Taylor-Robinson D, Morgan DJ, Ison C, Pearson J. Abnormal bacterial colonisation of the genital tract and subsequent preterm delivery and late miscarriage. BMJ 1994; 308: 295–298

38 Hillier SL, Nugent RP, Eshenback DA et al. Association between bacterial vaginosis and preterm delivery of a low birth weight infant. N Engl J Med 1995; 333: 1737–1742

39 Flynn C, Helwig A, Meurer L. Bacterial vaginosis in pregnancy and the risk of prematurity: a meta-analysis. J Fam Pract 1999; 48: 885–892

40 Lamont RF. Bacterial vaginosis. In: Studd JWW, Jardine-Brown C. (eds) The Yearbook of the Royal College of Obstetricians & Gynaecologists 1994. London: Parthenon, 1995; 149–160

41 Carey JC, Klebanoff MA, Hauth JC et al. Metronidazole to prevent preterm delivery in pregnant women with asymptomatic bacterial vaginosis. National Institute of Child Health and Human Development. Network of maternal fetal medicine? N Engl J Med 2000; 342: 534–540

42 Ugwumadu J, Manyonda I, Reid F, Hay P. Effect of early oral clindamycin on late miscarriage and preterm delivery in asymptomatic women with abnormal vaginal flora and bacterial vaginosis a randomised controlled trial. Lancet 2003; 361: 983–988

43 Lamont RF, Duncan SLB, Mandal D, Bassett P. Intravaginal clindamycin to reduce preterm birth in women with abnormal genital tract flora. Obstet Gynecol 2003; 101: 516–522

44 Hauth JC, Goldenberg RL, Andrews WW, DuBard MB, Copper RL. Reduced incidence of preterm delivery with metronidazole and erythromycin in women with bacterial vaginosis. N Engl J Med 1995; 333: 1732–1736

45 King J, Fenady V. Prophylactic antibiotics for inhibiting preterm labour with intact membranes. Cochrane Database Syst Rev. 2002;(4):CD000246

46 Lamont RF. Can antibiotics prevent preterm birth – the pro and con debate. Br J Obstet Gynaecol 2005; 112 (Suppl 1): 67–73

47 Shennan A, Crawshaw S, Briley A et al. A randomised controlled trial of metronidazole for the prevention of preterm birth in women positive for cervicovaginal fetal fibronectin: the PREMET study. Br J Obstet Gynaecol 2006; 113: 65–74

48 Hardy P, Hardy J, Nell E *et al.* Prevalence of six sexually transmitted disease agents among pregnant inner city adolescents and pregnancy outcome. Lancet 1984; 2: 333–337

49 Andrew WW, Goldenberg RL, Mercer B *et al.* The Preterm Prediction Study: association of second-trimester genitourinary chlamydia infection with subsequent preterm birth. Am J Obstet Gynecol 2000; 183: 662–668

50 Carey JC, Klebanoff MA. National Institute of Child Health and Human Development Maternal-Fetal Medicine Units Network. Semin Perinatol 2003; 27: 212–216

51 Gyetvai K, Hannah ME, Hodnett ED, Ohlsson A. Tocolytics for preterm labour: a systematic review. Obstet Gynecol 1999; 94: 869–877

52 Royal College of Obstetricians and Gynaecologists Guideline. Tocolytic Drugs for Women in Preterm Labour 1 (B). London: RCOG, 2002

53 Royal College of Obstetricians and Gynaecologists guideline. Antenatal corticosteroids to prevent respiratory distress syndrome. London: RCOG, 2002

54 Baud O, Foix-L'Helias L, Kaminski M *et al.* Antenatal glucocorticoid treatment and cystic periventricular leukomalacia in very premature infants. N Engl J Med 1999; 341: 1190–1196

55 Crowley P. Antenatal corticosteroids – current thinking. Br J Obstet Gynaecol 2003; 110 (Suppl 20): 77–78

56 Crowley P. Prophylactic corticosteroids for preterm birth (Cochrane Review). In: Cochrane Database Syst Rev 2002; (4): CD000065

57 Blanks AM, Thornton S. The role of oxytocin in parturition. Br J Obstet Gynaecol 2003; 110 (Suppl 20): 46–51

58 Romero R, Sibai BM, Sanchez-Ramos L *et al.* An oxytocin receptor antagonist (atosiban) in the treatment of preterm labour: a randomised, double-blind, placebo-controlled trial with tocolytic rescue. Am J Obstet Gynecol 2000; 182: 1173–1183

59 Worldwide Atosiban versus Beta-agonists Study Group. Effectiveness and safety of the oxytocin antagonist atosiban versus beta-adrenergic agonists in the treatment of preterm labour. Br J Obstet Gynaecol 2001; 108: 133–142

60 King JF, Flenady V, Papatsonis D, Dekker G, Carbonne B. Calcium channel blockers for inhibiting preterm labour. Cochrane Database Syst Rev. 2002;(2):CD002255

61 King JF, Flenady V, Papatsonis D, Dekker G, Carbonne B. Calcium channel blockers for inhibiting preterm labour; a systematic review of the evidence and a protocol for administration of nifedipine. Aust NZ J Obstet Gynaecol 2003; 43: 192–198

62 Ducsay CA, Thompson JS, Wu AT, Novy MJ. Effects of calcium entry blocker (nicardipine) tocolysis in rhesus macaques: fetal plasma concentrations and cardiorespiratory changes. Am J Obstet Gynecol 1987; 157: 1482–1486

63 Coomarasamy A, Knox EM, Gee H, Khan K. Oxytocin antagonists for tocolysis in preterm labour – a systematic review. Med Sci Monit 2002; 8: RA268–RA273

64 Papatsonis D, Flenady V, Cole S, Loley H. Oxytocin receptor antagonists for inhibiting preterm labour. Cochrane Database Syst Rev 2005; (3): CD 004452

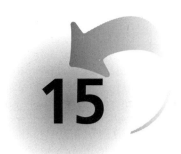

Wayne R. Cohen

Controversies in the assessment of labor

It is remarkable how limited is our understanding of a process as fundamental to the preservation and well-being of the human species as labor and birth. This is not for lack of trying; indeed, substantial progress in this regard has been made. We are now quite conversant with the anatomical, physiological, and biochemical features of uterine contractility. In some species, we have explained many of the intricacies involved in the initiation of labor, although this remains more mysterious in women. Despite our progress in unraveling the basic science that underlies parturition, the events that we observe and experience during human labor and birth (*i.e.* the development of co-ordinated uterine contractions that leads ultimately to expulsion of the wholly dependent fetus from the birth canal into the waiting world and relative independence) are understood primarily in descriptive clinical terms. The medical oversight of parturition is largely a matter of recognizing when abnormalities occur during what, for most women, is a normal physiological experience and a momentous and thrilling life event. Nevertheless, labor and delivery can confer harm, particularly when the process proceeds aberrantly.

When labor is abnormal and safe delivery of the fetus is thereby impeded, dystocia is said to be present. Humans may be unique among animals in that dystocia is a relatively frequent event; the evolutionary explanation for this fact is not certain.[1] Whatever the cause, it is clear that the outcome of labor and delivery can be improved through human intervention; but since interventions carry risk, the key to successful management is to intercede when the benefits of medical therapy are deemed to outweigh their potential harm. To make reasonable judgments in that regard it is obviously necessary to have a reliable and objective means to determine when labor has deviated from normal.

Wayne R. Cohen MD
Chairman of Obstetrics and Gynecology, Jamaica Hospital Medical Center, 89-06 135th Street, Suite 6A,
Jamaica, NY 11418, USA
E-mail: wcohen@jhmc.org

Controversies abound as to how best to manage labor and delivery in order to avoid fetal and maternal injury. The uncertainty about that issue is one of the forces that has propelled cesarean section rates in many parts of the world to previously unthinkable heights. Many obstetricians deem the risks of labor and delivery simply not worth taking, now that elective cesarean section is a readily performed operation with extremely low rates of serious morbidity and mortality. Whether a policy of near-universal cesarean delivery will really lead to improved short- and long-term outcome for mother and baby remains to be seen; such an approach should be viewed with earnest skepticism until its real consequences are understood.

In fact, the risks of parturition can be minimized through an objectified approach to the oversight of labor and delivery. This chapter will address some practical and clinically pertinent controversies regarding the assessment of labor. Are the Friedman labor curves still valid? Does the use of epidural anesthesia alter the course of labor adversely? Does dystocia confer any lasting adversity on the fetus? Is vaginal delivery a significant contributor to later life incontinence?

While the most obvious approach to the evaluation of labor is to study uterine contractions, this pathway has been unrewarding. Clearly, strong and co-ordinated uterine contractions are necessary to propel the fetus down the birth canal. While there are clinical methods to assess contractility (external tocodynamometry and intra-uterine pressure transducers) the information derived from them has done little to enhance our clinical decision-making. The problem is that the variability in measurable contractility among normal labors is so great that it cannot be used as a reliable or predictive tool to judge whether a labor is dysfunctional.[2,3] Recent work with uterine electro-myography seems to have potential in clinical management, but remains experimental.[4,5]

THE LABOR CURVES

The visionary work of Emanuel A. Friedman,[6-13] first published in the 1950s, elevated the management of labor from a rather subjective exercise informed mostly by an individual obstetrician or midwife's personal experience, to the status of evidence-based clinical evaluation. His first publication, describing graphic analysis of labor,[6] and many that followed over succeeding decades, created a legacy that was one of the most important contributions to obstetrics in the 20th century. He was the first to recognize the prognostic importance of quantifiable clinical observations in determining the likely need for cesarean or instrumental delivery. In his later work, he explored the potential for identifying long-term problems in offspring based on the type of labor and delivery that preceded birth.[14] Graphic analysis of labor progress raised the management of labor from a somewhat arbitrary exercise to one in which considerable scientific objectivity could be applied in concert with clinical art, an innovation that has served mothers and babies well.

The approach promulgated by Friedman has since been modified and re-interpreted by other workers for adaptation to specific populations or to unique circumstances.[15-27] Throughout its various permutations, the principal concept of evaluating progress by interpretation of the graphically expressed

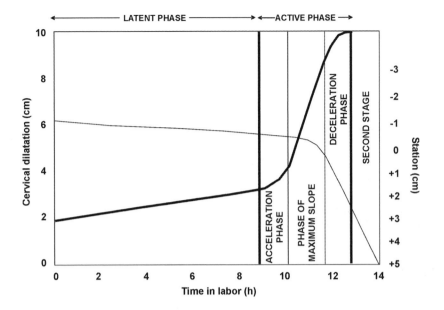

Fig. 1 Composite of cervical dilatation and fetal descent curves described by Friedman illustrating their interrelationship and their component phases. (From: Cohen WR, Friedman EA. Management of Labor. Rockville, MD: Aspen Publications, 1983; 13).

relation among cervical dilatation, fetal descent, and elapsed time in labor has been verified as a useful tool. In fact, it is the only extant system that allows a systematic, real-time measure of labor progress and provides an unequivocal language for communication about dysfunctional labor (Fig. 1).[28] Without the use of this uniform terminology, the study of labor and meaningful comparison of outcomes among obstetricians or institutions is impossible.

Recently, reasonable concerns have been expressed about whether data based on studies done more than a half century ago are still relevant to the early 21st century. In fact, some investigators have recently challenged the continuing validity of the labor curves and measures of abnormality that Friedman described.[29–31] Because these concerns disturb the bedrock of our diagnostic tactics for recognizing dysfunctional labor, it is important to address the soundness of our current working assumptions.

CORROBORATION OF THE FRIEDMAN DATA

Several investigators attempted to validate the observations made by Friedman during the decades following his seminal contribution. In most cases, his insights were verified. Although some argued that the latent phase was not really a part of labor, or that the deceleration phase did not really exist, almost all studies (done in a spectrum of patient populations) verified with close accord the rates of dilatation and descent described by Friedman, and the general concept that there is a uniform and predictable relationship between time elapsed during labor and progress in cervical dilatation and fetal descent (Fig. 2). Further, it became clear that deviations in patterns of cervical

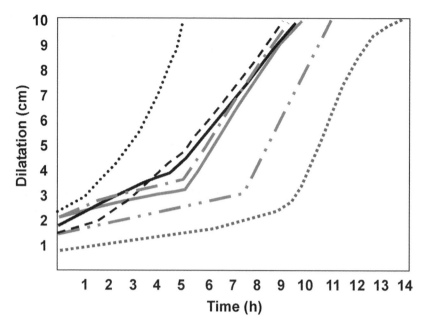

Fig. 2 A composite of cervical dilatation curves from several investigators demonstrating the uniformity of observed mean rates of cervical dilatation in the active phase. The Friedman curve is at the far right. Others come from references [17-22,59] (Modified from Williams Obstetrics, 21st edn. New York: McGraw-Hill, 2001; 429).

dilatation and fetal descent were useful to help predict the outcome of the labor and the need for operative intervention.

Work from the 1960s by Ledger and colleagues at two US institutions confirmed the presence of latent and active phases of labor, and verified the benefits of using the curves to diagnose abnormalities of the first stage of labor.[17-19] Data from the National Collaborative Perinatal Project, collected from a multicenter study in the US during the 1950s to 1970s (analyzed by Friedman) on more than 10,000 nulliparas was also confirmatory.[32]

Philpott and Castle[20,21] adapted the graphic analysis of labor to a population in Africa. Their focus was on active phase dilatation rates, which were determined to be similar to the original Friedman data. Their 'partogramme' added other useful information to the graphic display of dilatation (fetal heart rate, uterine contractions, membrane status, *etc.*), which served to emphasize that data in addition to the labor curves were important in making clinical decisions. Obstetric units in Britain,[22] Israel,[23,24] and other parts of the world[25-27] adopted the technique. Thus, an impressive volume of observations from many investigators over many decades have validated the general observations of Friedman concerning the expected patterns of cervical dilatation and (to a lesser extent because of more limited data) fetal descent during labor. Dissenting views have been relatively few, and have focused mainly on disagreement about whether the latent phase and deceleration phase exist.

Differences in many studies exist in the assessment of the duration of the latent phase. Given the frequent difficulty of ascertaining the exact time of labor onset, this is not surprising. Observations of the latent phase are important primarily for the recognition that there is a variable period of time (which may normally consume many hours) after the onset of labor during which little or no dilatation or descent takes place. Failure to recognize this, and rather to characterize a labor as abnormal simply because a certain number of hours has elapsed, has led to many unnecessary interventions during a normal latent phase. During this portion of labor, biochemical changes occur in the cervix that serve to increase its compliance (primarily through degradation of collagen and changes in ground substance), changes necessary to allow the subsequent rapid dilatation that characterizes the active phase.

The deceleration phase noted in Friedman's graphic depictions of dilatation refers to the apparent slowing of cervical dilatation during the terminal portions of the first stage of labor. Other investigators have suggested that dilatation is linear throughout the active phase, and that the observed deceleration is an artifact arising from the infrequency of examinations during labor. In other words, patients are not necessarily examined precisely at the time the cervix reaches full dilatation, and the longer the interval between complete dilatation and the examination that records its occurrence, the longer will appear the graphed deceleration phase. This deception can, in fact, occur; a true deceleration phase has, however, been observed in several studies, and was seen by Friedman in some early data in which a mechanical cervimeter was used to provide continuous evaluation of dilatation.[7,33,34]

The deceleration phase is widely misunderstood, and its proper assessment is a vital part of labor evaluation. Advancement in cervical dilatation is in fact linear from the end of the acceleration phase to full dilatation; but the nature of our clinical examination technique creates the apparent slowing. During all of dilatation, the cervix retracts along the surface of the presenting part; the separation of the edges of the cervix from each other is therefore curvilinear. During most of the active phase, however, the dilatation occurs sufficiently close to the transverse plane of the body that the examining fingers detect true dilatation. As full dilatation approaches, separation of the edges of the cervix occurs more in a cephalad than a transverse direction as the cervix retracts around the presenting part. Consequently, the transverse change in dilatation does slow, accounting for the deceleration phase (Fig. 3). Careful and frequent examination will reveal an obvious deceleration in most patients. It may be very short (and undetectable) when the cervix is dilating rapidly.

The importance of the deceleration phase is that the terminal events of cervical dilatation will generally not occur without some descent taking place. Thus, the attainment of complete dilatation is actually an important milestone in descent; when the initiation of descent is delayed at this point in labor, cephalopelvic disproportion, abnormalities of the second stage, and shoulder dystocia occur frequently.[34,35]

A recent challenge to the continuing validity of the Friedman curves arose from evaluation of a retrospective analysis of a data base of 1329 nulliparas.[29] These data showed a much slower rate of active phase dilatation than most previous studies, and no discernible deceleration phase. The latter might be attributable to an insufficient number of examinations in late first-stage labor; but the former observation is of more interest and potential importance. Why

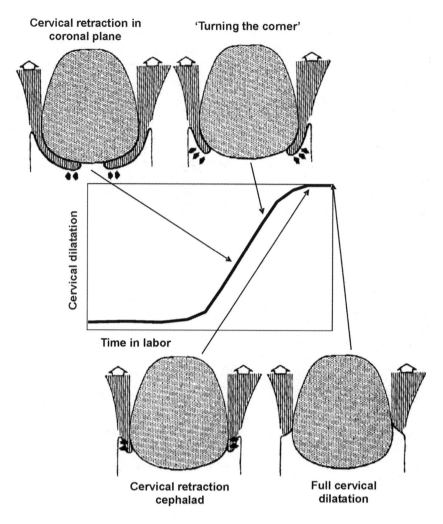

Fig. 3 Graphic explanation for the development of the deceleration phase. (From: Friedman EA. Labor: Clinical Evaluation and Management. New York: Appleton-Century-Crofts, 1978, 35).

would these contemporary data differ from those of Friedman and the many investigators who followed him? Should they lead us to change our approach to the recognition of dysfunctional labor?

If the new data are valid, and the classically defined patterns of normal labor no longer describe our obstetric populations, the discrepancy could exist for several reasons. The original data could be flawed, or their analysis specious; but this is unlikely given the similar findings of many studies and the vast numbers of cases in which they have been validated. The biological characteristics of human labor could have changed over 50 years; but this is too short a time for evolutionary changes. Modern obstetric interventions could have altered labor; but, if anything, contemporary use of analgesia, anesthesia and oxytocin are less likely to inhibit labor progress than in decades past. Most plausibly, the nature of the patient population has changed in ways that influence labor. The most evident demographic trends in this regard are a shift to more older nulliparas and a dramatic increase in maternal obesity. Both advancing age (via uncertain mechanisms) and obesity (probably through its association with larger fetal weights, but perhaps also in other ways) are known to affect labor progress adversely.[7,8,36,37]

If these factors have indeed had the effect of altering the patterns of labor curves, does this mean we should abandon the traditional measures of normality? If obesity leads to excess fetal growth and a consequent increase in the frequency of protraction and arrest disorders as classically defined, it would be hazardous to consider the new data to reflect normal expectations. The consequence of that approach would be to overlook labors that reflect an increased need for cesarean, and perhaps increased fetal risk. Rather than letting our changing population create new norms, we should use established norms to help us learn something about our changing population. The wheel need not be re-invented; in fact, it may prove particularly useful in identifying labors at risk as our population demographics change. The Friedman labor curves and their various derivative systems have provided a reliable chassis that has supported intrapartum care for many decades; there seems little reason to abandon them.

EXPECTATIONS OF GRAPHIC LABOR ANALYSIS

One of the reasons for the uncertainty about the validity of the curves is that there have sometimes been unreasonable expectations about what they can tell us. To assume the labor curves *per se* will always identify when a cesarean is necessary is an improbable expectation. The curves cannot be used in a clinical vacuum; rather, they are an important facet of the clinical evaluation of labor, which is essentially one of periodically estimating the likelihood of safe vaginal delivery. This determination is made by seriatim assessment of several streams of clinical information.

At each of many serial evaluations of the patient during labor, a number of facts are gathered. These relate not only to progress in dilatation and station. Pelvic architecture, uterine contractility, effects of anesthesia and other medications, as well as fetal molding, position, and attitude are all contributors to success of the labor process, and their sequential changes contribute importantly to clinical decision making about the need for intervention. The state of the mother's well-being and of fetal oxygenation are also taken into consideration, as is the presence of infection. At each evaluation, all of these separate but interrelated observations must be integrated by the obstetrician or midwife into a risk calculus. In other words, at each evaluation the attendant asks: 'based on the available information and the trends observed in the latest measured parameters, what is now the likelihood of a safe vaginal delivery?' This question, even if not asked explicitly, is implicit in rational decision-making during labor. Indeed, when the probability of a safe delivery becomes small, cesarean section (or, sometimes, instrumental vaginal delivery) should be employed to minimize fetal and maternal risks. All the clinical data used in reaching decisions about obstetric interventions (especially use of oxytocin, conduction anesthesia, cesarean section, and instrumental delivery) should be viewed from this perspective. Interpretation of the labor curves is a vital facet of this approach.

Unfortunately, the level of risk at which intervention is appropriate cannot always be determined with uniformity or precision. In fact, it should be considered as a variable influenced by many factors that bear upon the individual woman and her labor. Experience and judgment are important ingredients of clinical wisdom in these situations.

For example, consider a labor marred by a prolonged deceleration phase. A decision about whether or not to use oxytocin, observe for spontaneous progress, or intervene by cesarean section should be informed by several things. Based on the presence of the graphically determined dysfunction alone, there is at least a 50% probability of the patient needing to be delivered by cesarean. If the pelvic architecture were found to be normal, the fetal weight not excessive, molding minimal, and the head in normal position and attitude, oxytocin stimulation would be reasonable. If, however, the fetal weight were large and clinical cephalopelvimetry showed marked molding, a deflexed attitude, and a malposition, or if there were a history of a prior delivery with shoulder dystocia, prompt cesarean delivery would be more prudent. In either case, or in the more challenging situations that fall between these extremes, the probability estimate derived from graphic analysis is the foundation upon which the decision-making process is built.

INSIGHTS FROM LABOR GRAPHS

One of the reasons that some basic questions about the evaluation and management of labor remain enigmatic is that we have not adopted a uniform and unequivocal set of standards for the definition of labor dysfunction.[28] This is regrettable, but correctable if the uniform lexicon described by Friedman were adopted. Insightful analysis of labor curves has provided important insights into many common clinical problems. For example, from them we have learned that: (i) labors in multiparas who have had only cesareans in prior pregnancies act like those of nulliparas and should be judged by those criteria;[38] (ii) amniotomy is not generally an effective treatment for arrest of dilatation;[39,40] (iii) risks of precipitate labor are more closely related to the rate of dilatation and descent than to duration of labor;[41] (iv) the course of labor does not differ among ethnic groups;[42] (v) maternal age influences labor;[8,43] and (vi) newborn morbidity after a very long second stage is influenced by whether or not a graphic labor abnormality pattern was present.[44] Other important issues beg for attention, but the lack of an agreed upon nosology for dysfunctional labor makes creating uniform data bases of sufficient size for meaningful analysis difficult.

CONCERNS FOR THE PELVIC FLOOR

While anxieties about fetal welfare and the potential for long-term effects on the newborn drove most decisions about the need for cesarean delivery during the last half century, unease about the potential damage to the maternal pelvic floor from vaginal birth now inhabits our concerns about labor. There is particular uncertainty about whether abnormal labor might enhance the risk of pelvic floor injury and its possible consequences – genital prolapse, incontinence, and sexual dysfunctionality. These are legitimate worries, and deserve our attention. A full review of the topic is beyond the purview of this chapter, but one issue bears emphasis in our discussion of the pertinence of graphic analysis of labor to this topic.

While it is clear that vaginal delivery has the potential to injure the musculofascial supports of the pelvic floor, the extent to which such trauma contributes to incontinence and prolapse in later life is by no means certain. Other factors, including aging, smoking, and obesity may be more important; moreover, genetic influences may be paramount.[45] Until we understand how these factors interact, it will be difficult to arrive at a consensus concerning how to minimize risk. A thorough study of labor patterns will be important in that effort. The duration of the second stage, for example, has been variously shown to contribute to or not to influence the risk of urinary incontinence.[45,46] It may be that the rate of descent , irrespective of second stage duration, affects the chance of pelvic floor trauma; but this has never been studied. If we are not to abandon vaginal birth, we need to know whether maternal risks can be minimized by the intelligent and studied application of good labor management.

EFFECTS OF EPIDURAL ANESTHESIA

Epidural analgesia is now the most widely practiced mode of pain relief during labor in the industrialized world. As such, it is of obvious importance to know whether neuraxial medication influences the course of labor. The best way to ascertain this is to study the effects of epidural analgesia on progress in dilatation and descent and on rates of operative delivery.

Opinions about the effects of conduction anesthesia on labor have been many and varied since the technique came into widespread use beginning in the 1970s. Much of the information in the literature is difficult to interpret. For example, while some investigators have found cesarean rates to be increased when neuraxial anesthetics are given,[47,48] others have not.[49–51] One problem that defeats our efforts to understand the issue is that epidural analgesia is often studied in monolithic terms; but in fact its effects may vary considerably depending on the technique, the type and concentration of agent employed, on when in labor it is administered, and on other aspects of the extant obstetric situation. These are not always considered in planning, interpreting or comparing clinical studies. In addition, in some studies, the details of the analgesic were closely controlled, but the obstetric decision making was not, potentially confounding any conclusions about effects on operative delivery rates.

In some patients, epidural analgesia may lengthen the latent phase but, as long as there is no contra-indication to prolonging the labor modestly (infection, pre-eclampsia, *etc.*), this is a small price to pay for pain relief if it is needed early in labor. Neuraxial analgesics commonly lengthen the second stage, probably because their inhibition of motor function limits the force generated by bearing-down efforts. This prolongation of descent is also innocuous as long as the fetal condition is good.[52] A recent study of combined spinal-epidural analgesia showed no significant inhibition of labor progress in any phase of parturition.[53]

There is some evidence that neuraxial analgesia is more likely to slow progress if administered during the latent phase or in the presence of a dysfunctional active phase (protraction or arrest disorder).[7,8] That is not to imply that conduction anesthesia is always contra-indicated in such circumstances. On the contrary, it may be beneficial to the parturient who requires pain relief; but it should be employed with full cognizance that it might prolong the latent phase and create or abet an active phase abnormality, thus requiring administration of oxytocin.

The outcome of labors in which epidural analgesia is used depends in large measure on the clinical attitude of the obstetrician. For example, if the physician believes that the second stage of labor must always be terminated after 2 h, operative delivery would be more common in patients whose second stage is prolonged by epidural analgesia. However, a physician who understands that such prolongations are usually innocuous would not feel compelled to intervene. One can conclude from the available information that epidural analgesia administered with proper regard for the clinical situation will generally have no significant adverse impact on labor progress or mode of delivery.

EFFECTS OF LABOR ON THE FETUS

The question of whether labor, particularly dysfunctional labor, can affect the long-term health of offspring is a pivotal one. If being born after an abnormal labor, even if prolonged and neglected, does not confer risk, then prompt diagnosis and evidence-based management of abnormal labor is of no particular consequence, and discussions about how best to recognize and codify dysfunctional labor are moot. While there has long been suspicion in the clinical literature that abnormal labor can injure the fetus, most of the studies are hampered by small sample sizes or imprecise definitions of dystocia. Our understanding of this area is consequently incomplete and the conclusions of studies often conflicting or uninterpretable.

No one can really doubt that parturition can produce fetal and neonatal adversity; the appalling perinatal carnage engendered by prolonged and neglected labor in the non-industrialized world offers ample and convincing testimony to this fact. Whether labor and delivery that occurs in the context of competent and informed surveillance by health professionals causes enduring fetal injury is another matter, and one not readily answered.

There are evident difficulties in studying the influence of labor and delivery on offspring. Large samples sizes with meticulous long-term follow-up are necessary. It is, however, difficult and expensive to create large reliable data bases and to study them. Moreover, many environmental factors influence the performance of children on psychometric tests, and differences (or lack thereof) found many years after birth may reflect exposures and interventions that have influenced (positively or negatively) injury sustained during labor.

An important source of information is data from the National Collaborative Perinatal Project (NCPP), sponsored by the National Institutes of Health in the US.[14] These data have been analyzed exhaustively, and include records from a cohort followed for up to 7 years after birth. While almost unique in the thoroughness of both analysis of the events of parturition and the neuropsychological follow-up of children born to study mothers, legitimate questions about the current validity of the results have been raised, considering the substantial changes in obstetric and neonatal care that have occurred since the data were collected in 1958–1974. This reservation notwithstanding, the NCPP data are of considerable importance. They demonstrate remarkably uniform relations among several measures of outcome (perinatal mortality, Apgar scores, 3-year speech, language and hearing abilities, and Intelligence Quotients at 4 and 7 years of age) and events of labor and delivery.[14,54,55]

Specifically, prolonged latent phase was not associated with adverse outcome; but protraction and arrest disorders were, with arrested labor being the major contributor to childhood problems. A major portion of the demonstrable adversity associated with dysfunctional labors was attributable to the mode of delivery or to factors that led to the development of abnormal labor or the need for operative delivery. The use of midforceps conferred special risk to the fetus, especially when used in the wake of protraction and arrest disorders. It may be that the labor dysfunction may have somehow sensitized the fetal brain to injury during instrumental delivery or to the effects of oxytocin stimulation.

Other lines of evidence support the association of abnormal labor with adverse outcomes. In another analysis of the NCPP data, Nelson and Broman showed nearly 3 times the expected rate of arrest of dilatation in children with serious motor and mental handicap at age 7 years.[56] Roemer et al.[57] reported that the IQ of children delivered by cesarean after dysfunctional labor was significantly lower than that of their siblings delivered by elective cesarean without labor.

In the most recent analysis of this issue, Towner et al.[58] examined the frequency of neonatal intracranial hemorrhage according to delivery type in a sample of more than half a million cases. They found that, while instrumental delivery and cesarean done during labor were associated with higher rates of hemorrhage than was spontaneous vaginal delivery, the rate among babies delivered by cesarean before labor was not. In other words, their analysis strongly implicated abnormal labor (the reason for most operative deliveries) as the common risk factor for neonatal intracranial injury.

It is not likely that the controversy over the potential adverse effects of labor will soon be resolved to anyone's complete satisfaction. The issues are complex, and the ability to isolate labor as a contributing factor is limited. Moreover, it is quite likely that dysfunctional labor may act as an adversary of good outcome only when other factors are introduced, e.g. instrumental delivery, prolonged unrecognized arrest disorders, or undisciplined use of oxytocin. Also, it may be that when complex instrumental delivery is eschewed and dysfunctional labor is managed according to uniform and validated protocols, risks are minimized. This may explain why some contemporary data make dysfunctional labor seem less sinister than did earlier work. Wide-spread use of the labor curves may have reduced the number of dysfunctional labors that persist unrecognized and ignored, and that lead ultimately to fetal trauma.

There are many more questions than there are satisfying answers available in this regard. One thing is certain. If we are ever to answer compelling questions about abnormal labor and its effects on delivery outcome and long-term health, it can only be done in the context of our profession adopting a uniform system of diagnosing and a common lexicon for describing abnormal labor. Universal use of the same form of graphic labor analysis would be a good step in the direction of better understanding the processes and consequences of human labor and birth.

SUMMARY

The graphic method of labor analysis should be mastered and employed by all who care for women during labor. The Friedman labor curves are the best studied and most meaningful approach to the clinical analysis of dysfunctional labor. They have a value in predicting the need for operative delivery, and can alert us to potential long-term harm to the fetus.

This recommendation notwithstanding, it is vital to understand that labor curves provide information fundamental to clinical decision making, but which must be integrated with other obstetric data. Information obtained from the labor curves must be assessed in the context of that concerning obstetric history, prenatal events, cephalopelvic relationships, effects of medications, presence of infection, state of fetal oxygenation and maternal condition, among others, in order to make the most enlightened clinical judgments. A good outcome of every labor cannot be guaranteed; but disciplined use and interpretation of the labor curves can help bring us toward that ideal.

References

1 Roy RP. A Darwinian view of obstructed labor. Obstet Gynecol 2003; 101: 397–401
2 Schulman H, Romney S. Variability of uterine contractions in normal human parturition. Obstet Gynecol 1970; 36: 215–221
3 Jacobson JD, Gregerson GN, Dale S, Valenzuela GJ. Real-time microcomputer-based analysis of spontaneous and augmented labor. Obstet Gynecol 1990; 76: 755–758
4 Cohen WR, Pacheco C, Verdiales M, Karumanchi R, Rosenberg E. Uterine electromyography in latent and active phase labor. J Soc Gynecol Invest 2004; 119 (suppl): 73A
5 Garfield RE, Maner WI, MacKay LB, Schlembach D, Saade GR. Comparing uterine electromyography of antepartum patients versus term labor patients. Obstet Gynecol 2005; 193: 23–29
6 Friedman EA. The graphic analysis of labor. Am J Obstet Gynecol 1954; 68: 1568–1575
7 Friedman EA. Labor. Clinical Evaluation and Management. New York: Appleton-Century-Crofts, 1967
8 Friedman EA. Labor: clinical evaluation and management, 2nd edn. New York: Appleton-Century-Crofts, 1978
9 Friedman EA, Sachtleben MR. Dysfunctional labor: II. Protracted active phase dilatation in the nullipara. Obstet Gynecol 1961; 17: 566–578
10 Friedman EA, Sachtleben MR. Dysfunctional labor: III. Secondary arrest of dilatation in the nullipara. Obstet Gynecol 1962; 19: 576–591
11 Friedman EA, Sachtleben MR. Dysfunctional labor. I. Prolonged latent phase in the nullipara. Obstet Gynecol 1961; 17: 135–148
12 Friedman EA, Sachtleben MR. Station of the fetal presenting part: V. Protracted descent patterns. Obstet Gynecol 1970; 36: 558–567
13 Friedman EA, Sachtleben MR. Station of the fetal presenting part: VI. Arrest of descent in nulliparas. Obstet Gynecol 1976; 47: 129–132
14 Friedman EA, Neff RK. Labor and Delivery: Impact on Offspring. Littleton, MA: PSG Publishing, 1987

15 Drouin P, Nasah BT, Nkounawa F. The value of the partogramme in the management of labor. Obstet Gynecol 1979; 53: 741–745

16 Kwast BE, Lennox CE, Farley TMM. World Health Organization partograph in management of labour. Lancet 1994; 343: 1399–1404

17 Ledger WJ, Witting WC. The use of a cervical dilatation graph in the management of primigravidae in labour. J Obstet Gynaecol Br Commonw 1972; 79: 710–714

18 Ledger WJ. Monitoring of labor by graphs. Obstet Gynecol 1969; 34: 174–181

19 Schulman H, Ledger WT. Practical applications of the graphic portrayal of labor. Obstet Gynecol 1964; 23: 442–445

20 Philpott RH, Castle WM. Cervicographs in the management of labour in primigravidae. II. The action line and treatment of abnormal labour. J Obstet Gynaecol Br Commonw 1972; 79: 599–602

21 Philpott RH, Castle WM. Cervicographs in the management of labour in primigravidae: 1. The alert line for detecting abnormal labour. J Obstet Gynaecol Br Commonw 1972; 79: 592–598

22 Studd J. Partograms and nomograms of cervical dilatation in management of primigravid labour. BMJ 1973; 4: 451–455

23 Melmed H, Evans MI. Predictive value of cervical dilatation rates I. Primipara labor. Obstet Gynecol 1976; 47: 511–515

24 Evans MI, Lachman E, Kral S, Melmed H. Predictive value of cervical dilatation rates in labor in multiparous women. Isr J Med Sci 1976; 12: 1399–1403

25 Cardozo LD, Gibb DMF, Studd JWW, Vasant RV, Cooper DJ. Predictive value of cervimetric labour patterns in primigravidae. Br J Obstet Gynaecol 1982; 89: 33–38

26 Chen HF, Chu KK. Double-lined nomogram of cervical dilatation in Chinese primigravidas. Acta Obstet Gynecol Scand 1986; 65: 573–575

27 Poma PA. Use of labor graphs in a community hospital. Int Surg 1979; 64: 7–12

28 Schifrin BS, Cohen WR. Labor's dysfunctional lexicon. Obstet Gynecol 1989; 74: 121–124

29 Zhang J, Troendle JF, Yancey MK. Reassessing the labor curve in nulliparous women. Am J Obstet Gynecol 2002; 187: 824–828

30 Rinehart BK, Terrone DA, Hudson C, Isler CM, Larmon JE, Perry Jr KG. Lack of utility of standard labor curves in the prediction of progression during labor induction. Am J Obstet Gynecol 2000; 182: 1520–1526

31 Vahratian A, Zhang J, Troendle JF, Sciscione AC, Hoffman MK. Labor progression and risk of cesarean delivery in electively induced nulliparas. Obstet Gynecol 2005; 105: 698–704

32 Friedman EA, Kroll BH. Computer analysis of labor progression. II. Distribution of data and limits of normal. J Reprod Med 1971; 6: 20–25

33 Impey L, Hobson J, O'Herlihy C. Graphic analysis of actively managed labor: prospective computation of labor progress in 500 consecutive nulliparous women in spontaneous labor at term. Am J Obstet Gynecol 2000; 183: 438–443

34 Garrett K, Butler A, Cohen WR. Cesarean delivery during second stage labor: Characteristics and diagnostic accuracy. J Mat Fetal Neonat Med 2005; 17: 49–53

35 Hopwood HG. Shoulder dystocia: Fifteen years' experience in a community hospital. Am J Obstet Gynecol 1982; 144: 162–166

36 Vahratian A, Zhang J, Troendle JF, Savitz DA, Siega-Riz AM. Maternal prepregnancy overweight and obesity and the pattern of labor progression in term nulliparous women. Obstet Gynecol 2004; 104: 943–951

37 Cohen WR, Newman L, Friedman EA: Frequency of labor disorders with advancing maternal age. Obstet Gynecol 1980; 55: 414–416.

38 Chazotte C, Madden R, Cohen WR. Labor patterns in women with previous cesareans. Obstet Gynecol 1990; 75: 350–355

39 Laros RK, Work BA, Witting WC. Amniotomy during the active phase of labor. Obstet Gynecol 1972; 39: 702–704

40 Friedman EA, Sachtleben MR. Amniotomy and the course of labor. Obstet Gynecol 1963; 22: 755

41 Mahon T, Chazotte C, Cohen WR: Short Labor: Characteristics and outcome. Obstet Gynecol 1994; 84: 47–51

42 Duignan NM, Studd JWW, Hughes AO. Characteristics of normal labor in different racial groups. Br J Obstet Gynaecol 1975; 82: 593–601

43 Cohen WR, Mahon T, Chazotte C. Very long second stage of labor: characteristics and outcome. In: Cosmi EV. (ed) Labor and Delivery. Proceedings of the Second World Congress on Labor and Delivery. New York: Parthenon Publishing Group, 1998

44 Cohen WR, Newman L, Friedman EA: Frequency of labor disorders with advancing maternal age. Obstet Gynecol 1980; 55: 414–416.

45 Cohen WR, Romero R. Childbirth and the pelvic floor. In: Kurjak A, Chervenak F. (eds) Textbook of Perinatal Medicine, 2nd edn. London: Taylor and Francis, 2006

46 Van Kessel K, Reed S, Newton K, Meier A, Lentz G. The second stage of labor and stress urinary incontinence. Am J Obstet Gynecol 2001; 184: 1571–1575

47 Thorp JA, Hu DH, Albin RM et al. The effect of intrapartum epidural analgesia on nulliparous labor: a randomized, controlled, prospective trial. Am J Obstet Gynecol 1993; 169: 851–858

48 Lieberman E, Lang JM, Cohen A, D'Agostino Jr R, Datta S, Frigoletto FD. Association of epidural analgesia with cesarean delivery in nulliparas. Obstet Gynecol 1996; 88: 993–1000

49 Sharma SK, Sidawi JE, Ramin SM, Lucas MJ, Leveno KJ, Cunningham FG. Cesarean delivery: a randomized trial of epidural versus patient-controlled meperidine analgesia during labor. Anesthesiology 1997; 87: 487–494

50 Impey L, MacQuillan K, Robson M. Epidural analgesia need not increase operative delivery rates. Am J Obstet Gynecol 2000; 182: 358–363

51 Halpern SH, Leighton BL, Ohlsson A, Barrett JFR, Rice A. Effect of epidural vs parenteral opioid analgesia on the progress of labor. JAMA 1998; 280: 2105–2110

52 Cohen WR. Influence of the duration of second stage labor on perinatal outcome and puerperal morbidity. Obstet Gynecol 1977; 49: 266–269

53 Wong CA, Scavone BM, Peaceman AM et al. The risk of cesarean delivery with neuraxial analgesia given early versus late in labor. N Engl J Med 2005; 352: 655–665

54 Friedman EA, Sachtleben MR, Bresky PA. Dysfunctional labor. XII. Long-term effects on infant. Am J Obstet Gynecol 1977; 127: 779–783

55 Friedman EA. Patterns of labor as indicators of risk. Clin Obstet Gynecol 1973; 16: 172–183

56 Nelson KB, Broman SH. Perinatal risk factors in children with serious motor and mental handicaps. Ann Neurol 1977; 2: 371–377

57 Roemer FJ, Rowland DY, Nuamah IF. Retrospective study of fetal effects of prolonged labor before cesarean delivery. Obstet Gynecol 1991; 77: 653–658

58 Towner D, Castro MA, Eby-Wilkens BS, Gilbert WM. Effect of mode of delivery in nulliparous women on neonatal intracranial injury. N Engl J Med 1999; 341: 1709–1714

59 Hendricks CH, Brenner WE, Kraus G. Normal cervical dilatation pattern in late pregnancy and labor. Am J Obstet Gynecol 1970; 106: 1065–1082

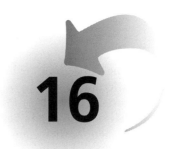

Gordon C.S. Smith

16

Delivery after caesarean section

As rates of primary caesarean increase, an increasing proportion of pregnant women have the complication of a previous caesarean delivery. One of the major issues among these women is the advisability and obstetric approach to attempting vaginal birth. The questions around this issue are informed almost exclusively by observational data which can be complex and subtle in their interpretation. Variability in the quality of data sources, in analytical approach and in interpretation has led to a large and often contradictory literature. The aim of the present article is to present an overview of this literature.

ASSESSING THE LITERATURE

Selection bias and RCTs

Theoretically, the ideal method for comparing the relative risk of vaginal birth after caesarean (VBAC) and planned repeat caesarean delivery (PRCD) would be a randomised, controlled trial. In practice, this is unlikely to occur since most women would not accept the choice being made in a random fashion. Further, many of the events of interest are relatively uncommon, such as uterine rupture, hysterectomy, perinatal or maternal death. Consequently, it is extremely unlikely that, if a trial was organised, it would be sufficiently powered to address the questions of central clinical interest. Moreover, one of the major concerns relating to PRCD is the potential for severe adverse effects on future pregnancies. For a trial to address this key issue, follow-up would be required for years after initial recruitment in a very large number of women and this is unlikely to be a practical proposition. Consequently, it is very likely that this debate will continue to be informed largely through observational data.

Gordon C.S. Smith MD PhD MRCOG
Professor and Head, Department of Obstetrics and Gynaecology, Cambridge University, Rosie Maternity Hospital, Robinson Way, Cambridge CB2 2QQ, UK
E-mail: gcss2@cam.ac.uk

The major weakness of observational studies is the issue of selection bias, *i.e.* that differences might be observed when comparing groups which are not due to the grouping but the factors that determined the grouping. The issue of selection bias is less problematic in the context of assessing potentially beneficial effects of PRCD. Women who have PRCD are systematically more likely to have complications such as pre-existing maternal disease, gestational diabetes and they are also older and shorter.[1,2] Selection of women for VBAC is likely to identify a healthy cohort. It follows that, if better outcomes are observed in observational studies among women having PRCD, the differences were observed despite (rather than because of) selection bias. However, it might be reasonably suggested that where the outcomes are equivalent between PRCD and VBAC or are better for VBAC, that selection bias may have contributed.

Influence of risk of emergency caesarean delivery

Many of the risks described for PRCD, such as infection and haemorrhage, are more common among women who attempt VBAC but require emergency caesarean delivery than among women who are delivered by PRCD.[3,4] It follows, therefore, that among groups who have a high risk of emergency caesarean section, comparison of outcomes of VBAC and PRCD are likely to favour the latter. The greater risk of adverse events following emergency than planned caesarean delivery[5] indicate that, at a certain level of risk of emergency caesarean delivery, a strategy of delivering all women by a planned procedure may actually carry a lower risk of adverse events directly attributable to surgery. The term breech trial, the largest RCT of planned caesarean section, confirmed this proposition demonstrating similar rates of maternal morbidity comparing those delivered by planned caesarean section and those where vaginal birth was attempted.[6] This paradoxical neutral rate of surgical complications despite close to 100% caesarean delivery in the intervention group reflects the 36% emergency caesarean section rate among those attempting vaginal breech birth. Similarly, comparisons of outcomes between women attempting VBAC and women having PRCD will differ according to the emergency caesarean delivery rate in the former group.

Relative and absolute risks

Medical research tends to follow an analytical paradigm inherited from the basic experimental sciences. The approach is to determine a measurable variable, to make a comparison between two groups and to determine whether the dependent variable differs in a way that exceeds what is consistent with chance. The focus on comparison rather than absolute risk lead to bizarre misinterpretation of the data. For instance, a meta-analysis of observational studies quoted absolute risks of perinatal death of 5.8 per 1000 for VBAC and 3.4 per 1000 for PRCD with an odds ratio of 1.7 for perinatal death in the VBAC group.[7] However, many of these deaths were not truly related to the chosen mode of delivery. A large-scale, retrospective, cohort study then described more accurate estimates of absolute risks of 1.2 per 1000 and 0.1 per 1000, respectively, with an odds ratio of approximately 12 for VBAC.[2] Despite the fact that the true absolute risk of VBAC described in that study was 5 times lower than previously described, the greater relative risk when compared with PRCD led to it being widely interpreted as justification of PRCD because of a much greater true relative risk.

Data sources

The sources of data used to compare outcomes between VBAC and PRCD are crucial for interpretation. The main qualities are the scale of the dataset, its content and whether it was collected prospectively or retrospectively. Many of the primary outcomes of interest are relatively rare. Small studies will inevitably yield negative results when comparing rare outcomes unless there are very considerable differences in the groups compared. Negative statements in relation to these comparisons must, therefore, be accompanied by confidence intervals in order to make explicit the magnitude of association that a given study is powered to exclude. The content of datasets is also clearly crucial. For example, when comparing perinatal mortality between VBAC and PRCD, the mode of delivery can only influence certain types of death. Analyses which fail to exclude deaths due to, for instance, lethal fetal abnormality will yield misleading comparisons. Many datasets lack detailed information on the cause of perinatal death.

A key determinant of data quality is whether a study was retrospective or prospective. Due to the issues of power, discussed above, many studies use routinely collected data. These data are often entered by non-medically qualified personnel. Moreover, there may be uncertainty in relation to a given outcome in the clinical case record due to poor documentation. The major strength of prospective studies is that they allow prior definition of events and standardised data collection. The problem with large-scale, prospective studies is that they are expensive. Fortunately, the NIH conducted such a study and in December 2004 reported outcomes comparing VBAC and PRCD among over 30,000 women with previous caesarean delivery studied prospectively.[4] Due to the inherent strengths of a prospective study design, the results of that study will be discussed in detail in the comparison of VBAC and PRCD. It is likely that further reports from that study will address other issues after publication of this review and interested readers are advised to search for these.

RISKS TO THE MOTHER

Maternal risks of attempting VBAC

Overall rates of maternal morbidity
The US prospective cohort study reported increased rates of severe maternal complications among women attempting VBAC (Table 1). Overall, there were significant maternal complications in 5.5% of women attempting VBAC compared with 3.6% of those delivered by PRCD. Although this study had the profound advantage of being prospective, the comparison between the VBAC and PRCD groups is biased. The PRCD group included all women who had had any number of previous caesarean deliveries, *i.e.* it included women who

Table 1 Maternal morbidity comparing women having a PRCD and those attempting VABC

Complication	Trial of labour (n = 17,898)	Elective repeated caesarean delivery (n = 15,801)	Odds ratio (95% CI)	P-value
	Number (%)			
Uterine rupture	124 (0.7)	0	–	< 0.001
Uterine dehiscence[a]	119 (0.7)	76 (0.5)	1.38 (1.04–1.85)	0.03
Hysterectomy	41 (0.2)	47 (0.3)	0.77 (0.51–1.17)	0.22}
Thrombo-embolic disease[b]	7 (0.04)	10 (0.1)	0.62 (0.24–1.62)	0.32
Transfusion	304 (1.7)	158 (1.0)	1.71 (1.41–2.08)	< 0.001
Endometritis	517 (2.9)	285 (1.8)	1.62 (1.40–1.87)	< 0.001
Maternal death	3 (0.02)	7 (0.04)	0.38 (0.10–1.46)	0.21
Other maternal adverse events[c]	64 (0.4)	52 (0.3)	1.09 (0.75–1.57)	0.66
One or more of the above	978 (5.5)	563 (3.6)	1.56 (1.41–1.74)	< 0.001

CI denotes confidence interval, and a dash not applicable.
[a]Not all women underwent examination of their scars after vaginal delivery.
[b]Thrombo-embolic disease includes deep venous thrombosis or pulmonary embolism.
[c]Other adverse events include broad-ligament haematoma, cystotomy, bowel injury, and ureteral injury.
Reproduced with permission from Landon *et al*. N Engl J Med 2004.[4] Copyright © 2004 Massachusetts Medical Society

were ineligible for an attempt at VBAC due to high numbers of previous caesarean deliveries. Since surgical complications become more common with the number of previous caesarean deliveries, it is likely that the outcomes among the PRCD group are worse than would have been anticipated if all the women who had attempted VBAC had been delivered by PRCD. Nevertheless, the data in Table 1 provide reasonable estimates of the absolute risks of major complications associated with VBAC and PRCD.

Risk of uterine rupture
One of the major determinants of severe adverse outcome associated with VBAC is whether uterine rupture occurs. The incidence of this is generally estimated to be in the region of 0.5–1.0%.[1,4,8–10] Many of these studies reported that the risk of uterine rupture is higher with VBAC than with PRCD. All but one of these studies was retrospective and employed routinely collected data. It is self-evident that uterine rupture will never truly be associated with a planned caesarean delivery. Many of the so-called ruptures will have been a uterine dehiscence. The single prospective study[4] demonstrated no true uterine ruptures among the PRCD group and a rate of 7 per 1000 in the VBAC group, and this is the most reliable estimate of the overall absolute risk of uterine rupture among women attempting VBAC.

Table 2 Maternal morbidity among women attempting VBAC in relation to whether the attempt was successful

Complication	Failed vaginal delivery (n = 4759)	Successful vaginal delivery (n = 13,139)	Odds ratio (95% CI)	P-value
	Number (%)			
Uterine rupture	110 (2.3)	14 (0.1)	22.18 (12.70–38.72)	< 0.001
Uterine dehiscence	100 (2.1)	19 (0.1)	14.82 (9.06–24.23)	< 0.001
Hysterectomy	22 (0.5)	19. (0.1)	3.21 (1.73–5.93)	< 0.001
Thrombo-embolic disease[a]	4 (0.1)	3 (0.02)	3.69 (0.83–16.51)	0.09
Transfusion	152 (3.2)	152 (1.2)	2.82 (2.25–3.54)	< 0.001
Endometritis	365 (7.7)	152 (1.2)	7.10 (5.86–8.60)	< 0.001
Maternal death	2 (0.04)	1 (0.01)	5.52 (0.50–60.92)	0.17
Other maternal adverse events[b]	63 (1.3)	1 (0.01)	176.24 (24.44–1271.05)	< 0.001
One or more of the above	669 (14.1)	309 (2.4)	6.81 (5.93–7.83)	< 0.001

CI denotes confidence interval.
[a]Thrombo-embolic disease includes deep venous thrombosis or pulmonary embolism.
[b]Other adverse events include broad-ligament haematoma, cystotomy, bowel injury, and ureteral injury.
Reproduced with permission from Landon et al. N Engl J Med 2004.[4] Copyright © 2004 Massachusetts Medical Society

Risks associated with failed VBAC

The major determinant of morbidity associated with a decision to attempt VBAC is whether the attempt is successful. Women who attempted VBAC and were successful had a 2.4% incidence of composite morbidity whereas those who attempted VBAC and failed (i.e. were ultimately delivered by emergency caesarean section during labour) had a 14.1% incidence of morbidity (Table 2).[4] Requirement for blood transfusion and endometritis made up the majority of these complications. These findings underline the importance of developing methods to predict the likelihood of success of a VBAC in relation to the maternal characteristics, and this is discussed below.

Long-term complications of VBAC

The data above primarily relate to short-term maternal complications of VBAC. There are a series of observational studies which suggest that vaginal birth may have adverse effects on the pelvic floor.[11–13] There are data from a single RCT, the term breech trial, which demonstrated a lower incidence of urinary incontinence in the planned caesarean delivery group at 3 months[14] but no difference at 2 years of follow-up.[15] However, the control group had an approximately 40% rate of caesarean delivery which complicates interpretation of that study.

Table 3 Association between number of previous caesarean deliveries and relative risk of placenta praevia

Number previous caesarean deliveries	Relative risk (95% CI)[a]
One	4.5 (3.6–5.5)
Two	7.4 (7.1–7.7)
Three	6.5 (3.6–11.6)
Four or more	44.9 (13.5–149.5)

[a]Relative to women with no previous caesarean deliveries.
Reproduced with permission from Ananth *et al*. Am J Obstet Gynecol 1997.[17]

Maternal risks of PRCD

Overall rates of morbidity

As discussed above, women having PRCD have an intermediate rate of complications (3.6%) which is higher than those women who attempt VBAC and succeed.[4] This is likely to be due, in part, to complications arising from caesarean section, primarily infection and necessity for blood transfusion. However, as stated above, the PRCD group in this study were much more likely to have had multiple previous caesarean deliveries and it is well recognised that the risk of complications increases with the number of prior caesarean sections. The true excess risk associated with a PRCD over a successful VBAC may be less than reported in that study.

Risk of future placental problems

Delivery by PRCD also carries long-term risks of complications, particularly placental problems. A meta-analysis of observational studies concluded that women with one or more prior caesarean deliveries had a 2.7-fold risk (95% CI 2.3–3.2) of placenta praevia in a subsequent pregnancy.[16] The risk of placenta praevia increased with the number of previous caesarean deliveries (Table 3).[17] Morbid adherence of the placenta, placenta accreta or percreta, is a rarer and still more serious complication of placentation which is associated with anterior placenta praevia among women with a previous caesarean delivery. The overall incidence of severe placenta accreta (defined as resulting in death, hysterectomy, blood transfusion, coagulopathy or being associated with placenta percreta) was estimated as 0.05% and the odds ratio for women with repeated caesarean deliveries is 3.3.[18] While the absolute risk of this event in future pregnancies is low, in the region of 1 in 1000, clearly the consequences can be severe. Moreover, among women with three or more previous caesarean deliveries, the risk exceeds 1% (Table 4).[19]

Future surgical complications

Current data suggest that the risk of surgical complications during repeat caesarean section increases with the number of previous caesarean deliveries and the absolute risks of these events estimated from a study are tabulated (Table 4). Multiple caesarean deliveries could, theoretically, also affect surgical procedures outside pregnancy, *e.g.* by increasing the likelihood of bladder

Table 4 Morbidity associated with number of prior caesarean deliveries

| Outcome | Number of previous caesarean sections | | | | | | P-value |
	1	2	3	4	5	6 and more	for 3–6 and more
Placenta praevia	34/882 (3.9)	23/722 (3.2)	45/889 (5.1)	31/447 (6.9)	16/170 (9.4)	13/77 (16.9)	0.005
Placenta accreta	0	0	10/890 (1.1)	5/447 (1.1)	9/170 (5.3)	5/77 (6.5)	0.001
Praevia with accreta	0	0	10/45 (22.2)	4/31 (12.9)	8/16 (50.0)	5/13 (38.5)	0.001
Severe adhesions	2/882 (0.2)	83/723 (11.5)	226/868 (26.0)	196/433 (44.8)	91/167 (54.5)	39/77 (50.6)	0.001
Hysterectomy	1/882 (0.1)	1/724 (0.1)	6/890 (0.7)	1/448 (0.2)	2/170 (1.2)	3/77 (3.9)	0.040
Bladder injury	0	2/724 (0.3)	7/890 (0.8)	6/448 (1.3)	4/170 (2.4)	3/77 (3.9)	0.020
Postoperative haemoglobin deficit	52/882 (5.9)	66/722 (9.1)	92/885 (10.4)	58/446 (13.0)	33/170 (19.4)	15/77 (19.5)	0.001
Blood transfusion	56/882 (6.3)	52/723 (7.2)	70/888 (7.9)	46/447 (10.3)	24/170 (14.1)	15/77 (19.5)	0.003
Prolonged hospital stay	25/882 (2.8)	33/724 (4.6)	46/889 (5.2)	40/448 (8.9)	17/169 (10.1)	13/75 (17.3)	0.012
Operating time (min)	44.2	50.3	53.6	54.0	61.6	64.6	0.001

Reprinted from Makoha et al. Int J Gynaecol Obstet 2004.[19] Copyright © 2004 wit permission from the International Federation of Gynaecology and Obstetrics.

trauma at the time of hysterectomy. A history of multiple previous caesarean deliveries is quoted as a relative contra-indication to vaginal hysterectomy. However, recent studies do not suggest either increased rates of complications overall or a trend of increasing risk of complications with the number of previous caesarean deliveries.[20,21]

Sub-fertility and early pregnancy loss

Observational studies have suggested that women delivered by caesarean section are more likely to experience difficulty in conceiving (OR = 1.5).[22] The implications of this for the decision between VBAC and PRCD are difficult to define. First, these women have already had a caesarean delivery and it is unclear whether there is a 'dose-response' relationship between number of caesarean deliveries and sub-fertility. Second, sub-fertility prior to the first birth is a risk factor for caesarean delivery[22] and it is questionable, therefore, whether the relationship between caesarean delivery and sub-fertility is causal. A recent study of over 100,000 first births has shown that there is no statistically significant association between first planned caesarean section for breech and the probability of a future pregnancy, which suggests that previous associations did not reflect a causal association but were due to confounding.[23] The same study also showed no association between caesarean section in the first pregnancy and the number of spontaneous early pregnancy losses between the first and second pregnancy.

Risks to infant associated with VBAC

Antepartum stillbirth

A study that utilised linked Scottish databases showed that women whose first birth was by caesarean section were at significantly increased risk of antepartum stillbirth in their second pregnancy compared to those women whose first birth was a vaginal delivery.[24] This additional risk was mainly due to an excess of unexplained stillbirths in the previous caesarean compared to vaginal delivery group, and this became significant after 34 weeks' gestation (Fig. 1). The absolute risk (expressed as the prospective risk of stillbirth – see Smith[25] for details) of antepartum stillbirth (all causes) from 39 weeks' gestation was 1.06 per 1000 for women who had had a previous caesarean section. It was concluded that 'an additional benefit of planned repeat caesarean delivery at 39 weeks' gestation may be to reduce the risk of unexplained stillbirth'. Commentators on the paper urged great caution prior to the finding being confirmed.[26] Subsequently, the large-scale, prospective, cohort study from the US reported very similar absolute risks of antepartum stillbirth. Among 15,338 attempting VBAC there were 16 antepartum stillbirths at or after 39 weeks, giving an approximate risk of stillbirth as 1.04 per 1000.

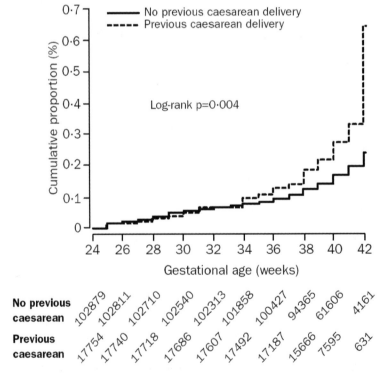

Fig. 1 Cumulative proportion of unexplained stillbirths per week of gestation. Hazard ratio for women with previous caesarean delivery with relative to women with a previous vaginal birth = 1·64 (95% CI 1·17–2·30). Reproduced with permission from Smith *et al.* Lancet 2003.[24]

Indeed, this figure is an underestimate since the denominator is all women delivering at or after 37 weeks rather than the correct denominator, *i.e.* women who delivered at or after 39 weeks. Overall (excluding malformations), there were 30 term antepartum stillbirths among 15,334 women attempting VBAC (2 per 1000) and 12 among 15,013 having a planned repeat caesarean section (0.8 per 1000; relative risk associated with VBAC 2.45; 95% CI 1.25–4.78; *P* = 0.007).[4]

Delivery-related perinatal death

One of the major areas of research into the management of women with a prior caesarean section is the way in which mode of delivery may influence the risk of death of the infant occurring as a complication of labour and delivery. Some early, large-scale studies had performed analyses which included preterm births.[27] Since these deaths account for the majority of neonatal deaths not due to congenital abnormality, inclusion of preterm deliveries may have masked the effect of VBAC and PRCD on truly delivery-related deaths. An analysis of record-linked data from Scotland described an approximately 12-fold excess of delivery-related perinatal death at term among women attempting VBAC compared with those having PRCD.[2] Nevertheless, the absolute risk of such deaths was relatively small. Among women attempting VBAC, the risk was about 1.3 per 1000 and this was comparable to the risk for nulliparous women attempting vaginal birth. Among women attempting VBAC, about one-third of deaths were due to uterine rupture (absolute risk of this event, approximately 1 in 2100), one-third were due to intrapartum anoxia due to other causes and one-third were not due to intrapartum anoxia.

The large-scale, prospective US cohort study demonstrated a lower absolute risk of delivery-related perinatal death due to uterine rupture – just 2 deaths among 15,338 women.[4] This study was conducted in large US teaching hospitals. A further study of data from Scotland has shown a negative association between the risk of delivery-related perinatal death due to uterine rupture and hospital through-put, from approximately 1 in 1000 in low through-put units to approximately 1 in 5000 in high through-put units.[9] It was speculated that in high through-put units, facilities were more likely to be immediately available for urgent delivery and resuscitation of an infant in the event that uterine rupture occurred. Consistent with this, the probability of survival following delivery associated with uterine rupture where the infant has a 5-min Apgar less than 4 increases with hospital through-put.[28] Taken as a whole, the data indicate that severe asphyxia accompanies about 10% of uterine ruptures. In large centres, this is more likely to lead to a survivor with hypoxic ischaemic encephalopathy whereas in smaller units it is more likely to lead to death of the infant.

Non-asphyxial neonatal morbidity

There are some observational data which indicate that complicated vaginal birth may be associated with an increased risk of intracranial haemorrhage. The rate of intracranial haemorrhage is lowest among infants delivered by planned caesarean section (about 1 in 2750) compared with those delivered by an operative vaginal method (range 1 in 600–900), caesarean section during labour (about 1 in 900) and those delivered spontaneously (about 1 in 2000). However, no informative data exist on long-term, neurodevelopmental outcome. Only 10% of cerebral palsy among infants born at term is thought to be related to intrapartum events.[29] The large number of cases of adverse neurological outcome which are determined independently of mode of delivery may, therefore, mask the effect of interventions, since the maximal effect, even of completely eliminating intrapartum events, would be a 10% reduction. Given the relative rarity of adverse neurological outcomes following birth at term, it is virtually inevitable that studies will be underpowered to detect any effect of elective caesarean delivery at term on long-term neurological outcome.

Risks to the infant associated with PRCD

Respiratory problems are the major cause of morbidity to the infant associated with planned caesarean section, principally transient tachypnoea of the newborn (TTN). More severe morbidity can also occur including both respiratory distress syndrome (RDS) and persistent pulmonary hypertension. Planned caesarean section is associated with about a 5-fold risk of TTN or RDS.[30] The risk is increased if caesarean delivery is performed before the onset of labour and if it is performed at earlier weeks of gestation, even at term.[31] The absolute risk of respiratory morbidity associated with term, planned caesarean section is in the region of 3–4%. It is well recognised that premature infants who suffer respiratory morbidity in the neonatal period are at increased risk of respiratory disease in childhood.[32] A more recent study linked birth data to infant hospital admissions for asthma and demonstrated a 2-fold risk of this event among infants born by caesarean section and diagnosed with TTN or RDS at birth.[30] A case series of infants with primary pulmonary hypertension reported that 12 infants out of 71 (17%) were delivered by planned caesarean section.[33] However, the study lacked a control group. A review of about 30,000 deliveries in single institution described a 4-fold excess of pulmonary hypertension among infants delivered by planned caesarean section.[34] However, there was limited adjustment for other factors which may have contributed to the condition. Moreover, the absolute risk of neonatal death at term among infants delivered by PRCD at term is extremely low.[2,4] A recent study has shown that the risk of respiratory morbidity associated with planned caesarean delivery at term may be reduced by antenatal administration of glucocorticoids.[35] However, given concerns about potential adverse long-term effects of fetal exposure to glucocorticoids, it remains to be determined whether this will be incorporated into routine clinical care.

ANTENATAL COUNSELLING

Overall success rates of VBAC

The typical overall reported success rate of trial of VBAC is 75%. Much of antenatal counselling involves discussion of the risks and benefits outline above. However, as discussed above, one of the primary determinants of adverse outcome is whether the attempt at VBAC is successful. Moreover, economic analyses demonstrate that when the caesarean section rate is 25–40%, VBAC and PRCD are economically equivalent.[36] It follows, therefore, that counselling regarding an attempt at VBAC starts with a discussion of the likelihood of success. Given that this is so crucial in counselling, it is perhaps surprising that there has been relatively little information until recently to inform this question.

Factors predicting successful VBAC

Many studies have addressed methods for identifying women at low and high risk of failure of an attempted vaginal birth after a prior caesarean. A recent systematic review reported that only two of the six available tools had been validated.[37] Both of these incorporated data which would only be available when a women presented in labour, such as the results of electronic fetal monitoring and cervical dilatation on admission.[38,39] Many models also incorporate birth weight as a predictive factor. This effectively makes estimation of risk using such a model impossible since the predictor is only known after the outcome has occurred!

A recent study has, however, addressed this question.[40] Data on approximately 24,000 women attempting VBAC at or after 40 weeks' gestation were analysed. The population was randomly split into model development and validation groups. The factors associated with emergency caesarean section were maternal age (adjusted odds ratio 1.22 per 5-year increase; 95% CI 1.16–1.28), maternal height (adjusted odds ratio 0.75 per 5-cm increase; 95% CI 0.73–0.78), male fetus (adjusted odds ratio 1.18; 95% CI 1.08–1.29), no previous vaginal birth (adjusted odds ratio 5.08; 95% CI 4.52–5.72), prostaglandin induction of labour (adjusted odds ratio 1.42; 95% CI 1.26–1.60) and birth at 41 weeks' (adjusted odds ratio 1.30; 95% CI 1.18–1.42) or 42 weeks' (adjusted odds ratio 1.38;, 95% CI 1.17–1.62) gestation compared with 40 weeks. When this model was used to predict the probability of caesarean section in the validation

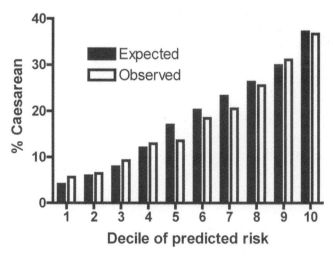

Fig. 2 Use of likelihood ratios to predict probability of caesarean section among women delivered at 37–39 weeks' gestation with a documented duration of labour of greater than or equal to 4 h. Probability estimated using likelihood ratios in Table 5 (excluding gestational age) and the prior odds of 0.22 (equivalent to background risk of caesarean section in this group). Reproduced with permission from Smith *et al.* PLoS Medicine 2005.[40]

group, 36% of the women had a low predicted risk of caesarean section (< 20%) and 16.5% of women had a high predicted risk (> 40%); 10.9% and 47.7% of these women, respectively, were actually delivered by caesarean section (Fig. 2).

A logistic regression model was then developed for the entire population and then converted into likelihood ratios. These are provided (Table 5) along

Table 5 Adjusted log likelihood ratios for maternal characteristics and fetal sex derived from logistic regression model fitted for the whole population

Age	ALLR	Height (cm)	ALLR	Previous vaginal birth	ALLR	Gestation (weeks)	ALLR	Method of induction	ALLR	Sex of infant	ALLR
18	0.62	143	2.68	Yes	0.30	40	0.88	None	0.93	Female	0.91
19	0.65	144	2.54	No	1.51	41	1.13	Non-prosta-glandin	0.99	Male	1.10
20	0.68	145	2.40			42	1.26	Prosta-glandin	1.37		
21	0.71	146	2.27								
22	0.74	147	2.15								
23	0.77	148	2.04								
24	0.81	149	1.93								
25	0.84	150	1.82								
26	0.88	151	1.72								
27	0.92	152	1.63								
28	0.96	153	1.54								
29	1.00	154	1.46								
30	1.04	155	1.38								
31	1.09	156	1.31								
32	1.13	157	1.24								
33	1.18	158	1.17								
34	1.23	159	1.11								
35	1.29	160	1.05								
36	1.34	161	0.99								
37	1.40	162	0.94								
38	1.46	163	0.89								
39	1.53	164	0.84								
40	1.59	165	0.80								
41	1.66	166	0.75								
42	1.74	167	0.71								
43	1.81	168	0.67								
		169	0.64								
		170	0.60								
		171	0.57								
		172	0.54								
		173	0.51								
		174	0.48								
		175	0.46								
		176	0.43								
		177	0.41								
		178	0.39								
		179	0.37								
		180	0.35								
		181	0.33								
		182	0.31								

Derived from the following logistic regression model: log odds (caesarean) = 5.091 + (0.043*age) + (−0.055*height) + (0.193*male) + (1.633*no previous vaginal birth) + (0.067*non-prostaglandin induction) + (0.393*prostaglandin induction) + (0.248*delivered at 41 weeks) + (0.355*delivered at 42 weeks), where age is expressed in years and height is expressed in cm and all other variables are yes = 1 and no = 0. ALLR denotes adjusted log likelihood ratio.
Reproduced with permission from Smith et al. PLoS Med 2005.[40]

> **Box** Sample calculation
> _____
>
> Background risk of caesarean section = 26%
> Convert into odds prior odds of caesarean section = 26/74 = 0.35
>
> Example: 37-year-old woman, 160 cm tall, no previous vaginal birth, male infant
> wishes to know probability of Caesarean section if she requires induction of
> labour at 41 weeks' gestation using prostaglandin
> Summary ALLR = 1.40 x 1.05 x 1.51 x 1.10 x 1.13 x 1.37 = 3.78
> Posterior odds = 0.35 x 3.78 = 1.32
> Chance of caesarean delivery = 1.32/(1+1.32) = 0.57 or 57%
>
> *(This is identical to the estimated risk using the logistic regression equation in
> the footnote of Table 5)*

with a sample calculation (Box 1). One of the advantages of a likelihood ratio based approach is that it is relatively easy to apply them to other cases with a lower prior risk. This study used the same table of likelihood ratios to predict the probability of caesarean section among women delivering between 37–39 weeks' gestation. These women had a background risk of caesarean of 18% compared with 26% among women at 40 weeks and beyond. When this was taken into account using the prior odds of 0.22 (*i.e.* 18/82), the model provided useful prediction (Fig. 2).

Despite a relatively simple series of predictors, this approach gave useful prediction for over half the population of women. Addition of other factors (such as body mass index [BMI],[41] indication for prior caesarean delivery[42]) would be very likely to improve prediction further. A key aspect of any future approach is to present models in such a way as to be understood by practising

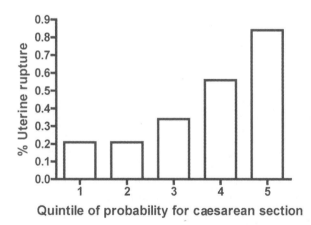

Fig. 3 Proportion of uterine ruptures in relation to the quintile of predicted probability of emergency caesarean delivery for the whole population (*n* = 23,286). *P* < 0.0001 (Chi square test for trend). Reproduced with permission from Smith *et al.* PLoS Medicine 2005.[40]

clinicians. One of the advantages of a likelihood ratio based approach is that it is already in wide-spread use in the context of Down's syndrome screening.

Factors predicting uterine rupture

One of the other principal concerns among women who have had a prior caesarean section is the risk of intrapartum uterine rupture. Even if a woman had a low risk of emergency caesarean section, she may chose to have a planned repeat caesarean section due to concerns about the possibility of uterine rupture. The modelling study found that women who were at low risk of emergency caesarean section were also at low risk of uterine rupture, including catastrophic rupture leading to perinatal death (Fig. 3). Among women with a predicted caesarean section risk of less than 20%, the incidence of uterine rupture was 2.0 per 1000 whereas among women with a caesarean section risk of greater than 40%, the incidence of uterine rupture was 9.1 per 1000. This association was also observed with the outcome of perinatal death due to uterine rupture. Since the association was also observed with these catastrophic ruptures, it cannot be explained by ascertainment bias (ascertainment bias in this context would be that a small dehiscence of the wound would only be noted among women having caesarean section – incorrect classification of dehiscence as a rupture would lead to an apparent association between any factor associated with caesarean delivery and the risk of uterine rupture). This demonstrates that the factors which determine a difficult and ultimately unsuccessful attempt at labour are related to the factors which determine rupture of the scar.

Other factors are also predictive of the risk of uterine rupture. Previous classical caesarean section is associated with a much greater risk of antepartum and intrapartum uterine rupture and is an indication for planned caesarean delivery at 36–37 weeks' gestation. In contrast, previous vertical lower uterine segment caesarean delivery does not appear to be associated with an increased risk of uterine rupture compared with a low transverse incision,[43] although this analysis is based on less than 400 women with such incisions. Single layer closure of a low transverse incision was associated with a 4–5-fold risk of uterine rupture after adjustment in multivariate analysis for a number of maternal and demographic factors.[44] A number of studies have demonstrated the risk of rupture varies inversely with the interval between the previous caesarean delivery and the next pregnancy.[44–47] Increased birth weight is also associated with an increased risk of rupture[48] but the clinical utility of this association in risk scoring is limited due to the inaccuracy of estimation of fetal weight.[49]

A number of studies have reported an increased risk of uterine rupture when labour is induced with prostaglandins.[1,4,9] The American College of Obstetricians and Gynecologists discourages the use of prostaglandin when inducing labour among women attempting VBAC.[50] Some studies have reported that the risk of uterine rupture is not increased when labour is induced with oxytocin when compared with women in spontaneous labour,[1,9] whereas others have also demonstrated an increased risk with oxytocin induction.[4] The overall absolute risk of uterine rupture was 0.2% among women with a previous vaginal birth, which was 5-fold lower than among women with no previous vaginal birth. The apparent protective effect was observed whether the vaginal births were before or after the caesarean delivery.[51] There is an association between the risk of uterine rupture or dehiscence and the thickness of the lower uterine segment measured using ultrasound.[52] However, this is not currently used in routine practice in the UK.

Future reproductive choices

Perhaps one of the key issues when deciding about mode of delivery in women with one previous caesarean section is the woman's aims regarding further pregnancies. The natural focus when making decisions regarding VBAC and PRCD is the possibility of serious adverse consequences in the current pregnancy. Although successful VBAC is associated with lower rates of non-life-threatening complications, the potential for catastrophic uterine rupture raises the possibility that PRCD may be associated with lower risks of severe maternal morbidity and mortality. This argument may not hold, however, in cases where the mother was planning many future births. Women who elect for PRCD and are planning future pregnancies must consider the additional future risks associated with multiple previous caesarean deliveries. In the context of complications likely to lead to severe maternal morbidity or death, the major factor is placenta praevia with accreta or percreta. It is currently very difficult to assess the balance of the risk of severe morbidity and mortality comparing VBAC and PRCD. These questions will only be addressed by high-quality observational studies using detailed and large-scale databases, probably involving record linkage to maternal death enquiry data and obstetric data. However, it is likely that the balance of risks and benefits favours an attempt at VBAC among women who may wish the option of many future pregnancies.

MANAGEMENT OF LABOUR

The management of labour in women attempting VBAC cannot be based on RCT evidence, since the trials have not been conducted – and almost certainly never will be conducted – that are powered to determine the effects of management on the risk of key events, such as perinatal death. Management must be guided, therefore, on the basis of understanding the risks of VBAC. Given the small, but finite, risks involved, a conservative approach is justified. Rejection of caution in this context on the basis that 'there is no evidence that demonstrates X is useful' is not justified when the issue is lack of evidence rather than convincing data that indicate no benefit.

Given that the absolute risk of uterine rupture is in the region of 0.5–1.0% and that it can result in rapid fetal demise and life-threatening maternal haemorrhage, it is advisable that VBAC should be attempted only in units where there is immediate access to facilities for the management of uterine rupture. This will usually require resident obstetric, anaesthetic and neonatology services with access to haematology and other support services. Uterine rupture is classically diagnosed by pain, vaginal bleeding, maternal hypotension or collapse. However, the earliest warning sign may be an abnormal CTG. Given this and the risk of intrapartum anoxia due both to the rupture and other events, continuous electronic fetal monitoring is advisable. As discussed above, the size of a unit may determine whether it results in death of the infant or delivery of a severely asphyxiated liveborn. This presents a dilemma in the practice of obstetrics in rural areas since smaller units may be unprepared to offer VBAC due to an inability to respond immediately in cases of suspected uterine rupture. This could, in practice, limit the availability of VBAC. This is not necessarily the safest thing for the mother particularly if she is planning a large family. The unavailability of VBAC may lead her to have large numbers of repeat caesarean sections which could place her at higher absolute risk of severe adverse events than attempting VBAC in a smaller unit. These issues underline the importance of developing quantitative methods of risk assessment in order to inform such questions.

Concerns that the symptoms of uterine rupture might be masked by epidural anaesthesia have not been sustained and use of epidural analgesia is appropriate when attempting VBAC.[53] The use of intra-uterine pressure catheters was previously wide-spread but this is no longer the case as they do not appear to indicate reliably the event of a uterine rupture and may, therefore, be falsely re-assuring.[54] Oxytocin as a means of inducing labour does not appear to be associated with an increased risk of uterine rupture compared with women in spontaneous labour.[1] However, oxytocin should be used extremely cautiously to augment women in labour. It should only be used when uterine activity is clearly inadequate. Regular cervical examinations should be performed in all cases and there should be a low threshold for emergency caesarean delivery when cervical dilation is inadequate in the presence of normal uterine activity. Postpartum examination of the uterine scar at the time of vaginal examination is no longer recommended since cases where surgical repair is required are almost invariably symptomatic.[55]

CONCLUSIONS

An increasing proportion of the population booking for antenatal care has had a previous caesarean delivery. These women are at increased risk of complications compared with other women. The primary choice for women in this situation is whether to have a repeat caesarean section or to attempt vaginal birth. Women have largely been encouraged to attempt vaginal birth. However, maternal morbidity is increased among women attempting VBAC principally due to complications among those who attempt VBAC and fail. The major obstetric drawback of planned repeat caesarean section is the risk of rare, but severe, adverse outcomes in future pregnancies. The two major clinical factors determining the choice for VBAC are, therefore, the likelihood of a successful attempt and the mother's plans for future pregnancies.

References

1 Lydon-Rochelle M, Holt VL, Easterling TR, Martin DP. Risk of uterine rupture during labor among women with a prior cesarean delivery. N Engl J Med 2001; 345: 3–8
2 Smith GC, Pell JP, Cameron AD, Dobbie R. Risk of perinatal death associated with labor after previous cesarean delivery in uncomplicated term pregnancies. JAMA 2002; 287: 2684–2690

3 McMahon MJ, Luther ER, Bowes Jr WA, Olshan AF. Comparison of a trial of labor with an elective second cesarean section. N Engl J Med 1996; 335: 689–695

4 Landon MB, Hauth JC, Leveno KJ et al. Maternal and perinatal outcomes associated with a trial of labor after prior cesarean delivery. N Engl J Med 2004; 351: 2581–2589

5 Lilford RJ, van Coeverden de Groot HA, Moore PJ, Bingham P. The relative risks of caesarean section (intrapartum and elective) and vaginal delivery: a detailed analysis to exclude the effects of medical disorders and other acute pre-existing physiological disturbances. Br J Obstet Gynaecol 1990; 97: 883–892

6 Hannah ME, Hannah WJ, Hewson SA, Hodnett ED, Saigal S, Willan AR. Planned caesarean section versus planned vaginal birth for breech presentation at term: a randomised multicentre trial. Term Breech Trial Collaborative Group. Lancet 2000; 356: 1375–1383

7 Mozurkewich EL, Hutton EK. Elective repeat cesarean delivery versus trial of labor: a meta- analysis of the literature from 1989 to 1999. Am J Obstet Gynecol 2000; 183: 1187–1197

8 Chauhan SP, Martin Jr JN, Henrichs CE, Morrison JC, Magann EF. Maternal and perinatal complications with uterine rupture in 142,075 patients who attempted vaginal birth after cesarean delivery: a review of the literature. Am J Obstet Gynecol 2003; 189: 408–417

9 Smith GC, Pell JP, Pasupathy D, Dobbie R. Factors predisposing to perinatal death related to uterine rupture during attempted vaginal birth after caesarean section: retrospective cohort study. BMJ 2004; 329: 375

10 Wen SW, Rusen ID, Walker M et al. Comparison of maternal mortality and morbidity between trial of labor and elective cesarean section among women with previous cesarean delivery. Am J Obstet Gynecol 2004; 191: 1263–1269

11 Farrell SA, Allen VM, Baskett TF. Parturition and urinary incontinence in primiparas. Obstet Gynecol 2001; 97: 350–356

12 Rortveit G, Daltveit AK, Hannestad YS, Hunskaar S. Urinary incontinence after vaginal delivery or cesarean section. N Engl J Med 2003; 348: 900–907

13 Handa VL, Harvey L, Fox HE, Kjerulff KH. Parity and route of delivery: does cesarean delivery reduce bladder symptoms later in life? Am J Obstet Gynecol 2004; 191: 463–469

14 Hannah ME, Hannah WJ, Hodnett ED et al. Outcomes at 3 months after planned cesarean vs planned vaginal delivery for breech presentation at term: the international randomized Term Breech Trial. JAMA 2002; 287: 1822–1831

15 Hannah ME, Whyte H, Hannah WJ et al. Maternal outcomes at 2 years after planned cesarean section versus planned vaginal birth for breech presentation at term: the international randomized Term Breech Trial. Am J Obstet Gynecol 2004; 191: 917–927

16 Faiz AS, Ananth CV. Etiology and risk factors for placenta previa: an overview and meta-analysis of observational studies. J Matern Fetal Neonatal Med 2003; 13: 175–190

17 Ananth CV, Smulian JC, Vintzileos AM. The association of placenta previa with history of cesarean delivery and abortion: a metaanalysis. Am J Obstet Gynecol 1997; 177: 1071–1078

18 Gielchinsky Y, Rojansky N, Fasouliotis SJ, Ezra Y. Placenta accreta – summary of 10 years: a survey of 310 cases. Placenta 2002; 23: 210–214

19 Makoha FW, Felimban HM, Fathuddien MA, Roomi F, Ghabra T. Multiple cesarean section morbidity. Int J Gynaecol Obstet 2004; 87: 227–232

20 Unger JB, Meeks GR. Vaginal hysterectomy in women with history of previous cesarean delivery. Am J Obstet Gynecol 1998; 179: 1473–1478

21 Poindexter YM, Sangi-Haghpeykar H, Poindexter AN et al. Previous cesarean section. A contraindication to vaginal hysterectomy? J Reprod Med 2001; 46: 840–844

22 Murphy DJ, Stirrat GM, Heron J. The relationship between caesarean section and subfertility in a population-based sample of 14 541 pregnancies. Hum Reprod 2002; 17: 1914–1917

23 Smith GCS, Wood AM, Pell JP, Dobbie R. First cesarean birth and subsequent fertility. Fertil Steril 2006; 85: 90–95

24 Smith GCS, Pell JP, Dobbie R. Caesarean section and risk of unexplained stillbirth in subsequent pregnancy. Lancet 2003; 362: 1779–1784

25 Smith GC. Estimating risks of perinatal death. Am J Obstet Gynecol 2005; 192: 17–22

26 Kurinczuk JJ, Gray R, Brocklehurst P. Risk of stillbirth after previous caesarean section. Lancet 2004; 363: 402

27 Rageth JC, Juzi C, Grossenbacher H. Delivery after previous cesarean: a risk evaluation. Swiss Working Group of Obstetric and Gynecologic Institutions. Obstet Gynecol 1999; 93: 332–337

28 Smith GC, Pell JP. Outcomes associated with a trial of labor after prior cesarean delivery. N Engl J Med 2005; 352: 1718–1720

29 Hankins GD, Speer M. Defining the pathogenesis and pathophysiology of neonatal encephalopathy and cerebral palsy. Obstet Gynecol 2003; 102: 628–636

30 Smith GC, Wood AM, White IR, Pell JP, Cameron AD, Dobbie R. Neonatal respiratory morbidity at term and the risk of childhood asthma. Arch Dis Child 2004; 89: 956–960

31 Morrison JJ, Rennie JM, Milton PJ. Neonatal respiratory morbidity and mode of delivery at term: influence of timing of elective caesarean section. Br J Obstet Gynaecol 1995; 102: 101–106

32 Ng DK, Lau WY, Lee SL. Pulmonary sequelae in long-term survivors of bronchopulmonary dysplasia. Pediatr Int 2000; 42: 603–607

33 Heritage CK, Cunningham MD. Association of elective repeat cesarean delivery and persistent pulmonary hypertension of the newborn. Am J Obstet Gynecol 1985; 152: 627–629

34 Levine EM, Ghai V, Barton JJ, Strom CM. Mode of delivery and risk of respiratory diseases in newborns. Obstet Gynecol 2001; 97: 439–442

35 Stutchfield P, Whitaker R, Russell I. Antenatal betamethasone and incidence of neonatal respiratory distress after elective caesarean section: pragmatic randomised trial. BMJ 2005; 331: 662

36 Clark SL, Scott JR, Porter TF, Schlappy DA, McClellan V, Burton DA. Is vaginal birth after cesarean less expensive than repeat cesarean delivery? Am J Obstet Gynecol 2000; 182: 599–602

37 Hashima JN, Eden KB, Osterweil P, Nygren P, Guise JM. Predicting vaginal birth after cesarean delivery: a review of prognostic factors and screening tools. Am J Obstet Gynecol 2004; 190: 547–555

38 Flamm BL, Geiger AM. Vaginal birth after cesarean delivery: an admission scoring system. Obstet Gynecol 1997; 90: 907–910

39 Troyer LR, Parisi VM. Obstetric parameters affecting success in a trial of labor: designation of a scoring system. Am J Obstet Gynecol 1992; 167: 1099–1104

40 Smith GC, White IR, Pell JP, Dobbie R. Predicting cesarean section and uterine rupture among women attempting vaginal birth after prior cesarean section. PLoS Med 2005; 2: e252

41 Goodall PT, Ahn JT, Chapa JB, Hibbard JU. Obesity as a risk factor for failed trial of labor in patients with previous cesarean delivery. Am J Obstet Gynecol 2005; 192: 1423–1426

42 Shipp TD, Zelop CM, Repke JT, Cohen A, Caughey AB, Lieberman E. Labor after previous cesarean: influence of prior indication and parity. Obstet Gynecol 2000; 95: 913–916

43 Shipp TD, Zelop CM, Repke JT, Cohen A, Caughey AB, Lieberman E. Intrapartum uterine rupture and dehiscence in patients with prior lower uterine segment vertical and transverse incisions. Obstet Gynecol 1999; 94: 735–740

44 Bujold E, Mehta SH, Bujold C, Gauthier RJ. Interdelivery interval and uterine rupture. Am J Obstet Gynecol 2002; 187: 1199–1202

45 Huang WH, Nakashima DK, Rumney PJ, Keegan Jr KA, Chan K. Interdelivery interval and the success of vaginal birth after cesarean delivery. Obstet Gynecol 2002; 99: 41–44

46 Shipp TD, Zelop CM, Repke JT, Cohen A, Lieberman E. Interdelivery interval and risk of symptomatic uterine rupture. Obstet Gynecol 2001; 97: 175–177

47 Esposito MA, Menihan CA, Malee MP. Association of interpregnancy interval with uterine scar failure in labor: a case-control study. Am J Obstet Gynecol 2000; 183: 1180–1183

48 Elkousy MA, Sammel M, Stevens E, Peipert JF, Macones G. The effect of birth weight on vaginal birth after cesarean delivery success rates. Am J Obstet Gynecol 2003; 188: 824–830

49 Smith GCS, Smith M-FS, McNay MB, Fleming J-EE. The relation between fetal abdominal circumference and birthweight: findings in 3512 pregnancies. Br J Obstet Gynaecol 1997; 104: 186–190

50 ACOG Committee opinion. Induction of labor for vaginal birth after cesarean delivery. Obstet Gynecol 2002; 99: 679–680

51 Zelop CM, Shipp TD, Repke JT, Cohen A, Lieberman E. Effect of previous vaginal delivery on the risk of uterine rupture during a subsequent trial of labor. Am J Obstet Gynecol 2000; 183: 1184–1186

52 Rozenberg P, Goffinet F, Phillippe HJ, Nisand I. Ultrasonographic measurement of lower uterine segment to assess risk of defects of scarred uterus. Lancet 1996; 347: 281–284

53 Flamm BL. Vaginal birth after caesarean (VBAC). Best Pract Res Clin Obstet Gynaecol 2001; 15: 81–92

54 Beckley S, Gee H, Newton JR. Scar rupture in labour after previous lower uterine segment caesarean section: the role of uterine activity measurement. Br J Obstet Gynaecol 1991; 98: 265–269

55 Silberstein T, Wiznitzer A, Katz M, Friger M, Mazor M. Routine revision of uterine scar after cesarean section: has it ever been necessary? Eur J Obstet Gynecol Reprod Biol 1998; 78: 29–32

George Condous   Tom Bourne

Post-partum uterine atony

Primary post-partum haemorrhage (PPH) is defined as the loss of greater than 500 ml of blood from the genital tract in the first 24 h following delivery.[1] PPH occurs in 2–11% of all deliveries;[1–3] however, when blood loss is quantitated objectively, the rate of PPH increases to 20%.[3] Fortunately, life-threatening PPH is rare and occurs with a frequency of 1 per 1000 deliveries in the industrialised world.[4] Massive PPH is a major cause of maternal mortality in the UK and world-wide.

In the most recent triennial report into *Why Mothers Die 2000–2002*, catastrophic obstetric haemorrhage was the second most common cause of direct maternal mortality.[4] The mortality rate per million maternities has more than doubled since the last report. There were 17 deaths from haemorrhage during 2000–2002 compared with seven in the previous triennium. While the numbers of deaths due to placental abruption and placenta praevia remain unchanged from the previous triennium, there was a striking increase in the numbers of deaths from PPH. As the number of caesarean sections increases so too does the number of placenta praevia/caesarean section hysterectomy deaths. Further research is needed to investigate the incidence of PPH in relation to previous caesarean section.

Uterine atony is responsible for up to 80% of primary PPH.[5] Uterine atony occurs when the uterine corpus does not contract appropriately, allowing continued blood loss from the placental site. In this chapter, we will discuss post-partum uterine atony. The other causes of primary PPH include retained

George Condous MRCOG FRANZCOG (for correspondence)
Clinical Research Fellow, Royal North Shore Hospital, University of Sydney, Department of Obstetrics
and Gynaecology, St Leonards, New South Wales 2065, Australia
E-mail: gcondous@hotmail.com

Tom Bourne PhD MRCOG
Consultant Gynecologist and Head of Unit, Early Pregnancy, Gynaecological Ultrasound and MAS Unit,
St George's Hospital Medical School, Blackshaw Road, London SW17 0QT, UK

placental tissue, uterine rupture, lower genital tract trauma, uterine inversion and consumptive coagulopathy and will not be covered here.

RISK FACTORS FOR UTERINE ATONY

Following the expulsion of the placenta from the uterus, myometrial fibres within the uterine corpus physiologically contract and retract causing kinking of the blood vessels at the placental site. This kinking effect results in cessation of blood flow to the placental site and consequently bleeding is controlled. Factors which compromise this physiological response can result in uterine atony and subsequent haemorrhage. These include prolonged first and/or second stage of labour, augmented labour, retained placenta and/or placenta accreta, overdistention of the uterus (*e.g.* multiple pregnancy, polyhydramnios) and, rarely, leiomyomata of the uterus. Previous history of PPH, multiparity and precipitate labour are also risk factors for uterine atony

PREVENTION OF UTERINE ATONY

Prevention of uterine atony is the key to reducing the incidence of PPH. The benefits of active management of the third stage of labour are well documented.[6-8] In a large, randomised, control trial (*n* = 1512) published in *The Lancet*, women were randomised to either active management of the third stage or expectant management. Active management of the third stage of labour included a prophylactic oxytocic given within 2 min of the baby's birth, immediate clamping and cutting of the cord, and delivery of placenta by controlled cord traction or maternal effort. The rate of PPH was significantly lower in the active management group (6.8% versus 16.5%; $P < 0.0001$).[9]

In a meta-analysis of seven randomised trials involving over 3000 women, the use of prophylactic oxytocin was compared to no uterotonic usage.[6] The former group demonstrated benefits with regard to both reduced blood loss and also the need for therapeutic oxytocics. There was, however, a non-significant trend towards more manual removals of the placenta.

In a randomised, double-blind, prospective study, intramuscular syntometrine (synthetic oxytocin 5 IU and ergometrine 0.5 mg) was a better choice than syntocinon (synthetic oxytocin) in the management of the third stage of labour.[7] Syntometrine not only reduced blood loss after delivery, but was associated with a 40% reduction in the risk of PPH and the need for repeat oxytocic injections. Its use, however, is contra-indicated in women with hypertensive disorders.

Ergometrine is comparable to oxytocin with regard to its haemostatic efficiency, but oxytocin seems to promote placental separation and expulsion better and, thereby, reduce the risk of retained placenta.[8]

Haemobate or carboprost, a 15-methyl analogue of prostaglandin F2α (PGF2α), is as effective as syntometrine in the prophylaxis of primary PPH, but there is a significant increase in diarrhoea with PGF2α medications.[10] Intramuscular haemobate is as effective as the intramyometrium route. These prostaglandins are also much more expensive than oxytocin or ergometrine.

Rectal or oral misoprostol (600 µg) are significantly less effective than oxytocin (10 IU) in the active management of the third stage of labour.[11-13] There are no data on the use of oxytocics versus expectant management in the treatment of PPH. More recently, buccal misoprostol (200 μg), when compared to placebo, reduced the need for additional uterotonic agents during caesarean section.[14]

MEDICAL MANAGEMENT OF UTERINE ATONY

If PPH occurs despite the use of prophylactic measures, the implementation of a PPH management plan is essential. The use of guidelines, staff education and the running of practice drills can successfully reduce the incidence of massive PPH.[15] This, in turn, can have a beneficial effect on maternal morbidity and potentially reduce mortality. All labour wards should have updated guidelines regularly disseminated to staff. This approach in conjunction with practice drills in labour ward emergencies, including massive PPH, should be the standard of care for all labour ward units.

There are two main aspects to the management of massive PPH – resuscitation and identification/management of the underlying cause. Establishing a cause should be done in parallel to resuscitation. The use of colloids is associated with an increase in the absolute risk of maternal mortality of 4% compared with crystalloids.[16] Thus crystalloids such as Hartmann's solution (compound sodium lactate intravenous solution) and 0.9% saline should be the first-line treatment in resuscitation. If colloids are given, the maximum volume should not exceed 1500 ml/day. Red cell transfusion is required where blood loss is in excess of 40% of the woman's blood volume. Since the approximate blood volume in litres of a woman is one-twelfth of the body weight in kilograms, the 40% estimated blood loss in an average woman would be more than 2000 ml. Cross-matched blood should be used wherever possible, but uncross-matched Group O Rhesus-negative blood can be used in life-threatening circumstances, when cross-matched blood is not readily available.

All other causes for PPH must be excluded before making a diagnosis of uterine atony. Examination of the upper and lower genital tract should be methodical and thorough. Identifying and removing retained placental tissue or repairing lower genital tract lacerations should be performed in the operating theatre if necessary. An empty uterus is paramount in order to facilitate not only physiological uterine contraction following delivery but also to maximise the pharmacological effect of uterotonics used in the event of PPH. If uterine atony is the underlying cause of the PPH, the bladder should be emptied, the uterine fundus rubbed and pharmacological agents (oxytocics) given to contract the uterus. While an infusion of oxytocin is being prepared (40 IU oxytocin in 500 ml of normal saline), a bolus of 250 μg of ergometrine should be administered intravenously. If the bleeding continues, a bolus of intravenous oxytocin 10 IU should be administered and bimanual compression of the uterus should be applied. If the haemorrhage continues, 15-methyl-prostaglandin F2α (haemobate) 250 μg can be administered either intramuscularly, repeated up to three more times at 15-min intervals, as necessary. For PPH unresponsive to oxytocin and/or ergometrine, or when ergometrine is contra-indicated, misoprostol 1000 μg administered rectally may have a role.

All units should have a 'massive obstetric haemorrhage' plan (Fig. 1). This not only mobilises the on-call obstetric consultant, but also the haematological unit. If bleeding still remains refractory despite the aforementioned therapies and other causes including retained placenta, lower genital tract trauma or an

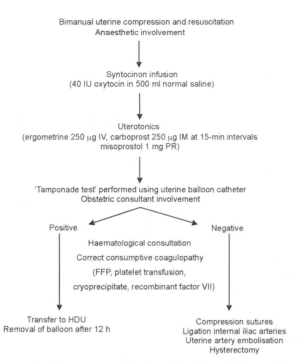

Bimanual uterine compression and resuscitation
Anaesthetic involvement

↓

Syntocinon infusion
(40 IU oxytocin in 500 ml normal saline)

↓

Uterotonics
(ergometrine 250 μg IV, carboprost 250 μg IM at 15-min intervals
misoprostol 1 mg PR)

↓

'Tamponade test' performed using uterine balloon catheter
Obstetric consultant involvement

Positive ← → Negative

Haematological consultation

Correct consumptive coagulopathy

(FFP, platelet transfusion,

cryoprecipitate, recombinant factor VII)

Transfer to HDU
Removal of balloon after 12 h

Compression sutures
Ligation internal iliac arteries
Uterine artery embolisation
Hysterectomy

Fig. 1 Flow diagram for the management of massive obstetric haemorrhage due to uterine atony. IV, intravenous; IM, intramuscular; PR, per rectum; FFP, fresh frozen plasma; HDU, high dependency unit.

underlying coagulopathy have been excluded, the use of balloon tamponade can be life saving.[17,18] The combination of refractory uterine atony and coagulopathy must always be considered in women with intractable haemorrhage. In such circumstances, the 'tamponade test' not only rapidly identifies those who will require a laparotomy but, when positive, arrests life-threatening haemorrhage and allows time to correct any consumptive coagulopathy.[19] Early consideration should be given to transferring the woman to an intensive care or high dependency unit.

Consumptive coagulopathy or disseminated intravascular coagulation (DIC) is a serious complication of massive PPH. This is a secondary phenomenon and management should concentrate on the removal or treatment of the underlying trigger. This involves maintaining circulating blood volume with appropriate fluid replacement. Rapid infusion of fresh frozen plasma (FFP) is recommended (15 ml/kg) with massive blood transfusion. One litre of fresh frozen plasma is recommended for every 6 units of blood transfused which equates to 4–5 bags of 200–250 ml of plasma to replace the lost clotting factors other than the platelets. The need for further FFP is dependent on the results of subsequent coagulation studies. Platelet transfusion should be given to maintain the platelet count $\geq 50 \times 10^9/l$, and cryoprecipitate should be given if the fibrinogen falls < 1 g/dl. The involvement of haematological colleagues is important in optimising the woman's haematological parameters. This is especially so with the more recent use of recombinant factor VII which has been shown to play a definitive role in the treatment of severe PPH associated with DIC.[20–24]

BALLOON TAMPONADE IN THE MANAGEMENT OF UTERINE ATONY

The successful use of the inflated stomach balloon of a Sengstaken-Blakemore oesophageal catheter (SBOC) as a therapy for obstetric haemorrhage has been previously reported.[25–27] Until recently, the use of the SBOC as a diagnostic test had not been reported. An inflated SBOC creates tamponade and identifies those women who will or will not need surgery.[19] The stomach balloon of the catheter is filled with 70–500 ml of warm saline until the distended balloon is palpable per abdomen and just visible at the cervical canal. Applying gentle traction at this stage confirms that the SBOC is firmly fixed *in situ* in the uterine cavity. If no or minimal bleeding is then observed through the cervix, or in the gastric lumen of the SBOC, the 'tamponade test' is considered to be positive and surgical intervention avoided. If significant bleeding continues through the cervix or the gastric lumen of the tube, the 'tamponade test' has failed and laparotomy is performed. This is the definition of the 'tamponade test'.[19]

The SBOC takes minutes to insert, is unlikely to cause trauma and it is possible to insert one with minimal anaesthesia, whilst removal is painless and easy. The tube is available in a pre-sterilised pack. Prior to insertion the distal end of the tube is cut off beyond the balloon to minimise the risk of perforation. The insertion is facilitated by grasping the anterior and lateral margins of the cervix with sponge forceps and placing the balloon into the uterine cavity with another sponge forceps. The procedure can be carried out by junior doctors in training whilst awaiting help from a senior colleague.

In the largest prospective study involving 16 women with intractable PPH due to uterine atony, 14 responded positively to balloon tamponade with a SBOC avoiding possible hysterectomy.[19] The efficacy of the SBOC was validated in this study of women whose intractable PPH condition was deteriorating such that surgical intervention was mandatory. It was at this predefined end-point that the 'tamponade test' was applied.[19] Fourteen of these women responded to the 'tamponade test' immediately following insertion of a SBOC, and arrest of the PPH was dramatic. Two failed the test and consequently went on to have surgical intervention. The insertion of the SBOC in those with massive PPH works very well and is associated with no significant complications. If bleeding continues despite insertion with a SBOC, this is prompt and noted either through the cervix or through the gastric lumen of the SBOC which is distal to the balloon. This diagnostic test not only rapidly identifies those women who require laparotomy but, when positive, allows time for correction of any consumptive coagulopathy.

The 'tamponade test' had a positive predictive value greater than 87% for successful management of PPH.[19] The Rusch urological hydrostatic balloon[28] and 'Bakri SOS' balloon[18] can be used for the 'tamponade test'. The Rusch catheter is significantly cheaper and has been shown to be effective in two cases.[28]

Although it is always a concern that a woman will bleed after removal of the balloon, this study had no cases of re-bleeding following removal of the SBOC. Should bleeding start, the balloon can be re-inserted to maintain the woman's stable condition whilst planning for the next step, which may include uterine arterial embolisation,[29–31] systemic devascularisation procedures,[32,33] compression sutures[34–40] or emergency hysterectomy.[41–43]

SURGICAL MANAGEMENT OF UTERINE ATONY

In the event that the above-mentioned measures are unsuccessful and potential causes of uterine bleeding other than uterine atony (such as retained products, soft tissue trauma, and coagulopathy) have been excluded, surgical intervention must be considered. This should involve input from a senior obstetrician. The choice of surgical procedure depends on the gravity of the situation, the age and parity of the mother, the underlying cause, the experience of the surgeon and the degree of radiological support.

Compression sutures

In recent years, interest in the surgical compression suture for the treatment of massive PPH secondary to uterine atony has surged.[34–40] This suturing technique involves a pair of vertical brace sutures around the uterus, apposing the anterior and posterior walls, resulting in continuous compression.[35] B-Lynch et al.[35] described a series of five women with intractable PPH where haemostasis was achieved by these sutures, thus avoiding difficult and hazardous pelvic surgery and potentially preserving fertility. A woman fulfils the criteria for the B-Lynch compression suture if, at laparotomy, bimanual compression decreases the amount of uterine bleeding on vaginal inspection.

Although originally described using No. 2 chromic catgut suture,[35] variations using 0 Vicryl (Ethicon, Somerville, NJ, USA) suture have been equally successful.[36] Modifications to the original B-Lynch suture may have the advantage of being simpler to perform without the need to open the uterus. More tension to appose the uterine walls can be achieved by two separate sutures rather than a single suture as described by B-Lynch.[37] Slippage of the uterine brace sutures is avoided by tying the loose ends of the brace sutures together at the uterine fundus.[37] When using the B-Lynch compression suture, we recommend using absorbable, as opposed to delayed absorbable, suture material. More recently, erosion of the suture through the uterine wall has been described,[44] but this should not discourage the use of the B-Lynch brace suture.

The brace suture probably works by direct application of pressure on the placental bed bleeding and also by reducing blood flow to the uterus. Horizontal, full-thickness, compression sutures without obliterating the cervical canal can provide a very effective means of controlling bleeding from the lower segment, especially when the latter was the site for placental insertion. In some cases of placenta praevia, both vertical and horizontal compression sutures may be needed to arrest haemorrhage.

The haemostatic 'multiple square' suturing technique, described by Cho et al.,[38] approximates the anterior and posterior uterine walls until no space is left in the uterine cavity, thus compressing and controlling bleeding secondary to uterine atony or placental site haemorrhage. The main advantages of this approach is that it is relatively safe to perform, there are no important structures such as ureters or great vessels in the vicinity, it can be performed by less-experienced surgeons and requires a short operating time.

Uterine and internal iliac artery ligation

As the uterus receives 90% of its blood supply from the uterine arteries, uterine artery ligation should be attempted prior to internal artery ligation if bleeding is from the uterus.[45] Uterine artery ligation is technically easier and associated with significantly less severe morbidity than internal iliac artery ligation. Ligation of the uterine vessels has been documented to be useful to control bleeding at caesarean section.[46]

Ligation of the internal iliac arteries for control of pelvic haemorrhage is performed in both obstetric and gynaecological cases.[47] Internal artery ligation helps to control uterine and vaginal bleeding from the vaginal branch of the internal iliac artery.[47] Bilateral internal iliac artery ligation results in 85% reduction in pulse pressure in the arteries distal to the ligation and reduces blood flow by 50% in the distal vessel.[48] The success of this procedure is reported to be 40–75%,[48] and by this stage the woman almost certainly will be compromised with a superimposed consumptive coaguloathy.[49] Tissue oedema and haematoma formation may further increase the morbidity of the procedure.

Complications of this procedure include long-term buttock pain due to inadvertent ligation of the artery above the point where the posterior branch comes off the internal iliac artery.[47] It can also result in ischaemic damage to the pelvis, laceration of iliac veins, accidental ligation of the external iliac artery and ureteric injury.[50] Fortunately, complications are infrequent.[49]

Uterine artery embolisation

Arterial embolisation requires appropriately trained interventional radiologists and thus is offered only in a small number of tertiary centres. The femoral artery is punctured and step-wise catheterisation of the internal iliac, uterine and ovarian arteries is performed.[29–31,51,52] Thereafter, by using contrast media and angiography, the active bleeding can be located. The feeding uterine artery is catheterised and embolised with pledgets of absorbable gelatine sponge, polyurethane foam or polyvinyl alcohol particles, which are usually resorbed within 10 days.[51] It may become necessary to embolise the ovarian vessels but, in order to prevent ischaemic bowel damage, the mesenteric artery needs to be identified.[52]

Success rates reported for arterial embolisation range from 85% to 95%,[30,31,53] with the time taken from the start of the procedure to the attainment of haemostasis averaging 1 h.[53] Failures have been reported in the case of cervical-vaginal tearing and abnormal placental insertion (placenta accreta).[54]

Pelage et al.[55] evaluated the effectiveness of selective uterine artery embolisation in 35 women with severe, intractable PPH. Bleeding was controlled in all but one woman, who required hysterectomy for re-bleeding 5 days later. Normal menstruation resumed in all women in whom embolisation was successful.

Interventional radiology in women with massive PPH is significantly less traumatic than surgical procedures, since it does not require laparotomy, the recovery time is more rapid, and fertility is retained. However, it is not without complications including haematoma,[56] pelvic infection,[57] tissue ischaemia,[58] and a theoretical risk of contrast nephrotoxicity.[56]

HYSTERECTOMY

When all medical and less radical surgical interventions have failed in the management of PPH secondary to uterine causes, emergency hysterectomy is the last resort.[5,41-43] Emergency hysterectomy will not be discussed in this review. We suggest performing a subtotal hysterectomy, as it is quicker, safer, simpler, and associated with less blood loss.[5] Total hysterectomy is needed where the bleeding is in the lower segment such as placenta praevia with accreta or tears in the lower segment.[59] There is no doubt that as the caesarean section rate increases so too will the rate of placenta accreta and subsequent caesarean hysterectomy.

CONCLUSIONS

Postpartum haemorrhage is one of the main causes of death associated with childbirth world-wide. The majority of deaths due to PPH are preventable by the active management of the third stage of labour and by following a logical management sequence. First, oxytocin as a bolus and as an infusion, along with prostaglandin analogues such as haemobate (carboprost), or rectal or oral misoprostol, arrests the haemorrhage in most cases. The action of these may be synergistic. Second, the 'tamponade test' which can be performed by obstetric registrars rapidly identifies those women who will require laparotomy. Third, women who fail the 'tamponade test' can be helped with uterine compression sutures, which are simple to use and quick to perform. Finally, if these conservative measures fail, internal iliac artery ligation or hysterectomy has to be considered.

Conservative techniques are attractive as they can be carried out quickly by junior medical personnel with minimal training and are successful in the vast majority of cases. The sequential approaches outlined in this chapter will help to reduce total blood loss, blood transfusions, hysterectomies, and maternal deaths.

KEY POINTS FOR CLINICAL PRACTICE

- Life-threatening primary post-partum haemorrhage (PPH) is rare and occurs with a frequency of 1 per 1000.

- In the most recent triennial report into *Why Mothers Die 2000–2002*, catastrophic obstetric haemorrhage was the second most common cause of direct maternal mortality.

- Uterine atony is responsible for up to 80% of primary PPH.

- Prevention of uterine atony is the key to reducing the incidence of PPH and the benefits of active management of the third stage of labour are well documented.

- All obstetric units should have a 'massive obstetric haemorrhage' plan.

- Resuscitation and identification/management of the underlying cause are the two main aspects to the management of massive PPH.

- Consumptive coagulopathy or DIC is a serious complication of massive PPH and the involvement of haematological colleagues is important in optimising the woman's haematological parameters.

KEY POINTS FOR CLINICAL PRACTICE (continued)

- More recently, the use of recombinant factor VII has been shown to play a definitive role in the treatment of severe PPH associated with DIC.

- The 'tamponade test' not only rapidly identifies those women who require laparotomy but, when positive, also allows time for correction of any consumptive coagulopathy.

- Between 70–500 ml of warm saline is required to fill the stomach balloon of the SBOC in order to create tamponade of the uterine cavity.

- Other balloons such as the Rusch urological hydrostatic balloon and the 'Bakri SOS' balloon can be used for the 'tamponade test'.

- A woman fulfils the criteria for the B-Lynch brace suture if, at laparotomy, bimanual compression decreases the amount of uterine bleeding on vaginal inspection.

- Haemostatic 'multiple square' sutures approximate the anterior and posterior uterine walls, compressing the uterus.

- Ligation of the internal iliac arteries for control of pelvic haemorrhage has a reported success of 40–75%.

- Success rates reported for uterine arterial embolisation range from 85–95%.

- When all medical and less radical surgical interventions have failed in the management of PPH secondary to uterine causes, emergency hysterectomy is the last resort.

- Delaying this decision is a recurring theme in confidential enquiries into maternal deaths.

References

1 Gilbert L, Porter W, Brown VA. Postpartum haemorrhage – a continuing problem. Br J Obstet Gynaecol 1987; 94: 67–71

2 Brant HA. Precise estimation of postpartum haemorrhage: difficulties and importance. BMJ 1967; I: 398–400

3 Newton M, Mosey LM, Egli GE et al. Blood loss during and immediately after delivery. Obstet Gynecol 1961; 17: 9–18

4 Lewis G, Drife J (eds). Why Mothers Die, Triennial Report 2000–2002. The sixth report of the confidential enquiries into maternal deaths in the United Kingdom. London: RCOG Press, 2004

5 Tamizian O, Arulkumaran S. The surgical management of postpartum haemorrhage. Best Pract Res Clin Obstet Gynaecol 2002; 16: 81–98

6 Elbourne DR, Prendiville WJ, Carroli G, Wood J, McDonald S. Prophylactic use of oxytocin in the third stage of labour. Cochrane Database Syst Rev 2001;(4):CD001808

7 Yuen PM, Chan NS, Yim SF, Chang AM. A randomised double blind comparison of Syntometrine and Syntocinon in the management of the third stage of labour. Br J Obstet Gynaecol 1995; 102: 377–380

8 Sorbe B. Active pharmacologic management of the third stage of labor. A comparison of oxytocin and ergometrine. Obstet Gynecol 1978; 52: 694–697

9 Rogers J, Wood J, McCandlish R, Ayers S, Truesdale A, Elbourne D. Active versus expectant management of third stage of labour: the Hinchingbrooke randomised controlled trial. Lancet 1998; 351: 693–699

10 Lamont RF, Morgan DJ, Logue M, Gordon H. A prospective randomised trial to compare the efficacy and safety of hemabate and syntometrine for the prevention of primary postpartum haemorrhage. Prostaglandins Other Lipid Mediat 2001; 66: 203–210

11. Gulmezoglu AM, Villar J, Ngoc NT *et al*. and WHO Collaborative Group To Evaluate Misoprostol in the Management of the Third Stage of Labour. WHO multicentre randomised trial of misoprostol in the management of the third stage of labour. Lancet 2001; 358: 689–695

12 Villar J, Gulmezoglu AM, Hofmeyr GJ, Forna F. Systematic review of randomized controlled trials of misoprostol to prevent postpartum haemorrhage. Obstet Gynecol 2002; 100: 1301–1312

13 Caliskan E, Meydanli MM, Dilbaz B, Aykan B, Sonmezer M, Haberal A. Is rectal misoprostol really effective in the treatment of third stage of labor? A randomized controlled trial. Am J Obstet Gynecol 2002; 187: 1038–1045

14 Hamm J, Russell Z, Botha T, Carlan SJ, Richichi K. Buccal misoprostol to prevent hemorrhage at cesarean delivery: a randomized study. Am J Obstet Gynecol 2005; 192: 1404–1406

15 Rizvi F, Mackey R, Barrett T, McKenna P, Geary M. Successful reduction of massive postpartum haemorrhage by use of guidelines and staff education. Br J Obstet Gynaecol 2004; 111: 495–498

16 Schierhout G, Roberts I. Fluid resuscitation with colloid or crystalloid solutions in critically ill patients: a systematic review of randomised trials. BMJ 1998; 316: 961–964

17 Mousa HA, Walkinshaw S. Major postpartum haemorrhage. Curr Opin Obstet Gynecol 2001; 13: 595–603

18 Bakri YN, Amri A, Abdul Jabbar F. Tamponade-balloon for obstetrical bleeding. Int J Gynaecol Obstet 2001; 74: 139–142

19 Condous GS, Arulkumaran S, Symonds I, Chapman R, Sinha A, Razvi K. The 'tamponade test' in the management of massive postpartum hemorrhage. Obstet Gynecol 2003; 101: 767–772

20 Brice A, Hilbert U, Roger-Christoph S *et al*. Recombinant activated factor VII as a life-saving therapy for severe postpartum haemorrhage unresponsive to conservative traditional management. Ann Fr Anesth Reanim 2004; 23: 1084–1088

21 Holub Z, Feyereisl J, Kabelik L, Rittstein T. Successful treatment of severe post-partum bleeding after caesarean section using recombinant activated factor VII. Ceska Gynekol 2005; 70: 144, 146–8

22 Ahonen J, Jokela R. Recombinant factor VIIa for life-threatening post-partum haemorrhage. Br J Anaesth 2005; 94: 592–595

23 Price G, Kaplan J, Skowronski G. Use of recombinant factor VIIa to treat life-threatening non-surgical bleeding in a post-partum patient. Br J Anaesth 2004; 93: 298–300

24 Boehlen F, Morales MA, Fontana P, Ricou B, Irion O, de Moerloose P. Prolonged treatment of massive postpartum haemorrhage with recombinant factor VIIa: case report and review of the literature. Br J Obstet Gynaecol 2004; 111: 284–7

25 Katesmark M, Brown R, Raju KS. Successful use of a Sengstaken-Blakemore tube to control massive postpartum haemorrhage. Br J Obstet Gynaecol 1994; 101: 259–260

26 Chan C, Razvi K, Tham KF, Arulkumaran S. The use of a Sengstaken-Blakemore tube to control postpartum hemorrhage. Int J Obstet Gynecol 1997; 58: 251–252

27 Condie RG, Buxton EJ, Payne ES. Successful use of a Sengstaken-Blakemore tube to control massive postpartum haemorrhage [Letter]. Br J Obstet Gynaecol 1994; 101: 1023–1024

28 Johanson R, Kumar M, Obhrai M, Young P. Management of massive postpartum haemorrhage: use of a hydrostatic balloon catheter to avoid laparotomy. Br J Obstet Gynaecol 2001; 108: 420–422

29 Chen C, Ma B, Fang Y. Transcatheter arterial embolization in intractable postpartum haemorrhage [In Chinese]. Zhonghua Fu Chan Ke Za Zhi 2001; 36: 133–136

30 Pelage JP, Laissy JP, College National des Gynecologues et Obstetriciens Francais; Agence Nationale d'Accreditation et d'Evaluation en Sante. Management of life-threatening postpartum hemorrhage: indications and technique of arterial embolisation. J Gynecol Obstet Biol Reprod (Paris) 2004; 33 (8 Suppl): 4S93–4S102

31 Tourne G, Collet F, Seffert P, Veyret C. Place of embolization of the uterine arteries in the management of post-partum haemorrhage: a study of 12 cases. Eur J Obstet Gynecol Reprod Biol 2003; 110: 29–34

32 AbdRabbo SA. Stepwise uterine devascularisation: a novel technique for management of uncontrolled postpartum hemorrhage with preservation of the uterus. Am J Obstet Gynecol 1994; 171: 694–700

33 Thomas JM. The treatment of obstetric haemorrhage in women who refuse blood transfusion [Letter]. Soc Obstet Gynaecol Can 1998; 20: 1051–1052

34 Smith KL, Baskett TF. Uterine compression sutures as an alternative to hysterectomy for severe postpartum haemorrhage. J Obstet Gynaecol Can 2003; 25: 197–200

35 B-Lynch C, Coker A, Lawal AH, Abu J, Cowen MJ. The B-Lynch surgical technique for the control of massive postpartum haemorrhage: an alternative to hysterectomy? Five cases reported. Br J Obstet Gynaecol 1997; 104: 372–375

36 Ferguson JE, Bourgeois FS, Underwood PB. B-Lynch suture for postpartum hemorrhage. Obstet Gynecol 2000; 95: 1020–1022

37 Hayman RG, Arulkumaran S, Steer PJ. Uterine compression sutures: surgical management of postpartum hemorrhage. Obstet Gynecol 2002; 99: 502–506

38 Cho JH, Jun HS, Lee CN. Haemostatic suturing technique for uterine bleeding during caesarean delivery. Obstet Gynecol 2000; 96: 129–131

39 Allam MS, B-Lynch C. The B-Lynch and other uterine compression suture techniques. Int J Gynaecol Obstet 2005; 89: 236–241

40 Pal M, Biswas AK, Bhattacharya SM. B-Lynch brace suturing in primary post-partum hemorrhage during cesarean section. J Obstet Gynaecol Res 2003; 29: 317–320

41 Baskett TF. Emergency obstetric hysterectomy. J Obstet Gynaecol Can 2003; 23: 353–355

42 Forna F, Miles AM, Jamieson DJ. Emergency peripartum hysterectomy: a comparison of cesarean and postpartum hysterectomy. Am J Obstet Gynecol 2004; 190: 1440–1444

43 Kwee A, Bots ML, Visser GH, Bruinse HW. Emergency peripartum hysterectomy: a prospective study in The Netherlands. Eur J Obstet Gynecol Reprod Biol 2006; 124: 187–192

44 Grotegut CA, Larsen FW, Jones MR, Livingston E. Erosion of a B-Lynch suture through the uterine wall: a case report. J Reprod Med 2004; 49: 849–852

45 Still DK. Postpartum haemorrhage and other third stage problems. In: James DK, Steer PJ, Weiner CP, Gonik B. (eds) High Risk Pregnancy – Management Options. London: WB Saunders, 1999

46 O'Leary JA. Uterine artery ligation in the control of postcesarean hemorrhage. J Reprod Med 1995; 40: 189–193

47 Nandanwar YS, Jhalam L, Mayadeo N, Guttal DR. Ligation of internal iliac arteries for control of pelvic haemorrhage. J Postgrad Med 1993; 39: 194–196

48 Burchell RC. Physiology of internal iliac ligation. J Obstet Gynaecol Br Commonwealth 1968; 75: 642–651

49 Das BN, Biswas AK. Ligation of internal iliac arteries in pelvic haemorrhage. J Obstet Gynaecol Res 1998; 24: 251–254

50 Rajaram P, Raghavan SS, Bupathy A, Balasubramanian SR, Habeebullah S, Umadevi P. Internal iliac artery ligation in obstetrics and gynecology. Ten years' experience. Asia Oceania J Obstet Gynaecol 1993; 19: 71–75

51 Yamashita Y, Harada M, Yamamoto H et al. Transcatheter arterial embolisation of obstetric and gynaecological bleeding: efficacy and clinical outcome. Br J Radiol 1994; 67: 530–534

52 Oei PL, Tan L, Ratnam SS, Arulkumaran S. Arterial embolisation for bleeding following hysterectomy for intractable haemorrhage. Int J Gynaecol Obstet 1998; 62: 83–86

53 Badawy SZ, Etman A, Singh M, Murphy K, Mayelli T, Philadelphia M. Uterine artery embolization: the role in obstetrics and gynecology. Clin Imaging 2001; 25: 288–295

54 Reyal F, Pelage JP, Rossignol M et al. Interventional radiology in managing post-partum hemorrhage. Presse Med 2002; 31: 939–944

55 Pelage JP, Le Dref O, Jacob O, Soyer P, Herbreteau D, Rymer R. Selective arterial embolisation of the uterine arteries in the management of intractable post-partum hemorrhage. Acta Obstet Gynecol Scand 1999; 78: 698–703

56 Pelage JP, Le Dref O, Jacob D et al. Uterine artery embolization: anatomical and technical considerations, indications, results, and complications. J Radiol 2000; 81: 1863–1872

57 Gilbert WM, Moore TR, Resnik R, Doemeny J, Chin H, Bookstein JJ. Angiographic embolization in the management of hemorrhagic complications of pregnancy. Am J Obstet Gynecol 1992; 166: 493–497

58 Cottier JP, Fignon A, Tranquart F, Herbreteau D. Uterine necrosis after arterial embolization for postpartum hemorrhage. Obstet Gynecol 2002; 100: 1074–1077

59 Kastner ES, Figueroa R, Garry D, Maulik D. Emergency peripartum hysterectomy: experience at a community teaching hospital. Obstet Gynecol 2002; 99: 971–975

18

Olanrewaju Sorinola

Severe obstetric injury causing anal sphincter damage, sexual dysfunction and fistulae

The earliest evidence of severe perineal injury sustained during childbirth is from the mummy of Henhenit, an Egyptian woman about 22 years of age from the harem of King Mentuhotep II of Egypt in 2050 BC. Henhenit's pelvis was in an abnormal shape and there was rupture of the vagina into the bladder, and bowel was found protruding from the anus. Nowadays, such severe perineal injury is uncommon in the industrialised world but parturition still has profound effects on the muscles of the pelvic floor. In most women this effect is transitory; however, in a few women permanent damage to the pelvic floor occurs, which is reflected by urinary/faecal incontinence, fistulae, and sexual problems.

Anal sphincter rupture occurs in 0.5–2% of vaginal deliveries. It is a serious complication with over 40% of the women having persistent defaecatory symptoms despite primary repair. More worryingly, 33% of women have structural damage to their anal sphincters on ultrasound after their first vaginal delivery which goes unrecognised.[1] Up to 10% of women develop symptoms of faecal urgency or incontinence after their first vaginal delivery.[2] Often very little attention is paid to these problems during postnatal visits and very few women volunteer information about this problem. Therefore, the true incidence of problems is unknown. It is important to identify the size of the problem, to increase awareness amongst obstetric staff, provide adequate services and explore ways of limiting pelvic floor damage during delivery.

The effect of parturition on pelvic floor damage has been well documented and protection against pelvic floor damage has recently become a more common reason cited for doing an elective caesarean section in some women. However, pregnancy itself affects pelvic floor function; therefore, there is a need for a more comprehensive evaluation of the relative effects of pregnancy on pelvic floor functions.

Olanrewaju Sorinola MRCOG MMedSc
Consultant Obstetrician and Gynaecologist, Warwick Hospital, Lakin Road, Warwick CV34 5BW, UK
E-mail: lanre.sorinola@swh.nhs.uk

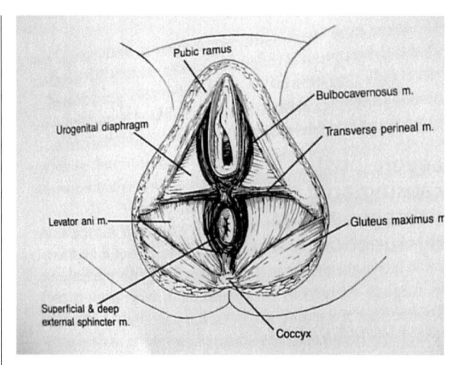

Fig. 1 Anatomy of the perineum. Note the close relationship of the bulbocavernosus, transverse perineal and external anal sphincter muscles. It is important to restore this anatomy during surgical repair to maintain continence.

ANATOMY OF THE PERINEUM

The levator ani muscles (sphincter vaginate, puborectalis, pubococcygeus, and ileococcygeus) and the coccygeus muscle with their respective fascial coverings make up the pelvic diaphragm. The levator ani forms a broad sling of musculature that originates from the posterior surface of the ischial spines, and from the obturator fascia in between. These muscles surround the vagina and the rectum, and occupy a median raphe between the vagina and rectum, and a raphe below the rectum, and into the coccyx (Fig. 1). The urogenital diaphragm lies external to the pelvic diaphragm in the triangle between the symphysis pubis and the ischial tuberosities. It is composed of the deep transverse perineal muscles, the urethra constrictor muscle, and the internal and external fascial coverings.

The anorectum is the most distal part of the gastrointestinal tract and consists of two parts – the anal canal and the rectum. The anal canal is about 3.5 cm in length and lies below the anorectal junction formed by the puborectalis muscle. The inner muscular tube, or internal anal sphincter, is a thickened continuation of the circular smooth muscle of the rectum while the external anal sphincter is made up of three parts (subcutaneous, superficial and deep) and is inseparable from the puborectalis posteriorly (Fig. 2). The perineal body is composed of fibres of the levator ani that unite in a median raphe between the vagina and rectum. This is re-inforced by the central perineal tendons, which are composed of fibres from the bulbocavernosus

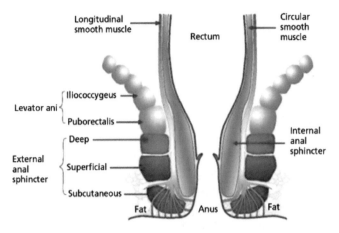

Fig. 2 Diagrammatic representation of the anal sphincter.

muscle, the deep transverse perineal muscles, and the external anal sphincter. These structures are often lacerated during vaginal delivery.

TYPES OF INJURIES

Perineal injury

Perineal injury remains the most common form of maternal obstetric injury and is classified as shown in Table 1. This classification removes any ambiguity and requires careful assessment of the injury as well as being clinically important for management purposes. Third and fourth degree tears constitute severe injuries as the anal sphincter mechanism is disrupted. Although the majority of perineal injuries are successfully repaired at the time of delivery, dehiscence of a repair can occur and can be associated with infection, abscess, sphincter disruption and fistula formation which commonly occur low in the rectovaginal septum but occasionally may extend much higher.

Uterine and cervical injury

Deep cervical lacerations are usually the result of instrumentation, especially forceps delivery. Such injuries may involve the vaginal vault and special care

Table 1 Classification of anal sphincter tears

Grade of tear	Classifying features
First degree	Laceration of the vaginal epithelium or perineal skin only
Second degree	Involvement of the perineal muscles but not the anal sphincter
Third degree	Disruption of the anal sphincter muscles and this should be further subdivided into three different grades (see below)
Grade 3a	< 50% thickness of external sphincter torn
Grade 3b	> 50% thickness of external sphincter torn
Grade 3c	Internal sphincter also torn
Fourth degree	A third-degree tear with disruption of the anal epithelium

has to be taken to avoid damage to the bladder in anterior tears or the ureter in lateral tears. Lacerations involving the uterus are rare and are usually the result of rotational Kjelland forceps. Injury to the uterine artery or vessels at the base of the broad ligament can cause haemorrhage or may result in a haematoma. Uterine rupture is usually associated with the rupture of a previous uterine scar with upper uterine segment scar presenting a greater risk.

Genital haematoma

A concealed persistently bleeding vessel adjacent to the genital tract will form a haematoma and depending on its site, can present in its mildest form as a vulva swelling or in the other extreme as third stage collapse and shock.[3] There are two main causes: (i) an incomplete repair and obliteration of the dead space; or (ii) disruption of the paravaginal plexus of veins with an intact perineum. The haematoma can be above or below the levator ani. A supralevator haematoma forms in the broad ligament and could be due to an extension of a tear in the cervix, vaginal fornix, or uterus. As the haematoma distends, it displaces the uterus contralaterally and bulges into the upper vagina. An infralevator haematoma collects in the region of the vulva, perineum and lower vagina.

Lower urinary tract injury

Direct lacerations involving the bladder and urethra are not common; when they do occur, they are usually associated with the use of high forceps or rotational forceps especially if the bladder has not been emptied. Direct injury to the bladder and ureter can also occur during caesarean section or peripartum hysterectomy.

Fistulae

The vast majority of fistulae that occur in non-industrialised countries are caused by obstetric trauma with prolonged obstructed labour being the most important cause. Prolonged impaction of the presenting part against a distended oedematous bladder eventually leads to pressure necrosis and fistula formation.

Table 2 Causes of obstetric genito-urinary fistulae

Non-industrialised countries
Prolonged obstructed labour
Instruments used to dismember and deliver stillborn infants
Trauma from forceps
Trauma from surgical abortions
Symphysiotomy
Gishiri cuts – an incision on the anterior vaginal wall made for a variety of obstetric and gynaecological disorders
Industrialised countries
Caesarean delivery including infection or urinoma following bladder trauma
Peripartum hysterectomy especially in the presence in the presence of distorted anatomy, *e.g.* fibroids
Trauma from forceps

Other causes are as listed in Table 2. In modern obstetrics, most of these conditions do not exist; however, genito-urinary fistulae still occur for the reasons listed in Table 2. Apart from urinary fistulae, rectovaginal fistula (RVF) can also occur following trauma to perineum, anal sphincter tear or direct injury.

RISK FACTORS FOR SEVERE OBSTETRIC INJURY

Perineal injury

Most authors[3-7] agree that the following factors are associated with an increased risk.

Maternal factors
Nulliparity increases the risk of perineal injury by up to 4%. The relative inelasticity of the perineum in nulliparae may be responsible.

Fetal/perinatal factors
Increased birth weight (4 kg or more) is associated with perineal injury. This may be attributed to a larger head circumference, difficult delivery, disruption of the fascial supports of the pelvic floor, and stretch injury to the pelvic and pudendal nerves. Even after safe delivery of the head, shoulder dystocia is associated with anal sphincter injury. Persistent occipito-posterior position at delivery has a larger presenting diameter and the risk of a third or fourth degree tear is increased by up to 3%.

Labour/delivery factors
Precipitate labour is associated with cervical, perineal, labial, and urethral injury. This is due to the lack of time available for the maternal tissues to adjust to delivery forces and allow a controlled delivery. A prolonged second stage of labour (i.e. second stage of labour longer than 1 h) increases the risk of severe perineal injury by up to 4%. More recently, it has been argued that the duration of bearing down (or active pushing), rather than the total duration of second stage of labour, is more important as it causes pudendal nerve damage. Epidural analgesia may be a confounding factor by prolonging the second stage of labour and increasing the risk of perineal injury by 2%. However, others argue that by relaxing the perineal muscles it is actually protective.

Mode of delivery
Instrumental vaginal delivery, especially forceps delivery, increases the risk of severe perineal injury by up to 7%. Forceps occupy an extra 10% space in the pelvis; the shanks stretch the perineum and can cause injury to the anal sphincter when pulling in the posterior direction to encourage flexion of the head.

Perineal factors
Lack of visualisation of the perineum, severe perineal oedema, and lack of manual protection of the perineum increases the risk and can be just as important in sphincter tears.

Episiotomy
The role of episiotomies in anal sphincter injury is not clear. Episiotomy is said to be the over-riding determinant of anal sphincter injury and perineal

laceration length, adding an extra 3 cm length to lacerations.[8] It has been shown that women who underwent episiotomy have a significantly decreased maximum anal squeeze pressure and are prone to develop anal incontinence symptoms.[9] On the other hand, large studies[4,5] of singleton deliveries have shown that there is no significant relation between third degree tear and episiotomy. Others have tried to differentiate between the effects of midline and mediolateral episiotomy, with midline episiotomy said to have a greater tendency to involve the anal sphincters and cause injury. Mediolateral episiotomy, more common in British obstetric practice, causes fewer tears into the rectum when compared to midline incision; however, it is not protective as it has also been found to increase the incidence of anal tears. The conclusion is that neither midline nor mediolateral episiotomy seem to fulfil their intended role of protecting the pelvic floor from injury with a slightly increased tendency to increased anal sphincter injury.

Fistulae

Urinary
Fistulae following caesarean section are usually due to incomplete reflection of the bladder or blind sharp dissection during bladder reflection. Incomplete bladder reflection results in a trapped knuckle in a suture line, which undergoes necrosis. Misplaced sutures passing through the bladder wall is another risk factor.

Rectovaginal fistula
The common underlying factor responsible for RVF formation include the breakdown of third- and fourth-degree perineal tears or from unrecognised injury at the time of forceps or precipitous delivery. Midline episiotomy commonly performed in the US is complicated in up to a quarter of cases by rectal tear or anal sphincter disruption. Up to 1.5% of such women who undergo an episioproctotomy develop a rectovaginal fistula.

Urinary incontinence

Pre-pregnancy body mass index
An increase in pre-pregnancy BMI of 1 kg/m^2 is associated with a 7% increase in the incidence of urinary incontinence in the post natal period.

Parity
Vaginal delivery appears to be associated with the development of urinary incontinence in a proportion of women. Foldspang et al.[10] showed a strong relationship between parity and urinary incontinence, especially stress incontinence. Thomas et al.[11] found that nuliparous women were less likely to report urinary incontinence than primiparous women. Prevalence of incontinence was highest for women who had four or more vaginal deliveries, but there was no difference in prevalence between women having one, two or three deliveries.

Obstetric factors
Other factors with development of post-partum stress incontinence were prolonged active second stage of labour, large birth weight and large head circumference.[12]

Faecal incontinence

Parity
Ryhammer *et al.*[13] reported an increasing risk of anal incontinence after three or more deliveries, but the results were not adjusted for potential confounding factors, *e.g.* age. However, it has generally been suggested that childbirth is a major cause of anal incontinence.

Age
An age > 30 years is associated with an increased risk of flatus incontinence and an age > 35 years significantly increased the risk compared with women aged 25–29 years.

Anal sphincter injury
Anal sphincter tear is a major risk factor with a risk 6 times as high for anal incontinence in women with tears compared to women with intact sphincter.

Birthweight
On its own, a birthweight of > 4 kg is an independent risk factor for developing flatus incontinence[14] even in those with intact anal sphincter.

Mechanism
There appears to be two separate mechanisms which result in faecal incontinence. The first is damage to the innervation of the pelvic floor muscles. Vaginal delivery has been shown to be associated with significant prolongation of pudendal nerve terminal motor latency and pelvic floor descent in the postnatal period.[15] The second is direct damage to the anal sphincter and with the advent of anal endosonography (Fig. 3) this is considered to be the major cause of faecal incontinence.[16,17] More significantly, endo-anal ultrasound has

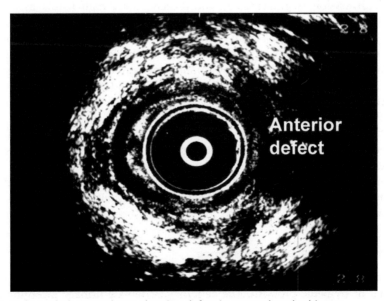

Fig. 3 Endo-anal ultrasound scan showing defect in external anal sphincter.

shown that some women who subsequently develop faecal incontinence after childbirth have unsuspected defects in their anal sphincters,[18] with defects found in over one-third of all primiparturients.[1]

SEQUELAE OF SEVERE OBSTETRIC INJURY

Fistulae

Vesicovaginal (VVF)

VVF is an epithelial tract between the bladder and the vagina. Patients with genito-urinary fistulae present in many ways. Most patients have urinary incontinence or persistent vaginal discharge. If the fistula is very small, leakage may be intermittent, occurring only at maximal bladder capacity or with particular body positions. Other signs and symptoms include: unexplained fever; haematuria; recurrent cystitis or pyelonephritis; vaginal, suprapubic or flank pain; and abnormal urinary stream. Obstetric genito-urinary fistula tends to present around 2 weeks while postsurgical fistulae usually present 7–21 days after surgery.

Vesico-uterine (VUF)

VUF deserves special mention as it used to be the least common of all genito-urinary fistulae constituting about 4% of this group; with a rising caesarean section rate, this may change. There are three common presentation of VUF following Caesarean section: (i) urinary incontinence with cyclical haematuria; (ii) urinary incontinence alone; and (iii) Youssef's syndrome,[19] i.e. amenorrhoea and menouria (menstruation through the bladder) in the absence of urinary incontinence. Presentation depends on the level of the fistula. Those arising above the isthmus will present as Youssef's syndrome. The cervical isthmus acts as a sphincter that will only relax if it is distended with menstrual fluid but such distension is prevented in the presence of a high fistula as a lower pressure route of exit into the bladder is available. Likewise, the isthmic sphincter prevents urine from entering the vagina, hence these women are continent. Fistulae arising below the level of the isthmus can present with incontinence alone or with menouria; some menstruation still occurs vaginally.

Rectovaginal (RVF)

RVF is an epithelial tract between the rectum and the vagina. Symptoms include passage of flatus or stool through the vagina. Occasionally, the presenting complaint is a recurrent vaginal or bladder infection, the result of faecal soilage. A small fistula may be symptomatic only when loose or liquid stool is passed. Usually, with obstetric injury, the circumference of the anorectal ring is disrupted. This defect may be felt during digital rectal examination.

Urinary and faecal incontinence

Urinary incontinence is defined as the involuntary loss of urine which is a social or hygienic problem. The aetiology of female urinary incontinence is multifactorial, but damage to the pelvic floor innervation during childbirth is thought to play a major part.[20] Although urinary incontinence has been reported in 20–30% of women at 3 months' postpartum,[21] the peak incidence is still during pregnancy.[22] In a study of 305 primigravid women, 4% reported stress incontinence prior to pregnancy, 32% developed stress incontinence during pregnancy and 7% developed stress incontinence after delivery. Stress incontinence is the commonest type of incontinence reported (54%), followed by mixed (30%) then urge urinary incontinence (16%).[21]

Faecal incontinence is defined as the involuntary loss of flatus, liquid or solid faeces. Faecal incontinence has a prevalence of about 1% in the general population. Although faecal incontinence can affect both sexes, in younger people it is much more common in women than men. Obstetric injury is thought to be the cause of faecal incontinence in most healthy women.[23] Episodes of incontinence or urgency following delivery have been reported in 4–10% of primiparous women,[15,24] with the lower percentage representing frank faecal incontinence and the higher percentage flatus incontinence or urgency. However, in women who have sustained anal sphincter injury, these figures are considerably higher, 20–50%.[3,25] It is likely that there is considerable under-reporting of faecal incontinence because of the patient's reluctance to volunteer the information and doctor's reluctance to ask. Very few women report symptoms (Table 3) at the postnatal visit, and of those that are symptomatic, only one-third had ever discussed the problem with a physician.[26] Leigh and Turnberg,[27] in 1982, reported that many women do not seek medical attention for faecal incontinence because of the embarrassment engendered by this 'taboo' symptom. Many years later, the situation remains the same. A UK Department of Health consultation document[28] reported that women are easily discouraged from discussing faecal incontinence.

Psychosexual dysfunction

Postpartum sexual dysfunction has not been explored in detail by most authors. Sexual function is altered in a significant number of women with severe obstetric injury with decrease in sexual frequency, appetite, and pleasure. Resumption of sexual intercourse following delivery depends on a variety of factors, both physical and emotional. Women who deliver with an intact perineum resume sexual activity sooner than women who have an episiotomy or perineal laceration.[29] Similarly, pain experienced on first intercourse is less in women who deliver with an intact perineum.[29] Other factors which may influence sexual function include urinary and faecal incontinence or the fear of inadvertent

Table 3 Faecal incontinence symptoms

• Poor flatal control
• Faecal staining
• Frank incontinence
• Faecal urgency (< 5 min)
• Defaecatory straining
• Defaecatory pain
• Bleeding on defaecation

incontinence during intercourse.[30] Gjessing et al.[31] reported that 17% of women suffered from anal incontinence during sexual intercourse, following their third degree perineal repair. This is quite depressing for most women and embarrassment is one of the major reasons given for not seeking help despite having a poor quality of life. A woman in a letter to the Continence Foundation[32] described 'the eternal shame of being with another person when the worst occurs'. This is usually in total contrast to the expectations of these women as majority of them are unaware of the possibility of incontinence following primary repair of their perineal tears.

MANAGEMENT

Severe perineal injury

Anal sphincter tears

Repair should be performed according to strict guidelines. Repair should be performed only by a doctor experienced in anal sphincter repair or by a trainee under direct supervision. The repair should be conducted in an operating theatre with access to good lighting, appropriate equipment and aseptic conditions. General or regional anaesthesia is needed for muscle relaxation to retrieve the ends of the torn sphincter. Careful evaluation of the extent of the injury should be carried out by vaginal and rectal examination. If the anal epithelium is torn (fourth degree tear), a 3-0 interrupted polyglactin suture (Vicryl) should be used for repair. The sphincter muscle is repaired with 3-0 monofilament polydioxalone sulphate (PDS) suture using the overlap or end-to-end method. Even though there is no evidence to date that indicates any significant difference in short-term outcome between end-to-end approximation and overlap repair, the current trend is to do an overlap repair. This is because overlapping allows for a greater surface area of contact between muscles compared with incomplete apposition more likely to occur with end-to-end repair. If further retraction of the of the overlapped muscle ends were to occur, it is more likely that muscle continuity will be maintained in overlap repair compared with end-to-end. The perineal muscles should be reconstructed with interrupted Vicryl suture to provide support to the sphincter repair. A vaginal and rectal examination should be done to confirm complete repair and to ensure all swabs are removed. A comprehensive record and pictorial representation are useful for auditing and medicolegal purposes. Antibiotic cover, stool softener, and adequate analgesia should be given as well as a follow-up appointment with a senior obstetrician in about 8 weeks or more.

Cervical and uterine injury

Deep cervical lacerations involving the vaginal vault should be repaired in the operating theatre with regional or general anaesthesia. Care must be taken to avoid insertion of sutures into the bladder in anterior tears or the ureter with lateral cervical tears. The uterine artery or the vessels at the base of the broad ligament can also be injured leading to haemorrhage or haematoma. The management options following tears and ruptures include repair of the tear, hysterectomy, internal iliac artery ligation and the B-Lynch repair technique.

Genital haematoma

Management depends on the level of the haematoma. A large infralevator haematoma usually requires surgical exploration and the insertion of deep sutures at the base of the haematoma as the actual bleeding point is rarely identified. In contrast, the management of the supralevator haematoma is largely conservative as surgical exploration is usually very frustrating as the bleeding point cannot be identified and the ureter can be injured with the insertion of deep sutures. The options include: (i) conservative approach with evacuation of the clot and packing the cavity for 24 h with blood transfusion as necessary; (ii) performing an internal iliac artery ligation; and (iii) embolisation of the bleeding vessel under radiographic control by an interventional radiologist, if available.

Fistulae

The management depends on the type of fistula and its location but there are some key principles that apply to all repairs – accurate diagnosis, timing of repair, appropriate expertise, and detailed postoperative care with follow-up. Examination under anaesthesia, dye test (methylene blue), cystoscopy, cystogram (Fig. 4) and/or intravenous urography are important diagnostic investigations. An IVU is useful where there is suspicion of a ureteric fistula, while the cystogram can diagnose VVF. Accurate diagnosis establishes that the discharge is urinary and the leakage is extra-urethral; it also identifies the site of leakage and identifies or excludes multiple/complex tracks. The timing of repair is critical, particularly in non-industrialised countries. A 2–3 month wait is common to eradicate infection and for the tissues to become healthier and less friable. However, in the industrialised world, repairs can usually be done after a few weeks.

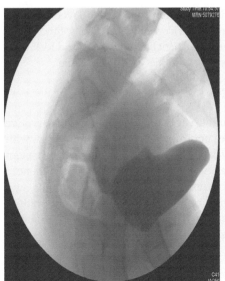 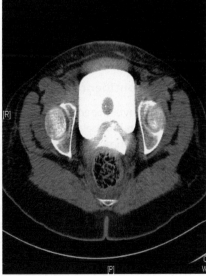

Fig. 4 Vesicovaginal fistula. The plain film on the left shows a lateral view of a cystogram showing the leakage of dye into the vagina while the CT cystogram demonstrates the fistulous tract from the left side of the bladder into the vagina.

Ureteric fistula

Though rare, spontaneous healing can occur, especially where there has been incomplete division of the ureter and where it has been possible to pass a ureteric catheter. Re-implantation of the ureter is usually done via an abdominal transperitoneal approach. A psoas hitch and/or a Boari flap may be necessary to re-implant the ureter without tension.

Vesico-uterine fistula

Ureteric catheterisation via cystoscopy followed by an abdominal transperitoneal repair in which the bladder is opened and the fistulous tract excised. The defects in the uterus and bladder are repaired using absorbable sutures and omentum interposed between them. Postoperatively, the bladder is drained via a urethral catheter for 14 days.

Vesicovaginal fistula

Spontaneous healing of small fistulae can occur following continuous free catheter drainage for 3–4 weeks. If this fails, an abdominal or vaginal approach will be chosen according to the practice of the operator and the site of the fistula. Gynaecologists tend to prefer a vaginal approach and this is usually acceptable for a low VVF. Following ureteric catheterisation, a classic VVF repair involves split-flap dissection, mobilisation of tissue planes, absolute haemostasis, and closure without tension. Occasionally, a supporting graft, the Martius pedicle graft of fibrofatty tissue is brought down from one labium majus to cover and re-inforce the repaired fistula and provide increased vascularity. Post-operative care is the same as in VUF repair.

Rectovaginal fistula

A temporary colostomy is useful when managing a high RVF, but low- and mid-RVFs can be managed without colostomy. Adequate pre-operative bowel preparation is essential. The same basic principles as in VVF repair apply, *i.e.* adequate mobilisation so that the fistula can be repaired in two layers without tension using interrupted inverting mattress 2-0 Vicryl sutures. If anal sphincter tear is present, it is repaired as described above. If a patient has both a VVF and RVF, both can be repaired at the same operation, usually with the VVF repaired first.

Urinary incontinence

Management will depend on the type and severity of incontinence. Conservative measures including pelvic floor exercises and bladder retraining in women with stress incontinence, frequency/urgency have been shown to prevent persistent urinary incontinence in 10% of women with postnatal urinary incontinence.[5] Medical options include anticholinergics for overactive bladder symptoms, and duloxetine for stress incontinence. Surgical options will include the mid-urethral tapes and injectables. These procedures have a good success rate in experienced hands and women should be referred appropriately.

Faecal incontinence

Conservative

Pelvic floor exercises might help to alleviate some of the symptoms. Sander *et al.*[33] found only 7% flatus incontinence and no faecal incontinence in women with third-degree tear following 1 year of pelvic floor exercises. Dietary advice, bulking agents, medications to produce well-formed, solid stools, enemas, anal plug to prevent leakage of stools, and biofeedback. All these measures have been used with varying success according to severity of symptoms.

Surgical

The success rates of secondary repairs carried out by colorectal surgeons months or years later vary between 75–90%.[34] It has been suggested that the functional result of delayed anal sphincter repair after obstetric lesions is partly dependent upon whether the nerve supply is intact. This is because in some patients with faecal incontinence there is additional weakness of the anal sphincter muscles from damage to the innervation of these muscles during delivery. Pre-operative physiological evaluation has been suggested to provide some information on the probability of a successful surgical result.

Gracilis muscle transposition aims to mobilise the gracilis muscle and use it to re-inforce the damaged external anal sphincter muscle, thereby improving the muscle bulk. Varying success has been quoted.

Artificial bowel sphincter can be employed as a last resort if there is no other viable alternative.

PREVENTIVE MEASURES

Prevention of perineal injury

The risk factors identified above cannot readily be used to prevent the occurrence of anal sphincter tear. Most factors are unavoidable. Investigators continue to search for innovative methods of preventing anal sphincter injury. Perineal massage, which was thought to be of benefit[35] has now been shown in a randomised trial[36] not to reduce the risk of pain, dyspareunia, urinary or faecal problems, nor increase the likelihood of an intact perineum. Other preventive measures suggested including manual perineal protection and visualisation of the perineum during the last phase of bear-down, need further evaluation before wide-spread practice. The reality is that the search is still on for effective preventive measures.

Caesarean section

Caesarean section appears to protect against development of urinary stress incontinence,[22] but the protection is not complete as 10% of women undergoing elective caesarean section develop urinary incontinence and 38% of nuns develop urinary incontinence.[3,16] With regards to faecal incontinence, it has been shown that there is no evidence of mechanical or neurological damage after elective caesarean section and anorectal physiology remains unchanged. While no structural anal sphincter damage occurred after emergency caesarean section, caesarean section performed late in labour (cervical dilatation of 8 cm or more), even in the absence of attempted vaginal delivery, is not protective. This is because prolonged pudendal nerve latencies, reduction in anal squeeze pressures, and significant perineal descent occurs after such emergency caesarean section. Pregnancy itself whether via hormonal, physiological or mechanical effects do alter pelvic floor functions which might negate the protective effect of caesarean section and alter our views on mode of delivery.

Screening for sphincter damage

A normal perineum on clinical examination does not exclude underlying sphincter damage. Perineal sonography has been suggested as a feasible alternative to anal endosonography for screening in women, as it is more acceptable and provides good information on external anal sphincter defects. This will be useful including those with occult tears. Magnetic resonance imaging with an endo-anal coil reveals the integrity and bulk of individual muscle components of the anal sphincter. The high resolution obtained with an endo-anal coil allowed differentiation of the various muscle components of the anal sphincter complex. Hopefully, this will provide a better understanding of the pelvic floor and anal sphincter complex and help plan future approach to repair techniques.

Education

Bowel or urinary symptoms are not currently included in the routine questions asked at the booking clinic in early pregnancy, nor is there education or information given regarding possible anal sphincter injury or bowel symptoms following vaginal deliveries. Therefore, women with pre-existing symptoms are not identified, nor do women know what to expect in the postnatal period. This practice needs to be changed with proper documentation of pre-pregnancy symptoms and education about possible symptoms after delivery. This information should be given at the beginning of pregnancy and taught at antenatal classes. This will go a long way in re-educating the public and removing the stigma associated with this condition.

Counselling about recurrence risk and subsequent delivery

It has been shown that a prior third-degree or fourth-degree perineal tear is associated with a 3.4-fold increased risk of a recurrent severe obstetrical laceration[37] and women should be advised about this. There are no Cochrane reviews or randomised controlled trials to suggest the best method of delivery following a previous sphincter tear. Studies[38,39] have shown that 17–24% of women develop worsening faecal symptoms after a second vaginal delivery. This seemed to occur particularly if there had been transient incontinence after the index delivery. The conclusion is that subsequent vaginal delivery may worsen anal incontinence symptoms. All women with previous anal sphincter injury should be counselled at the booking visit regarding this risk and the mode of delivery. If symptomatic or with abnormal endo-anal ultra-sonography (large defect of more than one quadrant) or abnormal manometry (squeeze pressure increment of less than 20 mmHg), it is advisable to offer them an elective caesarean section, even in the absence of symptoms. This should be clearly documented. Asymptomatic women who do not have compromised anal sphincter function can be advised to undergo vaginal delivery by an experienced accoucher. Women who have had a previous successful secondary sphincter repair or successful fistulae repair should be delivered by caesarean section.

MEDICOLEGAL

There has been an increase in litigation related to anal sphincter injury, fistulae with urinary and/or faecal incontinence resulting from childbirth. The majority relate to failure to identify the injury after delivery, leading to subsequent anal incontinence, rectovaginal fistulae or genito-urinary fistulae. At present, the occurrence of a third-degree tear is not considered substandard care because it is a known complication of vaginal delivery. Liability issues include:[40,41]

1. Failure to recognise anal sphincter damage and to carry out a proper repair.

2. Failure of repair due to poor technique, poor materials, or poor healing. This is a training issue. The importance of clear documentation is vital.

3. Failure to inform and counsel the woman, inappropriate follow-up and failure to inform the general practitioner.

4. Failure to carry out a vaginal and rectal examination so as to exclude a misplaced suture. Whilst inadvertently incorporating the rectal wall when repairing a tear may not amount to substandard treatment in itself, failure to diagnose a misplaced suture, which can lead to a rectovaginal fistula, is liable.

5. Delivery or subsequent delivery should have been by caesarean section. A common and alarming theme to these cases is a failure to acknowledge the significance of a complaint of incontinence of flatus or faeces following a first delivery. Women are frequently re-assured by their medical advisers that incontinence will resolve with time and so advice is not given in relation to the management of subsequent deliveries.

Damages

Faecal and or urinary incontinence is a devastating complication for a young mother; it can often result in a series of surgical interventions. It is a humiliating problem, which affects the mother psychologically as well as physically. It is sometimes difficult for the sufferer to work or to lead any kind of social life, puts a severe strain on personal relationships, and often there are significant psychosexual sequelae.

It is, therefore, not surprising that the amounts awarded for damages in these cases are rising. Commonly evidence is obtained not only from an obstetrician and colorectal surgeon, but often from a psychiatrist specialising in birth trauma, a clinical psychologist, a gastro-enterologist, and a stoma care nurse as necessary.

KEY POINTS FOR CLINICAL PRACTICE

• The risk factors for severe obstetric injury are many; while some are preventable, the majority are not. Women should be informed and advised of the relevant risks and for those unfortunate enough to sustain severe injury, prompt attention to their symptoms and early referral for specialist management and support is crucial.

• Primary anal sphincter repair is inadequate in most women who sustain third or fourth degree tears, with more than half still experiencing significant anal incontinence symptoms. Symptomatic women have poor quality of life and significant sexual dysfunction. A multidisciplinary approach to the management of these women is essential.

• At present, the advice offered to women regarding their next delivery is inadequate. A better approach is for all women with anal sphincter damage to undergo endo-anal ultrasonography and anal manometry studies, with elective caesarean section offered to those at risk. Women who have had successful secondary anal sphincter repair or successful fistulae repair should be offered caesarean section.

• Education is the key for both clinicians and the public. Pre-existing bowel and urinary symptoms should be identified, documented, and all women educated about possible postnatal symptoms and how to seek help.

References

1   Sultan AH, Kamm MA., Hudson CN, Thomas JM, Bartram CI. Anal-sphincter disruption during vaginal delivery. N Engl J Med 1993; 329: 1905–1911

2. Sultan AH. Anal incontinence after childbirth. Curr Opin Obstet Gynecol 1997; 9: 320–324

3   Sultan AH, Fernando R, Maternal obstetric injury. Current Obstet Gynecol 2001; 11: 279–284

4   Shihadeh AS, Nawafleh AN. Third degree tears and episiotomy. Saudi Med J 2001; 22: 272–275

5   Buekens P, Laggase R, Draimaix M, Wollast E. Episiotomy and third-degree tears. Br J Obstet Gynaecol 1985; 92: 820–823

6   Wood J, Amos L, Rieger N. Third degree anal sphincter tears: risk factors and outcome. Aust NZ J Obstet Gynaecol 1998; 38: 414–417

7   Samuelsson E, Ladfors L, Wennerholm UB et al. Anal sphincter tears: prospective study of obstetric risk factors. Br J Obstet Gynaecol 2000; 107: 926–931

8   Nager CW, Helliwell JP. Episiotomy increases perineal laceration length in primiparous women. Am J Obstet Gynecol 2001; 185: 440–450

9   Tetzschemer T, Sorenson M, Rasmussen OO, Lose G, Christiansen J. Pudendal nerve damage increases the risk of faecal incontinence in women with anal sphincter rupture after childbirth. Acta Obstet Gynecol Scand 1995; 74: 434–440

10 Foldspang A, Mommsen S, Lam GW, Elving L. Parity as a correlate of adult female urinary incontinence prevalence. J Epidemiol Community Health 1992; 46: 595–600

11 Thomas TM, Plymat KR, Blannin J, Meade TW. Prevalence of urinary incontinence. BMJ 1980; 281: 1243–1245

12 Dimpfl T, Hesse U, Schussler B. Incidence and cause of postpartum urinary stress incontinence. Eur J Obstet Gynecol Reprod Biol 1992; 43: 29–33

13 Ryhammer AM, Bek KM, Lauberg S. Multiple vaginal deliveries increase the risk of permanent incontinence of flatus urine in normal premenopausal women. Dis Colon Rectum 1995; 38: 1206–1209

14 Hojberg KE, Salvig JD, Winslow NA, Bek KM, Lauberg S, Secher JN. Flatus and faecal

incontinence: prevalence and risk factors at 16 weeks of gestation. Br J Obstet Gynaecol 2000; 107: 1097–1103

15 Sultan AH, Hudson CN. Pudendal nerve damage during labour: prospective study before and after childbirth. Br J Obstet Gynaecol 1994; 101: 22–28

16 Sultan AH, Stanton SL. Preserving the pelvic floor and the perineum during childbirth – elective caesarean section? Br J Obstet Gynaecol 1996; 103: 731–734

17 Sultan AH, Kamm MA, Hudson CN, Bartram CI. Third degree obstetric anal sphincter tears: risk factors and outcome of primary repair. BMJ 1994; 308: 887–891

18 Burnett SJD, Spence-Jones C, Speakman CTM, Kamm MA, Hudson CN, Bartram CI. Unsuspected sphincter damage following childbirth revealed by anal endosonography. Br J Radiol 1991; 64: 225–227

19 Youssef AF. Menouria following lower segment caesarean section. A syndrome. Am J Obstet Gynecol 1957; 73: 759

20 Benson JT. Neurophysiology of the female pelvic floor. Curr Opin Obstet Gynecol 1994; 6: 320–323

21 Glazener CMA, Herbison PG, Wilson DP et al. Conservative management of persistent postnatal urinary and faecal incontinence: randomised controlled trial. BMJ 2001; 323: 593–596

22 Viktrup L, Lose G, Rolff M, Barfoed K. The symptom of stress incontinence caused by pregnancy or delivery in primiparas. Obstet Gynecol 1992; 79: 945–949

23 Kamm MA. Obstetric damage and faecal incontinence. Lancet 1994; 344: 730–733

24 MacAthur C, Bick DE, Keighley MRB. Faecal incontinence after childbirth. Br J Obstet Gynaecol 1997; 104: 46–50

25 Johanson JF, Lafferty J. Epidemiology of faecal incontinence: the silent affliction. Am J Gastroenterol 1996; 91: 33–36

26 Zetterson JP, Lopez A, Anzen B, Dolk A, Norman M, Mellgren A. Anal incontinence after vaginal delivery: a prospective study in primiparous women. Br J Obstet Gynaecol 1999; 106: 324–330

27 Leigh RJ, Turnberg LA. Faecal incontinence: the unvoiced symptoms. Lancet 1982; 1: 1349–1351

28 Department of Health. Consultation document. London: Department of Health, 2000

29 Klein MC, Gauthier RJ, Robbins JM et al. Relationship of episiotomy to perineal trauma and morbidity, sexual dysfunction, and pelvic floor relaxation. Am J Obstet Gynecol 1994; 171: 591–598

30 Wyman JF. The psychiatric and emotional impact of female pelvic floor dysfunction. Curr Opin Obstet Gynecol 1994; 6: 336–339.

31 Gjessing H, Backe B, Sahlin Y. Third degree obstetric tears; outcome after primary repair. Acta Obstet Gynaecol Scand 1998; 77: 736–740

32 The Continence Foundation. Incontinence: a challenge and an opportunity for primary care. In: The Continence Foundation Information leaflet. London: The Continence Foundation, 2000

33 Sander P, Bjarnesen J, Mouritsen L, Fuglsang-Frederiksen A. Anal incontinence after obstetric third/fourth-degree laceration. One-year follow-up after pelvic floor exercises. Int Urogyn J Pelvic Floor Dysfunction 1999; 10: 177–181

34 Engel AF, Kamm MA, Sultan AH et al. Anterior anal sphincter repair in patients with obstetric trauma. Br J Surg 1994; 81: 1231–1234

35 Shipman MK, Boniface DR, Tefft ME, McCloghry F. Antenatal perineal massage and subsequent perineal outcomes: a randomised controlled trial. Br J Obstet Gynaecol 1997; 104: 787–791

36 Stamp G, Kruzins G, Crowther C. Perineal massage in labour and prevention of perineal trauma: a randomised controlled trial. BMJ 2001; 322: 1277–1280

37 Payne TN, Carey JC, Rayburn WF. Prior third or fourth-degree perineal tears and recurrence risks. Int J Obstet Gynaecol 1999; 64: 55–57

38 Bek KM, Laurberg S. Risks of anal incontinence from subsequent vaginal delivery after a complete obstetric anal sphincter tear. Br J Obstet Gynaecol 1992; 99: 724–726

39 Fynes M, Donnelly V, Behan M, O'Connell PR, O'Herlihy C. Effect of second vaginal delivery on anorectal physiology and faecal incontinence. Lancet 1999; 354: 983–986

40 Sultan AH. Obstetrical perineal injury and anal incontinence. Clin Risk 1999; 5: 193–196

41 Eddy A. Litigating and quantifying maternal damage following childbirth. Clin Risk 1999; 5: 178–180

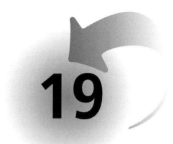

Sapna Shah   Margaret Johnson

Gynaecological issues in human immunodeficiency virus (HIV) infected women

Since 1981 when the first case of acquired immune deficiency syndrome (AIDS) was described in the US, the world has seen a huge surge in the number of people diagnosed with AIDS. The causative agent of AIDS, human immunodeficiency virus (HIV), was identified in 1983.

By the end of 2004, the United Nations Programme on HIV/AIDS[1] estimated there to be 39.4 million people living with HIV world-wide. In 2004 alone, the AIDS epidemic claimed 3.1 million lives and an estimated 4.9 million people acquired the virus. Globally, 17.6 million women are living with HIV and of the 14,000 new HIV infections a day in 2004, 50% are estimated to be in women. The majority of the women living with HIV/AIDS are of reproductive age; figures from the US estimate that about 80% of those living with HIV/AIDS are aged 15–44 years. Over 2 million children under the age of 15 years are living with HIV and over 90% of these have been infected through mother-to-child transmission (MTCT). The epidemic has already altered population structures in many countries and has created a large number of AIDS orphans. Whilst the burden of the epidemic remains focused within Africa, in particular sub-Saharan Africa which is home to about 65% of the people living with HIV, the number of infections in other regions is also increasing, particularly Asia.

The UK Public Health Laboratory Service[2] data suggest that by the end of 2003, 53,000 adults over the age of 15 years were living with HIV in the UK, of whom 27% were unaware of their infection. Women represent a growing proportion of those infected with the total number of women infected having

Sapna Shah BSc MBBS DFFP (for correspondence)
Clinical Research Fellow in HIV & Women's Health, Royal Free and University College Medical School, Hampstead Campus, Rowland Hill Street, London NW3 2PF, UK
E-mail: s.shah@pcps.ucl.ac.uk

Margaret Johnson MD FRCP
Consultant in Thoracic/HIV Medicine and Medical Director, Royal Free Hospital, Pond Street, London NW3 2QG, UK

doubled from 14% of all new diagnoses in 1990 to 35% in 2000. A total of 850 HIV-positive women gave birth in the UK in 2003; about 60% of these births occurred in inner London. As a result of the growing MTCT rates, the rising trend of HIV in women is of concern.

In 1988, heterosexual transmission exceeded injecting drug use as the primary source of infection among women in the UK[3] and is currently the mode of transmission in 80% of all new diagnoses.[4] In sub-Saharan Africa, there are now more women infected with HIV than men. Social inequalities, poverty and a desire for a better life drive many young girls and women towards using sex as a commodity in exchange for money, goods or accommodation, often with older men. Women are also being infected at an earlier age than men although they often present later in the course of the disease and have been reported to be less likely to receive anti-retroviral treatment due to gender inequalities in access to healthcare.[5] This is probably a reflection of the cultural gender inequalities in access to care and treatment making women a particularly vulnerable group.

HIV is a retrovirus, so named because it encodes an enzyme, reverse transcriptase, which allows DNA to be transcribed from RNA. HIV becomes integrated within the host genome and the infected host cells are then used as a replicative factory producing multiple copies of the HIV genome as DNA. The main targets of the virus are the human CD4 'helper' lymphocytes, which start producing new virus particles, and thereby lose their central role in the immune response. In this way, HIV causes immunosuppression. HIV RNA levels (viral load) and CD4 cell counts in the peripheral blood are used to monitor the progression of the infection and help determine when antiretroviral treatment should be commenced. There are currently about 20 drugs licensed for the treatment of HIV with newer drugs in the pipeline. Three or more drugs, usually with different mechanisms of action, are often required to inhibit viral replication to below detectable levels; this is known as combination therapy or highly active anti-retroviral therapy (HAART). Since its introduction, the prognosis of those infected with HIV has improved dramatically.

HIV-infected women are likely to experience a similar range of gynaecological problems to HIV-uninfected women. They may also suffer from additional gynaecological problems that are a direct consequence of their HIV infection or of the antiretroviral drugs they may be receiving. However, gynaecological problems may be neglected, often as a consequence of more acute problems taking precedence, but sometimes because of a lack of understanding of the complex interactions of HIV infection in women. The clinical management of HIV infected women is often sub-optimal as it is usually largely based on research undertaken in men. This is despite reported gender differences in symptomatology, disease progression and HIV-related illnesses. A better understanding of the clinical manifestations of gynaecological disease is, therefore, essential in order to optimise patient care, particularly in light of the altered demographic characteristics of those infected.

Most of the research on gynaecological problems in HIV infected women has been concentrated on the effects of immunosuppression on cervical abnormalities. However, there are other important areas of the management of HIV-infected women that a gynaecologist needs to be aware of. Therefore, this chapter has been divided into the following topics: (i) HIV and cervical intra-epithelial neoplasia (CIN); (ii) HIV and contraception; (iii) HIV and subfertility; (iv) HIV and sexually transmitted diseases (STDs); and (v) HIV and menstrual dysfunction. It should be noted that while these topics have been treated separately in this review, in clinical practice these are rarely separate entities.

HIV AND CIN

Cervical cancer is the second most common cancer among women world-wide, with almost half a million new cases each year. Almost 80% of the women affected are in the non-industrialised world.[6] In the UK, it is the seventh most common cancer.[7] The vast majority of cervical cancers involve the squamous epithelium of the cervix that undergoes a pre-invasive stage, cervical intra-epithelial neoplasia (CIN) which can be detected and treated to prevent progression to cervical carcinoma. This led to the introduction of the cervical screening programme. In the UK, screening began in the 1960s and the National Health Service Cervical Screening Programme was set up in 1988 to ensure that all eligible women were screened with comprehensive follow-up. There has been a marked reduction in the incidence of cervical cancer since this time.

Infection with human papillomavirus (HPV) is the main risk factor for the development of CIN. Genital HPV is transmitted sexually and its prevalence is high. Currently, over 100 different HPV genotypes have been detected, of which 40 primarily infect the anogenital area.[8] These can be subdivided into low-risk genotypes (*e.g.* 6, 11, 42, 43 and 44) and high-risk/oncogenic types (*e.g.* 16, 18, 31, 33, 35, 39, 45, *etc.*). The presence of a high HPV load and persistence of infection with the oncogenic types are strongly associated with CIN.[9]

HIV has been recognised for many years to be an independent risk factor for the development of cervical abnormality[10] with the prevalence of abnormality increasing with advancing immunosuppression.[11,12] HIV-positive women are more likely to be infected with multiple,[13] frequently oncogenic,[14] HPV genotypes. They have also been shown to have a high cervical HPV viral load and persistence of HPV infections resulting in high-grade CIN lesions.[14] The pathogenesis of HPV in HIV-infected women is less clearly understood. Clinical expression of HPV infection is dependent on systemic and local cell-mediated immunity,[15] which are both suppressed in HIV infection. The higher and more persistent HPV DNA load that results from this may be one mechanism by which HIV infection increases the prevalence and progression of CIN.[11,16] However, this correlation has not been reported consistently.[17] High HIV RNA levels are independently associated with rapid progression of CIN suggesting that direct interactions between the viruses may also occur.[16,18]

As well as a more rapid progression, the likelihood of regression of CIN lesions is reduced in HIV-infected women.[16] They also experience an increased recurrence rate following treatment of CIN.[19] The most effective method of treatment of CIN lesions in this group is unclear but excisional procedures are generally preferred to ablative procedures as the former allows accurate histological diagnosis and surgical margin status to be obtained. However, there are conflicting data on whether surgical margin or immunological status has any effect on recurrence rates.[20–23] Complete excision of CIN lesions is less frequent in HIV-positive women (unpublished work) and this, together with an increased tendency for satellite lesions and multifocal disease involving the whole anogenital tract may partly explain the higher recurrence rate in this group.

The availability of HAART has lead to dramatic improvements in HIV-associated morbidity and mortality. It is hoped that HAART will have a beneficial effect on cervical disease by improving both the immunological and virological status of HIV-infected women, thus allowing more effective clearance of HPV infection. However, the effects of HAART on CIN are conflicting. Most studies have shown a beneficial effect of HAART on CIN prevalence,[24] progression[25] and regression.[26] Others, however, have showed persistence of HPV[24] and CIN despite HAART,[27] and an increase in the prevalence of CIN in those on HAART.[28] These conflicting data may be due to the use of different HAART regimens and varying lengths of follow-up between studies.

As a result of these inconsistent results, there remains uncertainty as to the most appropriate screening method and frequency for women with HIV, though there is general agreement that more intensive monitoring is necessary. In the UK, the Royal College of Obstetricians and Gynaecologists recommends that women without a history of cervical abnormality undergo annual cytology.[29] The NHSCSP guidelines state that: 'annual cytology should be performed with an initial colposcopy if resources permit'. Subsequent colposcopy for cytological abnormality should follow national guidelines. The age range screened should be the same as for HIV-negative women.[30] The guidelines recommend that high-grade CIN lesions should be managed according to national guidelines and low-grade lesions should be managed conservatively with regular cervical surveillance. The role of HPV testing and its effects on cervical screening in this high-risk population is, as yet, unclear.

At the Royal Free Hospital, there are currently about 500 HIV-positive women under active cervical screening follow-up in the joint HIV/gynaecology women's clinic. All women are offered cervical screening at presentation, which includes a cervical smear, colposcopy and biopsy if indicated. Women with negative smears/biopsy results are followed up with annual smears. Those with minor abnormalities undergo repeat smear and colposcopy at 6-monthly intervals and are referred for treatment, in the form of a laser loop excision of the transformation zone (LLETZ), if there is any progression. Women with CIN II/III are referred immediately for LLETZ, and then followed up at 6-monthly intervals with smears and colposcopy. Three consecutive negative smears at 6-monthly intervals are required after any treatment before reverting to annual follow-up. All cervical smears and colposcopy (± biopsy) are performed by BSCCP-accredited colposcopists or by those undergoing supervised BSCCP training.

HIV AND CONTRACEPTION

As in HIV-negative individuals, the choice of contraception and its effective use are related to a number of factors, which include the range of methods available, patient choice, religious beliefs, perceptions of the method safety, effectiveness, side effects, whether it is intercourse related, has any long-term effects on future fertility, is dependent on the user's memory and whether its effects are fully reversible.

With additional considerations, the range of contraceptives available to HIV-infected women are the same as those available to HIV-uninfected women. When compared to HIV-negative women, HIV-positive women are less likely to report consistent use of contraception, except for condom usage which is significantly higher amongst HIV-positive women.[31] Women who are HIV-positive are also less likely to report being sexually active. This increased abstinence may account for the reduced contraceptive usage amongst HIV-positive women. Other factors, however, such as AIDS, intercurrent illness, antiretroviral use, other drug treatments, particularly for tuberculosis, the serostatus of their partner, unequal access to contraceptive services particularly amongst women in power-imbalanced relationships, such as adolescents and those of minority groups, may also contribute to the reduced uptake and efficacy of contraceptives in HIV-positive women.

The implications of ineffective contraceptive usage are enormous. According to World Health Organization (WHO) estimates, half a million women die annually from complications of pregnancy or abortion, the majority of theses occurring in sub-Saharan Africa and Asia where there is an unmet need for contraceptive provision.[32] The implications of an unintended pregnancy are particularly complex for HIV-infected women, compounded by the risk of mother-to-child HIV transmission (MTCT), which occurs in 30–40% of pregnancies where interventions are not available (see below).[33]

HIV-positive women are strongly advised to use dual contraception or 'double dutch'. This involves a barrier method, to reduce the risk of sexual transmission of the virus or of virus resistance to a partner, used in combination with a more effective contraceptive method whether hormonal, intra-uterine or surgical.

Barrier methods

Male condom

Latex condoms are the most effective mechanical barrier to HIV infection, and they are the only recommended method for reducing HIV transmission.[34] When used consistently, they are estimated to provide about 87% protection against HIV transmission.[35] Most studies on condom use in HIV-positive women are encouraging, reporting a greater consistency of condom usage.[31,36,37] Condom accidents are reported in 1–2% of users,[33] and they have a contraceptive failure rate of 2–15%;[38] additional contraception should, therefore, be used to prevent pregnancy. Women opting to use condoms as their only method of contraception should also be made aware of emergency contraception. In sero-concordant couples, where both partners are HIV positive, condom use is still recommended not only to reduce the risk of an unwanted pregnancy and STIs, but also to reduce the risk of acquiring drug-resistant strains of HIV. In sero-discordant couples, where one partner is HIV positive and the other HIV negative, condom use is vital in reducing horizontal transmission of HIV. Transmission of HIV from men to women is more efficient than from women to men because of the large surface area of vaginal mucosa exposed to the virus. The theoretical per-exposure risk of HIV infection from unprotected sexual intercourse (UPSI) is 1:100 to 1:300.[39] Some units provide post-exposure prophylaxis on a case-by-case basis for condom accidents. The major drawback with condoms is that they require male participation which may be difficult for women to negotiate in power imbalanced relationships.

Female condom

The female condom or femidom has been shown to be an effective barrier to HIV in *in vitro* studies.[40] As it is less likely to leak or break than the male condom, the probability of vaginal exposure to semen is much less than with the male condom. However, there is a higher user and method failure rate of 5–21%.[33] Its use is independent of the male making it an ideal choice for women in relationships where there is difficulty in negotiating condom use; however, uptake of the femidom is poor, possibly due to a lack of awareness of its availability and knowledge of how to insert it.

Other barrier methods

The use of diaphragms, caps or other barrier methods are not recommended for HIV prevention as they leave large areas of the vaginal mucosa exposed and may result in microtrauma during their insertion.[33]

Hormonal methods

Combined oral contraception (COC)

Several studies have shown that the combined oral contraceptive pill (COCP) may increase HIV transmission. The mechanism by which this may occur is not clear but may involve a decrease in condom use by those using the COCP or an increased area of cervical ectropion resulting in an increased surface area for HIV transmission and increased genital tract shedding of HIV.[37] However, other studies have failed to show any such association between the COCP and HIV transmission.[41]

One of the major problems of using hormonal contraceptives in HIV-positive women are the drug interactions that may occur between the contraceptives and the other drugs that these women may be receiving which may alter the efficacy of the contraceptives. Individually, many of the antiretroviral drugs, particularly the protease inhibitors, induce or suppress the liver enzymes that are involved in the metabolism of the oestrogenic component of the COCP resulting in an decrease or increase in the levels of these hormones, respectively. The effect of these antiretroviral drugs on the liver enzymes when used in combination HAART regimens is not clear. Other factors that may reduce the efficacy of the COCP or may be a contra-indication to the use of the COCP in HIV-positive women include antiretroviral-associated gastrointestinal side effects, anti-tuberculous medication, liver damage from acute or chronic viral hepatitis and the chaotic life-styles of current drug and alcohol users.

Another disadvantage of the oral contraceptives is that they increase the pill burden and may, therefore, be less well accepted by HIV-positive women receiving HAART. This may be overcome by using the new weekly birth control patch called Evra, which, like the combined pill, contains oestrogens and progesterones.

Due to the difficulty in determining the efficacy of COCP in women receiving HAART, those wishing to use the COCP should be advised to use an additional barrier method. In those who experience break-through bleeding, the dose of oestrogen can be titrated by prescribing higher dose pills after excluding all other causes of break-through bleeding.

Progesterone only pill (POP)

The POP is not commonly used by HIV-positive women due to the strict dosing intervals and resultant menstrual irregularity. However, the POP is an alternative for women in whom oestrogen is a contra-indication. The new POP, Cerazette, may have a role in this population as it does not have such a strict dosing interval. Additional condom use must be emphasised.

Injectable contraceptives

Depo-provera and Noristat are injectable progesterone-only contraceptives. Depo-provera is a popular method of contraception amongst HIV-positive women in our clinic. The major non-contraceptive advantage of Depo-provera is its ability to induce amenorrhoea in around 35% of users. This not only has implications for reducing HIV transmission but also often provides symptomatic relief from menorrhagia secondary to fibroids, which are often seen in this population.

However, as with the COCPs, several studies have suggested that women using Depo-provera may be at increased risk of HIV acquisition, with one African study showing a 1.8-fold increased risk compared to women using no hormonal contraceptives.[42] The mechanism for this is unclear but it may be due to thinning of the vaginal epithelium as a result of the amenorrhoea and low oestrogen levels which then may result in increased trauma during sexual intercourse. Alternatively, lack of condom usage in hormonal contraceptive users may also account for the increased risk of transmission in those individuals. Although further work in this area is required, it highlights the importance of stressing concomitant condom use as the only means of preventing HIV transmission.

The injection interval in HIV-positive women had previously been reduced to 10 weeks due to the unknown effects of HAART on progesterone metabolism. However, this is now thought to be of less concern in the metabolism of injectable contraceptives. The Faculty of Family Planning has, therefore, issued a statement recommending that a reduction in the injection interval in those receiving HAART is probably unnecessary.[43]

Subdermal implant

These are progesterone-only contraceptives, which need to be inserted by a trained health professional and are effective for 3 years. They are a popular choice amongst HIV-positive women as they are very effective, non-user dependent, fully reversible and have the non-contraceptive advantage of inducing amenorrhoea in some women.[44] Although there are some concerns that subdermal implants may increase HIV transmission and enhance progression of HIV, there are no human studies that address these issues.[45] Once again, as with other hormonal contraceptives, the effects of HAART on their metabolism are unclear and, therefore, additional condom use must be advised.

Intra-uterine devices

Levonorgestrel intra-uterine system (IUS)

The IUS is a progesterone-releasing coil that acts locally by thinning the endometrium. It is a common choice of contraception amongst HIV-positive women due to its ability to reduce menstrual flow. The IUS, therefore, functions not only as a contraceptive but also as an effective treatment for menorrhagia. A further advantage of the IUS is its ability to reduce the risk of ectopic pregnancy and pelvic inflammatory disease (PID) compared to the copper intra-uterine devices (IUD).

Copper intra-uterine device (IUD)

The WHO and International Planned Parenthood Federation recommend that the IUD should not be used in HIV-positive women due to concerns about the increased risk of PID and pelvic abscesses in women using the IUD. This finding was challenged by an African study which found no significant difference in the rate of complications between HIV-positive and HIV-negative women using the IUD.[46] Although this study has flaws, it does suggest that IUDs may be used in HIV-positive women after exclusion of baseline cervical infection and in those with continued access to medical services. An additional disadvantage of the IUD, however, is its ability to increase the duration of menses. This has implications both for HIV transmission and for the use of the IUD in women prone to anaemia secondary to menorrhagia caused by fibroids.

Other methods

Male and female sterilisation

Female sterilisation was recommended as a contraceptive method in the past due to concerns about the high rates of vertical transmission. However, due to improvements in the prognosis of HIV-infected individuals and interventions to reduce vertical transmission, this is no longer an acceptable method of contraception unless specifically requested by the patient. In addition, tubal ligation has no effect on HIV transmission and vasectomy does not protect against HIV transmission because HIV is still present in the semen. A worrying finding from some studies is that sterilised couples are also less likely to use condoms.[42]

Emergency contraception

Two methods of emergency contraception exist, levonelle-2 (Levonelle is an identical over-the-counter product), a hormonal progesterone only method that is effective for up to 72 h after unprotected sexual intercourse (UPSI) and the IUD that can be used for up to 5 days after UPSI. Due to concerns that HAART may reduce the effectiveness of Levonelle-2, we advise women receiving antiretrovirals to take an additional tablet of Levonelle-2, although this is not licensed. Women using condoms alone for contraception must be advised about emergency contraception.

In summary, contraceptive messages should be provided in a culturally appropriate manner to ensure maximum uptake. A discussion of contraceptive options, safer sex and transmission risks should occur at each visit. Condoms are the only effective method in preventing HIV transmission but due to their failure rates, other methods should be used to prevent an unwanted pregnancy. Finally, the effect of HAART on contraceptive efficacy is unclear and should be considered when making contraceptive decisions.

HIV AND SUBFERTILITY

HIV-infected men and women desire and expect to have children,[47] and HIV-infected individuals unable to conceive may request advise and assistance with achieving a pregnancy safely. This has been the focus of much ethical debate although it is now beginning to be more accepted due to the improved HIV prognosis and reduced vertical transmission rates. Few centres are able to provide assisted conception techniques, however, due to the requirement for separate laboratory facilities to eliminate the risk of cross contamination of uninfected samples.

In the pre-HAART era, women with HIV were often discouraged from having children and may have been advised to undergo extreme procedures to ensure that they did not conceive, such as tubal ligation. There was widespread concern about the high rates of vertical transmission (~25% in the UK) and the potential for uninfected children to be left orphaned once their infected parents developed AIDS and died. With the introduction of HAART and the dramatic improvement in prognosis for HIV-infected individuals, such advice is no longer appropriate. The use of antiretroviral drugs during pregnancy and in the neonate, elective caesarean sections (or a well-managed vaginal delivery if the viral load is < 50 copies/ml) and avoidance of breast-feeding has resulted in a reduction in the vertical transmission rate to < 2%.

There is some evidence to suggest that pregnancy and birth rates among HIV-infected women are lower than those in the general population.[48] The reasons for this are multifactorial and may include increased rates of therapeutic abortion due to knowledge of HIV status, reduced sexual activity, weight loss, systemic illness, HIV effects on the hypothalamo–pituitary–gonadal axis, drug abuse, sexually transmitted infections and increased rates of spontaneous fetal loss.[49] HIV-infected individuals are, therefore, increasingly seeking fertility advice and assistance which should also consider horizontal transmission risk, general preconception care as well as appropriate fertility assessment for both partners. The British HIV Association (BHIVA) recommends fertility assessment if conception has not occurred after 6–12 months but sooner in women over 35 years, those with irregular cycles or a history suggestive of tubal disease.[39]

There are 3 possible scenarios to consider:

Serodiscordant couples   HIV-positive male + HIV-negative female
HIV-negative male + HIV-positive female

Seroconcordant couples   HIV-positive male + HIV-positive female

The serodiscordant couples may not have any problems achieving a pregnancy by UPSI; however, this would pose a risk of HIV seroconversion in the negative partner. In order to prevent this, numerous risk-reduction strategies exist but these are often expensive and time-consuming and are, therefore, not always accepted by the patients.

Discordant couples

For discordant couples in which the male partner is infected, the options for assisted conception/risk reduction include: (i) sperm washing; (ii) donor insemination; and (iii) timed unprotected intercourse. Timing unprotected intercourse during ovulation reduces, but does not eliminate, the risk of HIV transmission. Marina and colleagues[50] reported a seroconversion rate of 4.3% in HIV-negative women with HIV-positive partners trying to conceive through timed unprotected intercourse. All four women who were infected, however, reported inconsistent condom use by their partners at other times of the cycle. Donor insemination removes the possibility of genetic parenthood from the infected male but eliminates any risk of HIV transmission during conception.[40] Sperm washing is the most effective risk-reduction technique if genetic parenthood is desired by the infected male. It is a procedure in which spermatozoa, which do not carry HIV, are separated from HIV-contaminated seminal plasma and non-germinal cells using a density gradient and swim-up technique. The resulting sperm sample is then tested for HIV by PCR assays before being used for insemination or *in-vitro* fertilisation (IVF).[51] The technique was pioneered by Semprini and colleagues[52] who reported almost 1600 inseminations using sperm washing with no seroconversions in any of the mothers or children. Sperm washing is, however, expensive, is currently only provided by a few centres and is patient-funded in over 50% of cases.

Discordant couples in which the female partner is HIV-positive have the following options for assisted conception/risk reduction: (i) self-insemination of partner's semen; and (ii) timed unprotected intercourse. Timed unprotected intercourse should be avoided and quills, syringes, sterile containers or spermicide-free condoms should be provided for self-insemination during the fertile time of the cycle.

Concordant couples

For concordant couples, the options for assisted conception/risk reduction include: (i) sperm washing; and (ii) timed unprotected intercourse. Timed unprotected intercourse should be avoided to minimise the risk of transmitting a viral variant to the female partner and the future child. Sperm washing is, therefore, recommended.

At the Royal Free Hospital, couples wishing to conceive undergo baseline investigations to ensure they are able to conceive, as despite recommendations, many will engage in UPSI rather than risk-reduction techniques risking HIV transmission to the uninfected partner, or resistant virus transmission in seroconcordant couples. All couples are also referred to an HIV psychologist for counselling and discussion of the 'what if' scenarios.

HIV AND STDS

The prevalence of HIV and STDs among heterosexuals continues to rise. In order to address this, the UK Department of Health produced the National

Strategy for Sexual Health and HIV.[53] The principal aims of the strategy are to improve service provision, access to screening and to reduce the number of newly acquired infections by increasing awareness.

STDs, particularly ulcerative diseases, facilitate HIV transmission by augmenting HIV infectiousness and HIV susceptibility via a variety of biological mechanisms such as increased genital tract HIV shedding, increased recruitment of HIV susceptible inflammatory cells and disruption of mucosal barriers.[54] However, the effect of HIV on the acquisition and clinical course of STDs is less clear although there is some evidence that HIV-positive women may endure a more severe and complicated course of infection and this may be more pronounced in those with advanced immunosuppression.[55]

The high prevalence of STDs in seropositive women after HIV diagnosis (5%) reflects the continued sexual activity and inconsistent condom use in this group of women,[56] and re-inforces the need for the provision of adequate STD screening in this population. At the Royal Free Hospital, a detailed STD history is obtained during the gynaecological screen in all newly diagnosed women attending the women's clinic. A STD screen is then carried out on asymptomatic women and those at low risk using high vaginal swabs (HVS) to exclude *Candida* spp. and *Trichomonas vaginalis*, and endocervical swabs are taken to exclude *Neisseria gonorrhoea* and *Chlamydia trachomatis*. If endocervical swabs cannot be collected, a mid-stream urine sample is sent for chlamydia testing using strand displacement assays. Symptomatic women or those at high risk (< 25 years of age, new/multiple sexual partners or unprotected sexual intercourse) are referred to the sexual health clinic.

HIV AND MENSTRUAL DYSFUNCTION

Menstrual dysfunction in HIV-positive women is poorly understood. Most of the available data are conflicting and the few studies have involved small numbers of women.

No association was found between menstrual dysfunction, HIV infection and CD4 count in two studies,[57,58] while another study noted an increase in menstrual irregularity in HIV-positive women.[59] HIV-positive women with advanced disease (lower CD4, higher viral loads and taking antiretroviral therapy) have also been shown to experience either very short or very long menstrual cycles.[60] Clinical experience would certainly suggest an increase in the number of menstrual complaints in HIV-infected women. This may be the result of secondary acute or chronic illnesses complicating HIV disease or other independent social factors sometimes associated with HIV infection such as low socio-economic status, substance abuse or weight loss. Alternatively, it may a consequence of the fact that these women are already under medical care and may be more likely to report any problems to the doctor.

Anovulatory cycles are also thought to occur more frequently in HIV-positive women,[59] and are thought to be associated with older age and higher CD4 counts.[61]

In addition, HIV-infected women may experience the menopause earlier than HIV-uninfected women, although few are reported to receive hormonal replacement therapy (HRT), placing them at an increased risk of osteoporosis.[62] The effects of HIV on the hypothalamo–pituitary–gonadal axis are poorly understood. In HIV-seropositive men, a decrease in androgen level is associated with progressive immunosuppression, but limited information exists on the changes in endocrine function in women with HIV.

In our clinic, the most common menstrual problem seen is menorrhagia, usually secondary to fibroids. The management of these women is the same as for HIV-negative women. Many women opt to have the IUS inserted as it is not only an effective treatment for menorrhagia, but also has additional contraceptive benefits as well as reducing HIV transmission by reducing or obliterating cyclical bleeding. Uterine artery embolisation is another frequently used treatment option. It has been shown to be safe in HIV-positive women, although there may be a possible risk of developing post-procedural infection in those with a CD4 count < 200 cells/mm^3.[63]

SUMMARY

HIV-positive women have specific gynaecological needs that are often poorly addressed. Interest in this area is growing but further research is required to improve our understanding of HIV in women.

References

1 <http://www.unaids.org/html/pub/una-docs/q-a_ii_en_pdf.pdf>
2 <http://www.phls.co.uk/infections/default.htm>
3 Health Protection Agency: HIV/AIDS report 2003
4 <http://www.cdc.gov/hiv/pubs/facts/women.htm>
5 <http://www.un.org/events/women/iwd/2004/aids_backgrounder.pdf>
6 <http://www.who.int/reproductive-health/cancers/cervical_cancer_screening_in_dev_countries.pdf>
7 Parkin DM, Pisani P, Ferlay J. Estimates of the worldwide incidence of 25 major cancers in 1990. Int J Cancer 1999; 80: 827–841
8 Beerens E, Van Renterghem L, Praet M et al. Human papillomavirus DNA detection in women with primary abnormal cytology of the cervix: prevalence and distribution of HPV genotypes. Cytopathology 200; 16: 199–205
9 Flannelly G, Jiang G, Anderson D et al. Serial quantitation of HPV-16 in the smears of women with mild and moderate dyskaryosis. J Med Virol 1995; 47: 6–9
10 Ellerbrook TV, Chaisson MA, Bush TJ et al. Incidence of cervical squamous intraepithelial lesions in HIV-infected women. JAMA 2000; 283: 1031–1037
11 Heard I, Tassie J, Schmitz V et al. Increased risk of cervical disease among human immunodeficiency virus-infected women with severe immunosuppression and high human papillomavirus load. Obstet Gynecol 2000; 96: 403–409
12 Mandelblatt JS, Kanetsky P, Eggert L et al. Is HIV infection a cofactor for cervical squamous cell neoplasia? Cancer Epidemiol Biomarkers Prev 1999; 8: 97–106
13 Levi JE, Fernandes S, Tateno AF et al. Presence of multiple human papillomavirus types in cervical samples from HIV-infected women. Gynecol Oncol 2004; 92: 225–231
14 Sun X, Kuhn L, Ellerbrock TV et al. Human papillomavirus infection in women infected with the human immunodeficiency virus. N Engl J Med 1999; 337: 1343–1349
15 Minkoff H, Ahdieh L, Massad LS et al. The effect of highly active antiretroviral therapy on cervical cytologic changes associated with oncogenic HPV among HIV-infected women. AIDS 2001; 15: 2157–2164
16 Clarke B, Chetty R. Postmodern cancer: the role of human immunodeficiency virus in uterine cervical cancer. J Clin Pathol Mol Pathol 2002; 55: 19–24
17 Cardillo M, Hagan R, Abadi J et al. CD4 T-cell count, viral load and squamous intraepithelial lesions in women infected with human immunodeficiency virus. Cancer 2001; 93: 111–114

18 Minkoff H, Ahdieh L, Massad S *et al.* The effect of highly active antiretroviral therapy on cervical cytologic changes associated with oncogenic HPV among HIV-infected women. AIDS 2001; 15: 2157–2164

19 Tate DR, Anderson RJ. Recrudescence of cervical dysplasia among women who are infected with the human immunodeficiency virus: a case-control analysis. Am J Obstet Gynecol 2002; 186: 880–882

20 Holcomb K, Matthews RP, Chapman JE *et al.* The efficacy of cervical conization in the treatment of cervical intraepithelial neoplasia in HIV-positive women. Gynecol Oncol 1999; 74: 428–431

21 Heard I, Potard V, Foulot H *et al.* High rate of recurrence of cervical intraepithelial neoplasia after surgery in HIV-positive women. J AIDS 2005; 39: 412–418

22 Gilles C, Manigart Y, Konopnicki D *et al.* Management and outcome of cervical intraepithelial neoplasia lesions: a study of matched cases according to HIV status. Gynecol Oncol 2005; 96: 112–118

23 Nappi L, Carriero C, Bettocchi S *et al.* Cervical squamous intraepithelial lesions of low grade in HIV-infected women: recurrence, persistence, and progression, in treated and untreated women. Eur J Obstet Gynecol Reprod Biol 2005; 121: 226–232

24 Heard I, Schmitz V, Costagliota D *et al.* Early regression of cervical lesions in HIV seropositive women receiving highly active antiretroviral therapy. AIDS 1998; 12: 1459–1464

25 Minkoff H, Ahdieh L, Massad LS *et al.* The effect of highly active antiretroviral therapy on cervical cytologic changes associated with oncogenic HPV amongst HIV-infected women. AIDS 2001; 15: 2157–2164

26 Heard I, Jean-Michel T, Kazatchkine MD *et al.* Highly active antiretroviral therapy enhances regression of cervical intraepithelial neoplasia in HIV-seropositive women. AIDS 2002; 16: 1799–1802

27 Lillo FB, Ferrari D, Veglia F *et al.* Human papillomavirus infection and associated cervical disease in human immunodeficiency virus-infected women: effect of highly active antiretroviral therapy. J Infect Dis 2001; 184: 547–551

28 Moore AL, Sabin CA, Madge S *et al.* Highly active antiretroviral therapy and cervical intraepithelial neoplasia. AIDS 2002; 16: 927–929

29 The Royal College of Obstetricians and Gynaecologists. Working party report. HIV infection in maternity care and gynaecology. London: The Royal College of Obstetricians and Gynaecologists, 1997

30 Guidelines for the NHS cervical screening programme. NHSCSP publication No. 20, 2004

31 Wilson TE, Massad SL, Riester KA *et al.* Sexual, contraceptive, and drug use behaviours of women with HIV and those at high risk for infection: results from the Women's Interagency HIV Study. AIDS 1999; 13: 591–598

32 United Nations Population Division Statistics Department of Economics and Social Affairs. World contraceptive use, 2001

33 Mitchell HS, Stephens E. Contraception choices for HIV positive women. Sex Transm Infect 2004; 80: 167–173

34 World Health Organization. Effectiveness of male latex condoms in protecting against pregnancy and sexually transmitted infections. Geneva: World Health Organization. Fact sheet No. 243, 2000

35 Davis KR, Weller SC. The effectiveness of condoms in reducing heterosexual transmission of HIV. Fam Plan Perspect 1999; 31: 272–279

36 Magalhaes J, Amaral E, Giraldo PC *et al.* HIV infection in women: impact on contraception. Contraception 2002; 66: 87–91

37 Belzer M, Smith Rogers A, Camarca M *et al.* Contraceptive choices in HIV infected and HIV at-risk adolescent females. J Adolesc Health 2001; 29S: 93–100

38 Guillebaud J. (ed) Contraception Today, 4th edn. London: Dunitz, 2000

39 British HIV Association. Guideline for the management of HIV infection in pregnant women ant the prevention of mother-to-child transmission of HIV. British HIV Association, 2005

40 Howe JE, Minkoff HL, Duerr AC. Contraceptives and HIV. AIDS 1994; 8: 861–871

41 Mati J. Maggwa N, Hunter D *et al.* Reproductive events, contraceptive use, and HIV

infection among women users of family planning (FP) in Nairobi, Kenya. VII International Conference on AIDS. Florence, June 1991 [abstract WC3095]

42 Lavreys L, Chohan V, Overbaugh J et al. Hormonal contraception and risk of HIV-1 acquisition: results of a 10-year prospective study. AIDS 2004; 18: 695–697

43 FFPRHC Guidance: Drug interactions with hormonal contraception. J Fam Plan Reprod Health Care 2005; 31: 139–151

44 Taneepanichskul S, Intaraprasert S, Phuapradit W et al. Use of Norplant implants in asymptomatic HIV-1 infected women. Contraception 1997; 55: 205–207

45 Curtis KM. Safety of implantable contraceptives for women: data from observational studies. Contraception 2002; 65: 85–96

46 Morrison CS, Sekadde-Kingondu C, Sinei S et al. Is the intrauterine device appropriate contraception for HIV-1-infected women. Br J Obstet Gynaecol 2001; 108: 784–790

47 Chen JL, Philips KA, Kanouse DE et al. Fertility desires and intentions of HIV-positive men and women. Fam Plann Perspect 2001; 33: 144–152

48 Fylkesnes K, Ndhlovu Z, Kasumba K et al. Studying dynamics of the HIV epidemic: population-based data compared with sentinel surveillance in Zambia. AIDS 1998; 12: 1227–1234

49 Lo JC, Schambelen M. Reproductive function in human immunodeficiency virus infection. J Clin Endocrin Metab 2001; 86: 2338–2343

50 Marina S, Marina F, Alcolea R et al. Pregnancy following intracytoplasmic sperm injection from a HIV-1-seropositive man. Hum Reprod 1998; 13: 3247–3249

51 Ethics Committee of the American Society of Reproductive Medicine. Human immunodeficiency virus and infertility treatment. Fertil Steril 2002; 77: 218–222

52 Semprini AE, Levi-Setti P, Ravizza M et al. Assisted conception to reduce the risk of male-to-female sexual transfer of HIV in serodiscordant couples: an update [abstract]. Presented at the 1998 Symposium on AIDS in Women, Sao Paulo, Brazil, September 1998

53 Department of Health. Better prevention, better services, better sexual health – The national strategy for sexual health and HIV. London: Department of Health, 2001

54 Fleming DT, Wasserheit JN. From epidemiological synergy to public health policy and practice: the contribution of other sexually transmitted diseases to sexual transmission of HIV infection. Sex Transm Infect 1999; 75: 3–17

55 Cohen CR, Sinei S, Reilly M et al. Effect of human immunodeficiency virus type 1 infection upon acute salpingitis: a laparoscopic study. J Infect Dis 1998; 178: 1352–1358

56 Madge S, Phillips AN, Griffioen A et al. Demographic, clinical and social factors associated with human immunodeficiency virus infection and other sexually transmitted diseases in a cohort of women from the United Kingdom and Ireland. Int J Epidemiol 1998; 27: 1068–1071

57 Ellerbrook TV, Wright TC, Bush TJ et al. Characteristics of menstruation in women infected with human immunodeficiency syndrome. Obstet Gynecol 1996; 87: 1030–1034

58 Shah PN, Smith JR, Wells C et al. Menstrual symptoms in women infected by the human immunodeficiency virus. Obstet Gynecol 1994; 83: 397–400

59 Chirgwin KD, Feldman J, Muneyyirci-Delale O et al. Menstrual function in human immunodeficiency virus-infected women without acquired immunodeficiency syndrome. J AIDS Hum Retrovirol 1996; 12: 489–494

60 Harlow SD, Schuman P, Cohen M et al. Effect of HIV infection on menstrual cycle length. J AIDS 2000; 24: 68–75

61 Greenblatt RM, Ameli N, Grant RM et al. Impact of the ovulatory cycle on virologic and immunologic markers in HIV-infected women. J Infect Dis 2000; 181: 82–90

62 Clark RA, Cohn SE, Jarek C et al. Perimenopausal symptomatology among HIV infected women at least 40 years of age. J AIDS 2000; 23: 99–100

63 Prollius A, du Plessis A, Nel M. Uterine artery embolisation in HIV positive patients. Int J Gynecol Obstet 2005; 88: 67–68

Tanja Pejovic   Farr Nezhat

20

The adnexal mass

Anatomically, the adnexa consist of the ovaries, fallopian tubes, broad ligament, and the structures within the broad ligament. The differential diagnosis of the adnexal mass is complex because of the wide spectrum of the disorders that it encompasses and the numerous therapies that may be appropriate. The adnexal mass most frequently involves the ovary itself because of its propensity for neoplasia.[1] The magnitude of the problem is illustrated by the fact that an estimated 5–10% of women in the US will undergo a surgical procedure for a suspected ovarian neoplasm during their lifetime.[2] Although the majority of adnexal masses are due to benign processes, the primary goal of the diagnostic evaluation is the exclusion of malignancy.

DIFFERENTIAL DIAGNOSIS

The differential diagnosis of the adnexal mass varies with the age (Table 1). The age is also the most important factor in determining the potential for malignancy. In premenarchal and postmenopausal women, the presence of an adnexal mass should be considered highly abnormal and must be promptly evaluated.

Premenarchal patient

In prepubertal girls, most ovarian neoplasms are of germ cell origin and require immediate surgical exploration. Ehren *et al.*[3] reported a series of 63

Tanja Pejovic MD PhD
Department of Obstetrics and Gynecology, Oregon Health & Science University, Portland, Oregon, USA

Farr Nezhat MD FACOG (for correspondence)
Professor of Obstetrics and Gynecology, Division of Gynecologic Oncology, 1176 Fifth Avenue, Mount Sinai Medical Center, New York, NY 10029, USA
E-mail: farr.nezhat@mssm.edu

Table 1 Differential diagnosis of adnexal mass

Organ	Cystic	Solid

Ovary	Functional cyst
	Endometriosis
	Cystic neoplasm
	    benign
	    malignant
		Benign
		Malignant

Fallopian tube	Tubo-ovarian abscess or hydrosalpinx Paratubal cyst	Ectopic pregnancy Tubo-ovarian abscess Neoplasm
Uterus	Intra-uterine pregnancy	Myoma
Bowel	Distended colon with gas and/or feces	Appendicitis Diverticulitis Diverticular abscess Colon cancer
Other	Distended bladder	Abdominal wall hematoma or abscess Pelvic kidney Retroperitoneal neoplasm

patients with ovarian tumors of different histology. The final diagnosis was benign teratoma in 65% of the cases; in 21% of the patients, the removed tumor was malignant. All patients younger than 12 years had germ cell tumors, while one patient, a 4-year-old girl, had an epithelial tumor. Appendicitis was the most common misdiagnosis.

Abdominal pain was the most common presenting symptom; torsion was present in 22%. Other symptoms of adnexal mass may include precocious puberty, hirsuitism, urinary complaints, and primary or secondary amenorrhea. Palpable mass is found on examination in the majority of the patients.

Reproductive-age patient

The most common adnexal masses in reproductive-age women are benign functional cysts of the ovaries. These include follicular cysts, corpus luteum cysts, theca-lutein cysts and polycystic ovaries. Functional ovarian cysts are usually asymptomatic and tend to resolve spontaneously in 4–6 weeks. Occasionally, they may be accompanied with some degree of pelvic discomfort, pain or dyspareunia. In addition, the rupture of one of these cysts leads to peritoneal irritation and possibly hemoperitoneum. Functional cyst may also present with torsion and pain. The other benign conditions include endometriosis (with ovarian endometriotic cysts), inflammatory enlargements of the fallopian tubes and ovaries (hydrosalpinges, tubo-ovarian abscess) due to pelvic infection, ectopic pregnancy and trophoblastic disease.

True, benign, ovarian neoplasms could also cause adnexal enlargement. These include, most frequently, serous or mucinous cystadenoma and benign cystic teratomas (Table 2). It is unclear whether or not these are precursors of malignant neoplasms, although some changes may represent true ovarian intra-epithelial neoplasia. Other neoplastic processes include para-ovarian cysts, pedunculated fibroids, ovarian and fallopian tube cancers. In certain instances, the mass is clinically indeterminate and may be due to non-gynecological causes such as full bladder, stool in the colon, distended cecum, peritoneal cyst, appendiceal abscess, diverticular abscess, Crohn's disease, ectopic kidney, urachal cyst, abdominal wall tumor, lymphoma, retroperitoneal sarcoma, metastatic tumor to the ovaries, and malignant diseases of the gastrointestinal system (Table 1).

Postmenopausal patient

Any enlargement of the ovary is abnormal in postmenopausal women and should be considered malignant until proven otherwise. The postmenopausal ovary atrophies to 1.5 x 1.0. x 0.5 cm in size and should not be palpable on pelvic examination. Ovaries that are palpable must alert the physician to possible malignancy. The risk of malignancy in this age group is increased from 13% in premenopausal to 45% in postmenopausal women.[2] Still, 55% of postmenopausal women with palpable ovaries do have a benign tumor. The most common ovarian tumors in this age group include epithelial ovarian tumors followed by stromal tumors and sex-cord tumors (Table 2).

CLINICAL PRESENTATION AND EVALUATION

The majority of patients present with symptoms related to compression of the local pelvic organs due to adnexal mass. Less commonly, an ovarian mass is discovered during a routine pelvic examination in an asymptomatic patient. In

Table 2 Benign ovarian tumors

NON-NEOPLASTIC TUMORS
Inclusion cyst
Follicular cyst
Corpus luteum cyst
Pregnancy luteoma
Theca lutein cyst
Endometrioma
NEOPLASM ARISING FROM THE SURFACE EPITHELIUM OF THE OVARY
Serous cystadenoma
Mucinous cystadenoma
Mixed forms
NEOPLASMS OF STROMAL ORIGIN
Fibroma (Meigs' syndrome)
Brenner tumor
GERM CELL TUMORS
Dermoid tumor (mature cystic teratoma)

Table 3 Pelvic findings in patients with benign and malignant ovarian tumors

BENIGN	MALIGNANT
Unilateral	Bilateral
Cystic	Solid or complex
Mobile	Fixed
Smooth	Irregular
No ascites	Ascites
No growth	Rapid growth
Smooth rectovaginal septum	Nodularity of rectovaginal septum

patients with a malignant process, the most common clinical symptom is abdominal discomfort due to ascites. In several surgical series, the reported incidence of ovarian malignancy in patients with a pre-operative diagnosis of ovarian mass ranged from 13–21%. The most important predictor of malignancy is the age of the patient. In fact, the risk that an ovarian neoplasm is malignant increases 12-fold from ages 12–29 years to 60–69 years.[4] Again, even in postmenouspausal women, the majority of adnexal masses are benign (55%).[5]

The evaluation of a woman with a suspected adnexal mass consists of a clinical history, including a gynecological history and family history of ovarian or breast cancer. The physical examination should also include an abdominal, pelvic, and rectovaginal examination (Table 3). However, physical examination alone is often inaccurate in determining whether an adnexal mass is benign or malignant, unless there are associated findings of disseminated disease. Imaging studies including ultrasound and/or CT scans are usually required for further evaluation.

The roles of ultrasound and CT scan

Pelvic ultrasound is currently the most useful technique for diagnostic evaluation of the adnexal mass. Transvaginal ultrasound provides better resolution than abdominal ultrasound.[6] The parameters of significance for ultrasonographic evaluation of the adnexal mass are the size, number of loculi, overall echo density, presence of septations with flow within, presence of papillary or solid excrescences or nodules within the mass. There are no universally accepted criteria for the sonographic description of ovarian disease. However, the findings that suggest malignancy include size larger than 6 cm in postmenopausal and larger than 8 cm in premenopausal women, presence of thick septations, papillary projections within the lumen of the cyst, complexity (cystic and solid areas) of the mass, presence of the nodules within the wall. Although most comparison studies have found gray-scale sonography to be superior to Doppler sonography, or that Doppler offers no significant improvement over gray-scale sonography, a minority of studies report Doppler features to be superior. Most authors prefer pulsatility index (PI) as a standard and consider PI < 1.0 suggestive of malignancy; however, some authors use resistance index (RI) with values of 0.4–0.7 as indicators of malignancy.

The seminal work of Sassone *et al.*[7] evaluated an ultrasound scoring system to predict ovarian malignancy. Transvaginal sonographic pelvic images of 143 patients were correlated with surgicopathological findings. The variables in the scoring system included the inner wall structure of the adnexal cyst, wall thickness, presence and thickness of septa, and echogenicity. The scoring system was useful in distinguishing benign from malignant masses, with a specificity of 83%, sensitivity of 100%, and positive and negative predictive values of 37% and 100%, respectively. Subsequently, Alcazar and Jurado[8] developed a logistic model to predict malignancy based on menopausal status, ultrasound morphology and color Doppler findings in 79 adnexal masses. The authors derived a mathematical formula to estimate pre-operatively the risk of malignancy (or benignity) of a given adnexal mass in a simple and reproducible way. When this formula was applied prospectively, 56 of 58 (96.5%) adnexal masses were correctly classified.

In general, CT scan is not indicated routinely for the evaluation of the adnexal mass. However, it is indicated in the evaluation of a patient with a hard fixed lateralized mass, ascites, abnormal liver function tests or palpable abdomino-pelvic mass. In such cases, malignancy is suspected and CT can provide significant information about the spread and resectability of the disease. The major limitation of CT in other instances is its inability to detect early ovarian cancer or any lesion less than 2 cm in size.

MRI does not use ionizing radiation and it is, therefore, useful in evaluation of adnexal masses in pregnancy. It is also useful in further evaluation of adnexal masses detected by ultrasound and characterized as 'intermediate' in nature. Grab *et al.*[9] investigated the accuracy of sonography versus MRI and positron emission tomography (PET) in 101 patients with asymptomatic adnexal masses who subsequently underwent laparoscopy. Ultrasonography established the correct diagnosis in 11 of the 12 ovarian malignancies (sensitivity 92%), but the specificity was only 60%. With MRI and PET, specificity improved to 84% and 89%, respectively, but sensitivity declined. When all modalities were combined, specificity was 85%, sensitivity 92%, while accuracy was 86%. However, because negative MRI or PET does not rule out early ovarian cancer or borderline malignancy, ultrasound remains the most important tool in the evaluation of the adnexal mass.

Tumor markers

The most helpful laboratory studies in the evaluation of adnexal masses are the quantitative β-hCG, complete blood count (CBC) with differential and, in selected cases, tumor markers. The quantitative β-hCG is essential in ruling out ectopic pregnancy. CBC with differential is necessary when an infectious case is suspected. Serum tumor markers for malignant germ cell tumors, lactate dehydrogenase (LDH), β-hCG, and α-fetoprotein (AFP) should be obtained in the young patient with a cystic-solid or solid adnexal mass to evaluate the risk of germ cell tumor (Table 4). Serum CA-125 levels and CEA values should also be obtained in patients with suspected gynecologic or gastrointestinal cancers, respectively. However, CA-125 may be elevated to levels greater than normal (35 IU/ml) in about 1% of healthy individuals. Also, in premenopausal women, CA-125 is elevated in a variety of benign conditions and may cloud,

Table 4 Tumor markers in ovarian neoplasms

NEOPLASM	MARKER
Epithelial ovarian cancer	CA-125
Mucinous epithelial ovarian tumors	CA-19-9
Dysgerminoma	Lactate dehydrogenase
Endodermal sinus tumor	α-Fetoprotein
Choriocarcinoma	hCG
Placental site trophoblastic tumor	Human placental lactogen
Granulosa cell tumor	Inhibin A

rather than clarify, the differential diagnosis of ovarian masses. Benign conditions causing elevation of CA-125 include myoma, adenomyosis, benign ovarian tumors, pelvic inflammatory disease, liver disease, endometriosis, peritonitis, and pleural effusions. Normal pregnancy also causes elevated CA-125. Hypothyroidism is associated with slight elevation in CA-125.

Serum CA-125 is elevated in 80% of all patients with serous carcinoma of the ovary, but in only half of the patients with stage I disease, making it a poor screening tool for detection of ovarian cancer.[10] As a diagnostic aid, CA-125 is most useful in postmenopausal women with ultrasonographically suspicious pelvic mass. In that subgroup of patients, a level greater that 65 IU/ml has been shown to have a positive predictive value of 97%.[11] The most reliable use of CA-125 is in monitoring patients with ovarian cancers as an indicator for response to treatment or progression.[12]

MANAGEMENT

The crucial decisions regarding management of the reproductive age woman with an adnexal mass are 2-fold: (i) to observe the patient or proceed with surgical removal of the mass; and (ii) if surgical removal is indicated, when is a laparoscopic approach justified (Table 5).

During the reproductive years, cystic adnexal masses that are less than 8 cm in diameter could be followed expectantly in the asymptomatic patient, as 70% of these masses will resolve spontaneously. The patient should undergo repeat physical examination and pelvic ultrasound at a specified time interval. A common practice is to suppress ovulation with the oral contraceptive pill, but

Table 5 Adnexal mass: indications for surgery

Ovarian cystic structure > 6 cm without regression for 6–8 weeks
Any cystic structure > 10 cm
Any solid ovarian lesion
Ovarian lesion with papillary excrescences in the wall
Palpable adnexal mass in premenarchal or postmenopausal patient
Ascites

Table 6 Histological classification of malignant ovarian tumors

Epithelial ovarian cancer
        Serous
        Mucinous
        Endometrioid
        Clear cell
        Transitional cell carcinoma
        Undifferentiated carcinoma

Germ cell tumors
        Immature teratoma
        Malignant neoplasms arising within mature cystic teratoma
        Dysgerminoma
        Embryonal carcinoma
        Endodermal sinus tumor
        Choriocarcinoma
        Gonadoblastoma

Sex-cord stromal tumors
        Granulosa cell tumor (adult and juvenile types)
        Sertoli-Leydig tumors (arrhenoblastoma and Sertoli tumor)

Neoplasm derived from non-specific mesenchyme
        Sarcoma
        Lymphoma

Metastatic tumors to the ovary
        Gastrointestinal tumors (Krukenberg)
        Breast
        Uterus

the value of this strategy remains unproven. Indications for surgery include persistence of the mass, change in ultrasonic characteristics to a more complex appearance, solid enlargement or evidence of ascites. However, if the mass remains less than 8 cm, simple on ultrasound appearance, and causing no symptoms, continued follow-up is a reasonable option. In the reproductive age, woman with an adnexal mass greater than 8 cm in diameter, solid appearance on ultrasound, bilaterality, and presence of ascites, surgical evaluation is indicated.[1] In the premenarchal and postmenopausal patient, the presence of adnexal mass of any size is considered an indication for surgical removal of the mass. Classification of malignant ovarian tumors is given in Table 6.

Once surgery is decided upon, accurate diagnosis at surgery is a key in the management of adnexal masses. Many surgeons are now using the laparoscopic approach for the management of the adnexal mass in reproductive age women. In a 1990 survey by the American Association of Gynecologic Laparoscopists, operative laparoscopy was accomplished in most patients and there were only 53 cases of unsuspected ovarian cancer in a total of 13,739 cases (0.04%).[13] The benefits of laparoscopic surgery include shorter length of hospital stay, decreased postoperative pain and recovery time, and probably reduced cost.[14–17] However, there are understandable persisting concerns about the laparoscopic management of adnexal masses. These include the failure to diagnose ovarian malignancies, tumor spillage, and inability to proceed immediately with a staging procedure and delay in therapy. In the largest series of laparoscopically managed adnexal masses in reproductive age women, Nezhat et al.[18] reported that the most reliable indicators of malignancy were the combination of laparoscopic visualization of the whole peritoneal cavity and frozen section analysis. Chapron et al.[19] examined the accuracy of frozen section analysis in 228 patients of whom 26 had suspicious adnexal masses at the time of laparoscopy. In all 26 patients, frozen sections showed benign results, and in each case definitive histological diagnosis was confirmatory.[19] Dottino et al.[20] found discrepancy between the frozen section and final pathology in 3% of the cases. However, in a study of 149 patients with macroscopically suspicious ovarian masses, Canis et al.[21] found the frozen section to be accurate in 93% of the cases involving tumors smaller than 10 cm and in 74% of larger tumors. Intra-operative pathological diagnosis was accurate in 77.8% of low malignant potential tumors.[21]

Therefore, the two important exceptions to the high accuracy of frozen section are in very large tumors or tumors with borderline characteristics. The accuracy in these instances depends on the relative sample bias. The solution to this problem should be in removing the entire adnexa and allowing pathological, rather than surgical, sampling. If a malignant ovarian neoplasm is discovered at the time of laparoscopy, the current standard of care is the performance of a comprehensive surgical staging procedure, followed in most cases by adjuvant chemotherapy.

On balance, laparoscopic surgery can be attempted for selected patients requiring operative treatment of an adnexal mass provided there is no evidence of metastatic disease, frozen section diagnosis is available, and the patient has consented to comprehensive surgical staging for ovarian cancer, including laparotomy. Postoperatively, the patient should follow-up with the physician to determine the need for further therapy based on the results of full pathological evaluation of the surgical specimen.

The standard operative approach to adnexal masses in postmenopausal women has been explorative laparotomy to ensure adequate exposure for the treatment of ovarian cancer. However, because the observation that even in this group of the patient benign adnexal tumors are more frequent than malignant, some authors justify starting the surgical procedure laparoscopically. In the only prospective study, Dottino et al.[20] reported that nearly 90% of cases were managed laproscopically. The same principles of careful visualization of the entire peritoneal cavity and obtaining pelvic washings and biopsies for the diaphragm, paracoloc gutters, and pelvis should be undertaken. Cystectomy is not recommended in postmenopausal women; removal of the entire adnexa with frozen section diagnosis is warranted.[22] Removal of a normal appearing contralateral ovary should be performed according to pre-operative consultation and past medical history. Initial laparoscopic approach with the removal of the adnexa with the mass accompanied with careful inspection of the peritoneal cavity, generous biopsies, availability of frozen section and respecting the principles of cancer surgery are essential in management of the adnexal masses in premenarchal patient and the exclusion of the germ cell malignancy is a requirement.

ADNEXAL MASS IN PREGNANCY

Adnexal masses are frequently observed in gravid women, complicating as many as one in 190 pregnancies.[23] The risk of malignancy in pregnant woman with adnexal mass is 5%.[24] At least one-third of adnexal masses discovered during pregnancy are found during routine obstetrical ultrasonography, as both benign and malignant ovarian masses tend to be asymptomatic in pregnant women. Careful evaluation is necessary to differentiate between benign and malignant processes. It this regard, the sonographic appearance of the mass may be helpful. Simple cystic structures are most consistent with physiological cysts. Most of the physiological cysts resolve spontaneously by the end of the first trimester. Failure of simple cyst to resolve by this time may be indication for surgery. Other indications for surgery include tumor size greater than 6 cm, a solid or complex sonographic appearance of the mass, and the presence of bilateral abnormalities. Doppler ultrasound is potentially useful in differentiating high- and low-risk ovarian masses. Regardless of size, adnexal masses with blood flow characterized by a high resistive index appear to carry little risk, even when these masses fail to resolve by the second trimester. Magnetic resonance imaging may be helpful in situations where ultrasound is equivocal or the mass cannot be distinguished from the uterine neoplasm.

Most ovarian cancers complicating pregnancy are either borderline malignant epithelial ovarian tumors or germ cell tumors.[1] The latter observation reflects the younger age of pregnant women when compared to the typical ovarian cancer patient. Dysgerminomas are the most common ovarian germ cell tumors complicating pregnancy, followed by endodermal sinus tumors. Sex cord or stromal tumors may also occur during pregnancy. Great care must be taken to differentiate sex cord-stromal tumors from luteoma of the pregnancy, ovarian decidualization, or benign granulosa cell tumor proliferations observed with the pregnancy. Although elevated levels of tumor markers are helpful in establishing diagnosis in non-pregnant woman, elevations of these markers for reasons not related to malignancy reduces their diagnostic potential. For example, elevations of α-fetoprotein and human chorionic gonadotropin can be effective markers for follow-up of endodermal sinus tumor and gestational trophoblastic tumors, respectively (Table 4). However titers of all these markers as well as CA-125 are routinely elevated in pregnancy for reasons unrelated to malignancy. Their levels may be misleading even when normalized as a multiple of the mean for prenatal patients.

Only 3–5% of adnexal masses in pregnancy will ultimately prove to be malignant. Thus, most may be managed conservatively, provided that patient's symptoms and characteristics of the mass are consistent with benign etiology. Because adnexal masses are more likely to undergo torsion during pregnancy, explorative laparotomy may be necessary when torsion is suspected in the patient with severe or intermittent abdominal pain, nausea and vomiting. If possible, surgical intervention should be delayed until the second trimester to reduce the risk of pregnancy loss. When first trimester exploration and ovarian resection are necessary, supplementary progesterone has been administered to decrease the likelihood of pregnancy loss. The efficacy of this treatment remains, however, unproven. Several reports have suggested the safe use of laparoscopy in the management of adnexal masses in the first and second pregnancy trimester. The conclusion was made that laparoscopic management by an experienced team is a safe and effective procedure that allows for reduced rate of postoperative complications and a decreased maternal and fetal morbidity.[25,26]

In rare cases of ovarian cancer, complete surgical staging should be performed in a manner similar to that in the non-pregnant woman. Although the gravid uterus makes assessment of the retroperitonum more difficult, every effort should be made to remove tumor intact. The remaining ovary should be carefully inspected and biopsied, if suspicious. Because germ cell tumors are almost invariably unilateral, it is not necessary to remove both ovaries. The exception is dysgerminoma, which may be bilateral in 20% of the cases and may be present in grossly normal contralateral ovary. Even in this situation, it is not absolutely necessary to remove the entire ovary. However, if the both ovaries are involved but malignancy, and the gestation, has reached the second trimester, both ovaries should be removed as the pregnancy no longer requires the hormonal support from corpus luteum. Because dysgerminomas spread to para-aortic lymph nodes, every effort should be made to sample these nodes. An omentectomy and peritoneal biopsies along with cytological assessment of peritoneal cavity should be routinely performed.

Pregnant patients with stage Ia or Ib ovarian cancer can be managed conservatively with surgery and allowed to continue to term. The need for further chemotherapy is dictated by histological type of the tumor and its invasiveness. Cytotoxic chemotherapy should be avoided in the first trimester; however, it may be used in the second and third trimester with little harm, if any, to the fetus. For these reasons, women with stage IC and greater ovarian cancer or with high-grade tumors should be given the opportunity to receive chemotherapy without terminating the pregnancy.

KEY POINTS FOR CLINICAL PRACTICE

- Of women in the US, 5–10% will undergo surgery for suspected ovarian neoplasm. Of these, 13–21% will be found to have ovarian cancer.

- Age is the most important factor in determining the risk of malignancy.

- In reproductive-age women, functional cysts are the most frequent findings. These may be managed conservatively as most disappear within 4–6 weeks.

- Any cystic ovarian enlargement greater than 8 cm, the presence of solid mass is indication for surgery in reproductive-age woman.

- Solid mass of any size is indication for surgery in prepubertal girls. Abdominal pain and abdominal mass are the two most frequent presenting symptoms in children. Malignant neoplasms are found in 8% of children undergoing surgery for adnexal mass. Germ cell tumors are the most frequent malignant tumor in children.

KEY POINTS FOR CLINICAL PRACTICE *(continued)*

• Ovaries should not be palpable in postmenopausal women. Any ovarian enlargement in this age group is suggestive of malignancy until proven otherwise. Up to 40–45% of these patients who undergo surgery would be found to have malignant tumor. However, the most frequent finding is a benign ovarian neoplasm (fibroma or Brenner tumor).

• Fibromas are benign and associated sometimes with right-sided pleural effusion (Meigs' syndrome).

• A combination of history, physical examination, tumor marker analysis and pelvic ultrasound are all used in the evaluation of adnexal mass. While pelvic ultrasound remains the best imaging tool for evaluation of ovarian pathology, MRI is useful in diagnosis of endometriotic and hemorrhagic cysts; CT is useful in evaluating the extent of ovarian cancer.

• The surgical approach to the adnexal mass has traditionally been via laparotomy. With the advancements in laparoscopy, more surgeons initially approach adnexal masses laparoscopically. The laparoscopy offers better visualization, shorter hospital stay and lower rate of complications in comparison with laparotomy. The availability of frozen section diagnosis and ability to obtain immediate gynecological oncology assistance in cases malignant disease is found is essential.

• The adnexal mass is found in 1 in 190 pregnancies. The most frequent adnexal tumors in pregnancy are dysgerminoma and borderline ovarian tumors. The adnexal mass can be safely removed surgically during the second trimester of pregnancy. Surgeons with extensive laparoscopic experience can safely approach these masses laparoscopically.

References

1 Disaia PJ, Creasman WT. The adnexal mass and early ovarian cancer. In: Clinical Gynecologic Oncology, 6th edn. St Louis, MO: Mosby, 1997; 253–281

2 Curtin JP. Management of the adnexal mass. Gynecol Oncol 1994; 55: S42–S46

3 Ehren IM, Mahour GH, Isaacs H. Benign and malignant ovarian tumors in children and adolescents. Cancer 1984; 147: 339–343

4 Koonings PP, Campbell DR, Mishell JR Grimes DA. Relative frequency of primary ovarian neoplasms: a 10-year review. Obstet Gynecol 1989; 74: 921–926

5 Shalev E, Eliyahu S, Peleg D, Tsabari A. Laparoscopic management of adnexal cystic masses in postmenopausal women. Obstet Gynecol 1994; 83: 594–596

6 Kurjak A, Predanic M, Kupresic-Urek S, Jukic S. Transvaginal color and pulsed Doppler assessment of adnexal tumor vascularity. Gynecol Oncol 1993; 50: 3–8

7 Sassone A, Timor-Tritch I, Artner A *et al*. Transvaginal sonographic characterization of ovarian disease: evaluation of a new scoring system to predict ovarian malignancy. Obstet Gynecol 1991; 78: 7–11

8 Alcazar JL, Jurado M. Prospective evaluation of a logistic model based on sonographic morphologic and color Doppler findings developed to predict adnexal malignancy. J Ultrasound Med 1999; 18: 837–843

9 Grab D, Flock F, Stohr I. Classification of asymptomatic adnexal masses by ultrasound, magnetic resonance imaging, and positron emission tomography. Gynecol Oncol 2000; 77: 454–459

10 Jacobs I, Davies AP, Bridges J et al. Prevalence screening for ovarian cancer in postmenopausal women by CA125 measurement and ultrasonography. BMJ 1993; 306: 1030–1032

11 Brooks SE. Preoperative evaluation of patients with suspicious ovarian cancer. Gynecol Oncol 1994; 55: 80–90

12 Meyer T, Rustin GSJ. Role of tumor markers in monitoring epithelial ovarian cancer. Br J Cancer 2000; 82: 1535–1538.

13 Hulka JT, Parker WH, Surrey MH, Phillips JM. Management of ovarian masses. AAGL 1990 survey. J Reprod Med 1992; 37: 599–602

14 Mais V, Ajossa S, Piras B et al. Treatment of nonendometriotic benign adnexal cyst. A randomized trial to evaluate benefits in early outcome. Am J Obstet Gynecol 1996; 174: 654–658

15 Davison J, Park W, Penney L. Comparative study of operative laparoscopy vs. laparotomy: analysis of financial impact. Reprod Med 1993; 38: 357–360

16 Lundorff PJ, Thorburn J, Hahlin M et al. Adhesion formation after laparoscopic surgery in tubal pregnancy: a randomized trial versus laparotomy. Fertil Steril 1991; 55: 911–915

17 Maruiri F, Azziz A. Laparoscopic surgery for ectopic pregnancies: technology assessment and public health implications. Technol Steril 1993; 59: 487–498

18 Nezhat FR, Nezhat CH, Welander CE, Benigno B. Four ovarian cancers diagnosed during laparoscopic management of 1011 women with adnexal masses. Am J Obstet Gynecol 1992; 167: 790–796

19 Chapron C, Dubuisson JB, Kadoch O et al. Laparoscopic management of organic ovarian cysts: is there a place for frozen section in the diagnosis. Hum Reprod 1998; 13: 324—329

20 Dottino PR, Levine DA, Ripley DL, Cohen CJ. Laparoscopic management of adnexal masses in premenopausal and postmenopausal women. Obstet Gynecol 1999; 93: 223–228

21 Canis M, Mashiach R, Wattiez A et al. Frozen section in laparoscopic management of macroscopically suspicious ovarian masses. J Am Assoc Gynecol Laparosc 2004; 11: 365–369

22 Pejovic T, Nezhat F. Laparoscopic management of adnexal masses. The opportunities and the risks. Ann NY Acad Sci 2003; 943: 255-268.

23 Whitecar MP, Turner S, Higby MK. Adnexal masses in pregnancy: a review of 130 cases undergoing surgical management. Am J Obstet Gynecol 1999; 181: 19–24

24 Schnee DM. The adnexal mass in pregnancy. Mo Med 2004; 101: 42–45

25 Mathevet P, Nessah K, Dargent D, Mellier G. Laparoscopic management of adnexal masses in pregnancy. A case series. Eur J Obstet Gynecol Reprod Biol 2003; 108: 217–222.

26 Yen PM, Ng PS, Leung PL, Rogers MS. Outcome in laparoscopic management of persistent adnexal mass during the second trimester of pregnancy. Surg Endosc 2004; 18: 1354–1357

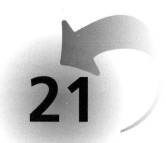

Alaa A. El-Ghobashy   Abeer M. Shaaban
Sue M. Calvert

Borderline ovarian tumours: a continuing dilemma

Ovarian tumours are traditionally classified into benign and malignant groups with a third group in which the prognosis is intermediate between benign and malignant tumours. The latter group is referred to as borderline tumours and was introduced by the World Health Organization (WHO) and International Federation of Gynecology and Obstetrics (FIGO) in 1971. The introduction of this entity represented a great advancement since it separated a group of ovarian tumours with a much better prognosis, stage-for-stage, from conventional ovarian carcinomas.[1] It was recognised, at that time, that this category probably represents a heterogeneous group and that subsequent refining of criteria for diagnosis was expected. The designation borderline ovarian tumours (BOTs) refers to ovarian epithelial neoplasms that demonstrate higher proliferative activity when compared with benign neoplasms but do not show stromal invasion.

Others synonyms include low malignant potential and atypical proliferative tumours. The most recent WHO classification[2] recommended 'borderline ovarian tumours' as the preferred terminology and 'tumours of low malignant potential' as an accepted synonym.

EPIDEMIOLOGY

Borderline ovarian tumours are uncommon tumours with an incidence of 2.5/100,000 women-years.[3] Borderline ovarian tumours account for about

---

Alaa A. El-Ghobashy MD MRCOG (for correspondence)
Specialist Registrar in Obstetrics and Gynaecology, St James's University Hospital, Leeds, UK
E-mail: ghobashy@doctors.org.uk

Abeer M. Shaaban PhD MRCPath
Consultant Histopathologist/Honorary Senior Lecturer, Leeds General Infirmary, Leeds, UK

Sue M. Calvert MRCOG
Consultant in Obstetrics and Gynaecology, Bradford Royal Infirmary, Bradford, UK

10–15% of all epithelial ovarian cancers in Caucasians.[4] Previous epidemiological studies indicate common risk factors for invasive epithelial ovarian cancers and borderline tumours. It remains unclear whether these tumours represent a continuum to invasive cancers or are a separate disease entity.

Risk factors

A Swedish case-control study examined the risk factors for epithelial BOTs. Increasing parity and lactation were found to be associated with a reduction in the risk of BOTs in women aged 50–74 years. No protection was noticed following the use of oral contraceptives. Hormonal factors such as the use of unopposed oestrogen and obesity might increase the risk of serous BOTs.[5,6]

Age

The mean age at diagnosis ranges from 38–56 years (10 years younger than for malignant tumours of the ovary).[4] Age-specific incidence rates for BOTs increase into the sixth decade of life and then stabilise, possibly declining among women in the ninth decade. Although rates for serous BOTs are slightly higher than those for mucinous BOTs, the overall age-specific patterns are similar. In contrast, rates of serous and mucinous carcinomas continue to increase for approximately 2 decades after menopause.[3] An Australian study showed that the later the age at menarche was associated with increasing risk of mucinous BOTs (odds ratio, 3.8; 95% confidence interval, 1.3–11.4 for those with age at menarche $\geq$ 14 years compared with those < 12 years; $P = 0.003$). Women with mucinous BOTs were significantly younger than women diagnosed with invasive cancers (mean 44 versus 57 years; $P < 0.0001$).[7]

Infertility

Borderline tumours are encountered more often in patients who suffer from infertility. It was suggested that the recurrent microtraumas associated with multiple induced ovulations might be responsible for the higher risk of malignancies. Ness et al.[8] showed that the use of fertility drugs in nulligravid women was associated with BOTs (OR, 2.43; 95% CI, 1.01–5.88) but not with any of the invasive histological subtypes. Nevertheless, another study revealed an equal increase in the incidence of BOTs in groups of patients suffering from infertility without any treatment, as in those being treated.[9,10] Further investigations are needed to prove that ovulation-inducing medications are implicated in the genesis of BOTs.

Racial susceptibility

Rates of BOTs are lower in black than in white women.[11] Mucinous tumours, both borderline and invasive, were reported to be more common in Asian women than in Caucasians and other ethnic groups.[12] However, another study found similar rates of ovarian carcinoma in Asian women born in the US and those born in Asia and for both groups, lower rates than those for whites in the US. Data from this study suggest the presence of either genetic or epigenetic

Table 1 Classification of borderline epithelial tumours (WHO classification)

Serous tumours
  Papillary cystic tumour
  Surface papillary tumour
  Adenofibroma, cystadenofibroma
Mucinous tumours
  Intestinal type
  Endocervical-like
Endometrioid tumours
  Cystic tumour
  Adenofibroma and cystadenofibroma
Clear cell tumours
  Cystic tumour
  Adenofibroma and cystadenofibroma
Transitional cell tumours
  Borderline Brenner tumour (proliferating variant)

factors that could be prevalent among Asians, which protect them from ovarian carcinoma.[13]

Genetic susceptibility

Although the incidence of BOTs may not be increased in patients with hereditary breast-ovarian cancer syndrome (HBOC) and those who carry cancer-associated BRCA1 and BRCA2 mutations, these individuals could be susceptible to malignant progression of borderline lesions of the ovaries and peritoneum.[14]

Other factors

In a population-based, case-control study, women who had ever smoked cigarettes were more likely to develop ovarian cancer than women who had never smoked. Risk was greater for BOTs (OR, 2.4; 95% CI, 1.4–4.1) than for invasive tumours (OR, 1.7; 95% CI, 1.2–2.4). The histological subtype most strongly associated was the mucinous subtype among both current smokers (OR, 3.2; 95% CI, 1.8—5.7) and past smokers (OR, 2.3; 95% CI, 1.3–3.9).[15]

PATHOLOGY

The great majority of BOTs are of serous and mucinous types. Borderline ovarian tumours also exist for endometrioid, clear, transitional cell (Table 1) but those tumours have been so rare for clinicopathological characterisation. Therefore, in this review, only the borderline serous and mucinous variants will be discussed.

Serous borderline tumours

These are the most common type of BOTs. These tumours occur across the age spectrum including young women. This is of particular significance since

Table 2 TNM and FIGO classification of tumours of the ovary[2]

T – Primary tumour		
TNM categories	FIGO stages	
TX		Primary tumour cannot be assessed
T0		No evidence of primary tumour
T1	I	Tumour limited to the ovaries
T1a	IA	Tumour limited to one ovary; capsule intact, no tumour on ovarian surface; no malignant cells in ascites or peritoneal washings
T1b	IB	Tumour limited to both ovaries; capsule intact, no tumour on ovarian surface; no malignant cells in ascites or peritoneal washings
T1c	IC	Tumour limited to one or both ovaries with any of the following: capsule ruptured, tumour on ovarian surface, malignant cells in ascites or peritoneal washings
T2	II	Tumour involves one or both ovaries with pelvic extension
T2a	IIA	Extension and/or implants on uterus and/or tube(s); no malignant cells in ascites or peritoneal washings
T2b	IIB	Extension to pelvic tissues; no malignant cells in ascites or peritoneal washings
T2c	IIC	Pelvic extension (2a or 2b) with malignant cells in ascites or peritoneal washings
T3 and/ or N1	III	Tumour involves one or both ovaries with microscopically confirmed peritoneal metastasis outside the pelvis and/or regional lymph node metastasis
T3a	IIIA	Microscopic peritoneal metastasis beyond the pelvis
T3b	IIIB	Macroscopic peritoneal metastasis beyond the pelvis
T3c and/ or N1	IIIC	Peritoneal metastasis beyond pelvis more than 2 cm in greatest dimension and/or regional lymph node metastasis
M1	IV	Distant metastasis (excludes peritoneal metastasis)

Note: liver capsule metastasis is T3/stage III, liver parenchymal metastasis M1/stage IV. Pleural effusion must have positive cytology for M1/stage IV.

N – Regional lymph nodes*

	NX	Regional lymph nodes cannot be assessed
	N0	No regional lymph node metastasis
	N1	Regional lymph node metastasis

M – Distant metastasis

	MX	Distant metastasis cannot be assessed
	M0	No distant metastasis
	M1	Distant metastasis

Stage grouping

Stage IA	T1a	N0	M0
Stage IB	T1b	N0	M0
Stage IC	T1c	N0	M0
Stage IIA	T2a	N0	M0
Stage IIB	T2b	N0	M0
Stage IIC	T2c	N0	M0
Stage IIIA	T3a	N0	M0
Stage IIIB	T3b	N0	M0
Stage IIIC	T3c	N0	M0
	Any T	N1	M0
Stage IV	Any T	Any N	M1

Note: a help desk for specific questions about the TNM classification is available at <http://tnm.uicc.org>.
**The regional lymph nodes are the hypogastric (obturator), common iliac, external iliac, lateral sacral, para-aortic and inguinal nodes.*

decisions regarding fertility preservation, premature hormonal deprivation and adjuvant chemotherapy are particularly pertinent.

These tumours exhibit a papillary growth pattern with fibrous stalks and secondary papillae or micropapillae. The papillae are covered by serous-type epithelium showing nuclear tufting, stratification and cytological atypia.

All BOTs should be sampled thoroughly by pathologists and at least one section per centimetre of maximal tumour diameter should be taken. The macroscopic description should include the presence of exophytic growth, intracystic growth pattern and state of the capsule. Staging of BOTs is crucial for adequate management (Table 2). If there is evidence of capsular rupture, then sections should be taken from the immediate vicinity for histological examination.

Micropapillary serous borderline tumour

This category was first characterised by Burks et al.[16] in 1996 and was designated as 'micropapillary carcinoma'. These tumours are thought to have a more aggressive clinical course than the typical serous BOTs. Six series of micropapillary serous tumours have been described; almost all reported series show higher rates of exophytic growth, extra-ovarian peritoneal implants and bilaterality.[17–19] The most recent study of 276 patients with more than 5-year follow-up,[20] confirmed the higher incidence of bilaterality and peritoneal implants with papillary or cribriform patterns but the differences were not statistically significant. In this study, micropapillary serous BOTs were also more frequently associated with invasive implants as defined by Bell et al.[21] and decreased survival. However, a micropapillary architecture did not have significant effect on survival when controlled for implant type; neither was there significant difference between the two types of serous BOTs with respect to recurrent disease.

Surface serous borderline tumours

Fine papillae with features of BOTs occupy the outer surface of the ovary.

Serous borderline adenofibroma and cystadenofibroma

In this variant, there are glands and cysts lined by atypical epithelium with borderline morphology. The epithelium is set in a dense fibrous stroma.

Peritoneal implants

Two types of peritoneal implants associated with BOTs are recognised – non-invasive and invasive implants. The former almost have no negative influence on the prognosis of BOTs whereas the latter is associated with a poor prognosis (more than 50% have recurrences and the 10-year survival is about 35%). Non-invasive implants are further divided into desmoplastic and epithelial subtypes (Table 3).

Serous borderline tumours with micro-invasion

This category is also called serous tumour of borderline potential, serous tumour of borderline malignancy with micro-invasion. It is an ovarian serous tumour showing early invasion characterised by the presence in the stroma of individual or cluster of neoplastic cells cytologically similar to those of the

Table 3 Classification of peritoneal implants of serous borderline ovarian tumours (modified from Tavassoli and Devilee[2])

Non-invasive implants

Extension into fibrous tissue septa of the omentum
Lacks disorderly infiltration of underlying tissue

Desmoplastic type
Proliferation is localised to peritoneal surface
Predominant > 50% demoplastic stroma (fibroblastic or granulation tissue) containing atypical cells, glands or papillae

Epithelial type
Fills submesothelial spaces
Exophytic proliferation of hierarchical branching papillae
Composed predominantly of epithelial cells without a stromal reaction
Frequent psammoma bodies

Invasive implants

Haphazardly distributed glands invading normal tissue
Predominantly epithelial
Stromal reaction without significant inflammation
Irregular borders
Aneuploidy

---

non-invasive tumour. These invasive cells generally have abundant oesinophilic cytoplasm. One or more foci might be present, none of which should exceed 10 mm^2. The behaviour of this category is similar to that of serous borderline tumours without micro-invasion. Unilateral salpingo-oophorectomy is currently acceptable therapy for young women wishing to preserve fertility.

Mucinous borderline tumours

Mucinous BOTs are divided into endocervical-like (mullerian) and intestinal subtypes, which differ in their morphological appearances and clinical behaviour.[22] The intestinal-type tumours are by far the most common. These tumours are commonly heterogeneous in that they often co-exist with benign and malignant elements.[23]

Several comments on the mucinous BOTs were made by experts in the field who participated in the Borderline Ovarian Tumour Workshop held in Bethesda in 2003. The intestinal (gastrointestinal) type tumours are usually large and unilateral with a smooth capsule, lined by tufted epithelium showing mild-to-moderate cytological atypia. Based on studies published between 1973 and 2002 specific aspects of these tumours were summarised:[24]

1. The vast majority of borderline mucinous ovarian tumours of intestinal type are stage I.

2. Of more than 500 reported stage I cases, approximately 1% were shown to have a fatal outcome (patients died of the disease). Most of these tumours, however, had inadequate or an unknown degree of sampling.

3. A small number (about 100) of the 'advanced borderline tumours' has been reported to have nearly 50% mortality rate. However, 85% of these tumours were associated with the clinical syndrome of pseudomyxoma

peritonei. The latter is currently established to be a complication of an appendiceal primary. Therefore, the existence of an advanced stage borderline mucinous tumour is questionable. When these questionable advanced stage tumours are removed from the primary borderline category, the overwhelming majority will be stage I tumours with favourable outcome.

The mucinous BOTs of endocervical type comprise 10–15% of mucinous BOTs. The mucinous epithelial cells resemble endocervical epithelium. They may be associated with abdominal or pelvic implants, some of which may be invasive. However, in the few reported cases, the behaviour has been indolent.

Mucinous borderline ovarian tumours with intra-epithelial carcinoma

The histological appearances are similar to the intestinal type borderline mucinous tumour but, in addition, there are foci of malignant nuclei often with highly stratified, solid or cribriform areas.

Pseudomyxoma peritonei

It is a clinical term that has traditionally been recognised as a complication of mucinous tumours of the ovary. It used to describe the finding of abundant mucinous or gelatinous material in the pelvis or abdominal cavity surrounded by fibrous tissue. Recent evidence, however, show that ovarian lesions are metastatic from an appendiceal primary.[25,26] A high index of suspicion is required by pathologists to diagnose metastatic tumour to the ovary accurately as such, and not to misdiagnose them as ovarian primaries. Features suggestive of metastatic tumours include: bilaterality, garland pattern of necrosis and prominent vascular invasion. Secondary ovarian tumours are usually of higher stage. A history of a primary mucinous carcinoma elsewhere is helpful. Immunohistochemical staining for several antibodies can be applied to aid in the differential diagnosis although none is specific.[27] The majority of metastatic carcinomas are cytokeratin 7 negative.

In the presence of any epithelial cells within the mucinous material, the pathology report should comment on the degree of epithelial atypia (benign, borderline, malignant) as well as on whether the mucin dissects into tissue with a fibrous response or is merely on the surface. Pseudomyxoma peritonei with benign or borderline epithelium has been termed 'disseminated peritoneal adenomucinosis' which is usually associated with benign or protracted course.[25] The term 'peritoneal mucinous carcinomatosis' has been applied to malignant epithelial cells in pseudomyoma peritonei and the clinical course has usually been fatal, the source being generally the appendix or colon.

It is of note that involvement of the peritoneum, mucinous ascites and superficial organising intra-abdominal mucin that contains tumour cells should not be considered as metastasis from the ovarian tumour. In cases where the tumour is thought to be primary ovarian, the tumour should be placed in the FIGO Ic stage (TNM T1c) in the absence of more advanced disease. On the other hand, if the peritoneal disease is secondary to an appendiceal primary, the tumour should be in the TNM T4 stage. Dissecting mucin with fibrosis places an ovarian tumour in the FIGO stage 2 or 3 (TNM T2 or T3) and makes an intestinal tumour TNM stage 4.[28]

DIAGNOSIS

Clinical presentation

Some BOTs are diagnosed accidentally during investigations for other diseases. This could be due to the indolent nature of these tumours in comparison with invasive ovarian cancers.

A retrospective review of women with stages I and II ovarian cancer or BOTs identified that 78% of the patients were symptomatic. The most common symptoms were abdominal or pelvic pain (34.7%), bloatedness (31.9%) and vaginal bleeding (19.4%). Similar symptoms were reported among women with BOTs and those with cancer with a higher proportion of BOTs patients reporting no symptoms (31.8% versus 18.0%, respectively). Women with BOTs had a significantly longer average time interval between symptoms and diagnosis than women with ovarian carcinoma (8.0 ± 7.7 months versus 3.4 ± 3.7 months, respectively; $P = 0.03$).[29]

In another prospective study, Vine et al.[30] confirmed the above findings using a standardised in-person interview to obtain different symptoms. Women with BOTs had a longer duration of symptoms than women with ovarian carcinoma (median duration of symptoms 6 months versus 4 months, respectively).

Biochemical markers

Cancer antigen 125 (CA 125) is a high molecular weight antigenic glycoprotein. A monoclonal antibody recognises and allows the measurement of CA 125 expression in serum. CA 125 is frequently elevated in serous tumours of the ovary, with significant levels in borderline and malignant ovarian tumours. Cancers of the breast, gastrointestinal tract, and kidney occasionally show increased levels of CA 125. Moreover, some normal tissues like those derived from coelomic epithelia show high levels of CA 125. CA 125 is a tumour-associated rather than a tumour-specific marker.[31] In one study, serous BOTs were found to be associated with high levels of CA 125 in 75% of cases prior to surgery compared with only 30% of mucinous tumours ($P = 0.004$). CA 125 was elevated in 35% of stage IA serous tumours (mean, 67 IU/ml) compared with 89% of tumours with advanced stages (mean, 259 IU/ml; $P = 0.001$).[32]

Other useful tumour markers include: CEA, CA 19-9, CA 15-3, CA 72-4, OVX1, and macrophage-colony stimulating factor (M-CSF). The combination of tumour markers has the advantage of increasing the sensitivity of detection of borderline tumours.[33,34]

Engelen et al.[35] studied the clinical significance of CA 125, CA 19-9 and CEA in borderline ovarian tumours. The authors showed elevated preoperative levels of CA 125 in 8 of 33 (24%), CEA in 3 of 32 (9%), and CA 19-9 in 11 of 24 (46%) cases. In patients with mucinous tumours, the pre-operative CA 19-9 level was more frequently elevated (8/14, 57%) than CA 125 (3/20, 15%; $P = 0.02$) or CEA (2/18, 11%).[35]

Imaging

Ultrasound scanning, especially with the transvaginal approach, detects the ovarian pathology with a high sensitivity (87–95%) depending on the experience of the operator.[36] Different parameters could be assessed by ultrasound scanning including cyst diameter, thickness and regularity of the cyst wall, complexity of the cyst content (septa, solid elements, intracystic projections and vegetations) and the presence of ascites. Colour Doppler ultrasound allows examination of the intracystic blood flow. It has a high sensitivity in differentiating malignancies from benign tumours.[37]

Computerised tomography (CT) is required for adequate staging of suspected ovarian tumour. Full evaluation of the lesion and other abdominal and pelvic structures is feasible using CT with contrast medium. This allows a closer evaluation of the limits of the disease. Detection of omental and lymph node involvement and ascites is also possible using this technology.

Malignant and borderline ovarian tumours are formed of cells that contain high amounts of triglyceride in their membrane and, therefore, show a characteristic spectrum in magnetic resonance imaging (MRI). MRI is a useful technique for predicting malignancy and invasion within ovarian cysts and peritoneal implants. Enhancing endocystic vegetations, local masses within a cyst and irregular thick walls of a large multicystic tumour are important MRI findings of BOTs.[38] MRI was found to have a high specificity in detecting malignancy of an ovarian mass in comparison with the ultrasound scan (84% versus 60%).[39] A Japanese group tested the use of contrast-enhanced MRI in the diagnosis of BOTs. The findings were similar to those previously reported for invasive ovarian cancers.[40]

MANAGEMENT

Management of BOTs is individualised depending on the age of the patient, the stage of the disease, the potential desire for pregnancy and the nature of the peritoneal implants. It is important to establish the borderline nature of the disease prior to contemplating any form of conservative surgery.

Frozen-section evaluation of ovarian tumours can be used to establish pathological diagnosis and guide surgeons to perform a more appropriate intervention. In a study by Houck et al.,[41] the diagnoses of borderline tumours by frozen section and by final pathology were concordant in 60% of cases. Frozen section interpreted a benign lesion as malignant in 10.7% of cases, and interpreted a malignant lesion as benign in 29.3%.[41] Similarly, Gol et al.[42] found that the sensitivity of frozen section in detecting benign, malignant, and BOTs were 98%, 88.7%, and 61%, respectively. The diagnosis of BOTs is sometimes difficult, mainly due to their heterogeneity in appearance, especially in large tumours of mucinous histological type.[43] More recently, a systematic review revealed that diagnostic accuracy rates for frozen-section diagnosis are high for malignant and benign ovarian tumours, but the accuracy rates in BOTs remain relatively low.[44]

Early stage (stage I) BOTs

The majority of mucinous (90%) and serous (65–70%) BOTs present early as stage I disease. Many patients are wishing to preserve their fertility. In carefully staged cases with a borderline lesion confined to one ovary, a more conservative treatment is possible. A unilateral oophrectomy or salpingo-oophrectomy preserves fertility, leaving one functional ovary and the uterus. Several groups have reported pregnancies after such treatment.[45,46] Ovarian cystectomy (either uni- or bilaterally), unilateral salpingo-oophrectomy and contra-lateral ovarian cystectomy have also been reported in the management of BOTs with an increasing risk of recurrence (10–15%). Ovarian tissue preservation and *in vitro* fertilisation is another option that has to be discussed with the patient prior to contemplating surgery.[47] A limited number of stimulation cycles is acceptable in such patients.[48]

Re-operation after a diagnosis of recurrence is possible and another conservative surgery might be appropriate in some cases. Pregnancy outcome and tumour recurrence were evaluated in 44 women treated conservatively (unilateral adnexectomy or cystectomy) for BOTs. There were 17 reported pregnancies; 15 were spontaneous, one after treatment with clomiphene citrate and one after *in-vitro* fertilisation (IVF). The recurrence rate after adnexectomy and cystectomy was 15.1% and 36.3%, respectively. Five patients underwent second, fertility-sparing operations, without relapse during follow-up.[49]

Laparoscopic surgery has been suggested as a limited approach in the management of BOTs. In a study by Seracchioli *et al.*,[50] laparoscopic cystectomy or unilateral salpingo-oophorectomy was evaluated in 19 young women with adnexal masses proved to be BOTs on subsequent histological examination. Peritoneal washings, targeted peritoneal biopsies and biopsy of the other ovary were performed. A second-look laparoscopy was arranged for all cases between 6 and 12 months. One recurrence was observed in a patient who underwent cystectomy at a mean follow-up of 42 (±19) months. There were six spontaneous pregnancies, and all went to term.[50]

Adequate follow-up and removal of the preserved ovary should be carried out after completion of family in order to reduce the risk of ovarian tumour recurrence.[51]

Advanced stage (stages II–IV) BOTs

Extra-ovarian spread is encountered in 30% of serous BOTs. These lesions should be treated more aggressively than the localised, early-stage disease. A laparotomy through a midline incision is ideal for complete surgical staging. This could be extended, cephalically if required, to complete the procedure. Ascitic fluid should be obtained for cytological examination. Otherwise, a generous peritoneal washing of the pelvis, bilateral para-colic gutters as well as sub-diaphragmatic area should be performed. Generally, total abdominal hysterectomy with bilateral salpingo-oophrectomy is the standard procedure together with omentectomy. Removal of all visible disease should be attempted to a maximum of less than 1-cm residuals. Lymph node sampling is proposed by some surgeons in the management of advanced stage BOTs although its role has not yet been established.[47]

The rate and the clinical outcome of lymph node involvement in patients treated for BOTs were assessed in 42 patients. Twenty-four patients had pelvic lymphadenectomy, 6 had para-aortic lymphadenectomy, and 12 had both procedures. Eight patients were found to have lymph node involvement related to the BOTs, all were patients with serous BOT with peritoneal implants. Neither cases with mucinous tumours nor those with early-stage disease (without peritoneal disease) had nodal involvement. None of the patients with nodal involvement died of the borderline tumour. The authors concluded that routine lymphadenectomy is not justified in patients with early-stage disease. This procedure should be performed in cases with serous tumour that are associated with enlarged lymph nodes.[52]

Occasionally, in carefully selected young cases, a more conservative approach might be attempted in order to preserve fertility. Camatte *et al.*[53] reported that of 17 women with stage II or III borderline ovarian tumour treated with fertility preserving surgery, only two tumours recurred and there were no deaths at a median follow-up of 60 months.

Disseminated mucinous BOTs (pseudomyxoma peritoneii) requires repeated surgical removal of the tumour tissue (de-bulking) and mucinous ascites. The prognosis of this form is relatively poor, when compared to simple mucinous BOTs, even after optimal surgical management. Appendicectomy and careful examination of the gastrointestinal tract should be performed.[1]

There is no consensus on the role of adjuvant therapy in cases of BOTs. Observational studies showed that more patients with BOTs die as a result of complications after chemo- or radiotherapy than from progression to invasive ovarian cancer. A Swedish study revealed that, in radically operated patients with low-risk borderline tumours, the prognosis is very good and there is no indication for adjuvant therapy.[54] Chemotherapy is only indicated in the more aggressive BOTs, *e.g.* serous invasive implants and eventually pseudomyxoma peritonei.[55] Generally, these adjuvant modalities are less effective in tumours with cellular proliferation lower than the normal bone marrow.[56]

PROGNOSIS AND FOLLOW-UP

Women with well-sampled borderline serous tumours of FIGO stage Ia and Ib, with or without micro-invasion, have a 5-year survival rate close to 100% and have a very low recurrence rate.[57] However, the exact number of years of follow-up, necessary to consider these patients cured, is still rather controversial. Recent reviews of the literature and Surveillance and Epidemiology End Result (SEER) data[58] confirm lack of adverse events in these patients during a 10-year follow-up period. Among six trials on 373 patients, there were no tumour deaths. A literature review of more than 2000 patients showed survival rates exceeding 95.5%.[59] There are no definitive studies reporting on the significance of a small proportion of borderline morphology in an otherwise benign ovarian tumour.[57]

In another study, Trope *et al.*[60] reported that the 5-year survival for women with stage I BOTs was about 95–97% but, because of late recurrence, the 10-year survival was only 70–95%. The 5-year survival for stage II–III patients was 65–87%. Independent prognostic factors for patients with BOTs without residual disease after primary surgery were: DNA ploidy, morphometry, FIGO stage, histological type, and age.

The prognosis of mucinous BOTs has been shown, in several studies, to be dependent on their stage. The cumulative 5-year survival figures in published series are 95% for stage I tumours and 32% for higher stages.[28,61] The behaviour of mucinous BOTs is summarised in Table 4.

In 1998, Gershenson *et al.*[62,63] observed that approximately 30% of women with either invasive or non-invasive implants had progression or recurrence of disease, with a median time from date of diagnosis of 24 months for those with invasive implants and 7.1 years for those with non-invasive implants.

Follow-up is critically important in women treated conservatively for BOTs as recurrences occur in up to 36% of these cases. Zanetta *et al.*[36] evaluated three different modalities for following up patients after fertility sparing surgery

Table 4 Behaviour of mucinous borderline tumours

Tumour	Tumour type	Extra-ovarian disease	Prognosis
intestinal type	Without intrepithelial carcinoma	None Invasive implants without PP (rare)	Excellent Poor prognosis invasive implants are likely to be due to unsampled invasive areas in the ovarian tumours
Intestinal type	With intrepithelial carcinoma	Invasive implants without PP	Same as above
Any MBT		PP (often primary appendiceal tumour)	Variable depending on degree of atypia of epithelial cells in PP
Endocervical-type		None Invasive or non-invasive implants	Excellent Benign

MBT, mucinous borderline tumour; PP, pseudomyxoma peritonei.

including physical examination, pelvic ultrasonography, and serum CA 125. Patients were assessed every 3 months for the first 2 years and then every 6 months thereafter. Recurrences were observed in 28/164 (17%) women. In 14 patients, there was a palpable mass on pelvic examination. CA 125 levels were elevated in eight patients. Ultrasound revealed an adnexal mass in 23 women and persistent free pelvic fluid in one woman. The study concluded that transvaginal scanning is an effective method for the follow-up of patients treated conservatively for early BOTs.[36]

KEY POINTS FOR CLINICAL PRACTICE

- Borderline ovarian tumours (BOTs) account for 10–15% of all ovarian tumours.
- It remains unclear whether these tumours represent a continuum to invasive cancers or are a separate disease entity.
- The majority of BOTs are of serous and mucinous types.
- Surgery remains the most effective treatment for patients with BOTs.
- In carefully staged cases with BOTs confined to one ovary, a more conservative fertility sparing surgery could be considered.
- Chemotherapy is only indicated in serous BOTs with invasive implants and in cases of pseudomyxoma peritonei.
- Studies have consistently demonstrated the favourable prognosis of these tumours.
- BOTs with invasive implants are associated with recurrence in more than 50% of cases and the 10-year survival is approximately 35%.

References

1 Prat J. Ovarian tumors of borderline malignancy (tumors of low malignant potential): a critical appraisal. Adv Anat Pathol 1999; 6: 247–274

2 Tavassoli FA, Devilee P. World Health Organization Classification of Tumours. Pathology and Genetics of Tumours of the Breast and Female Genital Organs. Lyon: IARC Press, 2003

3 Sherman ME, Berman J, Birrer MJ et al. Current challenges and opportunities for research on borderline ovarian tumors. Hum Pathol 2004; 35: 961–970

4 Auranen A, Grenman S, Makinen J, Pukkala E, Sankila R, Salmi T. Borderline ovarian tumors in Finland: epidemiology and familial occurrence. Am J Epidemiol 1996; 144: 548–553

5 Riman T, Dickman PW, Nilsson S et al. Risk factors for epithelial borderline ovarian tumors: results of a Swedish case-control study. Gynecol Oncol 2001; 83: 575–585

6 Wright JD, Powell MA, Mutch DG et al. Relationship of ovarian neoplasms and body mass index. J Reprod Med 2005; 50: 595–602

7 Jordan SJ, Webb PM, Green AC. Height, age at menarche, and risk of epithelial ovarian cancer. Cancer Epidemiol Biomarkers Prev 2005; 14: 2045–2048

8 Ness RB, Cramer DW, Goodman MT et al. Infertility, fertility drugs, and ovarian cancer: a pooled analysis of case-control studies. Am J Epidemiol 2002; 155: 217–224

9 Gotlieb WH, Flikker S, Davidson B, Korach Y, Kopolovic J, Ben-Baruch G. Borderline tumors of the ovary: fertility treatment, conservative management, and pregnancy outcome. Cancer 1998; 82: 141–146

10 Mosgaard BJ, Lidegaard O, Kjaer SK, Schou G, Andersen AN. Ovarian stimulation and borderline ovarian tumors: a case-control study. Fertil Steril 1998; 70: 1049–1055

11 Mink PJ, Sherman ME, Devesa SS. Incidence patterns of invasive and borderline ovarian tumors among white women and black women in the United States. Results from the SEER Program, 1978–1998. Cancer 2002; 95: 2380–2389

12 Tung KH, Goodman MT, Wu AH et al. Reproductive factors and epithelial ovarian cancer risk by histologic type: a multiethnic case-control study. Am J Epidemiol 2003; 158: 629–638

13 Herrinton LJ, Stanford JL, Schwartz SM, Weiss NS. Ovarian cancer incidence among Asian migrants to the United States and their descendants. J Natl Cancer Inst 1994; 86: 1336–1339

14 Casey MJ, Bewtra C. Peritoneal carcinoma in women with genetic susceptibility: implications for Jewish populations. Fam Cancer 2004; 3: 265–21

15 Green A, Purdie D, Bain C, Siskind V, Webb PM. Cigarette smoking and risk of epithelial ovarian cancer (Australia). Cancer Causes Control 2001; 12: 713–719

16 Burks RT, Sherman ME, Kurman RJ. Micropapillary serous carcinoma of the ovary. A distinctive low-grade carcinoma related to serous borderline tumors. Am J Surg Pathol 1996; 20: 1319–1330

17 Deavers MT, Gershenson DM, Tortolero-Luna G, Malpica A, Lu KH, Silva EG. Micropapillary and cribriform patterns in ovarian serous tumors of low malignant potential: a study of 99 advanced stage cases. Am J Surg Pathol 2002; 26: 1129–1141

18 Gilks CB, Alkushi A, Yue JJ, Lanvin D, Ehlen TG, Miller DM. Advanced-stage serous borderline tumors of the ovary: a clinicopathological study of 49 cases. Int J Gynecol Pathol 2003; 22: 29–36

19 Prat J, De Nictolis M. Serous borderline tumors of the ovary: a long-term follow-up study of 137 cases, including 18 with a micropapillary pattern and 20 with microinvasion. Am J Surg Pathol 2002; 26: 1111–1128

20 Longacre TA, McKenney JK, Tazelaar HD, Kempson RL, Hendrickson MR. Ovarian serous tumors of low malignant potential (borderline tumors): outcome-based study of 276 patients with long-term (≥ 5-year) follow-up. Am J Surg Pathol 2005; 29: 707–723

21 Bell DA, Weinstock MA, Scully RE. Peritoneal implants of ovarian serous borderline tumors. Histologic features and prognosis. Cancer 1988; 62: 2212–2222

22 Siriaunkgul S, Robbins KM, McGowan L, Silverberg SG. Ovarian mucinous tumors of low malignant potential: a clinicopathologic study of 54 tumors of intestinal and mullerian type. Int J Gynecol Pathol 1995; 14: 198–208

23 Hart WR. Mucinous tumors of the ovary: a review. Int J Gynecol Pathol 2005; 24: 4–25

24 Ronnett BM, Kajdacsy-Balla A, Gilks CB *et al*. Mucinous borderline ovarian tumors: points of general agreement and persistent controversies regarding nomenclature, diagnostic criteria, and behavior. Hum Pathol 2004; 35: 949–960

25 Ronnett BM, Kurman RJ, Zahn CM *et al*. Pseudomyxoma peritonei in women: a clinicopathologic analysis of 30 cases with emphasis on site of origin, prognosis, and relationship to ovarian mucinous tumors of low malignant potential. Hum Pathol 1995; 26: 509–524

26 Young RH, Gilks CB, Scully RE. Mucinous tumors of the appendix associated with mucinous tumors of the ovary and pseudomyxoma peritonei. A clinicopathological analysis of 22 cases supporting an origin in the appendix. Am J Surg Pathol 1991; 15: 415–429

27 Hart WR. Diagnostic challenge of secondary (metastatic) ovarian tumors simulating primary endometrioid and mucinous neoplasms. Pathol Int 2005; 55: 231–243

28 Lee KR, Scully RE. Mucinous tumors of the ovary: a clinicopathologic study of 196 borderline tumors (of intestinal type) and carcinomas, including an evaluation of 11 cases with 'pseudomyxoma peritonei'. Am J Surg Pathol 2000; 24: 1447–1464

29 Eltabbakh GH, Yadav PR, Morgan A. Clinical picture of women with early stage ovarian cancer. Gynecol Oncol 1999; 75: 476–479

30 Vine MF, Ness RB, Calingaert B, Schildkraut JM, Berchuck A. Types and duration of symptoms prior to diagnosis of invasive or borderline ovarian tumor. Gynecol Oncol 2001; 83: 466–471

31 Welander CE. What do CA 125 and other antigens tell us about ovarian cancer biology? Acta Obstet Gynecol Scand Suppl 1992; 155: 85–93

32 Gotlieb WH, Soriano D, Achiron R *et al*. CA 125 measurement and ultrasonography in borderline tumors of the ovary. Am J Obstet Gynecol 2000; 183: 541–546

33 Schutter EM, Davelaar EM, van Kamp GJ, Verstraeten RA, Kenemans P, Verheijen RH. The differential diagnostic potential of a panel of tumor markers (CA 125, CA 15-3, and CA 72-4 antigens) in patients with a pelvic mass. Am J Obstet Gynecol 2002; 187: 385–392

34 van Haaften-Day C, Shen Y, Xu F *et al*. OVX1, macrophage-colony stimulating factor, and CA-125-II as tumor markers for epithelial ovarian carcinoma: a critical appraisal. Cancer 2001; 92: 2837–2844

35 Engelen MJ, de Bruijn HW, Hollema H *et al*. Serum CA 125, carcinoembryonic antigen, and CA 19-9 as tumor markers in borderline ovarian tumors. Gynecol Oncol 2000; 78: 16–20.

36 Zanetta G, Rota S, Lissoni A, Meni A, Brancatelli G, Buda A. Ultrasound, physical examination, and CA 125 measurement for the detection of recurrence after conservative surgery for early borderline ovarian tumors. Gynecol Oncol 2001; 81: 63–66

37 Zanetta G, Vergani P, Lissoni A. Color Doppler ultrasound in the preoperative assessment of adnexal masses. Acta Obstet Gynecol Scand 1994; 73: 637–641

38 Van Vierzen PB, Massuger LF, Ruys SH, Barentsz JO. Borderline ovarian malignancy: ultrasound and fast dynamic MR findings. Eur J Radiol 1998; 28: 136–142

39 Grab D, Flock F, Stohr I *et al*. Classification of asymptomatic adnexal masses by ultrasound, magnetic resonance imaging, and positron emission tomography. Gynecol Oncol 2000; 77: 454–459

40 Takemori M, Nishimura R, Hasegawa K. Clinical evaluation of MRI in the diagnosis of borderline ovarian tumors. Acta Obstet Gynecol Scand 2002; 81: 157–161

41 Houck K, Nikrui N, Duska L *et al*. Borderline tumors of the ovary: correlation of frozen and permanent histopathologic diagnosis. Obstet Gynecol 2000; 95: 839–843

42 Gol M, Baloglu A, Yigit S, Dogan M, Aydin C, Yensel U. Accuracy of frozen section diagnosis in ovarian tumors: Is there a change in the course of time? Int J Gynecol Cancer 2003; 13: 593–597

43 Acs G. Intraoperative consultation in gynecologic pathology. Semin Diagn Pathol 2002; 19: 237–254

44 Medeiros LR, Rosa DD, Edelweiss MI *et al*. Accuracy of frozen-section analysis in the diagnosis of ovarian tumors: a systematic quantitative review. Int J Gynecol Cancer 2005; 15: 192–202

45 Morice P, Leblanc E, Rey A *et al*. Conservative treatment in epithelial ovarian cancer: results of a multicentre study of the GCCLCC (Groupe des Chirurgiens de Centre de Lutte Contre le Cancer) and SFOG (Societe Francaise d'Oncologie Gynecologique). Hum Reprod 2005; 20: 1379–1385

46 Boran N, Cil AP, Tulunay G *et al*. Fertility and recurrence results of conservative surgery for borderline ovarian tumors. Gynecol Oncol 2005; 97: 845–851

47 Gershenson DM. Clinical management potential tumours of low malignancy. Best Pract Res Clin Obstet Gynaecol 2002; 16: 513–527

48 Camatte S, Rouzier R, Boccara-Dekeyser J *et al*. [Prognosis and fertility after conservative treatment for ovarian tumors of limited malignity: review of 68 cases]. Gynecol Obstet Fertil 2002; 30: 583–591

49 Morice P, Camatte S, El Hassan J, Pautier P, Duvillard P, Castaigne D. Clinical outcomes and fertility after conservative treatment of ovarian borderline tumors. Fertil Steril 2001; 75: 92–96

50 Seracchioli R, Venturoli S, Colombo FM, Govoni F, Missiroli S, Bagnoli A. Fertility and tumor recurrence rate after conservative laparoscopic management of young women with early-stage borderline ovarian tumors. Fertil Steril 2001; 76: 999–1004

51 Morice P, Camatte S, Wicart-Poque F *et al*. Results of conservative management of epithelial malignant and borderline ovarian tumours. Hum Reprod Update 2003; 9: 185–192

52 Camatte S, Morice P, Atallah D *et al*. Lymph node disorders and prognostic value of nodal involvement in patients treated for a borderline ovarian tumor: an analysis of a series of 42 lymphadenectomies. J Am Coll Surg 2002; 195: 332–338

53 Camatte S, Morice P, Pautier P, Atallah D, Duvillard P, Castaigne D. Fertility results after conservative treatment of advanced stage serous borderline tumour of the ovary. Br J Obstet Gynaecol 2002; 109: 376–380

54 Hogberg T, Glimelius B, Nygren P. A systematic overview of chemotherapy effects in ovarian cancer. Acta Oncol 2001; 40: 340–360

55 Camatte S. [Management of borderline ovarian tumours]. Rev Prat 2004; 54: 1770–1776

56 Kurman RJ, Trimble CL. The behavior of serous tumors of low malignant potential: are they ever malignant? Int J Gynecol Pathol 1993; 12: 120–127

57 Silverberg SG, Bell DA, Kurman RJ *et al*. Borderline ovarian tumors: key points and workshop summary. Hum Pathol 2004; 35: 910–917

58 Trimble CL, Kosary C, Trimble EL. Long-term survival and patterns of care in women with ovarian tumors of low malignant potential. Gynecol Oncol 2002; 86: 34–37

59 Seidman JD, Kurman RJ. Ovarian serous borderline tumors: a critical review of the literature with emphasis on prognostic indicators. Hum Pathol 2000; 31: 539–557

60 Trope CG, Kristensen G, Makar A. Surgery for borderline tumor of the ovary. Semin Surg Oncol 2000; 19: 69–75

61 Watkin W, Silva EG, Gershenson DM. Mucinous carcinoma of the ovary. Pathologic prognostic factors. Cancer 1992; 69: 208–212

62 Gershenson DM, Silva EG, Levy L, Burke TW, Wolf JK, Tornos C. Ovarian serous borderline tumors with invasive peritoneal implants. Cancer 1998; 82: 1096–1103

63 Gershenson DM, Silva EG, Tortolero-Luna G, Levenback C, Morris M, Tornos C. Serous borderline tumors of the ovary with noninvasive peritoneal implants. Cancer 1998; 83: 2157–2163

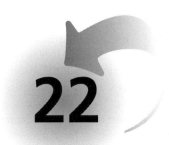

Aradhana Khaund Mary Ann Lumsden

Fibroid embolisation

Uterine leiomyomata are the most common benign tumours of the female genital tract. Many women with fibroids are asymptomatic and do not require clinical intervention. However, it is estimated that 25% of women during reproductive life and over 40% of women above the age of 50 years are affected by these tumours.[1]

The malignant potential of fibroids is less than 1% and thus the main aim of treatment is to provide relief of symptoms and improve quality of life. Symptoms can often be distressing and include menorrhagia, reproductive dysfunction and bulk-related problems such as urinary frequency and pelvic pain.

The traditional treatment of symptomatic fibroids is surgical, namely hysterectomy and myomectomy. Hysterectomy ensures complete resolution of menstrual symptoms and is associated with a high patient satisfaction rate. However, it is also associated with significant morbidity, a relatively long hospital stay and guarantees infertility.[2,3] Myomectomy, whilst aiming to preserve fertility, is also associated with morbidity, a hospital stay of a few days and carries the risk of proceeding to emergency hysterectomy. In addition, it may further compromise reproductive potential and provide clinicians with difficulties in long-term management owing to the high recurrence rate of fibroids and adhesion formation.[4]

Medical treatments such as the levonorgestrel intra-uterine system (Mirena IUS) and gonadotrophin-releasing hormone (GnRH) analogues have also been

Aradhana Khaund MRCOG (for correspondence)
Specialist Registrar in Obstetrics and Gynaecology, South Glasgow University Hospitals NHS Trust, Southern General Hospital, 1345 Govan Road, Glasgow G51 4TF, UK
E-mail: aradhana@postmaster.co.uk

Mary Ann Lumsden MD FRCOG
Professor of Reproductive and Maternal Medicine, Division of Developmental Medicine, Glasgow Royal Infirmary, 10 Alexandra Parade, Glasgow G31 2ER, UK
E-mail: M.A.Lumsden@clinmed.gla.ac.uk

used to treat fibroid-associated menorrhagia and pain, with limited success. The Mirena IUS is only useful if the fibroids are small and there is minimal distortion of the uterine cavity.[5] GnRH analogues, whilst proven to be effective in shrinking fibroids and greatly improving menstrual symptoms, are limited by their side-effect profile, in particular, osteoporosis and unpleasant menopausal symptoms. Even when used in conjunction with add-back therapy, they are only a short-term treatment solution for symptomatic fibroids. Analogues are, however, useful in reducing peri-operative blood loss, when administered for short periods of time pre-myomectomy.[6]

With the evolution of minimally invasive surgical and non-surgical techniques, and changing attitudes towards uterine preservation, the popularity of conservative treatment options has escalated over the last decade. Uterine artery embolisation (UAE) is a minimally invasive angiographic procedure which is increasingly being used as an alternative to surgery for symptomatic fibroids. Other conservative therapies include laparoscopic myolysis, MRI-guided percutaneous laser ablation, interstitial laser photocoagulation and high-intensity focused ultrasound energy. The latter modalities are relatively new and, therefore, the data on their clinical outcomes are limited.[7–10]

UAE has been used in the management of acute pelvic haemorrhage for more than two decades. Its use, however, in the treatment of symptomatic fibroids, was first reported in France by Ravina and colleagues, in 1995.[11] Since then, thousands of UAE procedures have been performed in the UK and it is now estimated that more than 50,000 have been carried out world-wide. With increasing experience of fibroid embolisation, there is a greater understanding of the indications, patient selection, pre- and post-procedural imaging, potential risks and clinical outcomes associated with this technique.

PATIENT SELECTION

Optimal pre-procedural selection of women is vital for high clinical success rates and avoidance of complications following UAE. Women who have symptomatic fibroids in the absence of other pelvic pathology are suitable candidates. Exclusion of women with adenomyosis is necessary as this particular uterine pathology responds less well than fibroids to embolisation.[12] Those with pedunculated subserosal fibroids should also be excluded owing to the risk of ischaemic necrosis and potential for the fibroid to disintegrate and become free in the abdomen. The latter may be further complicated by causing peritoneal irritation, infection and possibly even bowel adhesions.[13]

Confirmed or suspected pelvic infection, an undiagnosed pelvic mass, the immunocompromised and severe contrast allergy are other contra-indications. Previous pelvic irradiation or surgery and coagulopathies are relative contra-indications to the procedure. UAE is particularly useful in women who are not ideal candidates for surgery. Such patients include the morbidly obese, diabetic and those with multiple medical problems. Embolisation is also a useful alternative to surgery in women who refuse blood transfusions. These women, however, must be counselled about the risk of emergency hysterectomy.

Pregnancy is an absolute contra-indication to UAE and, until the effects of embolisation on reproductive potential have been fully established, the procedure should be offered to women who desire future fertility with much caution.

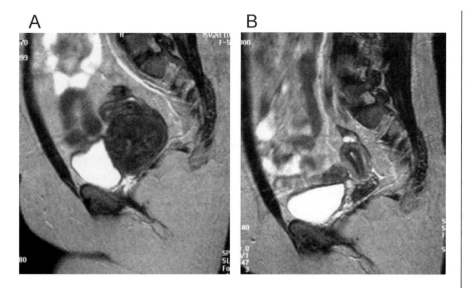

Fig. 1 (A) Pre-embolisation MRI. Sagittal T1-gadolinium enhanced sequence. Normal sized uterus displaced upwards by large cervical fibroid which shows good enhancement. (B) Post-embolisation MRI. Sagittal T1-gadolinium enhanced sequence. Note marked reduction in cervical fibroid volume and the return of the body of the uterus to its correct anatomical site.

PRE-PROCEDURAL EVALUATION

Detailed gynaecological and general medical histories should be taken and a gynaecological examination performed. All women should have separate consultations with a gynaecologist and interventional radiologist. This team approach is the key to a successful outcome. Baseline full blood count, ferritin levels and a coagulation screen should be performed. A hormone profile should also be considered, to provide information about ovarian reserve. Ideally, women should be screened for infection, with vaginal swabs and a serum C-reactive protein estimation. Endometrial biopsy should be performed where appropriate, to exclude endometrial hyperplasia and malignancy. For example, women with irregular cycles, constant or intermenstrual bleeding and those with prolonged menses or mennorhagia above the age of 45 years, should all undergo endometrial evaluation prior to UAE. This can be done with an out-patient pipelle endometrial biopsy or during formal hysteroscopy and endometrial biopsy.

Uterine imaging must be performed, first to confirm the diagnosis of fibroids, and second to provide information on their location, size and number. It also assists in excluding other pelvic pathology which may be responsible for a woman's symptomatology. Imaging should also assess the viability of the fibroid. Those tumours with a poor blood supply (*e.g.* calcified fibroids or degenerative fibroids with cystic or haemorrhagic necrosis) are more likely to respond poorly to embolisation.[14,15] Whilst Doppler ultrasound is used in some centres to fulfil these tasks, most radiologists prefer to use contrast-enhanced magnetic resonance imaging (MRI) where available (Fig. 1A).

A 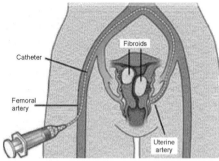 B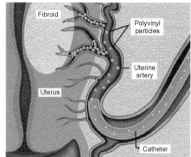

Fig. 2 (A) Transfemoral catheterisation of the uterine arteries. (B) Injection of poly-vinylalcohol particles into the circulation to effect embolisation.

PROCEDURE

Bilateral UAE is performed by appropriately trained interventional radiologists using a standard technique. The procedure is usually carried out under conscious sedation, although spinal or epidural anaesthesia have been used as alternatives. Anti-emetics are administered and local anaesthetic is infiltrated into the groin prior to percutaneous catheterisation of each of the femoral arteries. Thereafter, both internal iliac arteries are selectively catheterised in turn, allowing catheterisation of their respective uterine arteries (Fig. 2A). The latter is facilitated by contrast enhancement and digital fluoroscopy (Fig. 3A). Once catheter placement is confirmed and the vascular supply to the fibroids and uterus demonstrated, multiple small particulate emboli in the form

A 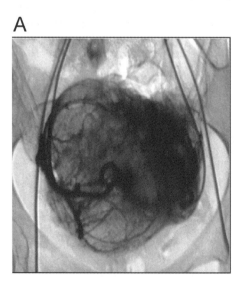 B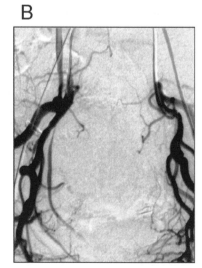

Fig. 3 (A) Pre-embolisation angiogram demonstrating simultaneous catheterisation of both uterine arteries and the tortuous branches of the uterine arteries supplying the fibroid uterus. (B) Post-embolisation angiogram showing virtually no demonstrable flow in the distal uterine arteries, thus highlighting that the embolic procedure is complete.

of polyvinyl alcohol particles (PVA, 500–710 μm in diameter) are then injected into the circulation (Fig. 2B). The aim of the embolic material is to occlude both uterine arteries selectively, resulting in fibroid devascularisation and subsequent fibroid shrinkage. Owing to the rich pelvic collateral circulation, however, the normal myometrial tissue revascularises. Initially, embolisation was considered complete when there was virtually no demonstrable flow in the distal uterine artery (Fig. 3B).[11,13,16] With increasing experience and the evolution of embolic materials, the degree of arterial occlusion has become more precise and most radiologists aim to achieve arterial blushing rather than stasis, where the main arterial trunk is left patent at the end of the procedure.[17] This improved precision allows more targeted fibroid embolisation with concurrent reduced unnecessary devascularisation of the myometrium and ovarian vessels.

Individual procedures take about 45 min to complete and every effort is made to keep the total fluoroscopy time and number of image sequences taken to a minimum, thus reducing the radiation penalty to the ovaries.

POST-PROCEDURAL EVALUATION

Most patients experience a degree of pain after the second uterine artery is embolised. This may be accompanied by nausea and vomiting which responds to intravenous anti-emetics. Pelvic or abdominal pain usually peaks at 6–12 h post-procedure and it tends to be self-limiting over a further 12 h. For this reason, most women undergo this procedure either as a day-case or with a single overnight hospital stay where they can receive adequate pain control. A clear pain management protocol should be in place to facilitate this. A combination of oral non-steroidal anti-inflammatory drugs and a paracetamol/codeine-based preparation can provide adequate pain relief post-embolisation, but usually, opiate analgesia is required in the immediate postoperative period.

It is common to experience mild lower abdominal cramps for the next 7–14 days and most women return to normal activities within a couple of weeks. They should be made aware of all potential complications and side effects of the procedure and have an emergency contact number in their possession, prior to discharge from hospital.

All women should undergo postembolisation uterine imaging, usually with contrast-enhanced MRI (Fig. 1B). This is to assess fibroid shrinkage and vascularity, and tends to be performed 6 months after the procedure. In addition, women should be reviewed by both gynaecologist and interventional radiologist within the 6-month postembolisation period.

COMPLICATIONS AND SIDE EFFECTS

Contrast allergy

Allergy to the contrast medium used during MRI is rare and occurs in about 1% of patients.

Puncture site

Complications in this area include bleeding, haematoma formation and infection. They occur in less than 1% of women.

Radiation exposure

The radiation penalty to the ovaries appears to be minimal and occurs during digital fluoroscopy at the time of arterial catheterisation. Radiologists aim to keep individual fluoroscopic time to a minimum with a radiation dose which is similar to that of a barium enema.[18]

Non-target embolisation

Misembolisation may occur either as a result of poor technique or due to the presence of aberrant arteries. It can cause premature ovarian failure and ischaemia or necrosis of neighbouring organs.[19]

Postembolisation syndrome

This syndrome manifests as general malaise, a low-grade fever, pelvic pain, nausea and vomiting. It is associated with a leukocytosis and is difficult to distinguish from clinical infection. It occurs in up to 10% of women, typically 7–21 days after UAE. The syndrome is thought to result from the release of inflammatory mediators from fibroid tissue that has been rendered ischaemic. Management includes adequate pain control, hydration, prophylactic antibiotics and re-assurance.[16]

Fibroid expulsion

Transcervical fibroid expulsion has been reported in up to 5% of women.[20] This may occur as a result of uterine shrinkage forcing an intramural fibroid into the uterine cavity. Expulsion is more common in the presence of submucous fibroids. Intense abdominal pain can occur just prior to fibroid expulsion when the cervical canal is obstructed. Occasionally, fibroids are partially extruded and require hysterecopic myomectomy for complete removal.[21]

Persistent vaginal discharge

This occurs in approximately 4% of women after embolisation and may persist for a few weeks to many months.[16] It is due to the expulsion of fibroid necrotic tissue and if not self-limiting, may require antibiotic prophylaxis or (hysteroscopic) endometrial curettage.

Amenorrhoea and premature menopause

Transient amenorrhoea occurs in 5–10% of women after UAE. Permanent amenorrhoea occurs in up to 15% of women beyond the age of 45 years and in 1% of younger women. This is usually a consequence of embolic material entering the ovarian arterial circulation via uterine–ovarian anastomotic vessels.[22–24] The resultant reduced ovarian perfusion eventually leads to ischaemia. All women should be thoroughly counselled about this important potential side effect and its consequences, prior to undergoing embolisation.

Infection

Infection is potentially the most serious complication following UAE.[18,20,25] This may vary from mild infection requiring a course of oral or intravenous antibiotics, to pelvic sepsis, necessitating emergency hysterectomy. The latter occurs in less than 1% of cases and can be life-threatening. Two cases of death secondary to sepsis following UAE have been reported in the literature, to date.[26,27] Any patient, therefore, presenting with worsening pelvic pain, fever, vaginal discharge and leukocytosis following embolisation should be admitted as soon as possible. A full infection screen and uterine imaging should be performed urgently and the appropriate treatment administered promptly.

REPRODUCTIVE OUTCOME

The effect of embolisation on fertility and pregnancy is still not fully established. However, successful conceptions, pregnancies and deliveries have been reported in women following the procedure.[13,16,28,29]

It has been suggested by some authors that the rates of miscarriage, intra-uterine growth restriction, preterm delivery and post-partum haemorrhage are higher following UAE, all of which are complications thought to be due to alterations in uterine blood flow after the procedure.[28] It should also be borne in mind that women undergoing embolisation tend to be older and have large or multiple fibroids, factors which also influence fecundity.

Re-assuringly, MRI of the uterus performed 3–6 months postembolisation reveals rapid re-vascularisation of the normal myometrium and an essentially normal appearance of the endometrium.[15,30,31]

Whilst most women who undergo UAE have completed their family, the procedure may be offered to women who wish to retain their fertility with caution. The latter group of women must be thoroughly counselled about the potential risk of ovarian failure and be made aware that data on fertility and pregnancy remain limited.

CLINICAL OUTCOMES

The efficacy of uterine artery embolisation can be determined by the degree of improvement or resolution of symptoms. Most studies divide fibroid-associated symptoms into excessive menstrual bleeding, pelvic pain and bulk-related problems. Clinical success rates for treating these complaints range from 81–96%, 70–100% and 46–100%, respectively.[11,16,22]

Uterine volume reduction and thus fibroid shrinkage, can be measured by ultrasound or MRI. A 25–60% reduction in uterine volume has been reported between 3–6 months following UAE.[11,16,22] It should be noted, however, that reductions in fibroid volume do not always reflect an improvement in clinical symptoms.

A prospective observational study of 53 women undergoing UAE demonstrated a statistically significant reduction in objective menstrual blood loss following UAE using the alkaline haematin technique. This decline in blood loss was maintained up to 4 years after treatment (Fig. 4).[32,33]

Subjective assessments are also useful when evaluating the efficacy of a procedure or intervention. Health-related quality of life instruments such as the Short Form 36 (SF-36), assist in carrying out the latter as do menstrual questionnaires.[34,35] Satisfaction rates of 97% have been reported after embolisation and, in most cases, this tends to parallel improvements in

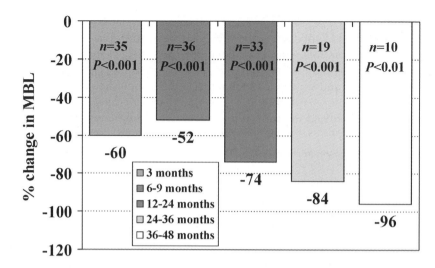

Post-treatment time intervals

Fig. 4 Median percentage reductions in MBL at all post-treatment time intervals.

symptoms.[16] Recently, a disease-specific questionnaire[36] has been created for fibroids which used in combination with a generic questionnaire such as the SF-36, provides further useful information regarding the efficacy of UAE. The fibroid specific UFS-QOL questionnaire aims to assess both symptom severity and quality of life, but as yet, has not been fully validated.

Three prospective clinical trials comparing the outcome of UAE and hysterectomy have been published to date.[37-39] UAE has been shown to be associated with a shorter hospital stay and recovery time when compared to hysterectomy. Whilst associated with a low complication rate, the higher re-admission rates after embolisation highlight the need for careful post-procedural follow-up.

The risks of major complications such as pelvic sepsis, emergency hysterectomy and premature ovarian failure are low. More evidence, however, is required on long-term outcomes following UAE and the effects of the procedure on both fertility and pregnancy. More prospective studies are also required to compare embolisation to myomectomy and hysterectomy.

KEY POINTS FOR CLINICAL PRACTICE

- Uterine artery embolisation (UAE) is both safe and efficacious and should be considered as an alternative to surgery, for women with symptomatic fibroids.

- A multidisciplinary approach is required for patient selection and follow-up with equal input and close liaison between gynaecologist and interventional radiologist.

- UAE is of proven benefit in women complaining of heavy menstrual loss.

KEY POINTS FOR CLINICAL PRACTICE

- UAE may be of limited value in women with large fibroids associated with only bulk-related symptoms, bearing in mind that mean fibroid shrinkage is less than 50%.

- All women undergoing UAE should be counselled thoroughly regarding the risk of ovarian failure.

- UAE should be used with caution in those women who wish to retain their fertility as its effects on fecundity and pregnancy have not been fully established.

- The incidence of fibroid recurrence following UAE is unknown.

- Studies are required comparing UAE to other uterine-sparing modalities.

- Long-term data on outcomes after UAE are not currently available.

References

1 Buttram VC, Reiter RC. Uterine leiomyomata: etiology, symptomatology and management. Fertil Steril 1981; 36: 433–445

2 Vessey MP, Villard-Makintosh L, Macpherson K, Coulter A, Yeates D. The epidemiology of hysterectomy: findings in a large cohort study. Br J Obstet Gynaecol 1992; 99: 402–407

3 Lumsden MA. Embolisation versus myomectomy versus hysterectomy – which is best, when? Hum Reprod 2002; 17: 253–259

4 Stewart EA. Uterine fibroids. Lancet 2001; 357: 293–298

5 Grigorieva V, Chen-Mok M, Tarasova M, Mikhailov A. Use of a levonorgestrel-releasing intra-uterine system to treat bleeding related to uterine leiomyomas. Fertil Steril 2003; 79: 1194–1198

6 Lethaby A, Vollhoven B, Sowter M. Pre-operative GnRH analogue therapy before hyster-ectomy or myomectomy for uterine fibroids. Cochrane Database Syst Rev 2000; (2): CD000547

7 Donnez J, Squifflet J, Polet R, Nisolle M. Laparoscopic myolysis. Hum Reprod Update 2000; 6: 609–613

8 Hindley JT, Law PA, Hickey M et al. Clinical outcomes following percutaneous magnetic resonance image guided laser ablation of symptomatic uterine fibroids, Hum Reprod 2002; 17: 2737–2741

9 Visvanathan D, Connell R, Hall-Craggs MA, Cutner AS, Brown SG. Interstitial laser photocoagulation for uterine myomas. Am J Obstet Gynecol 2002; 187: 382–384

10 Chan AH, Fujimoto VY, Moore DE, Martin RW, Vaezy S. An image-guided high intensity focused ultrasound device for uterine fibroids treatment. Med Phys 2002; 29: 2611–2620

11 Ravina JH, Herbreteau C, Ciraru-Vigneron N et al. Arterial embolisation to treat uterine myomata. Lancet 1995; 346: 671–672

12 Jha RC, Takahama J, Imaoka I et al. Adenomyosis: MRI of the uterus treated with uterine artery embolization. AJR Am J Roentgenol 2003; 181: 851–856

13 Pelage JP, Le Dref O, Soyer P et al. Fibroid-related menorrhagia: treatment with superselective embolization of the uterine arteries and midterm follow-up. Radiology 2000; 215: 428–431

14 Marret H, Tranquart F, Sauget S, Alonso AM, Cottier JP, Herbreteau D. Contrast-enhanced sonography during uterine artery embolization for the treatment of leiomyomas. Ultrasound Obstet Gynecol 2004; 23: 77–79

15 deSouza NM, Williams AD. Uterine arterial embolization for leiomyomas: perfusion and volume changes at MR imaging and relation to clinical outcome. Radiology 2002; 222: 367–374

16 Walker WJ, Pelage JP. Uterine artery embolization for symptomatic fibroids: clinical results in 400 women with imaging follow-up. Br J Obstet Gynaecol 2002; 109: 1262–1272

17 Pelage JP, Le Dref O, Beregi JP *et al.* Limited uterine artery embolization with tri-acryl gelatine microspheres for uterine fibroids. J Vasc Intervent Radiol 2003; 14: 11–14

18 Vilos GA. Side effects and complications of embolization. In: Tulandi T. (ed) Uterine Fibroids. Embolization and Other Treatments. Cambridge: Cambridge University Press, 2003; 111–117

19 Burbank F, Hutchins FL. Uterine artery occlusion by embolization or surgery for the treatment of fibroids: a unifying hypothesis-transient uterine ischaemia. J Am Assoc Gynecol Laparosc 2000; 7: S1–S4

20 Spies JB, Spector A, Roth AR *et al.* Complications after uterine artery embolization for leiomyomas. Obstet Gynecol 2002; 100: 873–880

21 Marret H, Keris YLB, Acker O *et al.* Late leiomyoma expulsion after uterine artery emboliz-ation. J Vasc Intervent Radiol 2004; 12: 1483–1485

22 Spies JB, Scialli AR, Jha RC *et al.* Initial results from uterine fibroid embolization for symptomatic leiomyomata. J Vasc Intervent Radiol 1999; 10: 1149–1159

23 Goodwin SG, McLucas B, Lee M *et al.* Uterine artery embolisation for the treatment of uterine leiomyomata: midterm results. J Vasc Intervent Radiol 1999; 10: 1159–1165

24 Tulandi T, Sammour A, Valenti D *et al.* Uterine artery embolization and utero-ovarian-collateral. J Am Assoc Gynecol Laparosc 2001; 8: 474

25 Pron G, Mocarski E, Cohen M *et al.* Hysterectomy for complications after uterine artery embol-ization for leiomyomata: results of a Canadian multicenter clinical trial. J Am Assoc Gynecol Laparosc 2003; 10: 99–106

26 Vashist A, Stuff J, Carey A, Burn P. Fatal septicaemia after fibroid embolization. Lancet 1999; 354: 307–308

27 Lanocita R, Frigerio LF, Patelli G, Di Tolla G, Spreafico C. A fatal complication of percutaneous transcatheter embolization for the treatment of uterine fibroids. Paper presented at Society for Minimally Invasive Therapy Meeting. 1999; Boston, MA, USA

28 Pron G, Mocarski E, Bennett J, Vilos G, Common A, Vanderburgh L. Pregnancy after uterine artery embolization for leiomyomata: the Ontario multicenter trial. Obstet Gynecol 2005; 105: 67–76

29 Carpenter TT, Walker WJ. Pregnancy following uterine artery embolisation for symptomatic fibroids: a series of 26 completed pregnancies. Br J Obstet Gynaecol 2005; 112: 321–325

30 Pelage JP, Guaou-Guaou N, Jha RC, Ascher SM, Spies JB. Uterine fibroid tumours: long-term MR imaging outcome after embolization. Radiology 2004; 230: 803–809

31 Katsumori T, Nakajima K, Tokuhiro M. Gadolinium enhanced MR imaging in the evaluation of uterine fibroids treated with uterine artery embolization. AJR Am J Roentgenol 2001; 177: 303–307

32 Hallberg L, Hogdahl AM, Nillson L, Rybo G. Menstrual blood loss – a population loss and uterine volume. Acta Obstet Gynecol Scand 1966; 45: 320–351

33 Khaund A, Moss JG, McMillan N, Lumsden MA. Evaluation of the effects of uterine artery embolisation on menstrual blood Br J Obstet Gynaecol 2004; 111: 700–706

34 Jenkinson C, Coulter A, Wright L. Short form 36 (SF 36) health survey questionnaire: normative data for adults of working age. BMJ 1993; 306: 1437–1441

35 Worthington-Kirsch RL, Popky GL, Hutchins FL. Uterine arterial embolisation for the manage-ment of leiomyomas: quality-of-life assessment and clinical response. Radiology 1998; 208: 625–629

36 Spies JB, Coyne KC, Guaou Guaou, N, Boyle D, Skyrnarz-Murphy K, Gonzalves SM. The UFS-QOL, a new disease-specific symptom and health-related quality of life questionnaire for leiomyomata. Obstet Gynecol 2002; 99: 290–300

37 Pinto I, Chimeno P, Roma A *et al.* Uterine fibroids: uterine artery embolization versus abdominal hysterectomy for treatment – a prospective, randomised and controlled clinical trial. Radiology 2003; 226: 425–431

38 Spies JB, Cooper JM, Worthington-Kirsch R *et al.* Outcome of uterine artery embolization and hysterectomy for leiomyomas; results from a multicenter study. Am J Obstet Gynecol 2004; 191: 22–31

39 Hehenkamp WJ, Volkers NA, Donderwinkel PF *et al.* Uterine artery embolization versus hysterectomy in the treatment of symptomatic uterine fibroids (EMMY trial): peri- and postprocedural results from a randomised controlled trial. Am J Obstet Gynecol 2005; 193: 1618–1629

Diaa M. El-Mowafi

Laparoscopic management of endometriosis

Endometriosis is a significant health problem for women of reproductive age. Defined as the presence of endometrial-like glands and stroma in any extra-uterine site, it is a disease that has fascinated gynecologists for more than a century.

INCIDENCE

Endometriosis occurs in 7–10% of women in the general population and up to 50% of premenopausal women,[1] with a prevalence of 38% (range, 20–50%)[2–4] in infertile women, and in 71–87% of women with chronic pelvic pain.[5–7] Contrary to much speculation, there are no data to support the view that the incidence of endometriosis is increasing, although improved recognition of endometriosis lesions[8] may have led to an increase in the rate of detection. There also appears to be no particular racial predisposition to endometriosis.

A familial association of endometriosis has been documented,[9] and patients with an affected first-degree relative have nearly a 10-fold increased risk of developing endometriosis.

ETIOLOGY

Although the pathogenesis of endometriosis remains unclear, leading theories include retrograde menstruation, hematogenous or lymphatic transport, and coelomic metaplasia. It has been suggested that virtually all women are potentially vulnerable to the development of the lesions of endometriosis, but

Diaa M. El-Mowafi MD
Professor, Obstetrics and Gynecology Department, Benha Faculty of Medicine, Egypt
Educator & Researcher, Wayne State University, Detroit, Michigan, USA
Fellow, Geneva University, Geneva, Switzerland
Consultant & Head of Obstetrics and Gynecology Department, King Khalid General Hospital,
Hafr El-Batin, Saudi Arabia
E-mail: dmowafi@yahoo.com

appropriate immunocompetency in most eradicates such lesions in a timely fashion, preventing clinical sequelae.[10] Menstrual flow that produces a greater volume of retrograde menstruation may increase the risk of developing endometriosis. Cervical or vaginal atresia with outflow obstruction also is linked with the development of endometriosis.[11] Early menarche, regular cycles (especially without intervening pregnancy-induced amenorrhea), and a longer and heavier than normal flow are associated with this disease.[12] Because endometriosis is an estrogen-dependent disease, factors that reduce estrogen levels, such as exercise-induced menstrual disorders, decreased body-fat content, and tobacco smoking, are associated with reduced risk of developing endometriosis.[12] The commonest sites for endometrial implantation within the pelvis are the ovaries, broad and round ligaments, Fallopian tubes, cervix, vagina and pouch of Douglas. The gastrointestinal tract may be involved in about 12% of cases and the urinary tract is affected in about 1%.

CLINICAL MANIFESTATIONS

The clinical manifestations of endometriosis are variable and unpredictable in both presentation and course. Dysmenorrhea, chronic pelvic pain, dyspareunia, uterosacral ligament nodularity, and adnexal mass (either symptomatic or asymptomatic) are among the well-recognized manifestations.[13–16] A significant number of women with endometriosis remain asymptomatic.

The association between endometriosis and infertility remains the subject of considerable debate.

Pelvic pain that is typical of endometriosis is characteristically described as secondary dysmenorrhea (with pain frequently commencing prior to the onset of menses), deep dyspareunia (exaggerated during menses), or sacral backache with menses. Endometriosis that involves specific organs may result in pain or physiological dysfunction of those organs, such as perimenstrual tenesmus or diarrhea in cases of bowel involvement or dysuria and hematuria in cases of bladder involvement.

The pain associated with endometriosis has little relationship to the type or location of the lesions that are visible at laparoscopy.[17]

DIAGNOSIS

Direct visualization confirmed by histological examination, especially of lesions with non-classical appearance,[18–20] remains the standard for diagnosing endometriosis. The presence of two or more of the following histological features is used as the threshold criteria for the diagnosis by a pathologist:[21] (i) endometrial epithelium; (ii) endometrial glands; (iii) endometrial stroma; and (iv) hemosiderin-laden macrophages.

Visual inspection as the sole means for making the diagnosis of endometriosis requires an experienced surgeon who is familiar with the protean appearances of endometriosis. Experience is associated with increased diagnostic accuracy,[8,18,19] but the correlation between visual inspection and histological confirmation of the presence of endometriosis in biopsy specimens is imperfect.[19] Although laparoscopy remains the investigation of choice in the diagnosis of endometriosis, imaging does play a significant role in its management.

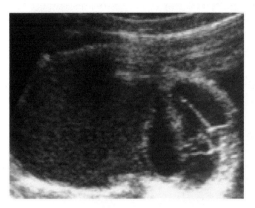

Fig. 1 Transabdominal ultrasound showing a multiloculated ovarian endometrioma containing low level echoes.

Currently available laboratory tests lack the necessary sensitivity and specificity to serve as reliable screening tests for endometriosis, although there is growing evidence that carcino-embryonic antigen CA125 may help to evaluate selected populations at risk, to follow the course of the disease and to monitor response to treatment.[22]

IMAGING STUDIES

Ultrasonography

High-resolution images may be obtained via the transvaginal approach using a 7.5 MHz probe. Sensitivity in the detection of focal endometrial implants is poor. However, the detection of endometriomas using ultrasound is excellent, with reports of 83% sensitivity and 98% specificity. Diagnostic accuracy may be enhanced by Doppler flow studies where blood flow in endometriomas is usually pericystic with a resistive index above 0.45.[23]

There is a broad range of ultrasound appearances of endometriomas. Diffuse, low-level internal echoes occur in 95% of endometriomas (Fig. 1). Hyperechoic wall foci and multilocularity also point towards an endometrioma.[24]

Computed tomography

Endometriomas may appear solid, cystic, or mixed solid and cystic, resulting in an overlap in the appearances with an abscess, ovarian cyst or even a malignant lesion (Fig. 2). Owing to the poor specificity and high radiation dose, use of CT in the evaluation of pelvic endometriosis has been replaced by MRI.

Magnetic resonance imaging

Identification of endometriomas by MRI relies on detection of pigmented haemorrhagic lesions. Signal characteristics vary according to the age of haemorrhage

1. Typically, lesions appear hyperintense on T_1-weighted spin echo (T1WSE)

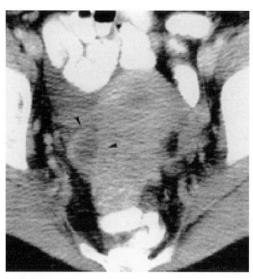

Fig. 2 Oral and intravenous contrast enhanced CT through the pelvis showing the endometrioma as a partly cystic mass posterior to the uterus and anterior to the rectosigmoid junction (arrow heads).

images and hypo-intense (shading) on T_2-weighted turbo spin echo (T2WTSE) images owing to the presence of deoxyhemoglobin and methemoglobin (Fig. 3 & 4).

2. Acute haemorrhage occasionally appears hypo-intense on T1WSE and T2WTSE sequences.

3. Old haemorrhage occasionally appears hyperintense on T1WSE and T2WTSE images.[23]

Endometrial implants are often small and express signal intensity similar to that of normal endometrium on both T1WSE and T2WTSE images.[24] Depending on hormonal influences, they exhibit varying degrees of haemorrhage.

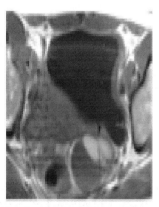
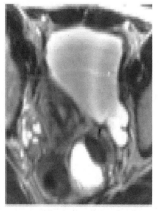

Fig. 3 Multiloculated left ovarian endometrioma showing (A) high signal intensity on T_1-weighted spin echo axial image and (B) low signal intensity on T_2-weighted turbo spin echo image (arrow heads), in keeping with the products of hemorrhage.

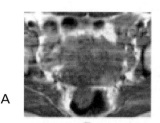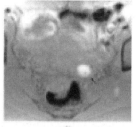

A   B

Fig. 4 The left pelvic endometrioma (arrow) is barely perceptible on the standard T_1-weighted spin echo (T1WSE) axial image (A), but is much better appreciated as an area of high signal intensity on the T1WSE fat suppressed sequence (B) owing to the presence of methemoglobin.

ENDOMETRIOSIS AND INFERTILITY

Treatment options for endometriosis-associated infertility include medical therapy, surgical intervention, and assisted reproduction. For endometriosis-associated infertility, medical therapy seems to have no value alone. Surgical therapy is beneficial for all stages of diseases, as well as assisted reproduction. The suggestion for the treatment of early-stage endometriosis is surgery and/or superovulation with intra-uterine insemination as first-line treatments. For more advanced disease, with tubal damage, surgery or *in vitro* fertilization are options. For the most advanced cases, *in vitro* fertilization preceded by 3 months of medical treatment of the endometriosis is advised.[25]

The goal of conservative surgery is to remove all apparent endometriosis from the abdomen and pelvis and restore normal anatomical relations. Actually, there is no proven difference in efficacy between open and endoscopic surgery for endometriosis.[26] However, the cost is lower, and the recovery time shorter with laparoscopy, even in women with advanced endometriosis.

A variety of instruments have been used in the treatment of endometriosis, ranging from scissors and monopolar cautery to multiple types of lasers and ultrasonic scalpels. There is no evidence that any of these instruments is superior to others in terms of efficacy in removing implants of endometriosis or lower frequency of complications.

Another pertinent issue involves the method of destruction of implants. Options include excision, vaporization, and the combination of fulguration and desiccation. These techniques have not been compared with one another in randomized trials, despite the fact that each approach has vocal proponents. In one retrospective study comparing the fertility rates in 101 women with early-stage disease treated by the excision of implants or by electrocoagulation, there was no difference between the two treatments.[27]

Laparoscopy versus laparotomy

The era of operative laparoscopy started in the 1980s and expanded to involve most of the previous traditional pelvic surgery. The advantages of endoscopic surgery are claimed to be reduction of hospital stay, postoperative pain, length of abdominal incision, and expense. One of the claims is the reduction of subsequent postoperative adhesion formation. This view is supported, in theory, by the concepts of lack of retractors and packs' usage at laparoscopy, maintaining a closed abdomen with presumed reduction in peritoneal drying, less likelihood of introduction of foreign bodies, decreased possibility of blind dissection of adhesions during abdominal exploration and less tissue damage at the abdominal wall incision(s) compared to that of laparotomy. Luciano and co-worker[28] have demonstrated no intra-abdominal adhesions in rabbits with the lesions created laparoscopically, whereas those lesions created at laparotomy were consistently followed by adhesion formation. Furthermore, the investigators then assigned those animals with adhesions to adhesiolysis at laparotomy or laparoscopy and demonstrated greater reduction in adhesion reformation following laparoscopic adhesiolysis. In their study, Nezhat and co-worker[29] reported no *de novo* adhesion formation at non-operated sites at a second look laparoscopy done 4–8 months after laser laparoscopy for the treatment of endometriosis associated infertility in 157 patients. An overall 60–79% reduction in adhesions in patients undergoing adhesiolysis was observed. Diamond and co-workers[30] described, in a multicenter study, a high (97%) incidence of adhesion reformation at early (90 days) second-look laparoscopy following laparoscopic adhesiolysis. Moreover, adhesion reformation occurred regardless of the consistency or vascularity of the initial adhesion. This incidence is consistent with that previously reported following adhesiolysis at laparotomy; therefore, they concluded that adhesion reformation would not be eliminated by utilization of endoscopic surgery *per se*. Their report also pointed to a 12% of patients who developed *de novo* adhesions.

At this time, it seems that there is no clear and convincing evidence that laparoscopic adhesiolysis in humans is superior to microsurgical lysis of adhesions at laparotomy in terms of adhesion reformation or subsequent pregnancy.

Open surgery

This is the usual method of approaching the more severe degrees of endometriosis, particularly where endometriomas are large and there is more extensive scarring involving the bowel and bladder.

Hysterectomy is an end-stage treatment for women who have completed their family and where endometriosis is severe. It is usual to suggest removal of the ovaries, particularly in a woman who is over the age of 40 years or where the disease is particularly severe. Hormone replacement therapy will protect the bones and avoid menopausal symptoms.

LAPAROSCOPIC MANAGEMENT

Laparoscopic appearance of endometriosis

Even an experienced laparoscopist who has treated hundreds of endometriosis patients can miss 7% or underdiagnose 50% of lesions.[31] The gross appearance of endometriosis is a result of several factors, including the relative proportion of glands and stroma, amount of scarring, intralesional bleeding and quantity of hemosiderin. While the relative contribution of the above factors results in a continuum of visual appearances, the most commonly described types of

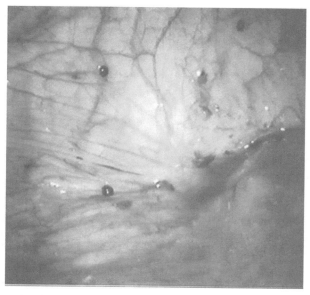

Fig. 5 Peritoneal endometriotic implants.

endometriosis include scarred white lesions, strawberry-like reddish lesions, red flame-like lesions, reddish polyps, clear vesicular lesions, adhesions, peritoneal defects, yellow-brown patches and black puckered lesions (Fig. 5). Histologically, lesions were confirmed in 90% of typical dark black lesions, 81% of white opacified, 75% of red-flame-like, 67% of glandular lesions, 50% of subovarian adhesions 48% of intra-ovarian cysts, 47% of yellow-brown patches, 45% of circular peritoneal defects, 33% of hemosiderin lesions, and 13–15% of normal peritoneum.[32]

The laparoscopic management of endometriosis usually includes: lysis of pelvic adhesions, dissection of ovaries from cul-de-sac or pelvic sidewall, tubes freed and chromopertubated, fulguration of endometrial implants, resection of endometriomas, and uterosacral nerve ablation or presacral nerve resection for chronic pelvic pain.

Lysis of pelvic adhesions

The bowel and omentum are carefully dissected from the parietal and visceral peritoneum. The large vessels are occluded using laparoscopic clips, electrosurgery, or laser. A 5-mm atraumatic grasping forceps is used to grasp either bowel or omentum, and then blunt dissection and aquadissection attempted. KTP laser may be used to vaporize thicker bands. If bleeding cannot be controlled with KTP laser, endoloop sutures or clips can be placed.

Resection of ovarian endometriosis

Endometrial implants or endometriomas less than 2 cm in diameter are coagulated, laser ablated or excised using scissors or biopsy forceps. For successful eradication, all visible lesions and scars must be excised from the

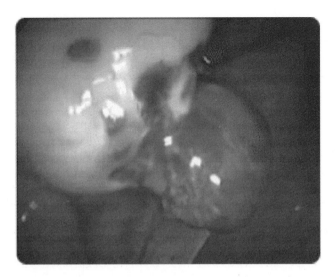

Fig. 6 Removal of chocolate cyst from the ovary.

ovarian surface. Endometriomas more than 2-cm diameter must be resected thoroughly to prevent recurrence. Draining the endometrioma or partial resection of its wall is inadequate because the endometrial tissue lining the cyst is likely to remain functional and can cause the symptoms to recur.[33] However, photocoagulation of the cyst wall has been equally therapeutic and occasionally less difficult.[34–36] For endometriomas over 2 cm in diameter, the cyst is punctured with the 5-mm trocar and aspirated with the suction probe. Using high pressure irrigation, at 500–800 mmHg, the cyst is irrigated, causing it to expand, and aspirated several times.[37] Following the repeated expansion and shrinkage with irrigation and suction, the cyst wall should separate from the surrounding ovarian stroma. If it does not, 5–20 ml of lactated Ringer's buffer is injected between the stroma and cyst wall.[37] The cyst wall is removed by grasping its base with laparoscopic forceps and peeling it from the ovarian stroma. If unsuccessful, the wall is separated from the ovarian cortex with forceps at the puncture site. A cleavage plane is created by pulling the two forceps apart and by cutting between the structures with laser or needle electrode (Fig. 6). The blood vessels supplying the endometrioma are usually small enough to be cut and coagulated simultaneously.

Cyst wall closure is not necessary according to animal experiments[38] and clinical experience.[39] For large defects that result from resecting endometriomas larger than 5 cm, the edges of the ovarian cortex are approximated with a single suture placed within the ovarian stroma. The knot is tied inside the ovary, so that no part of the suture penetrates the ovarian cortex or is exposed to the ovarian surface so as to minimize adhesion formation. Fibrin sealant has been described to atraumatically approximate the edges of large ovarian defects, without adhesion formation.[40]

In rare cases of unilateral ovarian affection, a unilateral salpingo-oophrectomy for the diseased ovary will decrease the recurrence rate and improve the fertility potential by limiting ovulation to the healthy ovary.[41]

The number of oocytes and embryos obtained was not significantly decreased by laparoscopic cystectomy, suggesting that, in experienced hands, this procedure may be a valuable surgical tool for the treatment of large ovarian endometriomas. However, great care must be taken to avoid ovarian damage.[42]

GENITO-URINARY ENDOMETRIOSIS

Involvement of the ureter in endometriosis was reported in 1–11% of patients.[43] Endometriosis of the urinary tract tends to be superficial but can be invasive and cause complete ureteral obstruction. Superficial implants over the ureter are generally treated by hydrodissection. Lactated Ringer's buffer (20–30 ml) is injected subperitoneally on the lateral pelvic wall to elevate the peritoneum and back it with a bed of fluid. The CO_2 laser is used to create a 0.5 cm opening on this elevation. The opening in the peritoneum is made anteriorly and laterally, close to corresponding round ligament. The hydrodissection probe is inserted into the opening and around 100 ml of lactated Ringer's solution is injected under 300 mmHg pressure into the retroperitoneal space along the course of the ureter. After creating the water bed, a CO_2 laser is used to vaporize or excise the lesion with a circumference of 1–2 cm .

Laparoscopic ureteroureterostomy was first performed for ureteral obstruction due to endometriosis by Nezhat and colleagues in 1990.[44] Under cystoscopic guidance, ureteral catheter is passed through the ureterovesical junction up to the level at which the CO_2 laser is used to open the ureter. Indigocarmine is injected intravenous to insure patency of the proximal ureter. The distal ureter was transected over the catheter , and the obstructed portion was removed. The ureteral catheter was introduced into the proximal ureter and advanced into the renal pelvis (Figs 7, 8). Finally, the edges of the ureter were re-approximated with four interrupted 4/0 polydioxanone sutures (PDSs).

Bladder endometriosis lesions are vaporized after hydrodissection if they are superficial. The lesion is circumcised with the laser and fluid is infused into the resulting defect. The lesion is grasped with forceps and dissected with the

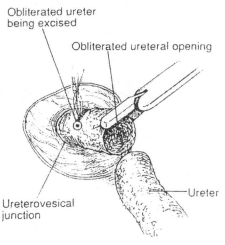

Obliterated ureter
being excised

Obliterated ureteral opening

Ureter

Ureterovesical
junction

Fig. 7 Excision of obliterated ureter

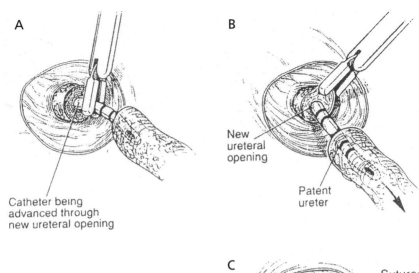

New
ureteral
opening

Catheter being
advanced through
new ureteral opening

Patent
ureter

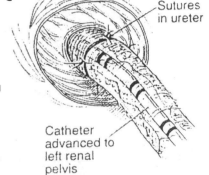

Sutures
in ureter

Fig. 8 Applying ureteral catheter and reanastomosis of the ureter. (A) Catheter being advanced through new ureteral opening. (B) The ureteral stent was introduced into the proximal ureter and advanced into the renal pelvis. (C) To perform anastomosis, four interrupted 4.0 polydioxanone sutures were placed at 6, 12, 9 and 3 o'clock to approximate the proximal and distal ureteral edges.

Catheter
advanced to
left renal
pelvis

laser. Traction allows the small blood vessels supplying the surrounding tissue to be coagulated as the lesion is resected (Fig. 9). Frequent irrigation is necessary to remove char, ascertain the depth of vaporization, and ensure that the lesion does not involve the mascularis and the mucosa.

Endometriosis extending to the muscularis but without mucosal involvement can be treated laparoscopically and any residual or deeper lesions may be treated successfully with postoperative hormonal therapy.[45] When endometriosis involves full bladder wall thickness, the lesion is excised and the bladder reconstructed. Simultaneous cystoscopy is performed and bilateral ureteral catheters are inserted. CO_2 gas distends the bladder cavity, allowing excellent observation of its interior. After again identifying the ureters and examining the bladder mucosa, the bladder is closed in with several interrupted 4-0 polydioxanone through-and-through sutures using extracorporal or intracorporeal knots.

GASTROINTESTINAL ENDOMETRIOSIS

The gastrointestinal tract is involved in 3–37% of cases with endometriosis.[46,47] This incidence can be increased to 50% if patients with serosal and subserosal lesions are included.[41] In cases of severe disease of the bowel wall, resection may be necessary. Pre-operative mechanical and antibiotic bowel preparation

A

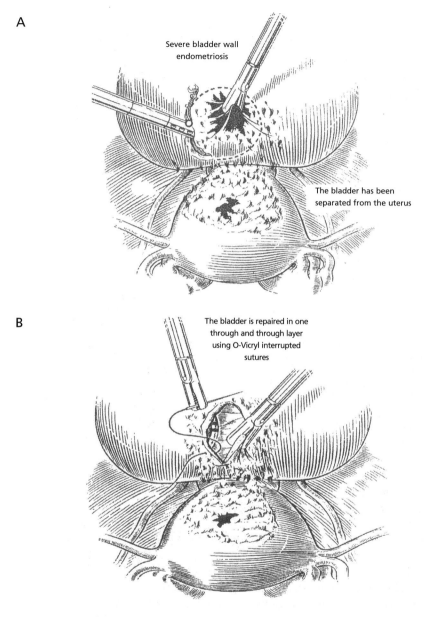

Severe bladder wall
endometriosis

The bladder has been
separated from the uterus

B

The bladder is repaired in one
through and through layer
using O-Vicryl interrupted
sutures

Fig. 9 Excision of endometriosis and repair of the bladder

is necessary. Three 5-mm suprapubic trocars are placed, one in the midline and
the others in the right and left iliac fossa, for the insertion of grasping forceps,
endoloop suture applicators, a suction irrigation probe, and a bipolar
electrocoagulator. The technique includes laparoscopic mobilization of the
lower colon, transanal prolapse, resection and anastomosis.

When the lesion involves only the anterior rectal wall near the anal verge,
the rectovaginal septum is delineated by simultaneous vaginal and rectal
examinations performed by an assistant. The rectum is mobilized along the

rectovaginal septum anteriorly to within 2 cm of the anus, using the CO_2 laser and hydrodissection. Mobilization continues along the left and right pararectal spaces by electrodessication and dividing branches of the hemorrhoidal artery, and partially posteriorly, as well. The lesion is excised using electrosurgery and rectal closure is confirmed by insufflating the rectum while the cul-de-sac is filled with lactated Ringer's solution.

In circumferential lesions, the entire rectum is mobilized and presacral space is entered. The rectum is transected proximal to the lesion, the rectal stump, containing the endometrial lesion, is prolapsed through the anal canal and transected using linear stapler. The rectal stump is replaced again into the pelvis and end-to-end anastomosis is done using the stapler. A proctoscope is used to examine the anastomosis for structural integrity and bleeding.

DIAPHRAGMATIC ENDOMETRIOSIS

Patients with diaphragmatic endometriosis may present with pleuritic, shoulder and upper abdominal pain occurring with menses. Laparoscopy is an excellent tool for diagnosis and treatment of endometriosis, which is difficult to reach through laparotomy. There is still a danger regarding possible injuries to the diaphragm, phrenic nerve, lungs or heart. So, other alternatives for management should be discussed with the patient.

In addition to the 10-mm umbilical port site for laparoscopy, three additional trocars are placed in the upper quadrant (right or left according to implant location), similar to the sites for laparoscopic cholecystectomy. Two grasping forceps are used to push the liver from the operative field. Lesions are removed using hydrodissection and vaporization or excision. If a diaphragmatic defect is formed, it is repaired with 4-0 PDS or staples.

UTEROSACRAL LIGAMENT

Uterosacral ligament can be resected for its involvement with endometriosis or transected for control of pain by laparoscopic uterine nerve ablation (LUNA). To resect the uterosacral ligament, incise the peritoneum lateral and parallel to it. This incision over the adjacent broad ligament results in spontaneous retraction of the peritoneum with the resultant visualization of the retroperitoneal structures. The ureter and uterine vessels can now be dissected bluntly laterally to ensure that they are not near the uterosacral ligament. The insertion of the uterosacral ligament into the posterior cervix is divided with unipolar coagulation current or with bipolar coagulation followed by scissors transection. For greater safety, a chemical laparoscopic presacral neurolysis was described by Soysal and colleagues.[48] A 10-mm umbilical port is used for the standard insufflation and video endoscopy. Two additional 5-mm subumbilical standard ports are created for diagnostic and therapeutic purposes. The peritoneum overlying the promontory is grasped and elevated by a grasper and from the other port, 5 ml of saline was injected retroperitoneally by the laparoscopic needle used for ovarian cyst puncture. This elevates the peritoneum and endopelvic fascia from the promontory. Furthermore, this space avoids inadvertent injection of phenol to vessels and backflow of phenol to the peritoneal space. Then 10 ml of phenol (10% in

Urografin, radiographic contrast medium; Schering AG, Germany) is injected slowly to the deeper part of the artificially created retroperitoneal space from another point of entry. Before withdrawing the needle, an additional 2 ml of saline was given to avoid intraperitoneal spillage of phenol during the withdrawal of the needle. Afterwards, a thorough pelvic lavage was done. The presacral neurolysis itself is a 2-min operation.

POSTOPERATIVE HORMONAL THERAPY

Combined surgery and medical therapy represents the best treatment for endometriosis according to various authors.[49-53] Theoretically, postoperative medical treatment may eradicate any foci of endometriosis remaining after surgery and this improves the results of the procedure. It may also stop the implantation and growth of endometriotic tissue disseminated at surgery and prevents recurrence. In spite of this, Bianchi et al.[54] reported that a 3-month course of danazol after laparoscopic surgery for stage III/IV endometriosis does not markedly improve the short-term reproductive prognosis or pelvic pain. Also, the study of Busacca et al.[55] did not support the routine postoperative use of a 3-month course of GnRH analogue in women with symptomatic stage III/IV endometriosis. However, larger series and longer follow-up periods are required to identify less important effects of treatment, in particular on the objective disease recurrence rate. Moreover, these data could not rule out that post-surgical GnRH analogue or other estrogen-lowering medical therapies may be of value in selected patients, particularly those in whom disease has not been completely extirpated.[55]

References

1 Wheeler JM. Epidemiology of endometriosis-associated infertility. J Reprod Med 1989; 34: 41–46
2 Rawson JM. Prevalence of endometriosis in asymptomatic women. J Reprod Med 1991; 36: 513–515
3 Strathy JH, Molgaard CA, Coulam CB, Melton 3rd LJ. Endometriosis and infertility: a laparoscopic study of endometriosis among fertile and infertile women. Fertil Steril 1982; 38: 667–672
4 Verkauf BS. Incidence, symptoms, and signs of endometriosis in fertile and infertile women. J Fla Med Assoc 1987; 74: 671–675
5 Carter JE. Combined hysteroscopic and laparoscopic findings in patients with chronic pelvic pain. J Am Assoc Gynecol Laparosc 1994; 2: 43–47
6 Koninckx PR, Meuleman C, Demeyere S, Lesaffre E, Cornillie FJ. Suggestive evidence that pelvic endometriosis is a progressive disease, whereas deeply infiltrating endometriosis is associated with pelvic pain. Fertil Steril 1991; 55: 759–765
7 Ling FW. Randomized controlled trial of depot leuprolide in patients with chronic pelvic pain and clinically suspected endometriosis. Pelvic Pain Study Group. Obstet Gynecol 1999; 93: 51–58
8 Ripps BA, Martin DC. Endometriosis and chronic pelvic pain. Obstet Gynecol Clin North Am 1993; 20: 709–717
9 Cramer DW. Epidemiology of endometriosis. In: Wilson EA. (ed) Endometriosis. New York: Alan R. Liss, 1987; 5–22
10 Vigano P, Vercellini P, Di Blasio AM, Colombo A, Candiani GB, Vignali M. Deficient antiendometrium lymphocyte-mediated cytotoxicity in patients with endometriosis. Fertil Steril 1991; 56: 894–899

11 Keltz MD, Berger SB, Comite F, Olive DL. Duplicated cervix and vagina associated with infertility, endometriosis, and chronic pelvic pain. Obstet Gynecol 1994; 84: 701–703

12 Cramer DW, Wilson E, Stillman RJ et al. The relation of endometriosis to menstrual characteristics, smoking and exercise. JAMA 1986; 255: 1904–1908

13 Adamson GD. Diagnosis and clinical presentation of endometriosis. Am J Obstet Gynecol 1990; 162: 568–569

14 The American Fertility Society. Management of endometriosis in the presence of pelvic pain. Fertil Steril 1993; 60: 952–955

15 Luciano AA, Pitkin RM. Endometriosis: approaches to diagnosis and treatment. Surg Annu 1984; 16: 297–312

16 Muse K. Clinical manifestations and classification of endometriosis. Clin Obstet Gynecol 1988; 31: 813–822

17 Demco L. Mapping the source and character of pain due to endometriosis by patient-assisted laparoscopy. J Am Assoc Gynecol Laparosc 1998; 5: 241–245

18 Martin DC, Hubert GD, Vander Zwaag R, el-Zeky FA. Laparoscopic appearances of peritoneal endometriosis. Fertil Steril 1989; 51: 63–67

19 Stripling MC, Martin DC, Chatman DL, Zwaag RV, Poston WM. Subtle appearance of pelvic endometriosis. Fertil Steril 1988; 49: 427–431

20 Jansen RP, Russell P. Non-pigmented endometriosis: clinical, laparoscopic, and pathologic definition. Am J Obstet Gynecol 1986; 155: 1154–1159

21 Pittaway DE. CA-125 in women with endometriosis. Obstet Gynecol Clin North Am 1989; 16: 237–252

22 Duleba AJ. Diagnosis of endometriosis. Obstet Gynecol Clin North Am 1997; 24: 331–346

23 Patel MD, Feldstein VA, Chen DC, Lipson SD, Filly RA. Endometriomas: diagnostic performance of US. Radiology 1999; 210: 739–745

24 Arrive L, Hricak H, Martin MC. Pelvic endometriosis: MR imaging. Radiology 1989; 171: 687–692

25 Olive DL, Lindheim SR, Pritts EA. Endometriosis and infertility: what do we do for each stage? Current Women's Health Reports 2003; 3: 389–394

26 Crosignani PG, Vercellini P, Biffignandi F. Laparoscopy versus laparotomy in conservative surgical treatment for severe endometriosis. Sterility 1996; 66: 706–711

27 Tulandi T, al-Took S. Reproductive outcome after treatment of mild endometriosis with laparoscopic excision and electrocoagulation. Sterility 1998; 69: 229–231

28 Luciano A, Maier DB, Kock EL et al. A comparative study of postoperative adhesions; laser surgery by laparoscopy versus laparotomy in the rabbit model. Obstet Gynecol 1989; 74: 220

29 Nezhat CR, Nezhat FR, Metzger DA, Luciano AA. Adhesion reformation after reproductive surgery by videolaseroscopy. Fertil Steril 1990; 53: 1008

30 Diamond MP, Daniell JF, Johns DA et al. Postoperative adhesion development after operative laparoscopy: evaluation at early second-look procedures. Fertil Steril 1991; 55: 700

31 Martin DC, Hubert GD, Vander Zwaag R, El-Zeky FA. Laparoscopic appearance of peritoneal endometriosis. Fertil Steril 1989; 51: 63–67

32 Nezhat CR, Nezhat FR, Luciano AA, Siegler AM, Metzger DA, Nezhat CH. Laparoscopic treatment of endometriosis. In: Operative Gynecologic Laparoscopy, Principles and Techniques. New York: MacGraw-Hill, 1995; 126–129

33 Hasson HM. Laparoscopic management of ovarian cysts. J Reprod Med 1991; 56: 349–352

34 Keye WR, Hansen LW, Astin M. Argon laser therapy of endometriosis: a review of 92 consecutive patients. Fertil Steril 1987; 47: 208–214

35 Brosens I, Puttemansi P. Double optic laparoscopy. Baillières Clin Obtet Gynecol 1989; 3: 595–598

36 Fayez JA, Collazo LM. Comparison between laparotomy and operative laparoscopy in the treatment of moderate and severe endometriosis. Int J Fertil 1990; 35; 272–276

37 Nezhat F, Nezhat C, Allan CJ, Metzger DA, Sears DL. A clinical and histologic classification of endometriomas: implications for a mechanism of pathogenesis. J Reprod Med 1992; 37: 771–776

38 Marana R, Luciano AA, Muzii L. Reproductive outcome after ovarian surgery: suturing versus nonsuturing of the ovarian cortex. J Gynecol Surg 1991; 7: 155–159

39 Nezhat C, Nezhat F. Postoperative adhesion formation after ovarian cystectomy with

and without ovarian reconstruction. Abstract O-012, 47th annual meeting of American Fertility Association, Orlando, FL, 1991

40 Donnez J, Nisolle M. Laparoscopic management of large ovarian endometrial cyst: use of fibrin sealant. Surgery 1991; 7: 163–168

41 Nezhat CR, Nezhat FR, Luciano AA, Siegler AM, Metzger DA, Nezhat CH. Laparoscopic treatment of endometriosis. In: Operative Gynecologic Laparoscopy, Principles and Techniques. New York: McGraw-Hill, 1995; 129–147

42 Canis M, Pouly JL, Tamburro S, Mage G, Wattiez A, Bruhat MA. Ovarian response during IVF–embryo transfer cycles after laparoscopic ovarian cystectomy for endometriotic cysts of > 3 cm in diameter. Hum Reprod 2001; 16: 2583–2586

43 Stanley EK, Utz DC, Dockerty MB. Clinical significant endometriosis of the urinary tract. Surg Gynecol Obstet 1965; 120: 491–496

44 Nezhat C, Nezhat F, Green B. Laparoscopic treatment of obstructed ureter due to endometriosis by resection and ureteroureterostomy: a case report. J Urol 1992; 148: 659–663

45 Busacca M, Somigliana E, Bianchi S et al. Post-operative GnRH analogue treatment after conservative surgery for symptomatic endometriosis stage III–IV: a randomized controlled trial. Hum Reprod 2001; 16: 2399–2402

46 Jenkinson EL, Brown WH. Endometriosis: a study of 117 cases with special reference to constricting lesions of the rectum and sigmoid colon. JAMA 1943; 122: 349–252

47 Samper ER, Sagle GW, Hand AM. Colonic endometriosis, its clinical spectrum. South Med J 1984; 77: 912–918

48 Soysal ME, Soysal S, Gurses E, Ozer S. Laparoscopic presacral neurolysis for endometriosis-related pelvic pain. Hum Reprod 2003; 18: 588–592

49 Buttram Jr VC. Use of danazol in conservative surgery. J Reprod Med 1999; 35: 82–84

50 Thomas EJ. Combining medical and surgical treatment for endometriosis: the best of both worlds? Br J Obstet Gynaecol 1992; 99 (Suppl. 7): 5–8

51 Malinak LR. Surgical treatment and adjunct therapy of endometriosis. Int J Gynaecol Obstet 1993; 40 (Suppl.): S43–S47

52 Muzii, L, Marana R, Caruana P, Mancuso S. The impact of preoperative gonadotropin-releasing hormone agonist treatment on laparoscopic excision of ovarian endometriotic cysts. Fertil Steril 1996; 65: 1235–1237

53 Rana N, Thomas S, Rotman C, Dmowski WP. Decrease in the size of ovarian endometriomas during ovarian suppression in stage IV endometriosis. Role of preoperative medical treatment. J Reprod Med 1996; 41: 384–392

54 Bianchi S, Busacca M, Agnoli B, Candiani M, Calia C, Vignali M. Effects of 3 month therapy with danazol after laparoscopic surgery for stage III/IV endometriosis: a randomized study. Hum Reprod 1999; 14: 1335–1337

55 Busacca M, Somigliana E, Bianchi S et al. Post-operative GnRH analogue treatment after conservative surgery for symptomatic endometriosis stage III–IV: a randomized controlled trial. Hum Reprod 2001; 16: 2399–2402

Michael Stark   Sandro Gerli
Gian Carlo Di Renzo

The Ten-Step Vaginal Hysterectomy

Vaginal hysterectomies were already being performed in the 19th century, the first by Langenbeck in 1813.[1,2] Since then, many modifications and variations have been reported. Most methods in use today, like the Porges,[3] Falk,[4] von Theobald,[5] Heaney,[6] Joel-Cohen[7] and the Chicago[8] methods, are carried out with defined sequences. These sequences result from personal interpretations of the pelvic anatomy and the individual experience of the authors.

Innovative procedures such as focused ultrasound[9] and cryomyolysis to reduce the size of fibroids[35] or endometrial resection and microwave treatment for endometrial ablation in uncontrolled vaginal bleedings[10] have reduced the number of all kinds of hysterectomies. These days, hysterectomies are often performed as laparoscopically assisted vaginal hysterectomies (LAVH), even for big uteri.[11] In a prospective, randomised study, no difference between vaginal hysterectomy and LAVH was found with respect to estimated blood loss, complications, hospital stay and period of convalescence. The costs of LAVH were, however, considerably higher.[12]

Even today, with hundreds of publications about laparoscopically assisted vaginal hysterectomy available, the vaginal route should always be considered when hysterectomy is indicated, because of the quick recovery, the lack of abdominal scar and the short hospital stay.[6,13] It seems that laparoscopically

Michael Stark MD (for correspondence)
President, The New European Surgical Academy (NESA) and Chairman of the Gynaecological Departments, HELIOS Hospitals Group, Karower Str 11, Haus 214, 13125 Berlin, Germany
E-mail: mstark@nesacademy.org

Sandro Gerli MD
Senior Gynaecologist, Department of Obstetrics and Gynaecology, Monteluce Hospital, University of Perugia, Italy

Gian Carlo Di Renzo MD PhD
Head, Department of Obstetrics and Gynaecology, Monteluce Hospital, University of Perugia, Italy/Italian Representative of the New European Surgical Academy (NESA)

assisted vaginal hysterectomy should not replace the vaginal but rather the abdominal hysterectomy when there are relative contra-indications for vaginal hysterectomy.[14] There are less and less contra-indications for vaginal hysterectomy,[15] and the operation can be performed with nulliparity[16] and with enlarged uterus.[17] Even uteri up to 982 g have been successfully removed vaginally.[18]

Therefore, in order to find out whether vaginal hysterectomies can still be optimised and simplified after so many years of practice and accumulated experience, a re-evaluation of the six mentioned methods was initiated. First, the steps common to all these methods were defined and analysed, then the steps were re-assessed and excluded if considered unnecessary. Thereafter, the ways of performing the essential steps were critically compared. As a result, only the re-evaluated and absolutely irreplaceable steps remained, sometimes with modifications. Finally, their logical sequence was defined and described.

The result is the so-called 'Ten-Step Vaginal Hysterectomy'. This method is logical, easy to learn, to perform and to teach.

METHOD DESCRIPTION

The operation steps, their alternatives, the underlying logic and the optimal way of performance will be described. The instruments and suture material needed for each step will be listed.

Vaginal hysterectomies have been recommended for treatment of endometrial cancer in elderly women,[19] but they are mostly performed for benign conditions. Therefore, endometrial malignancy should be excluded before starting the operation; if a diagnostic curettage was not performed before, a hysteroscopy should be done before starting the operation.

1.   INCISION OF THE VAGINAL WALL

The way in which the incision of the vaginal wall should be performed depends entirely on the individual anatomical conditions. Traditionally, most described methods start, where prolapse exists, with a circular incision around the cervix, extension towards the orificium urethrae externum and separation of the vaginal wall laterally, away from the bladder. This approach has already been challenged by Joel-Cohen.[7] He did the separation the other way around, starting it under the orificium urethrae externum continuing around the external os. We found this approach easy and logical, mainly in multiparae where one often finds adhesions around the external os; therefore, entering the right cleavage is easier upwards.

In a patient with a prolapsed uterus
The cervix is grasped with two single-toothed tenaculi. In a patient with a prolapsed uterus, the traditional incision around the cervix with a perpendicular extension and the separation of the vaginal wall from the midline to the side, as described above, has been changed into a drop-like

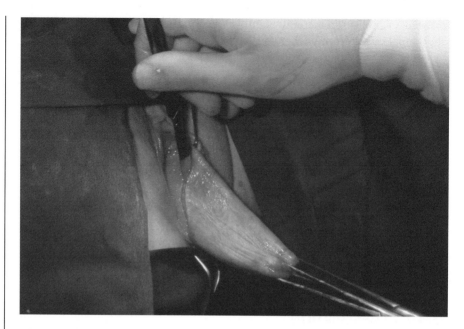

Fig. 1 A drop like incision around the cervix (Step 1).

incision of the vaginal wall starting under the urethra, continuing laterally and down, encircling the uterine cervix from behind and returning back to the starting point from the other side (Fig. 1). If the depth of the initial incision is correct and the right cleavage is reached, the vaginal wall will be easily separated laterally to the side of the uterus and downwards below the cervix by a gentle use of surgical forceps. This should be nearly bloodless and easier than separating the vaginal wall in the described traditional way. Doing so, the vaginal wall is already ready for the anterior wall colporrhaphy.

After this, the tip of the 'drop' still covering the bladder is pulled down, separating the vaginal wall from the bladder. Being in the right cleavage will also prevent unnecessary bleeding. This procedure, besides being, is performed in three main movements compared to six in all other methods.

INSTRUMENTS

Speculum, two single-toothed tenaculi, scalpel, surgical forceps.

In a patient without prolapse

The cervix is grasped with two single-toothed tenaculi. When no prolapse or just a minimal prolapse exists, the first step is a circular incision around the cervix about 5 mm above the external os, and then, being in the right cleavage, the vaginal wall should be separated from the cervix using surgical forceps; more vaginal retractors are sometimes needed in order to allow the surgeon to perform this manipulation under good vision.

The border between the anterior wall of the uterus and the bladder must be identified (curved scissors are sometimes needed). Then, by pushing the bladder up close to the uterus using a swab, it will separate from the uterus until the anterior peritoneum is exposed. No effort should be made to open the peritoneum. Opening the anterior peritoneum at this stage is not necessary and not recommended because it disturbs the dynamics of the operation and interrupts its continuity. It might cause damage to the bladder whenever the inter-anatomical relations between it and the peritoneum are not clear. Haemostasis should be done carefully. After the bladder has been pushed up, the swab stays between the anterior peritoneum and the bladder and should, therefore, be marked. Previous caesarean sections are not now considered a contra-indication for vaginal hysterectomy.[15]

> INSTRUMENTS
>
> Swab, Allis clamp, scalpel, optionally scissors

3. OPENING POSTERIOR PERITONEUM

To open the posterior peritoneum, the tenaculi holding the uterus should be pulled up by the assistant and the peritoneum should be grasped with surgical forceps while being cut and opened with scissors. The scissors are then

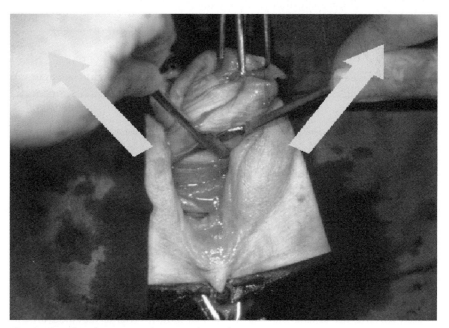

Fig. 2 Opening the post-peritoneum (Step 3).

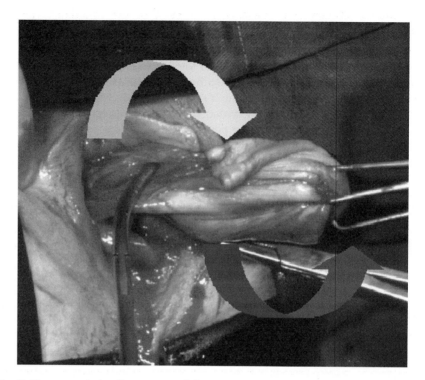

Fig. 3 The sacro-uterine ligaments and the paracervical tissues are grasped with one instrument (Step 3).

introduced into the Douglas cavity and, holding each blade with one hand, pulled out while they remain open, so that the back sides of the blades expose the insertions of the sacro-uterine ligaments (Fig. 2).[20,21]

> INSTRUMENTS
>
> Surgical forceps, scissors

4. DISSECTION OF THE LOWER PART OF THE UTERUS

In contradiction to the time-honoured, traditional anatomical approach which dealt with each anatomical structure separately, the sacro-uterine ligaments and the paracervical tissues, which are anatomically in different planes and directions, are clamped together. This is done by a designed manoeuvre: one blade of an open clamp is placed under the insertion of the sacro-uterine ligament, the instrument rotates towards the uterus while the uterus is being contrarotated (Fig. 3). Both anatomical structures are included between the blades of the instrument while it is being closed. Both structures, the relatively bloodless sacro-uterine ligament and the paracervical tissues, are cut and ligated leaving the suture material in its full length. This is repeated on the contralateral side. These steps are safe and, if correctly done, bloodless, dynamically correct and time-saving. In most of the traditional surgical methods for vaginal hysterectomy, both elements will anyway be sutured to each other at the end of the operation (there are exceptions, some surgeons perform vaginal hysterectomies without ligating the cervical ligaments).[20]

When done in a patient without a prolapsed uterus, this manoeuvre will instantly produce a significant descensus, and with a slight traction, the uterine arteries will be exposed.

> **INSTRUMENTS**
>
> Wertheim or Heaney clamp, needle holder, surgical forceps, scissors, two sutures

5. CUTTING AND LIGATING THE UTERINE ARTERIES

Both uterine arteries are clamped, cut and ligated.

> **INSTRUMENTS**
>
> Wertheim or Heaney clamp, needle holder, scissors, two sutures

6. OPENING THE ANTERIOR PERITONEUM

After both uterine arteries have been cut and ligated, the uterus is pulled down and two fingers are introduced behind the fundus to lift the anterior peritoneum which can be opened under vision with scissors. This will ensure the safety of the bladder, as its anatomical relations with the anterior peritoneum are not always clear, in particular after previous caesarean sections.

Access to the fundus in a myomatous uterus is sometimes difficult. In such a case, the surgeon should hold both tenaculi with the left hand while continuously and slowly pulling them down with rotating movements. Usually, the uterus is amenable and will descend until it is possible to insert the right index and middle fingers beyond the fundus and lift the anterior peritoneum. Occasionally, additional steps are necessary to separate the parametrium from the uterus. There is no risk of damaging the ovarian arteries with this rotating and pulling manoeuvre because the larger the uterus, the longer they are. It is amazing to realise how one can descend a large uterus with such a manoeuvre. The decision about the size of uterus that can be removed vaginally depends solely on the experience of the individual surgeon and should be taken before starting the operation. Morcellation of the uterus, which is safe and facilitates the removal of enlarged and well-supported uteri, may be performed where needed.[18] With increasing experience of this rotating manoeuvre, the less often morcellation becomes necessary. In experienced hands, a big uterus should not be a contra-indication for vaginal hysterectomy.[22,23]

INSTRUMENTS: scissors

7. DISSECTION OF THE UPPER PART OF THE UTERUS (AND APPENDAGES)

The round and ovarian ligaments and the blood vessels are clamped together and ligated. The ligature should be placed as lateral as possible away from the clamp, leaving the ovarian ligaments as long as possible. The uterus is cut away with scissors medial to the instrument. A transfiction suture is placed between the clamp and the ligature keeping the full length of the suture material. The ligature, which is placed before and lateral to the transfiction, will prevent bleeding, should this transfiction suture slip away or tear by traction. The same procedure should be done on the contralateral side.

INSTRUMENTS

Wertheim or Heaney clamp, scissors, needle holder, surgical forceps, four sutures

8. THE 'NON-STAGE' – LEAVING THE PERITONEUM OPEN

In 1980, Harold Ellis showed that closing the peritoneum at the end of abdominal surgery is not necessary.[24] The thin peritoneum, unlike skin, can not be adapted by placing its ends together. Vascular bridges over peritoneal sutures are a focus for ischaemia and adhesions. When peritoneum is left open, the coelum cells will produce a new peritoneum. Indeed, leaving peritoneum open in a caesarean section proved to cause less adhesions than when it was closed.[25] It was also shown that the peritoneal closure is not necessary for vaginal hysterectomy.[26,27] The British Royal College of Obstetrics and Gynaecology recommended in its guideline No. 15 in July 2002 to leave peritoneum open with evidence level Ib.[28]

The pelvic parietal peritoneum is attached to the pelvic ligaments. The ligation of the ligaments to each other (Step 9) will create a peritoneal sac between the ligaments and a closed peritoneum, with all consequences involved.

Another advantage of leaving peritoneum open is, therefore, the free drainage into the peritoneal cavity where blood can be absorbed by the peritoneum and lymph channels.

If an enterocoele has to be prevented or repaired, it should be done before continuing the operation.[29]

9.   RECONSTRUCTION OF THE PELVIC FLOOR

The left and right sacro-uterine ligaments with the paracervical tissues as well as the ovarian ligaments are ligated to each other respectively. An extra suture may be placed to join the sacro-uterine ligaments. The decision should be taken according to the individual anatomical relationships.

INSTRUMENTS

Scissors, needle holder, surgical forceps, optionally one suture

---

10.   CLOSING THE VAGINAL WALL

The vaginal wall is sutured continuously. It is recommended in sexually active women to close the vagina transversely. This will prevent dyspareunia as the suturing line will be on the upper side of the anterior wall.

INSTRUMENTS

Allis clamp, needle holder, surgical forceps, scissors, one suture.

COMPARATIVE RESULTS

In a study in two hospitals, 96 women with prolapse II or III underwent vaginal hysterectomy, 52 with the Heaney method and 44 with Ten-Step

Table 1 Prospective, randomised comparison of vaginal hysterectomies performed by the Heaney and the Ten-Step Vaginal Hysterectomy methods.

	Heaney method $n = 52$ Median (25th–75th percentile)	Ten-Step Vaginal Hysterectomy $n = 44$ Median (25th–75th percentile)
Age (years)	61.6 (46–75.9)	66.2 (53–77)
Operation time (min)	52.3 (23.3–90)	34.1 (20.5–50)*
Pain killers needed (h)	48.7 (19–86)	29.6 (8–75)*
Average hospital stay (range)	5.8 (4–8)	5.9 (4–8)

*Statistically significant difference ($P < 0.05$).

The data were stored in a database. The evaluation was done using SPSS for Windows. Frequencies and standard differences were calculated as mean variations.

Chi square analysis was used.

Vaginal Hysterectomy. There was no significant difference in both groups for age and parity. The women undergoing the Ten-Step Vaginal Hysterectomy had a significantly shorter operation time and shorter requirement of analgesics (Table 1).

DISCUSSION

As much as tradition is a benefit in cultural life, it might prevent new thinking and surgical developments if procedures are not constantly subjected to re-evaluation. No step of any operation should be a taboo. Each should always be examined in the light of new understanding of the pathology and physiology.

A surgical procedure should be evaluated by examining not only every single step but also their combinations and sequences. The necessity of each step and its exact way of performance should be critically assessed by comparing it to alternatives.

Each surgical procedure is composed of hundreds of movements. Each should have a defined purpose and a precise way of performance. Surgical steps and sequences often result from traditions and personal preference and are not necessarily based on randomised comparative and prospective studies.

Clinical studies concerning surgical procedures should take into account the early (febrile morbidity, analgesics needed, mobility) and late outcomes (adhesions, organ dysfunctions, chronic pains and life quality, next to the costs).

Many studies have compared the outcome of vaginal hysterectomy to abdominal or laparoscopically assisted vaginal hysterectomy. Campbell et al.[30] compared the three methods in 33,792 operations, analysing the duration of the hospital stay and the involved costs and concluded that 'vaginal hysterectomy provides the best patient outcomes, with the shortest hospital stays and lowest complication rates at the lowest cost'. The laparoscopically assisted vaginal hysterectomy is considered an alternative to abdominal hysterectomy.[31] Shorter hospital stay and less need of analgesia was reported in the laparoscopically assisted vaginal hysterectomy, but at the same time there was a higher rate of bladder injuries and a longer operation time when compared to vaginal hysterectomy.[32]

Only a few studies relate variations of single operative steps to the outcomes of vaginal hysterectomy. Leaving the parametrium unsutured resulted in a shorter operation time with no significant differences in other examined parameters.[20] Some advantages were reported where mass closure of the vaginal cuff was performed,[33] or when morcellation was practised.[23]

The vaginal route should always be considered when hysterectomy is indicated, because of a quicker recovery, lack of abdominal scar and shorter hospital stay. There is no justification for LAVH in the presence of significant uterine descent.[34]

The Ten-Step Vaginal Hysterectomy, which results from analyses of surgical steps used in different methods, is based, besides anatomical considerations, on up-to-date sound physiological principles. The result is a rational and simple operation which avoids unnecessary movements and follows rules of aesthetics and functional minimalism. Only ten instruments and ten sutures are needed and it was shown that this operation reduces the operation time and the use of pain killers. More randomised, prospective studies will be needed to evaluate the late outcome of this method.

References

1 Gray LA. Vaginal hysterectomy. Springfield, IL:Thomas, 1983
2 Leodolter S. The transvaginal surgical school in Austria. Retrospect-present-future. Gynaekol Geburtshilfliche Rundsch 1995; 35: 142–148
3 Paldi E, Filmar S, Naiger R, Weisseman A, Feldman EJ. Vaginal hysterectomy using the Porges method. Report on 100 cases. J Gynecol Obstet Biol Reprod 1988; 17: 233–236
4 Falk HC, Soichet S. The technique of vaginal hysterectomy. Clin Obstet Gynecol 1972; 15: 703–754
5 Von Theobald P. Simplified vaginal hysterectomy. J Chir 2001; 138: 93–98
6 Kalogirou D, Antoniou G, Zioris C, Fotopoulos S, Karakitsos P. Vaginal hysterectomy: technique and results in the last twenty years. J Gynecol Surg 1995; 11: 201–207
7 Joel-Cohen SJ. Abdominal and Vaginal Hysterectomy. New Techniques Based on Time and Motion Studies. London:Heinemann, 1972
8 Lash AF, Stepto RC. Chicago technique for vaginal hysterectomy at the Cook County Hospital. Clin Obstet Gynecol 1972; 15: 755–768
9 Tempany CM, Stewart EA, McDannold N, Quade BJ, Jolesz FA, Hynynen K. MR imaging-guided focused ultrasound surgery of uterine leiomyomas: a feasibility study. Radiology 2003; 226: 897–905
10 Cooper KG, Bain C, Lawrie L, Parkin DE. A randomised comparison of microwave endometrial ablation with transcervical resection of the endometrium; follow up at a minimum of five years. Br J Obstet Gynaecol 2005; 112: 470–475
11 Schutz K, Possover M, Merker A, Michels W, Schneider A. Prospective randomized comparison of laparoscopic-assisted vaginal hysterectomy (LAVH) with abdominal hysterectomy (AH) for the treatment of the uterus weighing > 200 g. Surg Endosc 2002; 16: 121–125
12 Summitt Jr RL, Stovall TG, Lipscomb GH, Ling FW. Randomized comparison of laparoscopy-assisted vaginal hysterectomy with standard vaginal hysterectomy in an outpatient setting. Obstet Gynecol 1992; 80: 895–901
13 Cravello L, Bretelle, F, Cohen D, Roger V, Giuly J, Blank B. Vaginal hysterectomy: apropos of a series of 1008 interventions. Gynecol Obstet Fertil 2001; 29: 288–294
14 Claerhout F, Deprest J. Laparoscopic hysterectomy for benign diseases. Best Pract Res Clin Obstet Gynaecol 2005; 19: 357–375
15 Doucette RC, Sharp HT, Alder SC. Challenging generally accepted contraindications to vaginal hysterectomy. Am J Obstet Gynecol 2001; 184: 1386–1389
16 Dhainaut C, Salomon LJ, Junger M, Marcollet A, Madelenat P. Hysterectomies in patients with no history of vaginal delivery. A study of 243 cases. Gynecol Obstet Fertil 2005; 33: 11–16
17 Li Z, Leng J, Lang J, Tang J. Vaginal hysterectomy for patients with moderately enlarged uterus of benign lesions. Chin Med Sci J 2004; 19: 60–63
18 Taylor SM, Romero AA, Kammerer-Doak DN, Qualls C, Rogers RG. Abdominal hysterectomy for the enlarged myomatous uterus compared with vaginal hysterectomy with morcellation. Am J Obstet Gynecol 2003; 189: 1579–1582
19 Susini T, Massi G, Amunni G et al. Vaginal hysterectomy and abdominal hysterectomy for treatment of endometrial cancer in the elderly. Gynecol Oncol 2005; 96: 362–367
20 Kudo R, Yamauchi O, Okazaki T, Sagae S, Ito E, Hashimoto M. Vaginal hysterectomy without ligation of the ligaments of the cervix uteri. Surg Gynecol Obstet 1990; 170: 299–305
21 Shef S, Studd J. Vaginal Hysterectomy. Berlin: Martin Dunitz, 2002
22 Harmanli OH, Gentzler CK, Byun S, Dandolu MH, Grody T. A comparison of abdominal and vaginal hysterectomy for the large uterus. Int J Gynaecol Obstet 2004; 87: 19–23
23 Switala I, Cosson M, Lanvin D, Querleu D, Crepin G. Is vaginal hysterectomy important for large uterus of more than 500 g? Comparison with laparotomy. J Gynecol Obstet Biol Reprod 1998; 27: 585–592

24 Ellis H. Internal overhealing: the problem of intraperitoneal adhesions. World J Surg 1980; 4: 303–306

25 Stark M. Clinical evidence that suturing the peritoneum after laparotomy is unnecessary for healing. World J Surg 1993; 17: 419

26 Janschek EC, Hohlagschwandtner M, Nather A, Schindl M, Joura EA. A study of non-closure of the peritoneum at vaginal hysterectomy. Arch Gynecol Obstet 2003; 267: 213–216

27 Lipscomb GH, Ling FW, Stovall TG, Summitt Jr RL. Peritoneal closure at vaginal hysterectomy : a reassessment. Obstet Gynecol 1996; 87: 40–43

28 Royal College of Obstetrics and Gynaecology. Peritoneal Closure Guideline No. 15. London: RCOG, 2002

29 Cruikshank SH, Kovac SR. Randomized comparison of three surgical methods used at the time of vaginal hysterectomy to prevent posterior enterocele. Am J Obstet Gynecol 1999; 180: 859–865

30 Campbell ES, Xiao H, Smith MK. Types of hysterectomy. Comparison of characteristics, hospital costs, utilization and outcomes. J Reprod Med 2003; 48: 943–949

31 American College of Obstetricians and Gynecologists. Appropriate use of laparoscopically assisted vaginal hysterectomy. Obstet Gynecol 2005; 105: 929–930

32 Meikle SF, Nugent EW, Orleans M. Complications and recovery from laparoscopy-assisted vaginal hysterectomy compared with abdominal and vaginal hysterectomy. Obstet Gynecol 1997; 89: 304–311

33 Miskry T, Magos A. Mass closure: a new technique for closure of the vaginal vault at vaginal hysterectomy. Br J Obstet Gynaecol 2001; 108: 1295–1297

34 Balfour RP. Laparoscopic assisted vaginal hysterectomy – 190 cases: complications and training. J Obstet Gynaecol 1999; 19: 164–166

35 Zupi E, Marconi D, Sbracia M et al. Directed laparoscopic cryomyolysis for symptomatic leiomyomata: one-year follow up. J Minim Invasive Gynecol 2005; 12): 343—346

Norma Pham   Peter E. Schwartz

Prophylactic oophorectomy in *BRCA* carriers

Breast cancer is the most common cancer affecting American women and is the second most common cause of death due to cancer in the US. The American Cancer Society estimates that 211,240 new cases of breast cancer will occur in 2005 and there will be 40,410 deaths from this disease.[1] Ovarian cancer is the fifth most common cancer and the fourth leading cause of death due to cancer, in the US. It is estimated that 22,220 new cases of ovarian cancer will occur and 16,210 deaths will be reported due to this disease.[1] While most cases of breast and ovarian cancers occur sporadically, 5–10% are due to a genetic predisposition.[2-4]

In the 1990s, two related genes, *BRCA1* and *BRCA2*, were found to be responsible for the majority of these hereditary forms of ovarian and breast cancer. Women with documented *BRCA1* and *BRCA2* mutations have a 15–65% life-time risk of developing ovarian cancer and a 60–85% risk of breast cancer.[2-4] This is compared to a 1.7% risk of ovarian cancer and 13% for breast cancer in the general population.[1] These mutations are found in 0.24% of the general population.[5] However, among the Ashkenazi Jewish population, the penetrance is approximately 2%[2] and accounts for 29–41% of all ovarian cancer cases.[6]

BRCA1 and *BRCA2* function as tumor suppression genes.[7] They encode proteins necessary for repair of DNA damage. It is thought that mutations in these genes lead to the uncontrolled cell growth responsible for cancers in the breast, ovary, fallopian tubes, and peritoneum. The penetrance of these mutations is incomplete, and depends on various factors such as the type of

Norma Pham MD
Chief Resident, Department of Obstetrics, Gynecology and Reproductive Sciences, Yale University School of Medicine, 333 Cedar Street, New Haven, CT 06510, USA

Peter E. Schwartz MD (for correspondence)
John Slade Ely Professor, Department of Obstetrics, Gynecology and Reproductive Sciences, Yale University School of Medicine, 333 Cedar Street, New Haven, CT 06510, USA
E-mail: peter.schwartz@yale.edu

mutation, the phenotype of the individual harboring the mutation and/or exogenous factors.[7] There are similar mutations found in different ethnic groups and are described as founder mutations. The most thoroughly studied are found in the Ashkenazi Jewish population. There has been a high prevalence of three mutations: the 85delAG and 5382insC in *BRCA1* and the 6174delT in *BRCA2*.[8–10] The risk of cancer conferred by a *BRCA* gene mutation is not the same in all women who have this genotype and depends mainly on the location and type of the mutation. For instance the Ashkenazi founder mutation discovered in *BRCA2* occurs in the ovarian cluster region of the gene. While mutations occurring outside of this region still carry an increased risk of ovarian cancer, it is, however, much lower.[11,12]

BRCA1 and *BRCA2* mutations most frequently produce ovarian cancers of the papillary serous (75%) histology. Endometrioid and Mullerian types are less commonly found and mucinous, clear cell types and borderline are rare or non-detected.[11,13,14]

Although *BRCA1 and BRCA2* mutations are similar with regards to the type of cancers they are associated with, they also exhibit many differences. Of *BRCA1*-related breast cancers, 90% were found to be estrogen receptor negative and 79% were found to be progestin receptor negative.[15] *BRCA2*, on the other hand, demonstrated the same amount of estrogen (65%), and progestin (40–60%) receptivity as matched controls.[16]

BRCA1-related gynecological cancers tend to occur on average 5–10 years earlier than those cancers due to *BRCA2* mutations.[11] For women with *BRCA1* mutations, the risk of developing ovarian cancer begins to rise in the late 30-year-olds and early 40-year-olds with the average age of diagnosis being 50.8 years. This is in contrast to the average age of onset of ovarian cancer of women with *BRCA2* mutations which is 59.2 years.[11] The life-time risk of ovarian cancer is 28–66% for a *BRCA1* mutation and 16–27% for a *BRCA2* mutation.[17] Fallopian tube cancer and primary peritoneal cancer have been included in the spectrum of *BRCA*-related gynecological cancers.[18] It is estimated that in women with BRCA mutations, the life-time risk of fallopian tube cancer is 0.6% and the life-time risk of primary peritoneal cancer is 1.3% which is still significantly higher than that of the general population. The age of diagnosis of these two cancers in individuals with BRCA mutations is approximately 10 years younger than that of patients without the mutation.[18]

This article will review the role of prophylactic oophorectomy in the management of women known to have *BRCA1* and *BRCA2* gene mutations.

PROPHYLACTIC BILATERAL SALPINGO-OOPHORECTOMY

As mentioned earlier, about 16,210 women are expected to die from ovarian cancer in the year 2005. This high mortality rate is attributed to 70% of ovarian cancers being found to be in an advanced stage at the time of diagnosis.[1] There is a lack of an effective screening tool to detect ovarian cancer at an early stage. With the inherent life-time risk of cancer and poor options for preventing or detecting these cancers at a curable stage, both the US National Institutes of Health (NIH) in 1995 and the Society of Gynecologic Oncologists (SGO) in 2005 in their committee statements recommend offering prophylactic surgery to *BRCA1* and *BRCA2* positive women.

The merits of these recommendations are largely based on the compelling evidence that prophylactic bilateral salpingo-oophorectomy (BSO) reduces the rates of subsequent ovarian, fallopian tube and breast cancers. Whether prophylactic BSO has any impact in the prevention of primary peritoneal carcinoma remains a controversial issue. Rebbeck *et al.*,[19] in 2002, retrospectively compared 259 women with *BRCA1* or *BRCA2* mutations who had undergone prophylactic oophorectomy to 292 women with *BRCA1* or *BRCA2* mutations who had not undergone surgery. Of the woman who had not undergone surgery, 58 cases of ovarian cancer were diagnosed. Of these 58 women, only six were stage I, underscoring again the lack of effective screening tools to detect early ovarian cancers. Among the surgery group, six cases of stage I ovarian cancer were identified at the time of surgery and two subsequent cases of peritoneal cancer were identified during the follow-up period.

Kauff *et al.*,[20] also in 2002, published evidence equally as supportive for the role of prophylactic BSO. They identified 170 *BRCA1* and *BRCA2* positive women and offered either risk-reducing surgery or surveillance. The surgery included BSO with or without hysterectomy. The surveillance group were advised to be monitored with gynecological examinations, transvaginal ultrasounds and serum CA125 levels. Thirteen cancers were subsequently diagnosed among the 78 women in the surveillance group, whereas in the surgery group, only four of the 94 participants developed breast cancer or *BRCA*-related gynecological cancers. Thus the 5-year cancer-free survival estimates for unaffected *BRCA1* and *BRCA2* carriers who underwent bilateral salpingo-oophorectomy was 94% compared to 69% in carriers who chose surveillance. Of note, 3 women in the prophylactic oophorectomy group were not included in the analysis because they were already found to have stage I gynecological cancer at the time of surgery.

In addition to preventing ovarian cancer, prophylactic oophorectomy serves the dual purpose in reducing the risk of breast cancer by removing an endogenous source of estrogen. By removing the ovaries, the risk of breast cancer decreased to 21% from 42% in women who had not undergone surgery.[19] This benefit reportedly extends to carriers who have already been diagnosed with breast cancer. In 2002, Møller *et al.*[21] found that the 5-year disease-free survival rate for women with *BRCA1/2*-associated breast cancer and negative nodes who underwent oophorectomy was 100% compared to 42% among women who had retained their ovaries. In the latter study, none of the 13 patients who underwent prophylactic oophorectomy within 6 months of the diagnosis recurred, but 14 of the 15 mutation carriers who kept their ovaries recurred.

Surgical technique

While the recommendations clearly advocate offering prophylactic oophorectomy to women with mutations in *BRCA1* and *BRCA2*, there is a lack of clear guidelines outlining precisely how and when this should be done.

There exists very little data regarding the preferred surgical technique for prophylactic salpingo-oophorectomy. In several of the studies, both laparotomy and the laparoscopic approach were utilized but there was no mention of the efficacy of one technique over the other.[22] A second area of controversy surrounds the type of surgery that should be performed. At a minimum, risk-reducing surgery should include bilateral oophorectomy. A population-based study of fallopian tube carcinoma has revealed the presence of BRCA1 and BRCA/2 germ-line mutation in over 15% of fallopian tube carcinomas.[23] Levine et al.[18] reported a mutation frequency of 17% and Brose et al.[24] found a 120-fold increased risk of fallopian tube carcinoma in BRCA1 mutation carriers. Compared to a risk in the general population of 0.025%, the cumulative age-adjusted life-time risk of fallopian tube cancer was 3.0%. Just as screening for ovarian cancer has many limitations, the same applies for fallopian tube carcinoma. Therefore, bilateral salpingectomy should be offered to reduce this risk and is now supported in the SGO consensus statement.

Currently, prophylactic surgery does not routinely incorporate a hysterectomy. Recently, there has been a suggestion that uterine papillary serous carcinomas (UPSCs) join the constellation of BRCA-related gynecological cancers. Lavie and colleagues[25] reported that 4 of 20 Jewish women with UPSC had germ-line founder mutations in BRCA1. Goldman et al.[26] reported that three of nine UPSC patients had germ-line BRCA2 mutations, but did not detect any BRCA1 mutations. On the contrary, Goshen et al.[27] retrospectively studied 56 unselected cases of UPSC and failed to find any correlation with the BRCA mutations.

Another argument for performing a hysterectomy is that it reduces the risk of leaving a residual fallopian tube behind at the time of a bilateral salpingo-oophorectomy (BSO).[28] The majority of fallopian tube carcinomas, however, occur in the more distal portions of the tube. Although, theoretically, malignant transformation of the remaining cells from the fallopian tube seems plausible, it has not yet been reported in the literature. Another important factor when considering hysterectomy in asymptomatic carriers of BRCA is that it eliminates the risk of developing uterine cancer conferred when taking HRT or tamoxifen. Due to conflicting evidence, the question of whether to perform hysterectomy during prophylactic surgery currently, however, remains unanswered.

For routine, benign, gynecological surgeries it is not routine to obtain peritoneal cytological washings. However, women undergoing risk-reducing surgery represent a unique subgroup of patients since they have no known evidence of tumor but merely are at higher risk for developing cancer. The question is, then, whether the surgical protocol in these cases should include routine peritoneal cytological sampling. Agoff et al.[29] found that in 5 women without suspicion of disease at the time of risk-reduction surgery, 2 had positive cytology. It was only after malignant cells were identified that the specimen was re-examined and the neoplasm found. Colgan et al.[30] reported 3 diagnoses of cancer based on peritoneal cytology collection among 35 women undergoing prophylactic oophorectomy. Since screening is unreliable in women who decline surgery, there may be a potential role for laparoscopic lavage or culdocentesis to aid in early detection.

Pathological examination

In addition to the lack of a consensus on surgical protocol, there is also no established pathological protocol to examine the specimens of apparently unaffected BRCA carriers. There have been several studies which have reported discovering occult carcinomas of the ovary and fallopian tube at the time of surgery. Colgan *et al.*[30] found carcinoma in 8.3% of a total of 60 specimens obtained from prophylactic BSO, while the study of Kauff *et al.*[20] demonstrated cancer in 3% and Rebbeck *et al.*[19] in 2.3% of specimens. On gross inspection, the majority of these specimens appeared normal and it was not until pathological examination that carcinoma was diagnosed. Powell *et al.*,[22] in an effort to implement a specific surgical–pathological protocol to detect malignancy in *BRCA* mutation carriers, found a 7-fold higher rate of cancer. The latter protocol incorporated a complete bilateral salpingo-oophorectomy either by laparotomy or laparoscopy, peritoneal washings, random peritoneal and omental biopsies, serial sectioning of the entire fallopian tubes and ovaries at 2-mm intervals and microscopic examination of all sections. They discovered 7 malignancies in 67 patients (17%), none of which exhibited gross tumor but instead were detected by pathological examination.

While removing the omentum and taking peritoneal biopsies are considered standard during an ovarian cancer staging procedure, it is uncertain whether omentectomy has a role in prophylactic surgery. In the Powell *et al.*[22] study, omentectomy for the most part was routinely performed. There were no detectable cancers in the omentum including specimens from patients found to have carcinomas arising in the ovaries or fallopian tube.

Optimal timing for risk-reduction surgery

For women who tested positive for the *BRCA* mutation and elect to reduce their risk of developing cancer, the appropriate timing of surgery becomes a delicate issue worthy of discussion. In *BRCA1* carriers, the risk of developing breast and ovarian cancer begins to rise in the late 30s to early 40s with 54% occurring before 50 years of age.[19,20] It seems reasonable to perform prophylactic oophorectomy at age 35 years or when childbearing is complete. However, there is a growing trend to delay childbearing into the late 30s and early 40s.[31] Women, knowing the rising risk of developing cancer, should be counseled that by postponing childbearing they are making themselves more susceptible to the perils their mutations afford them. In women with *BRCA2* mutations, on the other hand, the risk of developing ovarian cancer does not begin until 10 years later. While this may lend the opportunity to defer prophylactic bilateral salpingo-oophorectomy until closer to natural menopause, it is also important to remember that the risk of developing breast cancer by age 50 years is 26–34%.[20,32] Thus, by choosing to delay prophylactic surgery, the additive protection against breast cancer gained by oophorectomy may be lost.

Disadvantages of undergoing risk-reduction surgery

While there are many benefits to choosing prophylactic salpingo-oophorectomy, there are many disadvantages as well. Women undergoing risk-reduction surgery are subjected to the potential risk for surgical complications as well as the sequelae of premature menopause. The risks of surgery are mainly dependent on the skill of the surgeon, the type of surgery performed and the patient herself. The rate of major operative complications occurring during or after laparoscopy is about 1.9% and 4.5% of patients require conversion to laparotomy. The rate of injury and bleeding was found to be 9 times higher in women undergoing laparoscopic-assisted vaginal hysterectomy compared with laparoscopy without hysterectomy.[33] In the Kauff et al.[20] study, 4% of women undergoing prophylactic salpingo-oophorectomy developed surgical complications. Interestingly, none of the women who underwent concomitant hysterectomy developed surgical complication but the sample size was much smaller.[20]

Although there is a clear reduction in breast, ovarian and fallopian tube carcinomas after performing prophylactic BSO, there is still a risk of developing subsequent primary peritoneal carcinomas. Menczer et al.,[34] in a retrospective study, found that in Ashkenazi Jewish women with primary peritoneal cancer, 28% were carriers of the BRCA mutation. Recent data have estimated the risk of primary peritoneal cancers after prophylactic BSO to be 1–2%,[19,20] much lower than previously reported.[35]

Carriers of the BRCA mutations who elect prophylactic surgery at the earliest advisable age of 35 years, essentially become menopausal on average 16 years earlier than the general population. The associated risks for premature menopause include osteoporosis, vasomotor instability, a 2-fold increase in cardiovascular disease, decline in sexual drive, and changes in lipid profile.[36] While taking hormone replacement therapy (HRT) has become increasingly controversial in the general public, BRCA-positive women who have an already higher predisposition to developing cancer face even more of a conundrum. In a decision analysis, Armstrong et al.[36] looked at unaffected carriers who underwent prophylactic BSO both with and without hormone replacement therapy. Hormone replacement therapy after oophorectomy was associated with a relatively small decline in life expectancy when the treatment was stopped at age 50 years. BRCA1 germ-line mutations tend to be estrogen and progestin receptor negative while BRCA2 mutations are more likely to be estrogen and progestin receptor positive.[15,16] It would be logical, then, to assume that BRCA1 positive women would not be at increased risk for developing cancer by taking HRT. However, this hypothesis is suspect as prophylactic oophorectomy decreases the risk of breast cancer in both BRCA1 and BRCA2 mutation positive women.

SURVEILLANCE

Despite the reduction in breast cancer and BRCA-related cancers, 36–73% of carriers of the mutations opt for close surveillance.[37–39] For women who decline undergoing prophylactic salpingo-oophorectomy to reduce their risk of breast cancer and BRCA-related gynecological cancers, a standardized method of surveillance should be established. While mammography is the most commonly used screening tool to monitor unaffected BRCA carriers, there is no data regarding how frequently to obtain these images. Kauff et al.[40] recommended annual mammography in addition to monthly self breast examination and examination by a clinician 2–4 times per year. There is also limited data regarding the efficacy of screening mammography in this particular population. Unaffected carriers undergoing mammography are younger than the general population of women recommended for mammography. Breast tissue is much denser at a younger age making it more difficult for mammography to detect a malignancy. Similarly, it has been shown that breast tissue associated with BRCA mutations tends inherently to be denser, further decreasing the reliability of a mammogram.[41] Brekelmans *et al.*[42] reported results of mammographic screening of 128 BRCA mutation carriers, identifying nine cancers, five of which were associated with lymph node metastasis. Four of the nine tumors were so-called interval cancers detected between the screening examinations. There is growing evidence supporting the utility of MRI for screening in *BRCA1* and *BRCA2* carriers. Kuhl *et al.*[43] found the sensitivity of MRI to be 100% compared to 33% for mammography and 33%.

Surveillance strategies for the early detection of ovarian cancer also vary among institutions but typically entail serial serum CA125 levels and transvaginal ultrasound. The frequency of these measurements is also not universally specified. The Kauff *et al.*[20] study suggested twice yearly serum CA125 levels, transvaginal ultrasounds and bimanual examinations, while Vasen *et al.*[44] followed patients annually with gynecological examinations, transvaginal ultrasounds, and CA125. In both of these studies, ovarian cancer, when discovered, was advanced. Besides failure to detect early cancers, another disadvantage of surveillance in this population is the difficulty in interpreting abnormal results. Meeuwissen *et al.*,[45] in an attempt to evaluate the efficacy of surveillance, operated on 20 women with suspicious findings and found benign disease in 19 women. It can be argued, then, that establishing a protocol for the early detection of ovarian cancer in *BRCA*-positive women would be arbitrary since the efficacy of such screening is poor.

Other recommendations

For women who choose close surveillance, there are other options, besides the recommended risk-reducing bilateral salpingo-oophorectomy to decrease their risk of developing breast and *BRCA*-associated cancers.

Tamoxifen

Chemoprevention with tamoxifen is often used to decrease the incidence of breast cancer. King *et al.*[46] found that tamoxifen reduced the incidence of breast cancer in women with *BRCA2* mutations by 62% but had no effect for *BRCA1*. In a decision analysis by Grann *et al.*,[47] a 30-year-old *BRCA1* or *BRCA2* mutation carrier could prolong her survival by 1.8 years and her quality adjusted survival by 2.8 years by taking tamoxifen.

Oral contraceptives

In the general population, oral contraceptives offer protection against ovarian cancer. However, in mutation carriers, it is somewhat more complex. Earlier studies suggested there is a small increase in breast cancer in mutation carriers who took oral contraceptives, mostly in BRCA1 women.[48,49] However, a recent study by Milne *et al.*[50] showed that there was no evidence of increased risk of breast cancer when using low-dose oral contraceptives, which are more now more widely prescribed. The older studies were retrospective analyses and were based on life-time use of oral contraceptives. Milne et al.[50] ascribed the increased breast cancer risk seen in previous studies to be possibly a reflection of the high-dose formulations used before the mid-1970s.

There are conflicting data regarding the effect of oral contraceptives on prevention of ovarian cancer. Several studies have found that the use of oral contraceptives protected against ovarian cancer in both BRCA1 and BRCA2 carriers.[5,49] Modan et al.,[51] however, in 2001 found no added protection as typically seen in the general population. If, with the newer forms of oral contraceptives, there is no increased risk of breast cancer and possibly a decrease risk of ovarian cancer, the potential for chemoprevention seems promising, although further research in this area is warranted.

Pregnancy and breast-feeding

If women should choose prophylactic oophorectomy, the maximum benefit would be after the age of 35 years, when childbearing is complete. By delaying childbearing and thus prolonging surgery, there is some belief that the benefits associated with removing the ovaries will be lost with time. However, if a women should opt to retain her ovaries, the topic of reproduction becomes more intricate. Women with BRCA1 and BRCA2 mutations who have a full-term pregnancy are more likely to develop breast cancer before the age of 40 years.[52,53] Mothers who deliver at term before the age of 40 years have an increased odds ratio of 1.6 in BRCA1 and 2.1 in BRCA2 carriers.[52] In the general population, pregnancy offers protection against breast cancer occurring after age 40 years, but appears to increase the risk of very early onset breast cancer.[54]

In the general population, breast-feeding appears to decrease the risk of developing breast cancer. It has been thought that the mechanism is likely related to changes in mammary gland differentiation or the effect on estrogen levels in the breast.[52] Breast-feeding may decrease the level of estrogen in the breast directly or it may suppress ovulation itself. Jernstrom et al.,[52] in a large matched case control study in 2004, found that women with BRCA1 mutations who breast fed for more than a year had a significant reduction in the incidence of breast cancer.

Tubal ligation

Tubal ligation, similarly, reduces the risk of ovarian cancer in the general population. However, in a case-control study of Jewish BRCA1 carriers, there was no added protection.[55] There was, however, an associated decreased risk of ovarian cancer in women with BRCA1, but not BRCA2 gene mutations.[55] Thus, a strategy for evaluation and management of BRCA1 positive women who do not wish to lose their ovarian function upon completion of child-bearing would be to have them undergo a laparoscopic bilateral tubal ligation and perform peritoneal washings at the time of surgery to try to identify occult disease.

Proteomics

The concept of identifying abnormal serum proteins or altered levels of serum protein provides an excellent opportunity to detect preneoplastic changes in carriers of BRCA1 and BRCA2 gene mutation.[56] While the potential exists, the technology still lags behind but provides a promising option for the future.

CONCLUSIONS

Since the discovery of *BRCA1* and *BRCA2*, we can now identify women who are at greater risk for developing breast, ovarian, primary peritoneal, and fallopian tube carcinomas. However, the value of genetic testing is only beneficial if we have the ability to prevent or reduce this risk. By recommending prophylactic bilateral salpingo-oophorectomy, carriers of this germ-line mutation are able to increase the 5-year cancer-free survival rate from 69% to 94%.[20] Furthermore, women who take tamoxifen after an oophorectomy have a survival curve that is similar to that of non-carriers of the mutation.[47] However, this risk-reducing surgery is not without risk itself. Women must be counseled regarding the complications of surgery, albeit low, and the associated adverse effects of premature menopause. Unaffected carriers of *BRCA1* and *BRCA2* who choose close surveillance should also be offered alternatives such as bilateral tubal ligation and oral contraceptives to reduce their risk of breast cancer and *BRCA* related gynecological cancers. Until we have a more sensitive screening tool, women who harbor *BRCA1* and *BRCA2* mutations should be strongly encouraged to undergo prophylactic oophorectomy to decrease the risk of developing subsequent breast and *BRCA*-related gynecological cancers as well as to detect occult carcinomas at an early and potentially curable stage.

KEY POINTS FOR CLINICAL PRACTICE

- Women with *BRCA1* and *BRCA2* mutation should be offered a prophylactic bilateral salpingo-oophorectomy after the age of 35 years and/or after childbearing is complete.

- Risk-reducing surgery may be done either by laparotomy or laparoscopy and should at minimum include removing the ovaries and tubes and peritoneal washings.

- Specimens should be carefully reviewed by the pathologists who should already be alerted that the surgery is performed for 'unaffected' carriers of the *BRCA1* and *BRCA2* mutation. This may be an opportunity to detect occult disease at an early stage.

- Women who decline prophylactic surgery must be followed with close surveillance with CA-125 and transvaginal ultrasound although the frequency yet has not been established. These women should also be counseled that tubal ligation, breast-feeding and oral contraceptives may decrease their risk of ovarian cancer. However, each patient must be appropriately assessed.

References

1 Jemal A, Murray T, Ward E *et al*. Cancer statistics 2005. Ca Cancer J Clin 2005; 55: 10–30
2 Struewing JP, Hartge P, Wacholder S *et al*. The risk of cancer associated with specific mutations of BRCA1 and BRCA2 among Ashkenazi Jews. N Engl J Med 1997; 336: 1401–1408

3 Satagopan JM, Offit K, Foulkes W *et al*. The lifetime risks of breast cancer in Ashkenazi Jewish carriers of BRCA1 and BRCA2 mutations. Cancer Epidemiol Biomarkers Prevent 2001; 10: 467–473

4 Ford D, Easton DF, Stratton M *et al*. Genetic heterogeneity and penetrance analysis of the BRCA1 and BRCA2 genes in breast cancer families. The Breast Cancer Linkage Consortium. Am J Hum Genet 1998; 62: 676–689

5 Whittemore AS, Balise RR, Pharoah PD *et al*. Oral contraceptive use and ovarian cancer risk among carriers of BRCA1 or BRCA2 mutations. Br J Cancer 2004; 91: 1911–1915

6 Robles-Diaz L, Goldfrank DJ, Kauff ND, Robson M, Offit K. Hereditary ovarian cancer in Ashkenazi Jews. Fam Cancer 2004; 3: 259–264

7 Honrado E, Benitez J, Palacios J. The molecular pathology of hereditary breast cancer: genetic testing and therapeutic implications. Mod Pathol 2005; 18: 1–16

8 Struewing JP, Abeliovich D, Peretz T *et al*. The carrier frequency of the BRCA1 85delAG mutation is approximately 1 percent in Ashkenazi Jewish individuals. Nat Genet 1995; 11: 198–200

9 Roa BB, Boyd AA, Volcik K, Richards CS. Ashkenazi Jewish population frequencies for common mutations in BRCA1 and BRCA2. Nat Genet 1996; 14: 185–187

10 Oddoux C, Struewing JP, Clayton CM *et al*. The carrier frequency of the BRCA2 6174delT mutation among Ashkenazi Jewish individuals is approximately 1%. Nat Genet 1996; 14: 188–190

11 Moslehi R, Chu W, Karlan B *et al*. BRCA1 and BRCA2 mutation analysis of 208 Ashkenazi Jewish women with ovarian cancer. Am J Hum Genet 2000; 66: 259–272

12 Gayther SA, Warren W, Mazoyer S *et al*. Germline mutations of the BRCA1 gene in breast and ovarian cancer families provide evidence for a genotype–phenotype correlation. Nat Genet 1995; 11: 428–433

13 Risch HA, McLaughlin JR, Cole DE *et al*. Prevalence and penetrance of germline BRCA1 and BRCA2 mutations in a population series of 649 women with ovarian cancer Am J Hum Genet 2001; 68: 700–710

14 Werness BA, Ramus SJ, DiCioccio RA *et al*. Histopathology, FIGO stage, and BRCA mutation status of ovarian cancers from the Gilda Radner Familial Ovarian Cancer Registry. Int J Gynecol Pathol 2004; 23: 29–34

15 Lakhani SR, Van De Vijver MJ, Jacquemier J *et al*. The pathology of familial breast cancer: predictive value of immunohistochemical markers estrogen receptor, progesterone receptor, HER-2, and p53 in patients with mutations in BRCA1 and BRCA2. J Clin Oncol 2002; 20: 2310–2318

16 Armes JE, Trute L, White D *et al*. Distinct molecular pathogeneses of early-onset breast cancers in BRCA1 and BRCA2 mutation carriers: a population-based study. Cancer Res 1999; 59: 2011–2017

17 Satagopan JM, Boyd J, Kauff ND *et al*. Ovarian cancer risk in Ashkenazi Jewish carriers of BRCA1 and BRCA2 mutations. Clin Cancer Res 2002; 8: 3776–3781

18 Levine DA, Argenta PA, Yee CJ *et al*. Fallopian tube and primary peritoneal carcinomas associated with BRCA mutations. J Clin Oncol 2003; 21: 4222–4227

19 Rebbeck TR, Lynch HT, Neuhausen SL *et al*. Prophylactic oophorectomy in carriers of BRCA1 or BRCA2 mutations. N Engl J Med 2002; 346: 1616–1622

20 Kauff ND, Satagopan JM, Robson ME *et al*. Risk-reducing salpingo-oophorectomy in women with a BRCA1 or BRCA2 mutation. N Engl J Med 2002; 346: 1609–1615

21 Møller P, Borg A, Evans DG *et al*. Survival in prospectively ascertained familial breast cancer: analysis of a series stratified by tumour characteristics, BRCA mutations and oophorectomy. Int J Cancer 2002; 101: 555–559

22 Powell CB, Kenley E, Chen LM *et al*. Risk-reducing salpingo-oophorectomy in BRCA mutation carriers: role of serial sectioning in the detection of occult malignancy. J Clin Oncol 2005; 23: 127–132

23 Aziz S, Kuperstein G, Rosen B *et al*. A genetic epidemiological study of carcinoma of the fallopian tube. Gynecol Oncol 2001; 80: 341–345

24 Brose MS, Rebbeck TR, Calzone KA, Stopfer JE, Nathanson KL, Weber BL. Cancer risk estimates for BRCA1 mutation carriers identified in a risk evaluation program. J Natl Cancer Inst 2002; 94: 1365–1372

25 Lavie O, Hornreich G, Ben-Arie A. BRCA germline mutations in Jewish women with uterine serous papillary carcinoma. Gynecol Oncol 2004; 92: 521–524

26 Goldman NA, Goldberg GL, Runowicz CD. BRCA mutations in women with concurrent breast carcinoma and uterine papillary serous carcinoma. ASCO Proc 2002; 21

27 Goshen R, Chu W, Elit L *et al*. Is uterine papillary serous adenocarcinoma a manifestation of the hereditary breast-ovarian cancer syndrome? Gynecol Oncol 2000; 79: 477–481

28 Paley PJ, Swisher EM, Garcia RL *et al*. Occult cancer of the fallopian tube in BRCA-1 germline mutation carriers at prophylactic oophorectomy: A case for recommending hysterectomy at surgical prophylaxis. Gynecol Oncol 2001; 80: 176–180

29 Agoff SN, Mendelin JE, Grieco VS, Garcia RL. Unexpected gynecologic neoplasms in patients with proven or suspected BRCA-1 or -2 mutations: Implications for gross examination, cytology and clinical follow-up. Am J Surg Pathol 2002; 26: 171–178

30 Colgan TJ, Murphy J, Cole DE, Narod S, Rosen B. Occult carcinoma in prophylactic oophorectomy specimens: prevalence and association with BRCA germline mutation status. Am J Surg Pathol 2001; 25: 1283–1289

31 Hamilton LJ, Evans AJ, Wilson AR *et al*. Breast imaging findings in women with BRCA1- and BRCA2-associated breast carcinoma. Clin Radiol 2004; 59: 895–902

32 Struewing JP, Watson P, Easton DF, Ponder BA, Lynch HT, Tucker MA. Prophylactic oophorectomy in inherited breast/ovarian cancer families. J Natl Cancer Inst Monogr 1995; 17: 33–35

33 Mirhashemi R, Harlow BL, Ginsburg ES, Signorello LB, Berkowitz R, Feldman S. Predicting risk of complications with gynecologic laparoscopic surgery. Obstet Gynecol 1998; 92: 327–331

34 Menczer J, Chetrit A, Barda G *et al*. Frequency of BRCA mutations in primary peritoneal carcinoma in Israeli Jewish women. Gynecol Oncol 2003; 88: 58–61

35 Piver MS, Jishi MF, Tsukada Y, Nava G. Primary peritoneal carcinoma after prophylactic oophorectomy in women with a family history of ovarian cancer: A report of the Gilda Radner Familial Ovarian Cancer Registry. Cancer 1993; 71: 2751–2755

36 Armstrong K, Schwartz JS, Randall T, Rubin SC, Weber B. Hormone replacement therapy and life expectancy after prophylactic oophorectomy in women with BRCA1/2 mutations: a decision analysis. J Clin Oncol 2004; 22: 1045–1054

37 Schwartz MD, Kaufman E, Peshkin BN *et al*. Bilateral prophylactic oophorectomy and ovarian cancer screening following BRCA1/BRCA2 mutation testing. J Clin Oncol 2003; 21: 4034–4041

38 Meijers-Heijboer H, Brekelmans CT, Menke-Pluymers M *et al*. Use of genetic testing and prophylactic mastectomy and oophorectomy in women with breast or ovarian cancer from families with a BRCA1 or BRCA2 mutation. J Clin Oncol 2003; 21: 1675–1681

39 Botkin JR, Smith KR, Croyle RT. Genetic testing for a BRCA1 mutation: prophylactic surgery and screening behavior in women 2 years post testing. Am J Med Genet 2003; 118: 201–209

40 Kauff ND, Hurley KE, Hensley ML *et al*. Ovarian carcinoma screening in women at intermediate risk: impact on quality of life and need for invasive follow-up. Cancer 2005; 104: 314–320

41 Huo Z, Giger ML, Olopade OI *et al*. Computerized analysis of digitized mammograms of BRCA1 and BRCA2 gene mutation carriers. Radiology 2002; 225: 519–526

42 Brekelmans CT, Seynaeve C, Bartels CC *et al*. Effectiveness of breast cancer surveillance in BRCA1/2 gene mutation carriers and women with high familial risk. J Clin Oncol 2001; 9: 924–930

43 Kuhl CK, Schmutzler RK, Leutner CC *et al*. Breast MR imaging screening in 192 women proved or suspected to be carriers of a breast cancer susceptibility gene: preliminary results. Radiology 2000; 215: 267–279

44 Vasen H, Tesfay E, Boonstra H *et al*. Early detection of breast and ovarian cancer in families with BRCA mutations. Eur J Cancer 2005; 41: 549–554

45 Meeuwissen PA, Seynaeve C, Brekelmans CT, Meijers-Heijboer HJ, Klijn JG, Burger CW. Outcome of surveillance and prophylactic salpingo-oophorectomy in asymptomatic women at high risk for ovarian cancer. Gynecol Oncol 2005; 97: 476–482

46 King MC, Wieand S, Hale K *et al*. Tamoxifen and breast cancer incidence among women with inherited mutations in BRCA1 and BRCA2: National Surgical Adjuvant Breast and Bowel Project (NSABP-P1) Breast Cancer Prevention Trial. JAMA 2001; 286: 2251–2256

47 Grann VR, Jacobson JS, Thomason D, Hershman D, Heitjan DF, Neugut AI. Effect of

prevention strategies on survival and quality-adjusted survival of women with BRCA1/2 mutations: an updated decision analysis. J Clin Oncol 2002; 20: 2520–2529

48 Ursin G, Henderson BE, Haile RW *et al*. Does oral contraceptive use increase the risk of breast cancer in women with BRCA1/BRCA2 mutations more than in other women? Cancer Res 1997; 57: 3678–3681

49 Narod SA, Dube MP, Klijn J et al. Oral contraceptives and the risk of breast cancer in BRCA1 and BRCA2 mutation carriers. J Natl Cancer Inst 2002; 94: 1773–1779

50 Milne RL, Knight JA, John EM *et al*. Oral contraceptive use and risk of early-onset breast cancer in carriers and noncarriers of BRCA1 and BRCA2 mutations. Cancer Epidemiol Biomarkers Prevent 2005; 14: 350–356

51 Modan B, Hartge P, Hirsh-Yechezkel G *et al*. Parity, oral contraceptives, and the risk of ovarian cancer among carriers and noncarriers of a BRCA1 or BRCA2 mutation. N Engl J Med 2001; 345: 235–240

52 Jernstrom H, Lerman C, Ghadirian P *et al*. Pregnancy and risk of early breast cancer in carriers of BRCA1 and BRCA2. Lancet 1999; 354: 1846–1850

53 Johannsson O, Loman N, Borg A, Olsson H. Pregnancy-associated breast cancer in BRCA1 and BRCA2 germline mutation carriers. Lancet 1998; 352: 1359–1360

54 Narod SA. Hormonal prevention of hereditary breast cancer. Ann NY Acad Sci 2001; 952: 36–43

55 Narod SA, Sun P, Ghadirian P *et al*. Tubal ligation and risk of ovarian cancer in carriers of BRCA1 or BRCA2 mutations: a case-control study. Lancet 2001; 357: 1467–1470

56 Mor G, Visinti I, Lai Y et al. Serum protein markers for the early detection of ovarian cancer. Proc Natl Acad Sci USA 2005; 102: 7677–7682

Yatin Thakur   Rajiv Varma

New developments in the management of uterovaginal prolapse

Pelvic organ prolapse (POP) is an increasingly common condition for which women seek help and frequently undergo surgical treatment. The UK National Centre for Health Statistics[1] lists genital prolapse as the third most common reasons for a hysterectomy in women and the most common indication for hysterectomy in post-menopausal women. The cost of treating prolapse in the US annually is estimated to be around US$1 billion.

Prolapse is responsible for 20% of the waiting lists for major gynaecological surgery in the UK.[2] In the Oxford Family Planning Association study,[3] the incidence of hospital admission with a diagnosis of prolapse requiring surgical correction was 2.04/1000. The life-time risk of undergoing surgery for prolapse by age 80 years has been estimated as 11.1% and the likelihood of repeat surgery is as high as 29.2%.[4] With a gradual rise in life expectancy and resulting increase in an ageing population, there is likely to be an increase in the prevalence of pelvic organ prolapse. The demand for prolapse surgery, therefore, is likely to increase significantly in the next few decades.

DEFINITION

Despite the scale of the problem, the definition of prolapse requiring treatment remains vague. The US National Institutes of Health (NIH) in 2001 defined prolapse as the leading edge of any vaginal segment being ≥ -1 cm above the hymenal remnants. In 2002, the International Continence Society defined pelvic organ prolapse as the descent of one or more of vaginal segments – the

Yatin Thakur MD DNBE MRCOG (for correspondence)
Specialist Registrar, Basildon University Hospital, Nethermayne, Basildon, Essex SS16 5NL, UK
E-mail: yat@doctors.org.uk

Rajiv Varma FRCOG
Consultant Obstetrician and Gynaecologist, Basildon University Hospital, Nethermayne, Basildon, Essex SS16 5NL, UK

Table 1 Distribution of prolapse stage versus anatomical compartment

Prolapse stage	Anterior	Posterior	Apical
Stage 0	18%	19%	57%
Stage 1	14%	20%	17%
Stage 2	47%	45%	13%
Stage 3	13%	9%	6%
Stage 4	8%	6%	7%

Stage 2–4 POP in anterior compartment, 68%; apical compartment, 26%; and posterior compartment, 60%.

anterior, the posterior, and the apex of the vagina (cervix) or the vault (cuff) after hysterectomy. Thus, there are two definitions of prolapse from two significant institutions in urogynaecology; neither of these definitions are correct or clinically relevant. There is growing evidence that symptoms of prolapse are not described adequately by the anatomical arrangement of the lower genital tract organs.

PREVALENCE

The prevalence of prolapse to the level of the hymen varies from 2% to 48%.[5–8] This broad range is likely due to differences in sources of study populations, age, race, parity and examination techniques. There have been a few studies recently regarding the distribution of pelvic organ support in various populations. In the Women's Health Initiative (WHI) study, women with intact uterus, the rate of uterine prolapse, cystocoele and rectocoele were reported as 14.2%, 34.3% and 18.6%, respectively. In women who had undergone hysterectomy, the prevalence of cystocoele and rectocoele was 32.9% and 18.3%, respectively.[9] The overall distribution of pelvic organ prolapse by POP-Q system was found as stage 0, 6.4%; stage 1, 43.3%; stage 2, 47.7%; and stage 3, 2.6%.[6] In another study by Ellerkman et al.,[10] the distribution of prolapse stage with respect to anatomical compartment is shown in Table 1.

AETIOLOGY

The aetiology of POP is multifactorial. It is more common in women after a vaginal delivery as compared to a caesarean section.[11] All forms of caesarean delivery, especially prelabour caesarean section, is associated with less pelvic organ descent.[5] The strongest predisposing factor for prolapse is parity; following the birth of the first child, a woman is 4 times more likely to develop a prolapse. This risk then rises to 11 times with four or more deliveries; parity and obesity are strongly associated with increased risk for uterine prolapse, cystocoele, and rectocoele.[3] Samuelsson et al.[5] also found statistically significant associations of increasing parity and maximum birth weight with the development of POP. The other factors that are implicated are age, chronic cough, chronic constipation, previous hysterectomy and oestrogen deficiency. There are data that link clinical, laboratory, and genetic syndromes of abnormalities of collagen to pelvic organ prolapse.[12,13] In addition, POP in young women seems more common with a history of abdominal herniae, suggesting a possible connection with abnormal collagen.[14]

In recent years, imaging methods have contributed significantly to our understanding of the traumatic effects of childbirth on the pelvic floor. The changes in pelvic organ mobility and levator function following childbirth has been demonstrated on ultrasound imaging of the pelvic floor.[15,16]

PATHOPHYSIOLOGY

Neuromuscular injury has been proposed as an important factor predisposing to pelvic floor dysfunction. There are several neurophysiological studies that have used pudendal nerve latency or single fibre or concentric needle pelvic floor electromyography (EMG) to investigate the role of nerve injury in pelvic floor dysfunction. Histological studies have shown increased re-innervation, which occurs in response to denervation and is considered to be a marker for nerve injury. Progressive pelvic floor denervation is thought to lead to sagging of the levators, widening of the levator hiatus with loss of urethral and vaginal support leading to stress urinary incontinence and genital prolapse. Ageing and childbearing are the two major factors predisposing to pelvic floor denervation.[17] With increasing age, the connective tissue to muscle ratio is reduced and the hormonal changes during pregnancy or abnormal remodelling of collagen following pregnancy may be important in the development of these conditions in multiparous women.[18] Straining due to chronic constipation may also lead to atrophic damage to pelvic floor.

Collagen is the main constituent of endopelvic fascia and abnormalities in the quantity, type and quality of collagen have been observed in patients with both stress incontinence and genito-urinary prolapse.[18] A reduction in total collagen and increased turnover of collagen has also been identified in women with prolapse. Women with stress incontinence and prolapse have an increase in abdominal striae and increased incidence of joint hypermobility.[5]

ANATOMICAL CONSIDERATIONS

DeLancey,[19,20] in his famous work on cadaver dissection, divided the vaginal supports into three levels. Level 1 – superior attachment (cardinal/uterosacral ligament complex); Level 2 – lateral attachment (superolateral insertion points of the anterior vaginal wall, rectovaginal fascia); and Level 3 – distal attachment (perineal body, perineal membrane). Petros[21] confirmed these findings in his radiological study of 50 nulliparous females.

In normal women upright at rest, the proximal vaginal axis is almost horizontal, lying parallel to and on the levator plate. Colpographic studies have shown that as intra-abdominal pressure increases, the pelvic diaphragm contracts and maintains the position of the levator plate and horizontal vaginal axis.[22] As a consequence, uterus, vagina and rectum are pushed against the levator plate and not through the genital hiatus. Petros[21] demonstrated intact levator plate with obvious prolapse of the vagina and uterus on straining; hence, muscle damage alone cannot provide the entire explanation for the uterovaginal prolapse.

Uterovaginal prolapse is attributed to a break in the integrity of the uterosacral-ligament (USL) complex, weakening of the pelvic floor musculature and alteration of the normal vaginal axis. These are rarely found in isolation and tend to co-exist with defects in more than one compartment.

RECURRENCE AFTER SURGERY

Recurrent pelvic organ prolapse after surgical correction is one of the most vexing problems in reconstructive pelvic surgery. Nearly 30% of all surgery for prolapse and urinary incontinence performed in one US community-based sample was for recurrent problems.[4] The prevalence of re-operation in another community-based healthcare delivery system (Kaiser Permanente Northwest) was even higher (43–56%).[23] Yet, re-operation is not synonymous with recurrence, because many women do not seek repair of recurrent prolapse; thus, the prevalence of prolapse recurrence (depending on the definition) may be even higher. Despite the introduction of new and 'better' surgical tools and techniques, prolapse inevitably recurs in some women, and remarkably little is known about those factors that prevent or promote its occurrence. The recurrence of prolapse in individual compartments of the vagina is not well understood.

A recent study of recurrence showed that 1 year after surgery, 58% had recurrent prolapse (defined as stage II or worse). The most important finding of this study was in a population of women with prolapse who had vaginal surgery, aged < 60 years and more advanced prolapse (POP-Q stages III and IV) were associated with greater risk for recurrent prolapse at 1 year. At first, these findings seem contradictory because increasing age is a well-established risk factor for advancing prolapse. However, the idea that younger age may be associated with a higher risk of recurrent prolapse is consistent with certain pathophysiological concepts. A young woman with prolapse may have: (i) inferior tissue quality; (ii) greater nerve, muscle or fascial injury; or (iii) other factors relative to an older woman with the same degree of prolapse. These patients also have a life-style that is likely to predispose them to a higher risk of recurrence compared with older patients. This same trend was demonstrated by Nieminen et al.:[24] women younger than 73 years were more likely to experience recurrent prolapse after sacrospinous ligament fixation. Other factors associated with age (such as level of physical activity) may influence prolapse recurrence. This emphasises the point that prolapse repairs are compensatory at best and, by necessity, are applied empirically rather than designed to correct a specific pathophysiological abnormality.

However, what is success or failure with prolapse? In one sense, prolapse failure is purely anatomical, yet this ignores the fact that prolapse affects a woman's quality of life. Therefore, symptoms should be considered in the distinction between success and failure. However, the correlation between measured prolapse anatomy and patient-reported symptoms is poor.[25]

The anterior vagina is regarded as the site that is most prone to recurrent prolapse.[26] Challenges to providing a durable repair of anterior vaginal prolapse may include the relatively greater exposure to intra-abdominal strain.

Recurrent prolapse after surgery is a difficult and complicated problem and those factors that prevent or promote it are not well defined. A significant independent relationship between recurrent prolapse after vaginal prolapse repair and age < 60 years and greater prolapse severity has been demonstrated by the study by Whiteside et al.[27]

Quantification

Several systems to quantify POP objectively have been developed in recent years. The pelvic organ prolapse quantification (POP-Q) system introduced by Bump and colleagues[28] is now the only one that is widely accepted. It has also been objectively studied and proved to have good intra- and interexaminer reliability.[29] Three points (anterior, mid and posterior vaginal wall) are measured in centimetres during maximal straining, two points are measured externally along with the vaginal length under no strain. The anterior and posterior points may have positive or negative values, the negative values indicating a position proximal to the hymen. The size of genital hiatus is measured from external urethral orifice to hymen at 6-o'clock and the perineal body from the centre of the anus to the hymen. The anterior and posterior points form the basis of the staging. The staging system can have values from 0 to 4, 0 meaning excellent support of all compartments and 4 total uterine procidentia or vaginal vault prolapse (Fig. 1). The POP-Q system is a tool to quantify and stage results of physical examination at anterior, apical or posterior sites in the vagina, but it does not assign the specific location of fascial defects.

Pelvic floor imaging

Imaging studies might be useful for cases where the symptoms and signs of POP do not correlate with clinical findings or there are difficulties with differential diagnosis, when prior surgery has failed or in research settings. An examination under anaesthetic might be required for a few patients where none of these are helpful.

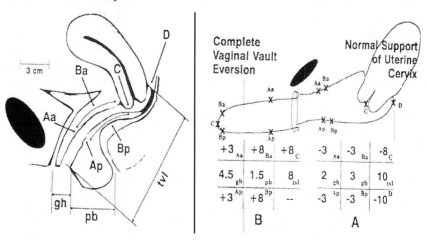

Fig. 1 Diagram of measurements taken for pelvic organ prolapse quantification (POPQ). Aa, 3 cm from the hymen on anterior vaginal wall; Ba, most distal point of upper interior vagina from hymen when compared to point A; C, lowest point of cervix; D, posterior fornix; Ap, 3 cm from the hymen on the posterior vaginal wall; Bp, most distal point of upper posterior vaginal when compared to point A; Pb, perineal body; gh, genital hiatus; tvl, total vaginal length. Adapted from Jackson *et al. The Obstetrician & Gynaecologist*, July 2000.

Ultrasound examination by transabdominal, endorectal, endovaginal, translabial or perineal approaches is an eminently suitable diagnostic tool for some forms of pelvic floor dysfunction.[30] It has been reported that women with a prolapse have greater bladder neck mobility than continent women and the extent of the movement correlates well with the anterior wall descent. A transrectal scan is found to be a useful tool in the diagnosis of enterocoele. A transperineal or a transvaginal approach has been described to image the levator ani muscle. With this technique, it is also possible to visualise lateral vaginal defects and the levator hiatus, which has been found to be larger in women with prolapse when compared to controls.[31]

Magnetic resonance imaging (MRI) has proven to be a more accurate imaging tool than clinical pelvic evaluation in diagnosing and grading functional disorders of the female pelvic floor and pelvic visceral prolapse. Quantification of the pelvic descent process with the use of dynamic MRI may be of value in surgical planning and post-surgical follow-up.[32] The advantages of MRI include lack of ionising radiation, depiction of the soft tissues of the pelvis, and multiplanar imaging capability.

In one small study on post-hysterectomy vault prolapse (13 patients), MRI was compared to intra-operative and ultrasound findings and showed no superiority towards planning a better repair.[33] In another study of 40 patients, dynamic MRI was found to be superior to fluoroscopic proctography because patients could be left in privacy while the images were continuously acquired without any concern for radiation exposure.[34] Another study of 125 POP patients staged by dynamic MRI prolapse was objectively graded; MRI staging was found accurate when compared with intra-operative findings, except for rectocoele.[35]

The importance of MRI in clinical work remains to be seen, the cost, however, prohibits its use in routine clinical practice and it is likely to remain a tool for research.

QUALITY OF LIFE IN POP

POP can severely affect the quality of life (QoL) of women, causing physical, social, psychological, occupational, domestic and/or sexual limitations to their life-styles. Some degree of prolapse is seen in 50% of parous women but only 20% of these women are symptomatic.[6] Women with prolapse can experience a variety of pelvic floor symptoms but few are specific to prolapse; it is often challenging for the clinician to determine which symptoms are attributable to the prolapse itself and will, therefore, improve or resolve once the prolapse is treated.

In recent years, there has been a considerable interest in the development of QoL tools or questionnaires. Historically, the development of generic and condition-specific questionnaires has been driven by a demand for reliable and valid outcome measures in research. Given some of the concerns surrounding the accuracy and reliability of the clinical interview, it may be appropriate to employ these instruments more routinely in clinical practice, taking account of patients' own views of their health and potentially improving the standard of care. In addition, the demands of clinical governance and evidence-based medicine mean that such measures will be increasingly required in order to evaluate the efficacy of medical interventions from the patient's perspective.

These tools are to provide a means of objectively identifying and quantifying symptoms that are produced by pelvic organ prolapse.[36]

Women who undergo surgical procedures for pelvic floor dysfunction have a variety of desired subjective outcomes. Goals that relate to social roles, sexuality, and self-image may take longer to achieve successfully than other types of goals. Hullfish et al.,[37,38] in their long-term follow-up study, reported 72% of goals were attained at short-term, and 68% attained at long-term follow-up at the individual goal level. At the person level, 45.8% of women reported achieving all listed goals in the short term, and 42.0% in the long term. Pre-operative assessment of goals is a useful addition to clinical and subjective data in the long-term management of women with pelvic floor disorders.

RECENT DEVELOPMENTS IN THE SURGICAL MANAGEMENT OF POP

The aim of surgery for prolapse is to correct anatomical defects, preserve the vaginal function, and improve patient symptoms with minimal morbidity and the least risk of recurrence in the long-term. The challenges in the management of POP are due to its high recurrence rates, paucity of randomised controlled trials and the poor definition of success/failure rates.

Use of prosthetic materials

There have been number of studies which have reported the use of prosthetic materials in an effort to reduce the high recurrence rates. Unfortunately, only a handful of these have been properly designed, randomised, control trials. The situation is made more difficult by the fact that there are many new materials, all claiming to be superior to each other. The material that has been studied most widely is the monofilament polypropylene mesh and there is emerging data that the repairs carried out using this might be more durable.

The mechanism and principles of surgical correction for vaginal prolapse are assumed to be the same as for the correction of abdominal wall hernia. Mesh used for hernia repair is buried under a tissue that is of a different composition and thickness when compared with vaginal skin. The introduction of minimally invasive sling techniques such as the tension-free vaginal tape (TVT) with minimal problems of erosion has played an important in role in the increased use of synthetic materials in prolapse surgery.[39]

We would like to caution against the routine use of mesh for repairs; we believe that use of a larger area of mesh compared with the small strip used for TVT is unlikely to behave in a similar manner. The use of some of newer prosthetic materials on the market should be limited to trial settings just as the TVT was in its early days. The use of mesh in the vagina is recommended in some patients who have recurrent prolapse. Mesh use in these patients is often difficult due to scar tissue and poor vaginal skin quality.

Classification of prosthetic grafts

A number of prostheses are currently available for use in reconstructive surgery. A working understanding of their inherent strengths, surgical

Table 2 Classification of prosthetic materials

SYNTHETIC	Component	Fibre type	Pore size
Type I	Polypropylene	Monofilament	Macro
	Polyglactin 910	Multifilament	Macro
Type II	Expanded PTFE	Multifilament	Micro
Type III	Polyethylene	Multifilament	Micro/Macro
Type IV	Polypropylene sheet	Monofilament	Submicro

BIOLOGICAL TYPE	Xenograft	Porcine small intestine
		Bovine pericardium
	Allograft	Dura mater
		Fascia lata
	Autologous	Rectus sheath
		Fascia lata
		Vaginal mucosa

Adapted from Birch and Fynes.[39]
PTFE, polytetrafluoroethylene; macro, > 75 µm; micro, < 75 µm.

handling, reaction within human tissues and potential morbidity is required to allow the appropriate selection. The ideal prosthesis should be biocompatible, inert, lack an allergic or inflammatory response, sterile, non-carcinogenic, resistant to mechanical stress or shrinkage and available in a convenient and affordable format for clinical use.

Prostheses may be classified as autologous, synthetic, allograft or xenograft (Table 2). Autologous grafts increase the risk of postoperative morbidity and may predispose to incisional hernia. Synthetic prostheses were developed to overcome these problems and may be classified into types I–IV according to the type of material, pore size and whether they are mono- or multifilament.

Vaginal vault or uterine prolapse (apical prolapse)

Traditionally, these two entities have been treated differently. Uterovaginal prolapse is treated using vaginal hysterectomy and repair. The treatment for post-hysterectomy prolapse has been to suspend the vaginal vault to sacrospinous ligament (sacrospinous fixation, infracoxccygeal sacropexy or posterior IVS) or to anterior periosteum of sacrum or sacral promontory (abdominal or laparoscopic sacrocolpopexy). Vault prolapse has long been assumed to be a long-term complication of hysterectomy without any real evidence.[40] The only study attempting to address this issue found an incidence of vaginal vault prolapse of 11.6% if the hysterectomy was performed for genital prolapse and 1.8% when it was for other benign diseases.[41] We believe that patients who go on to develop vaginal vault prolapse following a hysterectomy for conditions other than prolapse probably had some degree of pre-existing prolapse at the time of abdominal hysterectomy. These patients would have gone on to develop uterovaginal prolapse later in life even if the hysterectomy had not been performed.

Table 3 Results of various conservative surgeries for the uterine prolapse (published data)

Procedure	Reference	Patients (n)	Mean follow-up (months)	Success rate (%)
Laparoscopic sacral suture hysteropexy	Krause (2005)[46]	81	24	94.7
	Maher (2001)[47]	43	12	79
Sacrospinous cervicopexy	Hefni (2003)[45]	61	33	93.5
Abdominal sacrohysteropexy	Barranger (2003)[48]	30	44.5	93.4
Sacrospinous hysteropexy	Vaart (2003)[49]	44	–	89.6
Sacrohysteropexy – Teflon mesh	Stanton (2001)[50]	13	16	96.3
Retroperitoneal sacropexy – PTFE	Krantz (1991)[51]	147	60	93

Need for hysterectomy when treating uterovaginal prolapse?

At present, vaginal hysterectomy with or without pelvic floor repair is the commonest treatment of uterovaginal prolapse.[2] However, long-term follow-up of vaginal hysterectomy for correcting genital prolapse has shown very high incidence of vault prolapse.[3,41] Vaginal hysterectomy alone, therefore, not only fails to address the pathological deficiency of the uterosacral–cardinal ligament complex but also results in removal of non-diseased organ. There is mounting evidence that the use of hysterectomy might be inappropriate in the absence of uterine pathology and might add to the morbidity of the procedure without affecting the outcome of repair.

Vaginal hysterectomy concomitantly with the repair of sacrospinous ligament fixation is a recognised treatment for uterovaginal prolapse, particularly when the cardinal and uterosacral ligaments are attenuated.[42] More than one report has described the successful use of this technique with uterine conservation for primary treatment of uterovaginal prolapse in young women who want to preserve their fertility.[43,44] The report by Hefni et al.[45] concluded that sacrospinous cervicocolpopexy with uterine conservation was a safe and effective surgical option which could benefit elderly patients with uterovaginal prolapse. It avoids the potential morbidity of vaginal hysterectomy and had a high success rate. It remains to be assessed whether uterine conservation has, in addition, a long-term anatomical advantage through preservation of the integrity of the pericervical endopelvic fascia (Table 3).[45,48–51]

Posterior intravaginal slingplasty (infracoccygeal sacropexy) for uterovaginal prolapse

Petros[52] first reported this procedure in 1997 as a minimal invasive procedure for the treatment of vault prolapse. We have modified this technique for treating uterovaginal prolapse by attaching the polypropylene tape to the cervix instead of vaginal apex.

The aim of posterior intravaginal slingplasty procedure is to create neo-uterosacral ligaments using the polypropylene tape, thereby helping to relocate vaginal apex (level I support) to its original level above the levator plate and restore vaginal axis.[52]

Surgical technique

This involves the use of a multifilament polypropylene tape (recently monofilament tape has replaced this) 8 mm wide and 40 cm long (Tyco Health Care), inserted through two incisions lateral to the external anal sphincter via a disposable tunneller into the ischiorectal fossa and rectovaginal septum towards the cervix or vaginal vault. The inverted 'U'-loop of this tape is then secured to the cervix and fibrous encapsulation occurs through the knitted porous tape structure thereby suspending the cervix (Fig. 2).

Marcain (20 ml, 0.25%) with 1:100,000 adrenaline is injected just under the vaginal skin in the posterior vaginal fornix; this helps to reduce the bleeding and eases the dissection. A longitudinal incision is made in the vaginal skin in the posterior fornix beneath the cervix. Blunt dissection with the index finger is carried out in the pararectal space to reach the ischial spines bilaterally. The dissection is kept to minimum to just enable to create the path for the IVS tunneller.

Small transverse incisions are made 2 cm lateral to the external anal sphincter (EAS) at the 4- and 8-o'clock positions. The conical head of the tunneller is inserted parallel to the rectum into the ischiorectal fossa until it reaches 1–2 cm below the ischial spine. The index finger of the other hand inserted through the vaginal incision is placed on the ischial spine. The tunneller is then gently inclined medially and upwards towards the vaginal incision, the tunneller tip is railroaded

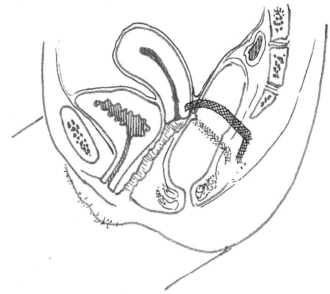

Fig. 2 Infracoccygeal sacropexy (posterior intravaginal slingplasty). The tape inserted through the levator muscle complex around the rectum before being anchored to the posterior cervical stroma.

with the tip of index finger of the other hand. The force needed for this manoeuvre is minimal. The tape is threaded in to the eye of the plastic insert and pulled through the tunneller and it is withdrawn at the same time.

The same manoeuvre is performed on the contralateral side and the medial end of tape is pulled out of the vaginal incision after inserting the inverted plastic insert through the distal end of the tunneller.

Our experience of using infracoccygeal sacropexy using the technique of posterior intravaginal slingplasty (PIVS) with uterine preservation has shown good medium-term results. In 137 patients with grade II and greater uterine prolapse, we carried out PIVS and achieved a 93% cure rate (median follow-up, 24 months). More importantly, the median length of stay in these patients was 4.5 h with very low pain scores as assessed by visual analogue charts.[53] In cases of elongated cervix, it is useful to carry out cervical amputation prior to posterior intravaginal slingplasty. We now recommend that an intravaginal cervix of 4 cm or longer should be shortened.

We are presently recruiting patients for a prospective, randomised study comparing the standard treatment (VH + repair) versus PIVS without a hysterectomy. This study will help to determine the need for hysterectomy when treating UV prolapse.

Anterior compartment

The standard anterior repair, *i.e.* anterior colporrhaphy with plicating sutures of pubocervical fascia, is the commonest surgery for anterior vaginal prolapse without urinary incontinence. The recurrence rate following this operation at 5 years is as high as 33% and up to 29% of women require further intervention.[4,54]

Prosthetic materials are used in order to reduce recurrences. A Cochrane systematic review suggested that the use of a polyglactin mesh overlay at the time of anterior vaginal wall repair may reduce the risk of recurrent cystocoele.[55] Vaginal mesh erosion is a significant complication (up to 13% of cases) but it is related to surgical experience, surgical technique and the synthetic material used. Most of these erosions can be cured by out-patient excision of the exposed mesh and suturing the undermining vaginal edges (Table 4).[56]

Table 4 Anterior repair – success rate and complications

Author	Repair	Patients (n)	Mean follow-up (months)	Success rate (%)	Compli- cations
Weber (2001)[57]	Standard anterior repair	33	23.6	30	
	Polyglactin 910	26	23.6	42	
	Ultralateral colporrhaphy	24	23.6	46	
De Tayrac (2005)[58]	Prolene mesh	63	37	89.1	Dyspareunia in 16.7%
Dwyer (2004)[59]	Polypropylene mesh	64	29	94	Mesh erosion in 9%
Adhoute (2004)[60]	Synthetic mesh	52	27	95	Mesh erosion in 3.8%
Milani (2005)[61]	Prolene mesh	63	17	94	Dyspareunia in 20%
Kuhn (2006)[62]	Standard anterior repair	68	30	87	–

Table 5 Comparison of results of fascial repairs of rectocoele in various published studies[64,65]

Reference	Patients (n)	Isolated rectocoele	Follow-up (months)	Anatomical cure (%)	Defaecation improvement (%)	Sexual dysfunction improvement (%)
Cundiff (1998)	69	5	12	82	63	66
Porter (1999)	125	8	6	82	44	73
Kenton (1999)	66	0	12	90	54	92
Glavind(0000)	67	29	3	100	85	75
Singh (2003)	26	–	18	92	65	38

For references, see Maher et al.[64] and Singh et al.[65]
Kahn (1999) reported worsening of defaecation and sexual function in 9% and 11% of patients, respectively.

Midvaginal sling (transverse strip technique)

This is a modification of the anterior mesh repair to reduce vaginal erosion, and is useful in central and lateral vaginal defects. A small strip of monofilament polypropylene mesh is inserted after creating a tunnel on either side of the vaginal bulge; depending on the size of the cystocoele, 1 or 2 strips of mesh can be used. In our own pilot study of 44 patients who underwent anterior repair for primary (35) or recurrent (9) cystocoele, use of a strip of polypropylene has shown very encouraging results.[63]

Posterior compartment

There has been reluctance to employ prosthetic material in the posterior compartment because of the risk of erosion and concerns regarding coital function. The use of mesh overlays has not improved the outcome of the rectocoele repair (level 1 evidence) and is associated with significant complications. The role of foreign body prosthesis in primary rectocoele repair would seem hard to justify but may have a role in recurrent rectocoele.

Fascial repairs have largely superseded the levator ani plication. The midline fascial plication may offer a superior anatomical and functional outcome compared to the discrete, site-specific fascial repair (level 2).

Abdominal rectopexy is usually undertaken for the correction of rectal prolapse using a suture suspension technique. More recently, a few studies have used prosthetic suspension, although there is no clear benefit in terms of surgical outcome (Table 5).[64]

Total vaginal mesh (TVM)

This is a new technique for urogenital prolapse repair using a one-piece synthetic mesh. The TVM Group selected a one-thread polypropylene mesh, Prolene Soft, which seemed the most appropriate for the transvaginal approach of prolapse surgical repair. The TVM technique for cystocoele repair uses anterior mesh transversally between arcus tendineus with two arms each side through obturator foramen. Rectocoele repair used posterior mesh anchored transversally between sacrospinal ligaments.

This technique should be reserved for the management of grade 3 and 4 prolapse, mainly as first-line management. The long-term results regarding its success and complications are awaited.[66]

Several modifications of TVM are now available. Prolift® mesh is obviously an improvement in pelvic organ prolapse surgery. Multicentre studies confirm its feasibility and short-term safety, but medium-term outcome is more disappointing. Mesh erosion remains significant (6.7%); similarly, high rates of recurrence (8.3%) at only 3.6 months question what the long-term anatomical results would be.[67]

The Perigee and Apogee is another modification of mesh repair to correct anterior, posterior vaginal wall defects and enterocoele. It is reported to be safe and effective in short-term studies; however, further investigation and follow-up is necessary to prove the long-term success and level of complications.[68]

KEY POINTS FOR CLINICAL PRACTICE

- There is an 11% life-time risk of undergoing surgery for prolapse and more than 30% require repeat surgery. There is a likelihood of an increase in prevalence of pelvic organ prolapse as a result of increasing life expectancy.

- The challenges in the management of pelvic organ prolapse are due to its high recurrence rates, lack of randomised controlled trials and poorly defined success and failure.

- A few highlights of advances in the field of pelvic floor surgery are: better understanding of the anatomy; objective and reproducible POP-Q classification; newer imaging techniques; and use of mesh or sling in the surgical treatment. In recent years, there has been considerable interest in the development of QoL tools or questionnaires that provide a means of objectively identifying and quantifying symptoms that are produced by pelvic organ prolapse and follow up to see its improvement.

- The role of vaginal hysterectomy for uterine prolapse in the absence of pathology is questionable. In recent years, there has been an increasing use of prosthetic materials in an effort to reduce the high recurrence rates associated with prolapse surgery. A well-designed, adequately powered, multicentre, prospective, randomised study including POP-Q classification and quality-of-life issues is required to confirm the benefits of various surgical techniques for the management of uterovaginal prolapse.

References

1 Popovic JR, Kozak LJ. National hospital discharge survey: annual summary. Vital Health Stat 148. 2000; 13: 1–19

2 Cardozo L. Prolapse. In: Whitfield CR. (ed) Dewhurst's textbook of obstetrics and gynaecology for postgraduates, 5th edn. London: Blackwell Science, 1995; 642–652

3 Mant J, Painter R, Vessey M. Epidemiology of genital prolapse: observations from the Oxford Family Planning Association Study. Br J Obstet Gynaecol 1997; 104: 579–585

4 Olsen AL, Smith VG, Bergstrom JO. Epidemiology of surgically managed pelvic organ prolapse and urinary incontinence. Obstet Gynecol 1997; 89: 501–506

5 Samuelsson EC, Victor FTA, Tibblin G et al. Signs of genital prolapse in a Swedish population of women 20 to 59 years of age and possible related factors. Am J Obstet Gynecol 1999; 180: 299–305

6 Swift SE. The distribution of pelvic organ support in a populationOf female subjects seen for routine gynecologic health care. Am J Obstet Gynecol 2000; 183: 277–285

7 Bland DR, Earle BB, Vitolins MZ, Burke G. Use of pelvic organ prolapse staging system of the International Continence Society, American Urogynecologic Society and Society of Gynecologic Surgeons in perimenopausal women. Am J Obstet Gynecol 1999; 181: 1324–1328

8 Progetto Menopausa Italia Study Group. Risk factors for genital prolapse in non-hysterectomized women around menopause results from a large cross-sectional study in menopausal clinics in Italy. Eur J Obstet Gynecol Reprod Biol 2000; 93: 125–140

9 Hendrix SL, Clark A, Nygaard I, Aragaki A, Barnabei V. Pelvic organ prolapse in the women's health initiative: gravity and gravidity. Am J Obstet Gynecol 2002; 186: 1160–1166

10 Ellerkmann RM, Cundiff G, Melick C et al. Correlation of symptoms with location and severity of pelvic organ prolapse. Am J Obstet Gynecol 2001; 185: 1332–1338

11 Degregorio G, Hillemans HG, Quass L, Mentzel J. Late morbidity following caesarean section: neglected factor. Geburtshilfe Frauenheilkd 1988; 48: 16–19

12 Al-Rawizs S, Al-Rawizs T. Joint hypermobility in women with genital prolapse. Lancet 1982; 326: 1439–1441

13 Marshman D, Percy J, Fielding I, Delbridge L. Rectal prolapse: relationship with joint mobility. Aust NZ J Surg 1987; 545: 827–829

14 Rinne KM, Kirkinen PP. What predisposes young women to genital prolapse? Eur J Obstet Gynecol Reprod Biol 1999; 84: 23–25

15 Dietz HP. Levator function before and after childbirth. Aust NZ J Obstet Gynaecol 2004; 44: 19–23

16 Dietz HP, Eldridge A, Grace M, Clarke B. Does pregnancy affect pelvic organ mobility? Aust NZ J Obstet Gynaecol 2004; 44: 517–520

17 Smith AR, Hosker GL, Warrell DW. The role of partial denervation of the pelvic floor in the aetiology of genitourinary prolapse and stress incontinence of urine. A neurophysiological study. Br J Obstet Gynaecol 1989; 96: 24–28

18 Hilton P, Dolan LM. Pathophysiology of urinary incontinence and pelvic organ prolapse. Br J Obstet Gynaecol 2004; 111: 5–9

19 Delancey JOL. Anatomical aspects of vaginal eversion after hysterectomy. Am J Obstet Gynecol 1992; 166: 1717–1728

20 DeLancey JOL. The anatomy of the pelvic floor. Curr Opin Obstet Gynecol 1994; 6: 313–316

21 Petros PE. Vault prolapse I: dynamic supports of the vagina. Int Urogynecol J 2001; 12: 292–295

22 Berglas B, Rubin IC. The study of the supportive structures of the uterus by levator myography. Surg Gynecol Obstet 1953; 97: 677–692

23 Clark AL, Gregory T, Smith VJ, Edwards R. Epidemiologic evaluation of reoperation of surgically treated pelvic organ prolapse and urinary incontinence. Am J Obstet Gynecol 2003; 189: 1261–1267

24 Nieminen K, Huhtala H, Heinonen PK. Anatomic and functional assessment and risk factors of recurrent prolapse after vaginal sacrospinous fixation. Acta Obstet Gynecol Scand 2003; 82: 471–478

25 Swift SE, Tate SB, Nicholas J. Correlation of symptoms with degree of pelvic organ support in a general population of women: what is pelvic organ prolapse? Am J Obstet Gynecol 2003; 189: 372–379

26 Shull BL, Bachofen C, Coates KW, Kuehl TJ. A transvaginal approach to repair of apical

and other associated sites of pelvic organ prolapse with uterosacral ligaments. Am J Obstet Gynecol 2000; 183: 1365–1374

27 Whiteside JL, Weber AM, Meyn LA, Walters MD. Risk factors for prolapse recurrence after vaginal repair. Am J Obstet Gynecol 2004; 191: 1533–1538

28 Bump RC, Mattiasson A, Brubaker LB *et al*. The standardization of terminology of female pelvic organ prolapse and pelvic floor dysfunction. Am J Obstet Gynecol 1996; 175: 10–17

29 Swift SE. Current opinion on the classification and definition of genital tract prolapse. Curr Opin Obstet Gynecol 2002; 14: 503–507

30 Stoker J, Halligan S, Bartram CI. Pelvic floor imaging. Radiology 2001; 218: 621–641

31 Karaus M, Neuhaus P, Wiedenmann TB. Diagnosis of enteroceles by dynamic anorectal endosonography. Dis Colon Rectum 2000; 43: 1683–1688

32 Yang A, Mostwin JL, Rosenshein NB, Zerhouni EA. Pelvic floor descent in women: dynamic evaluation with fast MR imaging and cinematic display. Radiology 1991; 179: 25–33

33 Tunn R, Paris ST, Taupitz M, Hamm B, Fischer W. MR imaging in posthysterectomy vaginal prolapse. Int Urogynecol J 2000: 11: 87–97

34 Gousse AE, Barbaric ZL, Safir MH *et al*. Dynamic half Fourier acquisition, single shot turbospin-echo magnetic resonance imaging for evaluating the female pelvis. J Urol 2000; 164: 1606–1613

35 Lamb GM, deJode MG, Gould SW *et al*. Upright dynamic MR defecating proctography in an open configuration system. Br J Radiol 2000; 73: 152–155

36 Digesu GA, Khullar V, Cardozo L, Robinson D, Salvatore S. P-QOL: a validated questionnaire to assess the symptoms and quality of life of women with urogenital prolapse. Int Urogynecol J 2005; 16: 176–181

37 Hullfish KL, Bovbjerg VE, Gibson J, Steers WD. Patient-centered goals for pelvic floor dysfunction surgery: what is success, and is it achieved? Am J Obstet Gynecol 2002; 187: 88–92

38 Hullfish KL, Bovbjerg VE, Steers WD. Patient-centered goals for pelvic floor dysfunction surgery: long-term follow-up. Am J Obstet Gynecol 2004; 191: 201–205

39 Birch C, Fynes M. The role of synthetic and biological prostheses in reconstructive pelvic floor surgery. Curr Opin Obstet Gynecol 2002; 14: 527–535

40 Varma R, Tahseen S, Lokugamage AU *et al*. Vaginal route as the norm when planning hysterectomy for benign conditions: change in practice. Obstet Gynecol 2001; 97: 613–616

41 Marchionni M, Bracco GL, Checcucci V, Carabaneanu EM, Mecacci F, Scarselli G. True incidence of vaginal vault prolapse. Thirteen years of experience. J Reprod Med 1999; 44: 679–684

42 Cruikshank SH, Cox DW. Sacrospinous ligament fixation at the time of vaginal hysterectomy. Am J Obstet Gynecol 1990; 162: 1811–1819

43 Richardson DA, Osteogard DR.Surgical management of uterine prolapse in young women. J Reprod Med 1989; 34: 388–392

44 Kovac SR, Cruikshank SH. Successful pregnancies and vaginal deliveries after sacrospinous uterosacral fixation in five of nine teen patients. Am J Obstet Gynecol 1993; 168; 1778–1786

45 Hefni M, El-Toukhy T, Bhaumik J, Katsimani E. Sacrospinous cervicocolpopexy with uterine conservation for uterovaginal prolapse in elderly women: an evolving concept. Am J Obstet Gynecol 2003; 188: 645–650

46 Krause HG, Goh JT, Sloane K, Higgs P, Carey MP. Laparoscopic sacral suture hysteropexy for uterine prolapse. Int Urogynecol J 2005; 30: 1–4

47 Maher CF, Carey M, Murrey C. Laparoscopic suture hysteropexy for uterine prolapse. Obstet Gynecol 2001; 97: 1010–1014

48 Barranger E, Fritel X, Pigne A. Abdominal sacrohysteropexy in young women with uterovaginal prolapse: long term follow up. Am J Obstet Gynecol 2003; 189: 1245–1250

49 Van Brummen HJ, van de Pol G, Aalders CI, Heintz AP, van der Vaart CH. Sacrospinous hysteropexy compared to vaginal hysterectomy as primary surgical treatment for a descensus uteri: effects on urinary symptoms. Int Urogynecol J 2003; 14: 350–355

50 Leron E, Stanton SL. Sacrohysteropexy with synthetic mesh for the management of uterovaginal prolapse. Br J Obstet Gynaecol 2001; 108: 629–633

51 Nyder TE, Krantz KE. Abdominal-retroperitoneal sacral colpopexy for the correction of vaginal prolapse. Obstet Gynecol 1991; 77: 944–949

52 Petros PE. Vault prolapse II: restoration of dynamic vaginal supports by infracoccygeal sacropexy, an axial day case vaginal procedure. Int Urogynecol J 2001; 12: 296–303

53 Varma R, Van den Hurk P, Ghosh A. Uterine preservation when treating primary uterovaginal prolapse. Use of modified posterior intravaginal slingplasty (MPIVS) a minimally invasive procedure. Abstract FIGO, San Diego 2003

54 Sand PK, Koduri S, Robert W *et al*. Prospective randomized trial of polyglactin 910 mesh to prevent recurrence of cystoceles and rectoceles. Am J Obstet Gynecol 2001; 184: 1357–1364

55 Maher C, Baessler K, Glazener CM, Adams EJ, Hagen S. Surgical management of pelvic organ prolapse in women. Cochrane Database Syst Rev. 2004; 18: CD004014

56 Milani R, Salvatore S, Solig M *et al*. Functional and anatomical outcome of anterior and posterior vaginal prolapse repair with prolene mesh. Br J Obstet Gynaecol 2004; 112: 107

57 Weber AM, Walters MD, Piedmonte MR, Ballard LA. Anterior colporrhaphy: a randomized trial of three surgical techniques. Am J Obstet Gynecol 2001; 185: 1299–1306

58 de Tayrac R, Deffieux X, Gervaise A, Chauveaud-Lambling A, Fernandez H. Long-term anatomical and functional assessment of trans-vaginal cystocele repair using a tension-free polypropylene mesh. Int Urogynecol J 2005; 17: 1–6

59 Dwyer PL, O'Reilly BA. Transvaginal repair of anterior and posterior compartment prolapse with Atrium polypropylene mesh. Br J Obstet Gynaecol 2004; 111: 831

60 Adhoute F, Soyeur L, Pariente JL, Le Guillou M, Ferriere JM. Use of transvaginal polypropylene mesh (Gynemesh) for the treatment of pelvic floor disorders in women. Prospective study in 52 patients. Prog Urol 2004; 14: 192–196

61 Milani R, Salvatore S, Soligo M, Pifarotti P, Meschia M, Cortese M. Functional and anatomical outcome of anterior and posterior vaginal prolapse repair with prolene mesh. Br J Obstet Gynaecol 2005; 112: 1164

62 Kuhn A, Gelman W, O'Sullivan S, Monga A. The feasibility, efficacy and functional outcome of local anaesthetic repair of anterior and posterior vaginal wall prolapse. Eur J Obstet Gynecol Reprod Biol 2006; 124: 88–92

63 Thakur Y, Varma R. Transverse strip technique: a novel minimally invasive method for anterior compartment repair using prolene mesh. Abstract International Continence Society meeting (ICS), Paris, 2004.

64 Maher C, Baessler K. Surgical management of posterior vaginal wall prolapse: an evidence-based literature review. Int Urogynecol J 2005; 17: 84–88

65 Singh K, Cortes E, Reid WM. Evaluation of the fascia technique for surgical repair of isolated posterior vaginal wall prolapse. Obstet Gynecol 2003; 101: 320–324

66 Debodinance P, Berrocal J, Clave H *et al* Changing attitudes on the surgical treatment of urogenital prolapse: birth of the tension-free vaginal mesh. J Gynecol Obstet Biol Reprod 2004; 33: 577–588

67 Cosson M, Caquant F, Collinet P *et al*. Prolift mesh (Gynecare) for pelvic organ prolapse surgical treatment using the TVM group technique: a retrospective study of 687 patients. ICS meeting 2005 Montreal, abstract 121

68 Gotze W, Melcher J, Stob V. A new option in the treatment of pelvic organ prolapse (POP) – Perigee Transobturator anterior prolapse repair system. ICS meeting Montreal 2005, abstract 607

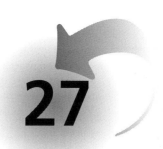

Sharif I.M.F. Ismail

Posthysterectomy vaginal vault prolapse

Vaginal vault (apical) prolapse refers to descent of the upper part of the vagina, which is distinct from an enterocele, where bowel bulges through the upper part of the posterior wall of the vagina.[1] It follows 11.6% of hysterectomies performed for prolapse and 1.8% for other benign diseases.[2] The incidence increases with time since the hysterectomy.[3] As hysterectomy is the commonest major gynaecological operation performed in the UK[4] and with increased life expectancy, the number of cases presenting with posthysterectomy vaginal vault prolapse is set to rise.[5] The condition can be distressing to patients, who may experience vaginal bulge, urinary and/or bowel symptoms, backache and limitation of movement as well as sexual function. These problems reduce the quality of life for elderly patients and are restricting for younger and more active ones.[6]

VAGINAL VAULT SUPPORT

DeLancy[7] provided a comprehensive analysis of vaginal vault support, recognising the value of ligaments, fascia as well as pelvic floor muscles. He described three levels of support, as shown in Table 1 and Figure 1.

Table 1 Vaginal vault support

Level	Type of support	Source of support
I	Suspension	Cardinal and uterosacral ligaments
II	Attachment	Arcus tendinous fascia and fascia over the pubococcygeus and iliococcygeus muscles
III	Fusion	Urogenital diaphragm and perineal body

Sharif I.M.F. Ismail MSc MBA MA MMedSci(Ed) LLM MD MRCOG
Locum Consultant Obstetrician and Gynaecologist, Royal Bournemouth Hospital, Bournemouth BH7 7DQ, UK. E-mail: sharif212121@yahoo.co.uk

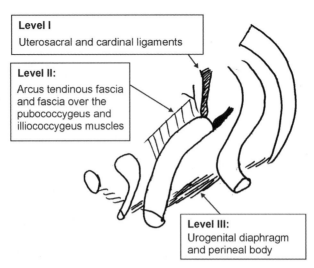

Level I
Uterosacral and cardinal ligaments

Level II:
Arcus tendinous fascia and fascia over the pubococcygeus and illiococcygeus muscles

Level III:
Urogenital diaphragm and perineal body

Fig. 1 Vaginal vault support.

PATIENT ASSESSMENT

Common symptoms and signs are outlined in Table 2. In recent years, special quality of life questionnaires have been developed for genital prolapse.[8]

It is important to examine all vaginal walls in addition to the vault, as vault prolapse is commonly associated with more generalised weakness.[9] Pelvic Organ Prolapse Quantification (PoP Q) is a scoring scheme introduced by the International Continence Society (ICS) to standardise description for more accurate comparison following surgery as well as for research purposes.[10] The

Table 2 History and examination in patients with posthysterectomy vaginal vault prolapse

- Age
- Parity

- Sense of pressure/vaginal fullness

- Stress incontinence, urge, urge incontinence
- Voiding problems, retention spells, incomplete emptying
- Constipation, digitation, anal incontinence
- Sexual activity/dysfunction

- Menstrual status, intake of hormone replacement therapy

- Occupation, heavy lifting

- Medical problems, asthma, cardiac, bone and/or joint disease

- Previous abdominal/vaginal surgery, previous continence or prolapse surgery
- Duration since hysterectomy

- Body mass index, chest and heart
- Abdominal scars, pelvi-abdominal masses

- Atrophy, ulceration
- Tone of pelvic floor muscles
- Stress incontinence

Anterior wall	Anterior wall	Cervix or cuff
Aa	**Ba**	**C**
Genital hiatus	Perineal body	Total vaginal length
gh	**pb**	**Tvl**
Posterior wall	Posterior wall	Posterior fornix
Ap	**Bp**	**D**

Fig. 2 Three-by-three grid for recording objective assessment of pelvic organ prolapse.

system is based on measuring the distance of specified points from the hymen as well as the length of vagina, genital hiatus and perineal body. The points are:

Point Aa – 3 cm proximal to the external urethral meatus.
Point Ba – most distal part of the anterior vaginal wall.
Point C – most distal part of the cervix or vaginal vault.
Point D – the posterior fornix, in those who still have their cervix.
Point Ap – 3 cm proximal to the hymen, on the posterior vaginal wall.
Point Bp – most distal part of the posterior vaginal wall.

All points and lengths are scored on a grid, as shown in Figure 2.
The prolapse is then staged as one of the following ordinal stages:

Stage 0   No prolapse. Points Aa, Ap, Ba and Bp are –3 and point C is between –TVL and –TVL-2 cm.

Stage 1   Most distal point < –1 cm (more than 1 cm above the hymen).

Stage 2   Most distal point ≥ –1 and ≤ 1 cm (between 1 cm above and 1 cm below the hymen).

Stage 3   Most distal point > 1 cm but < TVL-2 cm (more than 1 cm below the hymen, but at least 2 cm less than total vaginal length).

Stage 4   Most distal point > TVL –2 cm (complete vaginal eversion, with < 2 cm of the vaginal wall still above the hymen).

An illustration is shown in Figure 3.
It is also advisable to perform urodynamic assessment after reducing the prolapse with a pessary to detect occult stress incontinence. This might manifest after surgery, as a result of straightening the urethrovesical junction.[11]

PREVENTION

All patients with posthysterectomy vaginal vault prolapse had a prior hysterectomy, which was an opportunity to try to avoid such a problem. Vault prolapse should, therefore, be seen as potential consequence of hysterectomy, unless something is done to prevent it.

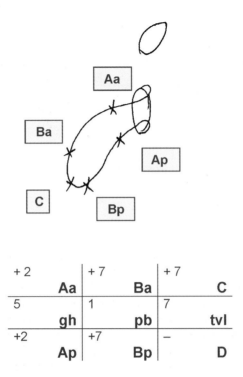

+2		+7		+7	
	Aa		Ba		C
5		1		7	
	gh		pb		tvl
+2		+7		−	
	Ap		Bp		D

Fig. 3 An illustration of stage 4 posthysterectomy vaginal vault prolapse.

McCall's culdoplasty has been recognised as a preventive measure during vaginal hysterectomy.[12] As shown in Figure 4, the technique entails obliteration of the posterior *cul-de-sac* by continuous sutures from the uterosacral ligament one side to that on the other side. It is important to identify the highest point of the sac so as to ensure its complete obliteration. The uterosacral ligaments are then approximated in the midline and fixed to the vaginal vault. It maintains vaginal length as well as the horizontal direction of its upper part,

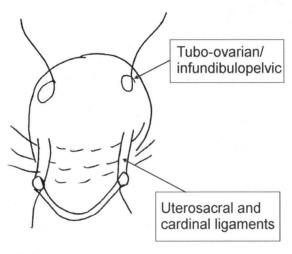

Tubo-ovarian/ infundibulopelvic

Uterosacral and cardinal ligaments

Fig. 4 McCall's culdoplasty.

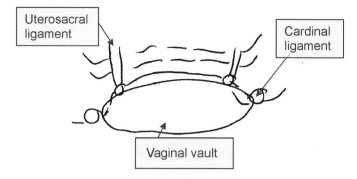

Fig. 5 Modified McCall's culdoplasty.

which ensures its closure under pressure. A prophylactic sacrospinous fixation is unnecessary, unless there is marked uterovaginal prolapse such that the uterosacrals are too weak to provide any support.[13]

A modified McCall's culdoplasty can be performed during abdominal hysterectomy.[14] As shown in Figure 5, this entails fixing the uterosacrals and cardinal ligaments to the vaginal vault, obliterating the posterior *cul-de-sac* and plicating both uterosacral ligament. It is important that the uterosacrals are identified prior to dividing them from the uterus, as they become difficult to discern after that. Whilst this can be done by suturing, it is probably better to clamp them separately close to the uterus; a step that also helps locating the posterior fornix.

MANAGEMENT

Pessaries control the prolapse, yet they require regular changing, which might be inconvenient for those leading an active life. They are, therefore, reserved

Table 3 Operations described for posthysterectomy vaginal vault prolapse

Type of surgery	Examples
Vaginal	Vaginal repair
	Sacrospinous/iliococcygeus fixation
	Uterosacral suspension
	Le Fort operation
	Colpocleisis/colpectomy/vaginectomy
Abdominal	Moschowitz/Halban procedure
	Sacrocolpopexy
	Rectus sheath colpopexy
Abdominoperineal	Zacharin's procedure
Tape	Posterior intravaginal slingoplasty (IVS)
Laparoscopic	Laparoscopic sacrocolpopexy
	Laparoscopic uterosacral suspension
	Laparoscopic sacrospinous fixation
	Laparoscopic paravaginal repair
Mesh	Prolift and Apogee

for elderly, frail patients, though spinal anaesthesia can be used in such patients.[15] Numerous operations have been described, as shown in Table 3. It is important, nowadays, not only to improve symptoms of prolapse, but also to restore sufficient vaginal length to preserve coital function. Operations like colpopectomy (vaginectomy), colpocleisis and Le Fort are, therefore, seldom performed. Similarly, abdomino-perineal operations, such as Zacharin's procedure, are complex and have a lower success rate than sacrocolpopexy.[16] Whilst it is important to identify and correct concomitant vaginal wall prolapse, an anterior and/or posterior repair alone is insufficient to support the vault. Similarly, associated urodynamic stress incontinence of urine, rectal prolapse and/or anal incontinence need to be addressed. Sacrospinous, or iliococcygeus, fixation as well as abdominal sacrocolpopexy are the commonly performed procedures and these are described in more detail here. An idea is also given about new tape and laparoscopic techniques.

Sacrospinous fixation

In this operation, the vaginal vault is fixed to the sacrospinous ligament, maintaining a horizontal position of the upper vagina on standing, as shown in Figure 6. This ensures compression, and thus closure, of the vagina against pelvic floor muscles during increase in intra-abdominal pressure.[17] Fixation needs to be at least 2 cm medial to the ischeal spines to avoid injuring the pudendal nerve and vessels as they course around the ischeal spines. It is also important to stay away from the upper border of the ligament, to avoid the sacral plexus, as well as the medial side, to avoid the presacral vessels.

The procedure is often done alongside a posterior repair, following an anterior repair, if one is required. The vaginal incision for the posterior repair is extended upwards till the vault and the lateral flap is dissected towards the ischeal spine on the right side, through the para-rectal space. Blunt dissection medially from the spine will expose the ligament, which can be palpated as a firm sliding band that widens towards the sacrum and feels stronger towards

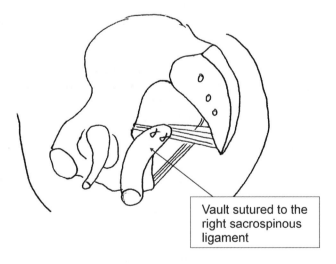

Vault sutured to the right sacrospinous ligament

Fig. 6 Sacrospinous fixation.

its upper border. A Miya hook ligature carrier is loaded with delayed absorbable suture, like PDS, and inserted just below the upper border, two fingers' breadth from the ischeal spines.

A pair of Breisky-Navratil retractors and a notched speculum are inserted to expose the suture after it passed through the ligament. They are held gently, to avoid injury to nearby structures, while the suture is retrieved using a nerve hook. The suture is divided in the middle, to create two supporting sutures. The free ends are loaded onto a Mayo needle and passed through the vaginal vault, a pair either side of the midline. The lower end of the each suture is passed twice through the vagina to act as a pulley, upon which the vault will be pulled up on tying both ends together at the end. This is usually done upon completion of posterior repair, as well as repair of enterocele, if required. A per rectal examination is important to detect injury and/or haematoma. The bladder is drained and the vagina is packed as usual.

Variations in the technique has been described, including the use of illuminated speculum[18] and anchoring device.[19] A unilateral procedure is commonly carried out on the right side to avoid injuring the sigmoid colon on the left.

Operative complications include bleeding, retention of urine, urinary tract infection, haematoma in the rectovaginal space[20] or ischeorectal fossa,[21] rectal perforation.[22] Early postoperative problems include detrusor overactivity and right buttock pain but both tend to resolve within 3 months.[22] Long-term success rates over 90% have been reported.[9,11,20,23]

In the long term, the direct recurrence of vault prolapse ranges from 5%[24] to 7%.[20] Vault infection is an important predisposing factor and should be avoided by providing antibiotic cover, pre-operative treatment of ulceration as well as good haemostasis. Indirect recurrence manifests through other vaginal wall defects. The anterior vaginal wall is more commonly affected than the posterior wall, due to the exaggerated retroversion of the vagina, as the vault is pulled backwards, exposing the anterior vaginal wall to more strain. However, such recurrence is not necessarily symptomatic.[20,24] Routine anterior repair at the time of sacrospinous fixation did not affect the incidence of this indirect recurrence.[20]

Iliococcygeus fixation

This technique entails the fixation of the vault to the iliococcygeus fascia, anterior to the ischeal spines.[25] Bilateral fixation is carried out and the technique is the same as sacrospinous fixation till the ischeal spines are reached. Subsequent dissection is directed forwards, exposing the iliococcygeus fascia, to which the vagina is fixed on both sides. The idea was to simplify the procedure and thus reduce the incidence of complications, such as bleeding and pain. It was also hoped that subsequent cystocele would be less frequent, by reducing the backward displacement of the vault. Comparative studies, however, showed no significant difference in operating time, postoperative complications, long-term recurrence of vault prolapse or subsequent development of cystocele.[26]

Sacrocolpopexy

The procedure was first described by Falk[27] who attached the vaginal vault directly to the sacrum. Subsequently, Lane[28] used mersilene vascular graft to bridge the gap

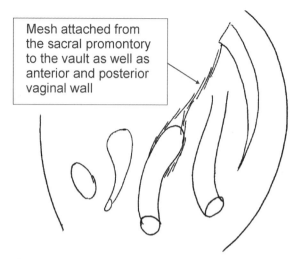

Mesh attached from the sacral promontory to the vault as well as anterior and posterior vaginal wall

Fig. 7 Sacrocolpopexy.

between the vault and the sacral promontory, as shown in Figure 7.

Since then, several types of mesh have been used, as outlined in Table 4. Whilst using an artificial material obviates the need to prepare another surgical site, as with fascia lata, it is fair to say that the ideal material is yet to be found. Autologous rectus sheath might be weak in those with prolapse. Fascia lata will require an additional incision, with its attendant complications. Allografts and xengrafts can cause reactions, which may lead to failure, and require special treatment to eliminate the risk of transmitting infection. Synthetic material has the risk of erosion. Type I mesh material, like prolene, is preferred, as it induces minimal reaction and allows granulation tissue growth, given its large pores. Type II material, like Gore-Tex, carries the risk of having to remove the mesh upon the occurrence of infection, as the pores are too small for inflammatory cells to enter so as eliminate the infection.

Patients are placed in a modified lithotomy (moderate Trendelenberg) position, as for Burch colposuspension. Catheterisation is carried out and a vaginal probe is inserted. Alternatively, the vagina can be packed with gauze. The abdomen is entered via a transverse or longitudinal incision, as appropriate, and any adhesions are divided to reach the vaginal vault, which is held on two

Table 4 The types of graft material used for abdominal sacrocolpopexy

Type of graft material			Examples
Natural			
	Human	Autologous	Rectus sheath, dermal graft, fascia lata
		Homograft	Dura mater, Lyodura
	Animal	Zenograft	Pelvicol
Synthetic		Type I	Marlex, Prolene
		Type II	Gore-Tex
		Type III	Teflon, Mersilene, Dacron, Propylene
		Type IV	Silastic sheets

Littlewood's forceps. Loops of intestine are packed away and self-retaining retractors are inserted as usual. A transverse incision is then made in the peritoneum overlying the vault, exposing the pubocervical and rectovaginal fascia. A longitudinal incision is made over the anterior surface of S1, exposing the anterior longitudinal ligament. Care is needed to avoid injuring the presacral vessels as well as the right common iliac vessels and ureters and the sigmoid colon. The vaginal pack is withdrawn at this stage, if inserted.

A piece of rectus sheath, or an alternative mesh, is attached to vaginal vault using delayed absorbable suture PDS (polydioxanone) or permanent sutures, like Ethibond. Inserting one's left hand in the vagina helps avoiding its penetration with sutures. Extending the mesh in front as well as behind the vagina has been applied to ensure closure of all vagina wall defects at the same time.[4] This requires skill and risks injuring the bladder and/or the rectum during the operation as well as mesh erosion into them later.[4,29] Indirect recurrence of anterior and/or posterior vaginal wall prolapse can still happen,[4,30,31] and there is no evidence to recommend this to a standard anterior and/or posterior fascial repair carried out at the same time. Broad attachment of the mesh to the vaginal vault avoids subsequent mesh avulsion and failure.[32] The mesh is then sutured to the anterior longitudinal ligament overlying S1, without being too tight. This will help maintaining a horizontal, rather than an upright, direction of the upper vagina on standing.

Peritonisation avoids intestinal adhesions to the mesh as well as obstruction, as a result of getting twisted around it.[32] Whilst some incise the peritoneum before inserting the mesh, it is easier to fix the mesh first, then pull the edge of the peritoneum overlying the vault on either side of the mesh, divide it towards the sacral promontory and suture it over the mesh. This helps avoiding ureteric injury.

As with sacrospinous fixation, it is important to address other vaginal wall defects as appropriate. If an anterior repair is needed, it is better done before the abdominal procedure, as fixing the vault may make it rather difficult. Posterior repair can be carried out either before or after the abdominal part. It is important to plicate the uterosacral ligaments using permanent suture to avoid future development of enterocele.[33]

Operative complications include bleeding from the presacral vessels, bowel as well as bladder injury and infection.[34] When artificial mesh material is used, erosion and infection can happen. Rates of erosion varied from 2.4%[35] to 12%.[36] Sacral osteomyelitis can also happen.[37] Reported long-term effectiveness varies from 93%[30] to 99%[32] and 100%.[35]

As with sacrospinous fixation, indirect recurrence affects the anterior vaginal wall more than the posterior wall[35] and is not necessarily symptomatic. The reason is the same, as a result of exposing the anterior vaginal wall to more strain with backward displacement of the vault. Long-term problems include incisional hernia,[38] to which patients with prolapse are prone.[39]

Tape procedures

Posterior intravaginal slingoplasty (Posterior IVS) was first described by Petros[40] and is the most known of tape procedures. It utilises the intravaginal slingoplasty technique using a multifilament prolene tape introduced using

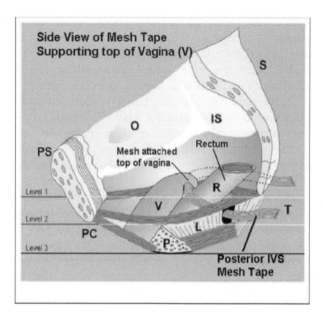

Fig. 8 Posterior intravaginal slingoplasty.

the IVS Tunneller used for stress incontinence of urine. It entails creating a new ligament that acts in a similar way to the uterosacral ligament (level I support) and repairing the rectovaginal fascia (level II support) as well as the perineal body (level III support), as shown in Figure 8.

At the beginning, a horizontal 4–5 cm incision is made in the vaginal vault, 1.5 cm below the hysterectomy scar line. Adherent rectocele and/or enterocele is identified through rectal examination and freed by dissection. A 0.5 cm incision is then made 2 cm posterolateral to the anus. The conical head of the device is inserted through this incision and passed for 4 cm in ischeorectal fossa, to reach the ischeal spine. Following this point, it is directed forwards and medially to emerge at the vaginal incision. The same sequence is repeated on the other side and the tape is threaded through the tunneller to complete a U shaped sling. All insertions are guided by the index finger in the vagina, to avoid rectal perforation. The head of the tape is the secured to the underneath of the vaginal vault.

After that, two longitudinal incisions are made from the vault incision down to 1 cm from the introitus. The lateral flaps are dissected exposing the rectovaginal fascia underneath. The epithelium of the vaginal bridge lying in the middle is then destroyed by diathermy and secured to the underneath of the upper vaginal flap and the perineal body below. Mattress sutures are then used to plicate the rectovaginal fascia, over the vaginal bridge, and the perineal body. The procedure ends by a Y-shaped closure of the vagina.

This is a short procedure that can be done as a day-case. Current evidence, which is limited to individual series,[40,41] shows subjective and objective cure rates well over 80%. As with other procedures that pull the vault backwards, there is a risk of subsequent anterior vaginal wall prolapse. Although the aim is to create a new uterosacral ligament, the tape only runs from the ischeal spines to the vault, resembling a sacrospinous fixation. The multifilament tape has been associated with more infections, requiring removal,[42] more defective vaginal healing[43] as well as more vaginal erosions[44] than the tension-free vaginal tape (TVT) sling. In addition, rejection can happen.[40] The value of using the vagina to support the rectovaginal fascia over a standard repair needs to be established.

The National Institute for Clinical Excellence advised special arrangements for consent, audit and research when using the technique.[45]

Laparoscopic sacrocolpopexy

Laparoscopic sacrocolpopexy was first described by Nezhat *et al.*[46] The procedure is carried out through a standard three-port laparoscopy, with the vaginal vault elevated using a probe or a swab on ring forceps. Care is needed to avoid bowel injury, especially with previous abdominal surgery, when Palmer point entry or open laparoscopy might be required to start with. Adhesions are divided to visualise the vault as well as the sacral promontory.

The peritoneum overlying the vault is divided, exposing the vaginal vault, which is sutured to the mesh, taking care not to injure the bladder, rectum or the ureters. Dissection can be extended anteriorly as well as posteriorly for mesh placement as with open sacrocolpopexy. The peritoneum over the promontory is divided, taking care not to injure the iliac vessels or the ureters. The mesh is then sutured or stapled over the promontory and the peritoneum as well as the posterior *cul-de-sac* are closed, as in open sacrocolpopexy.

The laparoscopic approach affords less scarring, and thus less pain, as well as shorter stay in hospital. By avoiding a long abdominal incision, the morbidity is reduced, which suits elderly patients. Complications of open sacrocolpopexy, including visceral injury, mesh erosion and osteomyelitis, can still be encountered. Operating time is longer, though it gets less with experience. The technique requires considerable skill that requires time to acquire. Current evidence is limited to small series suggest good outcome with success rates ranging from 100% at 1 year[47] to 93% at 5 years.[48]

Mesh procedures

A number of mesh procedures are being introduced, including Prolift and Apogee. These procedures entail the placement of a rectangular piece of mesh between the sacrospinous in the back and the pubic bone at the front. Some use sutures to secure the mesh in place[49] and newer techniques use needles in the same way as tape procedures. There are not enough data to enable judging these minimally invasive techniques at the moment, though they might become of more value in the future.

CHOICE OF SURGERY

Sacrocolpopexy is considered the gold standard approach, as outlined in a recent Cochrane review.[50] It maintains vaginal length and preserves coital function.[1] It is, however, an abdominal operation that entails a long incision, which may not be preferred in elderly patients. The laparoscopic approach may be suitable for these patients, though it requires experience. Although vaginal surgery allows repairing with other vaginal wall defects, such repair can be done alongside sacrocolpopexy, abdominally, laparoscopically or vaginally. Sacrospinous fixation requires long vagina for the vault to reach the sacrospinous ligament. Laparoscopic sacrocolpopexy and posterior intravaginal slingoplasty are new minimally invasive techniques that promise quicker recovery, though their value needs to be established through more research.

KEY POINTS FOR CLINICAL PRACTICE

- Posthysterectomy vaginal vault prolapse is a distressing and increasingly common problem.

- The vaginal vault is supported at a number of levels. These levels need to be maintained to prevent vault prolapse and restored to correct it.

- Patients with vault prolapse often have other vaginal wall defects. These defects should be identified and corrected alongside any surgical procedure for vault prolapse.

- Patients with vaginal vault prolapse may have occult stress incontinence. Urodynamic assessment after reducing the prolapse helps identifying the patients who might suffer from stress incontinence after corrective surgery. Concomitant continence surgery may avoid such a problem.

- Vault prolapse should be seen as a hazard whenever hysterectomy is performed. Securing the cardinal and uterosacral ligaments to the vaginal vault at the time of hysterectomy as well as plicating the uterosacral ligaments and obliterating the *cul-de-sac* should be performed to prevent such complication. Sacrospinous fixation might be considered if these ligaments are grossly weak.

- Sacrocolpopexy is regarded as the gold standard surgical procedure. It can be combined with vaginal wall repair to prevent future recurrence.

- Sacrospinous fixation is a popular procedure that can be combined with repair of vaginal wall prolapse.

- Laparoscopic sacrocolpopexy promises less scarring, and thus pain, as well as quicker recovery. However, it requires skill and takes time. Whilst current evidence is re-assuring, larger studies are awaited.

- Tape-based vaginal techniques are being introduced. Whilst early results might be encouraging, proper evaluation of safety and effectiveness is needed.

References

1 Birnbaum SJ. Rational therapy for prolapsed vagina. Am J Obstet Gynecol 1973; 115: 411–419

2 Marchionni M, Bracco GL, Checcucci V *et al*. True incidence of vaginal vault prolapse; thirteen years' experience. J Reprod Med 1999; 44: 679–684

3 Mant J, Painter R, Vessey M. Epidemiology of genital prolapse; observations from the Oxford Family Planning Association Study. Br J Obstet Gynaecol 1997; 104: 579–585

4 Marinkovic SP, Stanton SL. Triple compartment prolapse; Sacrocolpopexy with anterior and posterior mesh extensions. Br J Obstet Gynaecol 2003; 110: 323–326

5 Dunton JD, Mikuta J. Post hysterectomy vaginal vault prolapse. Postgrad Obstet Gynecol 1988; 8: 1–6

6 Lo T, Wang AC. Abdominal colposacropexy and sacrospinous ligament suspension for severe uterovaginal prolapse; a comparison. J Gynecol Surg 1998; 14: 59–64

7 DeLancy JO. Anatomic aspects of vaginal eversion after hysterectomy. Am J Obstet Gynecol 1992; 166: 1717–1728

8 Digesu GA, Khullar V, Cardozo L *et al*. P-QOL; a validated questionnaire to assess the symptoms and quality of life of women with urogenital prolapse. Int Urogynecol J 2005; 16: 176–181

9 Morely GW, DeLancey JL. Sacrospinous ligament fixation for eversion of the vagina. Am J Obstet Gynecol 1988; 158: 872–881

10 Bump RC, Mattiasson A, Bo K *et al*. The standardisation of terminology of female pelvic organ prolapse and pelvic floor dysfunction. Am J Obstet Gynecol 1996; 175: 10–17

11 Nicholas DH. Sacrospinous fixation for massive eversion of the vagina. Am J Obstet Gynecol 1982; 142: 901–904

12 McCall ML. Posterior culdoplasty: surgical correction of enterocele during vaginal hysterectomy; a preliminary report. Obstet Gynecol 1957; 10: 595–602

13 Cruikshank SH, Cox DW. Sacrospinous ligament fixation at the time of transvaginal hysterectomy. Am J Obstet Gynecol 1990; 162: 1611–1619

14 Wall LL. A technique for modified McCall culdoplasty at the time of abdominal hysterectomy. J Am Coll Surg 1994; 178: 507–509

15 Schettini M, Fortunato P, Gallucci M. Abdominal sacral colpopexy with prolene mesh. Int Urogynecol J 1999; 10: 295–299

16 Creighton MS, Stanton SL. The surgical management of vaginal vault prolapse. Br J Obstet Gynaecol 1991; 98: 1150–1154

17 Randall CL, Nichols DH. Surgical treatment of vaginal inversion. Obstet Gynecol 1971; 38: 327–332

18 Lantzsch T, Goepel C, Wolters M *et al*. Sacrospinous ligament fixation for vaginal vault prolapse. Arch Gynecol Obstet 2001; 265: 21–25

19 Lind LR, Choe J, Bhatia NN. An in-line suturing device to simplify sacrospinous vaginal vault suspension. Obstet Gynecol 1997; 89: 129–132

20 Meschia M, Bruschi F, Amicarelli P *et al*. The sacrospinous vaginal vault suspension; Critical analysis of outcomes. Int Urogynecol J 1999; 10: 155–159

21 Paraiso MFR, Ballard LA, Walters MD *et al*. Pelvic support defects and visceral and sexual function in women treated with sacrospinous ligament suspension and pelvic reconstruction. Am J Obstet Gynecol 1996; 175: 1423–1431

22 Sauer HA, Klutke CG. Transvaginal sacrospinous ligament fixation for treatment of vaginal prolapse. J Urol 1995; 154: 1008–1012

23 Imparato E, Aspesi G, Rovetha E *et al*. Surgical management and prevention of vaginal vault prolapse. Surg Gynecol Obstet 1992; 175: 233–237

24 Nieminen K, Huhtala H, Heinonen PK. Anatomic and functional assessment and risk factors of recurrent prolapse after vaginal sacrospinous fixation. Acta Obstet Gynecol Scand 2003; 82: 471–478

25 Shull BL, Capen CV, Riggs MW *et al*. Bilateral attachment of the vaginal cuff to iliococcygeus fascia; an effective method of cuff suspension. Am J Obstet Gynecol 1993; 168: 1669–1677

26 Maher CF, Murray CJ, Carey MP *et al*. Iliococcygeus or sacrospinous fixation for vaginal vault prolapse. Obstet Gynecol 2001; 98: 40–44

27 Falk HC. Uterine prolapse and prolapse of the vaginal vault treated by sacropexy. Obstet Gynecol 1961; 18: 113–115

28 Lane FE. Repair of post-hysterectomy vaginal vault prolapse. Obstet Gynaecol 1962; 20: 72–77

29 Cosson M, Debodinance P, Boukerrou M *et al.* Mechanical properties of synthetic implants used in the repair of prolapse and urinary incontinence in women; what is the ideal material? Int Urogynecol J 2003; 14: 169–178

30 Snyder TE, Krantz KE. Abdominal-retroperitoneal sacral colpopexy for the correction of vaginal prolapse. Obstet Gynecol 1991; 77: 944–949

31 Maher CF, Qatawneh AM, Dwyer PL *et al.* Abdominal sacral colpopexy or vaginal sacrospinous colpopexy for vaginal vault prolapse; a prospective randomised study. Am J Obstet Gynecol 2004; 190: 20–26

32 Timmons MC, Addison WA, Addison SB *et al.* Abdominal sacral colpopexy in 163 women with posthysterectomy vaginal vault prolapse and enterocele; evolution of operative technique. J Reprod Med 1992; 37: 323–327

33 Valaitis SR, Stanton SL. Sacrocolpopexy; a retrospective study of a clinician's experience. Br J Obstet Gynaecol 1994; 101: 518–522

34 Addison WA, Livengood CH, Sutton GP *et al.* Abdominal sacral colpopexy with Mersilene mesh in retroperitoneal position in the management of posthysterectomy vaginal vault prolapse and rectocele. Am J Obstet Gynecol 1985; 153: 140–146

35 Culligan PJ, Murphy M, Blackwell L *et al.* Long-term success of abdominal sacral colpopexy using synthetic mesh. Am J Obstet Gynecol 2002; 187: 1473–1482

36 Kohli N, Walsh PM, Roat TW *et al.* Mesh erosion after abdominal sacrocolpopexy. Obstet Gynecol 1998; 92: 999–1004

37 Weidner AC, Cundiff GW, Harris RL *et al.* Sacral osteomyelitis; an unusual complication of abdominal sacral colpopexy. Obstet Gynecol 1997; 90: 689–691

38 Costantini E, Lombi R, Micheli C *et al.* Colposacropexy with Gore-Tex mesh in marked vaginal and uterovaginal prolapse. Eur Urol 1998; 34: 111–117

39 Symmonds RE, Williams TJ, Lee RA *et al.* Posthysterectomy enterocele and vaginal vault prolapse. Am J Obstet Gynecol 1981; 140: 852–859

40 Petros PE. Vault prolapse II; restoration of dynamic vaginal supports by infracoccygeal sacropexy; An axial day-case vaginal procedure. Int Urogynecol J 2001; 12: 296–303

41 Fransworth BN. Posterior intravaginal slingoplasty (infracoccygeal sacropexy) for severe posthysterectomy vaginal vault prolapse; a preliminary report on efficacy and safety. Int Urogynecol J 2002; 13: 4–8

42 Bafghani A, Benizri EI, Trastour C *et al.* Multifilament polypropylene mesh for urinary incontinence; 10 cases of infections requiring removal of the sling. Br J Obstet Gynaecol 2005; 112: 376–378

43 Glavind K, Sander P. Erosion, defective healing and extrusion after tension-free urethropexy or the treatment of stress urinary incontinence. Int Urogynecol J 2004; 15: 179–182

44 Pifarotti P, Meschiaa M, Gattei U *et al.* Multicentre randomised trial of tension-free vaginal tape (TVT) and intravaginal slingoplasty (IVS) for the treatment of stress urinary incontinence in women. Neurol Urodyn 2004; 23: 494–495

45 National Institute for Health and Clinical Excellence. Posterior infracoccygeal sacropexy for vaginal vault prolapse, Interventional Procedure Guidance 125. London: NICE, 2005

46 Nezhat CH, Nezhat F, Nezhat C. Laparoscopic sacral colpopexy for vaginal vault prolapse. Obstet Gynecol 1994; 84: 885–888

47 Ross JW. Techniques of laparoscopic repair of total vault eversion after hysterectomy. J Am Assoc Gynecol Laparosc 1997; 4: 173–183

48 Ross JW, Preston M. Laparoscopic sacrocolpopexy for severe vaginal vault prolapse; five year outcome. J Min Invas Gynecol 2005; 12: 221–226

49 Shah DK, Paul EM, Rastinehad AR *et al.* Short-term outcome analysis of total pelvic reconstruction with mesh; the vaginal approach. J Urol 2004; 171: 261–263

50 Maher C, Bassler K, Glazener CMA *et al.* Surgical management of pelvic organ prolapse in women [Cochrane review]. In: The Cochrane Library, Chichester:Wiley, 2005

28

Jillian Noble   Gerald Gui

Hormone replacement therapy and breast cancer

Hormone replacement therapy (HRT) has been used for the treatment of menopausal symptoms for over 50 years. Historically, unopposed oestrogens were used to replace the production of hormones in postmenopausal women but when this resulted in an increase in endometrial carcinoma, oestrogen–progestogen combinations replaced unopposed oestrogens in women with a uterus. Recent media reports highlight trial data that suggest the risks of HRT exceed the benefits. The popularity of combined HRT has consequently declined. HRT was traditionally used in the treatment of menopausal symptoms including hot flushes, night sweats, vaginal atrophy, fatigue and also in women at risk of osteoporosis. As concerns have grown regarding the risks of HRT, alternative therapies are increasingly being sought. In this review, we consider the evidence linking HRT to breast cancer risk and the clinical management of oestrogen deprivation symptoms in breast cancer survivors.

The benefits of HRT have to be balanced against the recognised risks. This applies as much to women previously treated for breast cancer, where an early menopause may be induced as an effect of adjuvant chemotherapy or as part of intended adjuvant endocrine therapy. Menopausal-like symptoms may occur as an adverse effect of the selective oestrogen receptor modulators and aromatase inhibitors. The majority of breast cancers are influenced by oestrogen and progesterone and there is a natural tendency to be cautious. In this difficult area, evidence-based practice is as important as informed judgement and patient choice.

Jillian Noble MBChB MRCP(UK)
Specialist Registrar Medical Oncology, The Department of Academic Surgery (Breast Unit), Royal Marsden Hospital, Fulham Road, London SW3 6JJ, UK

Gerald Gui MS FRCS FRCS(Ed) (for correspondence)
Consultant Surgeon, The Department of Academic Surgery (Breast Unit), Royal Marsden Hospital, Fulham Road, London SW3 6JJ, UK
E-mail: gerald.gui@rmh.nhs.uk

BENEFITS OF HRT

Accepted indications for HRT are symptoms of oestrogen deprivation and the prevention and treatment of osteoporosis. Menopausal symptoms include hot flushes, night sweats, fatigue, insomnia, genito-urinary tract atrophy and depression. Randomised trial data including The Women's Health, Osteoporosis, Progestin, Estrogen (HOPE) study and the Women's Health Initiative (WHI) study both showed reduced severity of hot flushes in women taking HRT.[1,2] The HOPE study compared varying doses of conjugated equine oestrogens ranging from 0.3–0.625 mg/day of oestrogen-only and combined HRT for 1 year and reported improvement in hot flushes for all doses compared to placebo. The WHI trial found at 1-year follow-up, 76.7% of women in the oestrogen/progesterone group had improvement in hot flushes compared to 51.7% in the placebo group ($P < 0.001$). In the combined group, 71.0% of women had improvement in night sweats compared to 52.8% in the placebo group ($P < 0.001$). Sleep disturbance, fatigue and depression are known to be associated with hot flushes and also show improvement on commencement of HRT. The Heart and Estrogen/Progestin Replacement Study (HERS II) found that beneficial effects of hormone therapy were directly associated with the presence of menopausal symptoms.[3] Women with flushing at entry had improved mental health and fewer depressive symptoms with HRT while those without flushing had greater declines in physical measures and energy.

Genito-urinary tract atrophy and sexual dysfunction are also known to accompany the menopause in many women. The genito-urinary tract contains a large number of oestrogen receptors, which are thought to have a role in maintaining muscle tone and make this area particularly sensitive to decreasing levels of oestrogen. Levels of oestrogen have been correlated with vaginal dryness and dyspareunia and increasing serum oestrogen levels above 50 pg/ml is known to improve these symptoms.[4] As an alternative to oral HRT for the treatment of vaginal dryness without systemic features of oestrogen deprivation, topical oestrogens can be considered for maximal local effects. Oestriol is available as a cream while oestradiol is available as vaginal tablets. Topical treatments have the advantage of using lower overall doses of oestrogen with minimal systemic absorption.

Loss of ovarian hormone production puts menopausal women at increased risk of osteoporosis. The WHI study examined the risk of osteoporotic fractures and levels of bone mineral density in women taking combined HRT and placebo.[5] In the HRT group, 8.6% developed fractures compared to 11.1% in the placebo group. Bone mineral density increased 3.7% after 3 years of treatment in the HRT group compared to 0.14% in the placebo group, showing obvious benefits of HRT. Despite these benefits, HRT has recently fallen out of favour as a number of recent publications have highlighted the potential risks of HRT and suggested that these may outweigh the benefits. Alternatives to HRT in the maintenance of bone health are considered below.

HRT AND BREAST CANCER RISK

The pathogenesis of breast cancer and the presence of endogenous oestrogen are inextricably linked. Breast cancer risk rises after puberty but with the onset of menopause and the decline in sex hormones, the rise in breast cancer risk is less steep. Late menopause is known to confer increased risk and risk rises 3% with each year following menopause. In contrast, oophorectomy before the age of 35 years reduces breast cancer risk by approximately 40% compared to women who experience a natural menopause. In the light of these observations, it may be reasonable to assume that replacing oestrogen after the menopause may increase the risk of breast cancer.

Until recently, the trials regarding HRT and breast cancer risk were all observational. In 1997, the Collaborative Group on Hormonal Factors in Breast Cancer brought together over 90% of the epidemiological evidence on the relationship between HRT and breast cancer risk.[6] Data from more than 52,000 women with breast cancer and over 100,000 women without breast cancer from 51 studies were analysed. Among current or recent users of HRT, the relative risk of breast cancer increased in relation to prolonged duration of use but for past users there was no significant increase in relative risk of breast cancer. In current users, the relative risk of having breast cancer diagnosed increased by 2.3% per year, which is equivalent to the level of risk associated with delaying menopause. Relative risk also increased with increasing duration of HRT use. In western countries, approximately 45 women per 1000 aged between 50– 70 years are diagnosed with breast cancer. The excess number of breast cancers in women aged 50–70 years was 2 for 5 years of HRT use, 6 for 10 years and 12 for 15 years. The type of preparation used was only available for 39% of women in the study: 80% of those were oestrogen-only and 12% were combined oestrogen and progestagen. Approximately 18% of women in the study were defined as having an unknown age at menopause as they had previously undergone a hysterectomy without bilateral oophorectomy. These women were excluded from the final analysis since failure to account for time since the menopause leads to underestimation of breast cancer risk associated with HRT. There were no significant differences between HRT type or the doses used.

In recent years, a number of large trials have reported their results implicating HRT and breast cancer risk. The Women's Health Initiative Study (WHI) was a randomised controlled trial that enrolled 161,608 postmenopausal women aged 50–79 years between 1993 and 1998.[7] Patients were randomised to combined conjugated equine oestrogen plus medroxyprogesterone acetate or placebo. The primary outcome was coronary heart disease with the primary adverse outcome as invasive breast cancer. Other outcome measures were endometrial carcinoma, pulmonary embolism, stroke, hip fracture and colorectal cancer. This trial was stopped early after 5.2 years of follow-up as there were an excess of cardiovascular and breast cancer events and, therefore, the risks of HRT were felt to exceed the benefits. The hazard ratio (HR) for breast cancer in the HRT group compared to placebo was 1.26 (95% CI 1.00–1.59). Subgroup analysis of women who used HRT after the menopause had higher hazard ratios in excess of those who had never used postmenopausal hormones. There were several limitations of this study, the principal being the age of the cohort at study entry. The population recruited were between 50 and 79 years but only one-third of women were aged 50–59 years, the age group of women who most commonly take HRT. More than one-third of recruits were obese with a body mass index > 30 kg/m^2, which may have put them at increased risk of breast cancer prior to starting the study. The study also used oral continuous conjugated equine oestrogen combined with medroxyprogesterone acetate and it may be inappropriate to extrapolate these results to other formulations of HRT but also to other routes of administration such as the transdermal or topical route. Many women take HRT for a shorter period of time for relief of menopausal symptoms. In this study, women took HRT for 5 years and since we know increasing duration of use may be associated with increased risk it may not apply to shorter durations of use.

Further analyses of the WHI data were carried out to determine the relationship between HRT use and breast cancer characteristics.[8] Similar histology and grade was found between both groups but tumour size was slightly larger in women using HRT compared with placebo (1.7 cm versus 1.5 cm; $P = 0.04$) with a 10% greater incidence of regional spread (25.4% versus 16.0%; $P = 0.04$). After 1 year, the number of abnormal mammograms in the HRT group was substantially greater than in the placebo group. The rate of diagnosis of breast cancer in the HRT group was initially lower and subsequently increased. This may, in part, be due a predictable increase in mammographic density in women on HRT resulting in a higher false-positive recall rate and delayed breast cancer diagnosis.

The second significant trial was The Million Women Study published in *The Lancet* in 2003.[9] This cohort study was set up to investigate the effects of specific types of HRT on breast cancer incidence and mortality. More than a million women aged 50–64 years were recruited between 1996 and 2001. The average period of follow-up was 2.6 years for analyses of breast cancer incidence and 4.1 years for analyses of mortality. In all, 9364 cases of invasive breast cancer were reported and 50% of the study population had used HRT at some time. The risk of breast cancer was significantly higher among ever-users than never-users of HRT (RR 1.43; 95% CI 1.36–1.50; $P < 0.0001$). Current users of HRT were more likely than never users to develop breast cancer (RR 1.66; 95% CI 1.58–1.75; $P < 0.0001$) and past users who had discontinued HRT at least 5 years previously were not at increased risk (RR 1.01; 95% CI 0.94–1.09). Different preparations of HRT were compared and the risk was substantially greater for oestrogen–progestogen preparations (RR 2.00; 95% CI 1.88–2.12) than for oestrogen-only preparations (RR 1.30; 95% CI 1.21–1.40). There was little difference between specific oestrogen or progestogen types, nor was there any distinction between cyclical versus sequential regimens. Breast cancer risk increased with longer duration of HRT use. Oestrogen-only HRT taken for 5 years resulted in 2 more breast cancers by age 65 years per 1000 women; 10 years of HRT use resulted in 6 more breast cancers per 1000 and 15 years of use resulted in 12 more breast cancers per 1000 women users. In the oestrogen–progestogen group there were 5 more breast cancers in the 5-year group, 12 in the 10-year group and 19 in the 15-year group.

In the public eye, reporting of the previous two studies in the lay press has raised considerable concern on the safety of HRT. The clinical reality is that patient choice lies between the balance of benefits and risks. Despite benefits for many women in the relief of menopausal symptoms, the perceived risks may be felt by individual women to exceed these benefits. Current recommendations for HRT are that its use should be confined to severe menopausal symptoms in women adequately counselled and informed on the increased risk of breast cancer. If the benefit of HRT in these situations is felt to exceed the risks in individual cases, HRT could be prescribed on the basis of patient choice. Where indicated, it should be prescribed in the lowest possible dose for the shortest period of time to control symptoms.

More trials are needed to investigate shorter durations of use of HRT, varying doses and alternative means of administration other than the oral route. We may find 1–2 years of HRT use of, for example, a transdermal preparation, may result in significantly lower risks of breast cancer than portrayed in studies so far.

HRT after a diagnosis of breast cancer

The use of HRT for symptoms of oestrogen deprivation following a diagnosis of breast cancer remains controversial. As the number of breast cancer survivors rises due to the increasing incidence of breast cancer alongside a reduction in mortality from better treatment, the demand for HRT in women surviving breast cancer will also rise. As more women are diagnosed with early screen-detected cancers that have a good prognosis, quality of life after treatment for breast cancer becomes more important. A substantial number of women diagnosed with breast cancer are peri- or post-menopausal with a peak incidence in the 50–54 year age group. The treatment of breast cancer may render women prematurely menopausal. Cyclophosphamide is commonly used in many combination chemotherapy regimens for the adjuvant treatment of breast cancer and is known to cause amenorrhoea. More than 50% of women under the age of 40 years will become amenorrhoeic following CMF (cyclophosphamide, methotrexate, 5-fluorouracil), a standard adjuvant chemotherapy regimen for breast cancer.[10] Only 23% of these women will regain their fertility. For women over 40 years, the risk of infertility is more than 90%. The demand for relief from menopausal symptoms has consequently risen. Oestrogen has generally not been given following a diagnosis of breast cancer due to the belief that oestrogen promotes breast cancer growth. There is evidence to show some regression of metastatic breast cancer following withdrawal of HRT after diagnosis. It is, therefore, possible that oestrogen may stimulate any cancer cells left behind by primary treatment. There may also be an increased risk of contralateral breast cancer. HRT is known to increase the frequency of abnormal mammograms possibly by increasing mammographic density and this could lead to a delay in diagnosis of breast cancer recurrence or a new primary.

A recent review examined 11 studies on the risk of recurrence in breast cancer survivors.[11] Only four of the studies had control groups and included 214 women followed up for 30 months. Although 20% of patients were documented to be ER-positive and 16% were PGR-positive, the majority of cases were unknown. Of HRT users, 4.2% experienced a recurrence per year compared to 5.4% of controls. When they included all 11 trials in the analysis, the relative risk was 0.82 (95% CI 0.58–1.15). The wide confidence interval reported suggested no significant effect of HRT on risk of recurrence. In observational studies such as these, significant confounding factors no doubt exist. Women chosen to commence HRT may be women who have a favourable prognosis to start with. There may also be publication bias where

Table 1 Summary of systemic HRT effects from key HRT trials

Cardiovascular	
Study	HERS[40]
Design	Randomised
No. of patients	2763
Summary of results	No significant difference in myocardial infarction or death
Study	HERS II[41]
Design	Randomised
No. of patients	2321
Summary of results	No significant difference in myocardial infarction or death
Study	WHI[7]
Design	Randomised
No. of patients	161,608
Summary of results	Coronary heart disease – HR 1.29 (CI 1.02–1.63). Pulmonary embolism/deep vein thrombosis – HR 2.13 (CI 1.39–3.25). Stroke – HR 1.41 (CI 1.07–1.85)
Study	WEST[42]
Design	Randomised
No. of patients	664
Summary of results	No difference in incidence of stroke
Gynaecological malignancy	
Study	Swedish[43]
Design	Case-control
No. of patients	655 cases, 3899 controls
Summary of results	Increased risk with sequential but not continuous HRT preparation
Study	WHI[43]
Design	Randomised
No. of patients	161,608
Summary of results	Endometrial cancer – HR 0.81 (CI 0.48–1.36). Ovarian cancer – HR 1.58 (CI 0.77–3.24)
Cognitive function	
Study	WHI[44]
Design	Randomised
No. of patients	161,608
Summary of results	Dementia – HR 2.05 (CI 1.21–3.48). Mild cognitive impairment – HR 1.07 (CI 0.74–1.55)
Study	HERS[3]
Design	Randomised
No. of patients	2763
Summary of results	If menopausal symptoms – improved mental health. If no menopausal symptoms – decreased energy/increased fatigue
Colorectal	
Study	Grodstein et al.[45]
Design	Meta-analysis
No. of patients	18 studies
Summary of results	Colon cancer – RR 0.8 (CI 0.74–0.86). Rectal cancer – RR 0.81 (CI 0.72–0.92)
Study	WHI[7]
Design	Randomised
No. of patients	161,608
Summary of results	HR 0.63 (CI 0.43–0.92)

CHD, coronary heart disease; MI, myocardial infarction; HR, hazard ratio; RR, relative risk; CI, confidence interval.

trials suggesting an increase in recurrence rates tend not to be published. Good-quality, randomised, clinical trials can be the only intellectual approach but have been hindered by the findings of two Swedish trials.

In 2004, the HABITS trial began recruiting women experiencing menopausal symptoms who had received treatment for early stage breast cancer.[12] The intended sample size was 1300 women. Only 434 women were randomised to treatment with HRT or placebo for 2 years when the trial was terminated early as the hazard ratio crossed the pre-specified stopping parameter of 1.36 with a hazard ratio of 3.3 (95% CI 1.5–8.1). There were 26 new breast cancer events in the HRT group (11 local recurrences, 10 distant metastases and 5 contralateral breast cancers) compared to 8 in the control group (2 local recurrences, 5 distant metastases and 1 contralateral breast cancer). There were also 8 serious adverse events in the HRT group compared to 4 in the control group. A simultaneous trial in Stockholm found a hazard ratio of 0.8 for HRT but the combined analysis of both trials showed a significantly increased risk from HRT. The second trial was also stopped. Several important questions remain unanswered including the effects of short-term HRT use and the impact on ER-negative breast cancer survivors.

When considering HRT in women following treatment for breast cancer, it is important to consider both the advantages and disadvantages. Recent evidence on cardiovascular disease, gynaecological malignancy, cognitive effects and colorectal cancer also need to be taken into consideration to enable an informed decision to be made based on clinical parameters in the light of the available evidence. Established benefits of HRT need to be weighed against other risks of HRT and the level of risk acceptable to each patient carefully established.

Risks and benefits

Many body systems are affected by HRT and a number of trials have examined the effect of HRT on the cardiovascular system, gynaecological malignancy, cognitive function and colorectal cancer. Table 1 summarises the evidence to date in each of these areas. For cardiovascular disease, the HERS study found no significant difference in non-fatal myocardial infarction or death between women on HRT or placebo but the WHI study found a hazard ratio of 1.29. There is no strong evidence that the rate of gynaecological malignancy is affected by combined HRT based on the Swedish and WHI studies. An increased rate of dementia was seen in the WHI study but no effect on mild cognitive impairment. Several studies, including a large meta-analysis, have reported a decrease in colorectal cancer in women on HRT.

Management of women at risk or following breast cancer

There are no established guidelines for prescribing HRT to breast cancer survivors and, therefore, for each individual patient, the risks and benefits need to be carefully considered and an informed judgement made by consensus with the patient. A pragmatic approach to the management of common symptoms in breast cancer survivors follows.

Bone health

Osteoporosis causes considerable morbidity and mortality in the UK. It is responsible for over 200,000 fractures each year. Osteoporosis is defined by the World Health Organization as bone mineral density (BMD) T-score < –2.5 whereas osteopenia has a T-score between –1.0 and –2.5. The International Society for Clinical Densitometry (ISCD) recommends BMD be measured both at the lumbar spine and at the hip in all patients.[13] Osteoporosis is diagnosed based on the lowest T-score at either of these sites. This does not improve the prediction of fracture at any site but increases the number of patients selected.

Oestrogens act to inhibit bone resorption and, therefore, maintain bone mineral density. Menopause triggers an initial period of rapid bone loss followed by bone loss at a slower rate. HRT, as demonstrated by the WHI trial, is protective of bone mass.[5] HRT use without clear indication is not recommended for women at risk, or following a diagnosis, of breast cancer. Alternative treatment must, therefore, initially be sought. A further consideration for women receiving treatment for breast cancer is the effect of their antitumour therapy on bone health. Tamoxifen is a selective oestrogen receptor modulator (SERM) which prevents bone loss in postmenopausal women by an agonist effect on oestrogen receptors in bone.[14] In premenopausal women, tamoxifen has paradoxically been shown to enhance bone loss.[15] Tamoxifen may also hasten the onset of menopause.[16] The increasing use of the aromatase inhibitors in the treatment of breast cancer is a further cause for concern of osteoporosis risk. In postmenopausal women, aromatase inhibitors appear to accelerate bone loss due to their profound suppression of circulating levels of oestrogen. The ATAC trial comparing tamoxifen and anastrazole as adjuvant treatment for breast cancer found an increase in BMD in the tamoxifen group (+1.9% at the spine) but a decrease in the anastrazole group (–4.0% at the spine). Anastrazole was associated with a significant increase in fracture risk compared to tamoxifen.[17]

Clinical guidelines have been developed by the National Osteoporosis Foundation to address screening and treatment of osteoporosis and osteopenia in otherwise healthy women. The American Society of Clinical Oncology (ASCO) has also published guidance on bone health in women with breast carcinoma. In the latter document, specific attention is drawn to women receiving aromatase inhibitors and women with treatment-related early menopause. The ASCO guidelines recommend screening for all women over 65 years and women aged 60–65 years with a family history, weight < 70 kg and prior non-traumatic fracture. The recommendation also includes screening for premenopausal women with therapy-associated early menopause and postmenopausal women of any age receiving aromatase inhibitors.[18] No guidance, however, has been given on premenopausal women with a history of breast carcinoma.

Treatment for low bone mass in all women starts with a balanced diet and exercise. Calcium and vitamin D from diet or supplements can increase spinal BMD and reduce vertebral and non-vertebral fractures.[19] ASCO has published guidelines of thresholds for women with breast carcinoma for pharmacological intervention which includes women with a fragility fracture, women with a BMD < –2.5 and women with a borderline BMD score (< –1.0) and other risk factors.[18] The oral bisphosphonates (alendronate, risedronate and etidronate) are licensed in the UK for the prevention and treatment of osteoporosis. These drugs have been shown to increase BMD and reduce risk of fractures at vertebral and non-vertebral sites.[18,20]

Intravenous bisphosphonates are recommended by ASCO for use in women with bone metastases. Both pamidronate and zoledronic acid are recommended in the 2003 guidelines and have shown antiresorptive effects in women with metastatic breast cancer in randomised trials.[21] There are three prospective trials that address the role of adjuvant clodronate for women following treatment for breast cancer.[22–24] Two of these trials yielded favourable results while the third showed an adverse impact. It, therefore, remains uncertain whether bisphosphonates are beneficial in the adjuvant setting and will need further investigation. The NSABP B-34 trial, which is now closed to accrual, will determine whether clodronate for 3 years, alone or with chemotherapy and/or hormone therapy will improve disease-free survival in patients with early stage breast cancer.

The SERM raloxifene has also demonstrated efficacy in the treatment and prevention of postmenopausal osteoporosis but there are concerns over hormone manipulation in women following breast cancer. The Multiple Outcomes of Raloxifene Evaluation (MORE) study randomised 7705 postmenopausal women to raloxifene or placebo.[25] The main outcomes were vertebral and non-vertebral fracture and BMD. The frequency of vertebral fracture was reduced in the raloxifene group in which the BMD was also found to have increased. There was no significant effect on the non-vertebral fracture rate. The relative risk of breast cancer was also significantly reduced in the raloxifene group (RR 0.24; 95% CI 0.13–0.44). This benefit was seen for oestrogen receptor positive tumours but not for oestrogen receptor negative tumours.

Genito-urinary symptoms

Oestrogen deficiency is associated with genito-urinary symptoms related to urogenital atrophy. Topical oestrogens in the form of an oestriol ring or cream are often recommended for isolated genito-urinary symptoms and there was thought to be little systemic absorption. However, a recent study showed a reduction in total cholesterol, low-density lipoprotein and apolipoprotein B with topical oestriol suggesting substantial systemic effects.[26] If lipid profile is altered, the effect of topical oestrogen on breast cancer risk also raises concern. Ultra-low-dose oestrogen preparations such as Vagifem may be considered but extreme caution needs to be exercised when women are taking an aromatase inhibitor as part of their breast cancer treatment. Non-oestrogen based treatments such as K-Y jelly and vaginal moisturisers significantly reduce vaginal dryness and should be considered as first-line treatment in breast cancer survivors.

Menopausal symptoms can also occur as a result of anticancer treatment such as tamoxifen. Tamoxifen treatment can lead to endometrial thickening and symptoms such as bleeding in addition to vasomotor symptoms. The levonorgestrel-releasing intra-uterine device (Mirena) has been used successfully in a randomised trial and shown protective effects against the uterine effects of tamoxifen.[27]

Vasomotor symptoms

Vasomotor symptoms represent a much more common problem in breast cancer survivors than in an age-matched population. One alternative to combined HRT or unopposed oestrogen is progesterone which has been shown to reduce hot flushes substantially in clinical trials, but the use of any hormonal treatment is now controversial following the recent trials of HRT and breast cancer risk.[28]

Non-hormonal treatments for vasomotor symptoms include clonidine, selective-serotonin re-uptake inhibitors (SSRIs) and herbal or alternative remedies. Transdermal or oral clonidine has been shown to reduce the incidence of hot flushes effectively compared to placebo but the side-effects including dry mouth, drowsiness and constipation which limit its use.[29,30] SSRIs including venlafaxine and fluoxetine have both shown to be effective in reducing hot flushes in clinical trials and newer antidepressants such as citalopram and nefazadone are currently under evaluation.[31,32] SSRIs represent a reasonable first choice for vasomotor symptoms in breast cancer survivors. They may also be useful for the mood swings and depression often associated with menopause. Gabapentin, a gamma-amino butyric acid analogue, is also associated with a reduction in hot flushes.[33]

The use of herbal remedies in breast cancer survivors raises several issues. While the lack of clinical testing compared to conventional pharmacological agents is of concern, there are a number of oestrogen-like substances that may have a significant pharmacological effect. Black cohosh (*Cimicifuga racemosa*), a member of the buttercup family, has shown variable effectiveness in clinical trials although safety data are lacking.[34] Soy products containing isoflavones have also shown mixed activity.[35] The latter contain phytooestrogens and, therefore, their safety profile remains uncertain. Dong quai and vitamin E have not shown efficacy against hot flushes when subjected to clinical trials.[36,37] Acupuncture has been reported to be helpful in the treatment of menopausal symptoms with good effect but reports have only been based on anecdotal evidence.

Tibolone is a steroid compound that exerts oestrogenic, progestogenic and androgenic effects. It has beneficial effects on vasomotor symptoms as well as on the lower genital tract, mood and sexual well-being. The local progestogenic effect prevents endometrial stimulation. Tibolone stimulates apoptosis and reduces proliferation rate in normal human breast tissue *in vivo* as well as *in vitro*. Animal studies have shown that it does not stimulate mammary tissue and displays an antitumour effect on the breast similar to tamoxifen.[38] A small randomised study comparing tibolone to placebo in women receiving tamoxifen for breast cancer showed that tibolone prevented the increase in occurrence and severity of hot flushes and sweats associated with tamoxifen treatment.[39] Tibolone is also associated with a lower incidence of breast tenderness and does not increase mammographic density. The effect of tibolone on the breast recurrence rate in women with a history of breast cancer is currently being assessed in a large randomised, placebo-controlled trial. More research is needed in larger studies but tibolone looks promising as an alternative to combined HRT.

CONCLUSIONS

HRT was the mainstay of treatment for both menopausal symptoms and osteoporosis for many years. Evidence from recent randomised controlled trials now suggests that there is an increased risk of breast cancer associated with longer term use of combined HRT. HRT prescribing in healthy women should be restricted to those experiencing significant symptoms uncontrolled by other measures. When indicated, HRT should be given in the lowest possible dose for the shortest possible time to relieve symptoms. Osteoporosis in itself is no longer an indication for HRT as alternative treatments such as bisphosphonates are now available.

In survivors of breast cancer, the use of HRT remains controversial and until more trial data become available there currently is no definitive answer. Avoiding HRT in this situation where alternatives are available may be the safest solution. Many women continue to have significant symptoms and careful considered use of HRT with patient choice for an appropriate interval may provide for optimum quality of life. Clinicians caring for women undergoing treatment for breast cancer and patients previously treated for breast cancer should be aware of the options available to counsel patients on accepted risks and benefits to facilitate an informed judgement to be made.

References

1 Utian WH, Shoupe D, Bachmann G, Pinkerton JV, Pickar JH. Relief of vasomotor symptoms and vaginal atrophy with lower doses of conjugated equine estrogens and medroxyprogesterone acetate. Fertil Steril 2001; 75: 1065–1079

2 Hays J, Ockene JK, Brunner RL et al. Effects of estrogen plus progestin on health-related quality of life. N Engl J Med 2003; 348: 1839–1854

3 Hlatky MA, Boothroyd D, Vittinghoff E, Sharp P, Whooley MA. Quality-of-life and depressive symptoms in postmenopausal women after receiving hormone therapy: results from the Heart and Estrogen/Progestin Replacement Study (HERS) trial. JAMA 2002; 287: 591–597

4 Sarrel PM. Sexuality and menopause. Obstet Gynecol 1990; 75: 26S–30S, discussion 31S–35S

5 Cauley JA, Robbins J, Chen Z et al. Effects of estrogen plus progestin on risk of fracture and bone mineral density: the Women's Health Initiative randomized trial. JAMA 2003; 290: 1729–1738

6 Collaborative Group on Hormonal Factors in Breast Cancer. Breast cancer and hormone replacement therapy: collaborative reanalysis of data from 51 epidemiological studies of 52,705 women with breast cancer and 108,411 women without breast cancer. Lancet 1997; 350: 1047–1059

7 Rossouw JE, Anderson GL, Prentice RL et al. Risks and benefits of estrogen plus progestin in healthy postmenopausal women: principal results from the Women's Health Initiative randomized controlled trial. JAMA 2002; 288: 321–333

8 Chlebowski RT, Hendrix SL, Langer RD et al. Influence of estrogen plus progestin on breast cancer and mammography in healthy postmenopausal women: the Women's Health Initiative Randomized Trial. JAMA 2003; 289: 3243–3253

9 Beral V. Breast cancer and hormone-replacement therapy in the Million Women Study. Lancet 2003; 362: 419–427

10 Bines J, Oleske DM, Cobleigh MA. Ovarian function in premenopausal women treated with adjuvant chemotherapy for breast cancer. J Clin Oncol 1996; 14: 1718–1729

11 Col NF, Hirota LK, Orr RK et al. Hormone replacement therapy after breast cancer: a systematic review and quantitative assessment of risk. J Clin Oncol 2001; 19: 2357–2363

12 Holmberg L, Anderson H. HABITS (hormonal replacement therapy after breast cancer – is it safe?), a randomised comparison: trial stopped. Lancet 2004; 363: 453–455

13 Kanis JA, Seeman E, Johnell O, Rizzoli R, Delmas P. The perspective of the International Osteoporosis Foundation on the official positions of the International Society for Clinical Densitometry. Osteoporos Int 2005; 16: 456–459, discussion 479–480

14 Love RR, Mazess RB, Barden HS *et al.* Effects of tamoxifen on bone mineral density in postmenopausal women with breast cancer. N Engl J Med 1992; 326: 852–856

15 Powles TJ, Hickish T, Kanis JA, Tidy A, Ashley S. Effect of tamoxifen on bone mineral density measured by dual-energy X-ray absorptiometry in healthy premenopausal and postmenopausal women. J Clin Oncol 1996; 14: 78–84

16 Goodwin PJ, Ennis M, Pritchard KI, Trudeau M, Hood N. Risk of menopause during the first year after breast cancer diagnosis. J Clin Oncol 1999; 17: 2365–2370

17 Baum M, Budzar AU, Cuzick J *et al.* Anastrozole alone or in combination with tamoxifen versus tamoxifen alone for adjuvant treatment of postmenopausal women with early breast cancer: first results of the ATAC randomised trial. Lancet 2002; 359: 2131–2139

18 Hillner BE, Ingle JN, Chlebowski RT *et al.* American Society of Clinical Oncology 2003 update on the role of bisphosphonates and bone health issues in women with breast cancer. J Clin Oncol 2003; 21: 4042–4057

19 Dawson-Hughes B, Harris SS, Krall EA, Dallal GE. Effect of calcium and vitamin D supplementation on bone density in men and women 65 years of age or older. N Engl J Med 1997; 337: 670–676

20 Cranney A, Wells G, Willan A *et al.* Meta-analyses of therapies for postmenopausal osteoporosis. II. Meta-analysis of alendronate for the treatment of postmenopausal women. Endocr Rev 2002; 23: 508–516

21 Rosen LS, Gordon D, Kaminski M *et al.* Zoledronic acid versus pamidronate in the treatment of skeletal metastases in patients with breast cancer or osteolytic lesions of multiple myeloma: a phase III, double-blind, comparative trial. Cancer J 2001; 7: 377–387

22 Diel IJ, Solomayer EF, Costa SD *et al.* Reduction in new metastases in breast cancer with adjuvant clodronate treatment. N Engl J Med 1998; 339: 357–363

23 Saarto T, Blomqvist C, Virkkunen P, Elomaa I. Adjuvant clodronate treatment does not reduce the frequency of skeletal metastases in node-positive breast cancer patients: 5-year results of a randomized controlled trial. J Clin Oncol 2001; 19: 10–17

24 Powles T, Paterson S, Kanis JA *et al.* Randomized, placebo-controlled trial of clodronate in patients with primary operable breast cancer. J Clin Oncol 2002; 20: 3219–3224

25 Ettinger B, Black DM, Mitlak BH *et al.* Reduction of vertebral fracture risk in postmenopausal women with osteoporosis treated with raloxifene: results from a 3-year randomized clinical trial. Multiple Outcomes of Raloxifene Evaluation (MORE) Investigators. JAMA 1999; 282: 637–645

26 Naessen T, Rodriguez-Macias K, Lithell H. Serum lipid profile improved by ultra-low doses of 17 beta-estradiol in elderly women. J Clin Endocrinol Metab 2001; 86: 2757–2762

27 Gardner FJ, Konje JC, Abrams KR *et al.* Endometrial protection from tamoxifen-stimulated changes by a levonorgestrel-releasing intrauterine system: a randomised controlled trial. Lancet 2000; 356: 1711–1717

28 Bertelli G, Venturini M, Del Mastro L *et al.* Intramuscular depot medroxyprogesterone versus oral megestrol for the control of postmenopausal hot flashes in breast cancer patients: a randomized study. Ann Oncol 2002; 13: 883–888

29 Pandya KJ, Raubertas RF, Flynn PJ *et al.* Oral clonidine in postmenopausal patients with breast cancer experiencing tamoxifen-induced hot flashes: a University of Rochester Cancer Center Community Clinical Oncology Program study. Ann Intern Med 2000; 132: 788–793

30 Goldberg RM, Loprinzi CL, O'Fallon JR *et al.* Transdermal clonidine for ameliorating tamoxifen-induced hot flashes. J Clin Oncol 1994; 12: 155–158

31 Loprinzi CL, Kugler JW, Sloan JA *et al.* Venlafaxine in management of hot flashes in survivors of breast cancer: a randomised controlled trial. Lancet 2000; 356: 2059–2063

32 Loprinzi CL, Sloan JA, Perez EA *et al.* Phase III evaluation of fluoxetine for treatment of hot flashes. J Clin Oncol 2002; 20: 1578–1583

33 Loprinzi L, Barton DL, Sloan JA *et al.* Pilot evaluation of gabapentin for treating hot flashes. Mayo Clin Proc 2002; 77: 1159–1163

34 Lieberman S. A review of the effectiveness of *Cimicifuga racemosa* (black cohosh) for the symptoms of menopause. J Womens Health 1998; 7: 525–529

35 Van Patten CL, Olivotto IA, Chambers GK *et al.* Effect of soy phytoestrogens on hot flashes in postmenopausal women with breast cancer: a randomized, controlled clinical trial. J Clin Oncol 2002; 20: 1449–1455

36 Hirata JD, Swiersz LM, Zell B, Small R, Ettinger B. Does dong quai have estrogenic effects in postmenopausal women? A double-blind, placebo-controlled trial. Fertil Steril 1997; 68: 981–986

37 Barton DL, Loprinzi CL, Quella SK et al. Prospective evaluation of vitamin E for hot flashes in breast cancer survivors. J Clin Oncol 1998; 16: 495–500

38 Cline JM, Register TC, Clarkson TB. Effects of tibolone and hormone replacement therapy on the breast of cynomolgus monkeys. Menopause 2002; 9: 422–429

39 Kroiss R, Fentiman IS, Helmond FA et al. The effect of tibolone in postmenopausal women receiving tamoxifen after surgery for breast cancer: a randomised, double-blind, placebo-controlled trial. Br J Obstet Gynaecol 2005; 112: 228–233

40 Hulley S, Grady D, Bush T et al. Randomized trial of estrogen plus progestin for secondary prevention of coronary heart disease in postmenopausal women. Heart and Estrogen/progestin Replacement Study (HERS) Research Group. JAMA 1998; 280: 605–613

41 Grady D, Herrington D, Bittner V et al. Cardiovascular disease outcomes during 6.8 years of hormone therapy: Heart and Estrogen/progestin Replacement Study follow-up (HERS II). JAMA 2002; 288: 49–57

42 Viscoli CM, Brass LM, Kernan WN et al. A clinical trial of estrogen-replacement therapy after ischemic stroke. N Engl J Med 2001; 345: 1243–1249

43 Riman T, Dickman PW, Nilsson S et al. Hormone replacement therapy and the risk of invasive epithelial ovarian cancer in Swedish women. J Natl Cancer Inst 2002; 94: 497–504

44 Shumaker SA, Legault C, Rapp SR et al. Estrogen plus progestin and the incidence of dementia and mild cognitive impairment in postmenopausal women: the Women's Health Initiative Memory Study: a randomized controlled trial. JAMA 2003; 289: 2651–2662

45 Grodstein F, Newcomb PA, Stampfer MJ. Postmenopausal hormone therapy and the risk of colorectal cancer: a review and meta-analysis. Am J Med 1999; 106: 574–582

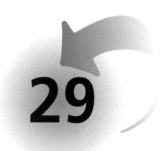

John Studd   Nick Panay

Hormones and depression in women

On Boxing Day 1851, Charles Dickens attended the patients' Christmas dance at St Luke's Hospital for the insane. On describing his visit in an article for *Household Words,* he commented that the experience of the asylum proved that insanity was more prevalent amongst women than men. Of the 18,759 inmates over the century, 11,162 had been women. He adds 'it is well known that female servants are more frequently affected by lunacy than any other class of persons'. Charles Dickens was as great an observer as any Nobel prize winner and indeed this passage is one of the very few references in Victorian literature that make the point between gender and depression but there are none to our knowledge relating reproductive function to depression. Jane Eyre's red room and Berthe Mason's monthly madness may be coded examples of this from Charlotte Bronte's pen.

Modern epidemiology confirms that depression is more common in women than men whether we look at hospital admissions, population studies, suicide attempts or the prescription of antidepressants.[1] The challenge remains to determine whether this increase in depression is environmental, reflecting women's perceived role in contemporary society or whether it is due to hormonal changes.

It is clear that this excess of depression in women starts at puberty and is no longer present in the 6th and 7th decade. The peaks of depression occur at times of hormonal fluctuation in: (i) the premenstrual phase; (ii) the postpartum phase; and (iii) the climacteric perimenopausal phase – particularly in the one or two years before the periods cease. This triad of

John Studd DS MD FRCOG (for correspondence)
Professor of Gynaecology, Chelsea & Westminster Hospital, 369 Fulham Road, London SW10 9NH, UK
E-mail: harley@studd.co.uk

Nick Panay BSc MRCOG MFFP
Consultant Obstetrician & Gynaecologist, Specialist in Reproductive Medicine & Surgery, Queen Charlotte's and Chelsea Hospital & Chelsea and Westminster Hospital, 369 Fulham Road, London SW10 9NH, UK.
E-mail: nickpanay@msn.com

hormone-responsive mood disorders, (HRMD) often occurs in the same vulnerable woman. The depression of these patients can be usually treated effectively by oestrogens, preferably by the transdermal route and in a moderately high dose. Transdermal oestrogen patches of 200 mcg has been the dose used in published placebo-controlled studies, but the 100 mcg dose is frequently effective.

The 45-year-old depressed perimenopausal woman who is still menstruating will often give a history of worsening premenstrual depression and also have physical manifestations of hormonal fluctuations such as menstrual migraine. She will have usually enjoyed very good mood during the latter half of pregnancy when hormonal levels were stable. Such a woman will often say that she last felt well during her last pregnancy. She then developed postnatal depression for several months. When the periods returned, the depression became cyclical and as she approached the menopause, the depression became more constant.

Reproductive events also affect the course of bipolar disorder in women; 67% of such women have a history of postpartum depression. Of these, all will have had episodes of depression after subsequent pregnancies. Subsequently, women who were not using hormone replacement therapy (HRT) were significantly more likely than those who were using HRT to report worsening of depressive symptoms during the perimenopause.

In spite of this clear clinical history of a woman who will probably respond to oestrogens, many psychiatrists believe that such patients are ideal for the use of antidepressants. This is because they identify that these women will have had a 'pre-morbid history of depression' and that they, therefore, must have a chronic relapsing depressive illness. However, the salient feature of the case history is that the depression is usually postnatal or premenstrual in timing. This key information often needs to be identified by direct, detailed enquiry otherwise the wrong conclusion can be drawn leading to sub-optimal therapy.

The clue to the use of oestrogens came with the important and somewhat eccentric paper by Klaiber and colleagues[2] who performed a placebo-controlled study of very high-dose oestrogens in patients with chronic relapsing depression. They had various diagnoses and were both premenopausal and postmenopausal. They were given Premarin 5 mg daily with an increase in dose of 5 mg each week until a maximum of 30 mg a day was used. There was a huge improvement in depression on these high doses but this work has not been repeated because of anxiety over high-dose oestrogens.

BIOLOGICAL PLAUSIBILITY

It is generally accepted that endogenous, oestrogenic steroids have a pivotal influence on the development of the female central nervous system (CNS) through genomic organisational effects in fetal life. Recent work has shown that not only α- but also β-oestrogen receptors are located in the hypothalamus and other parts of the CNS.[3] It is, therefore, not surprising that exogenous oestrogens may have benefits in controlling mood, cognition and neuronal health.

It has long been recognised that non-genomic activational effects can also be produced by the activation of the CNS neuroreceptors to alter the concentration of neurotransmitter amines such as serotonin and noradrenaline.[4]

Oestrogen can increase the level of serotonin in a number of ways: it can enhance the degradation of monoamine oxidase (which catabolises serotonin), it displaces tryptophan from its albumin binding sites, making more available for serotonin synthesis and it also enhances the transport of serotonin.[5] This explains how oestrogen can improve mood, when used in ovarian cycle stabilising doses, as depression is largely due to falling levels of serotonin.

PREMENSTRUAL SYNDROME

This condition is mentioned in the 4th century BC by Hippocrates but became a medical epidemic in the 19th century. Victorian physicians were aware of menstrual madness, hysteria, chlorosis, ovarian mania, as well as the more commonplace neurasthenia. In the 1870s, Maudsley,[6] the most distinguished psychiatrist of the time, wrote: 'The monthly activity of the ovaries which marks the advent of puberty in women has a notable effect upon the mind and body; wherefore it may become an important cause of mental and physical derangement'. This and other female maladies were recognised, rightly or wrongly, to be due to the ovaries. As a consequence, bilateral oophorectomy – Battey's operation[7] – became fashionable, being performed in approximately 150,000 women in North America and Northern Europe in the 30 years from 1870. Longo,[8] in his brilliant historical essay on the decline of Battey's operation, posed the question whether it worked or not. Of course they had no knowledge of osteoporosis and the devastation of long-term oestrogen deficiency, therefore, in balance the operation was not helpful as a long-term solution but it probably did, as was claimed, cure the 'menstrual/ovarian madness' which would be a quaint Victorian way of labelling severe PMS. The essential logic of this operation was to remove cyclical ovarian function but happily this can now effectively be achieved by simpler medical therapy.

Only in 1931 was the phrase 'premenstrual tension' introduced by Frank,[9] who described 15 women with the typical symptoms of PMS as we know it. Greene and Dalton[10] extended the definition to 'premenstrual syndrome' in 1953, recognising the wider range of symptoms.

Severe premenstrual syndrome (PMS) is a poorly understood collection of cyclical symptoms, which cause considerable psychological and physical distress. The psychological symptoms of depression, loss of energy, irritability, loss of libido and abnormal behaviour as well as the physical symptoms of headaches, breast discomfort and abdominal bloating may occur for up to 14 days each month. There may also be associated menstrual problems, pelvic pain, menstrual headaches and the woman may only enjoy as few as 7 good days per month. It is obvious that the symptoms mentioned can have a significant impact on the day-to-day functioning of women. It is estimated that up to 95% of women have some form of PMS but in about 5% of women of reproductive age they will be severely affected with disruption of their daily activities. Considering these figures it is disturbing that many of the consultations at our specialist PMS clinics start with women saying that for many years they have been told that there are no treatments available and that they should simply 'live with it'. In addition, many commonly used treatments of PMS, particularly progesterone or progestogens, have been shown by many placebo-controlled trials to be not only ineffective but they commonly make the symptoms worse as these women are progesterone or progestogen intolerant.

The exact cause is uncertain, but fundamentally it is due to hormonal fluctuations during the menstrual cycle and the resulting complex interaction between ovarian steroid hormones (*e.g.* progesterone or allopregnenalone) and central nervous system neurotransmitters, such as GABA and serotonin. These cyclical neuroendocrine changes produce the varied premenstrual symptoms in women who are genetically predisposed to the changes in their normal reproductive hormone levels.

OESTROGENS

PMS does not occur if there is no ovarian function.[11] Obviously, it does not occur before puberty, after the menopause or after oophorectomy. It also does not occur during pregnancy. It is, therefore, not surprising that hysterectomy with conservation of the ovaries does not cure PMS[12] as patients are left with the usual cyclical symptoms and cyclical headaches in spite of the absence of menstruation. This condition, best-called 'the ovarian cycle syndrome',[13] is usually not recognised to be hormonal in aetiology, as there is no reference point of menstruation. The failure to make this diagnosis is regrettable because these monthly symptoms of depression, irritability, mood change, bloating and headaches which might affect women for most days in the month, with only perhaps a good week each month, can easily be treated with transdermal oestrogens which suppress ovarian function and thus remove the symptoms.

A medical Battey's operation can be achieved by the use of GnRH analogues. Leather *et al.*[14] have demonstrated that 3 months of goserelin therapy cures all of the symptom groups of PMS. The long-term risk of goserelin therapy is bone demineralisation but the same group showed that add-back with a product containing 2 mg of oestradiol valerate and cyclical levonorgestrel (Nuvelle; Schering Health) maintains bone density at both the spine and the hip as well as alleviating vasomotor side effects.[15] Most PMS symptoms remain improved with this 'add-back' but bloating, tension and irritability can recur due to the cyclical progestogen. The tissue selective agent tibolone and low-dose, continuous, combined HRT are, therefore, better add-back preparations as these do not regenerate the hormonal fluctuations of the ovarian cycle.[16]

In a Scandinavian study, Sundstrom and colleagues[17] used low-dose GnRH analogues (100 µg buserelin) with good results on the symptoms of PMS, but the treatment still caused anovulation in as much as 56% of patients. Danazol is another method to treat PMS by inhibiting pituitary gonadotrophins, but it has side-effects including androgenic and virilising effects. When used in the luteal phase alone,[18] it only relieved mastalgia but not the general symptoms of PMS even though side-effects were minimal.

Greenblatt *et al.*[19] showed the effects of an anovulatory dose of oestrogen implants for the use of contraception and the first study for its use in PMS was by Magos *et al.*[20] using 100-mg oestradiol implants, the dose that had been shown to inhibit ovulation by using ultrasound and day-21 progesterone measurements in earlier studies by the same group. There was a big (84%) improvement with placebo implants but, despite this, the improvements of every symptom cluster was greater in the active oestradiol group. In addition, the placebo effect waned after a few months compared with a continued response to oestradiol. These patients were also given 12 days of oral progestogen per month to prevent endometrial hyperplasia and irregular bleeding.[21] It was clear that the addition of progestogen attenuated the beneficial effect of oestrogen. Subsequently, a placebo-controlled trial of cyclical norethisterone in well-oestrogenised, hysterectomised women reproduced the typical symptoms of PMS.[22] This study of cyclical oral progestogen in the oestrogen-primed woman was described as the model for PMS. It is also significant that progestogen intolerance is one of the principal reasons why older, post-menopausal women stop taking HRT,[23] particularly if they have a past history of PMS or progesterone intolerance. It is common for progestogens to cause PMS-like symptoms in these women in the same way endogenous cyclical progesterone secretion is the probable fundamental cause of premenstrual syndrome.

Although our group still uses oestradiol implants, often with the addition of testosterone for loss of energy and loss of libido, we have reduced the oestradiol dose, never starting with 100 mg because of concerns about tachyphylaxis. We will now insert pellets of oestradiol 50 mg or 75 mg with 100 mg of testosterone. These women must have endometrial protection by either oral progestogen or a Mirena (Schering Healthcare) levonorgestrel-releasing intra-uterine system (LNG IUS).[24] As women with PMS respond well to oestrogens, but are often intolerant to progestogens, it is common-place for us to reduce the orthodox 13-day course of progestogen to 10 or 7 days starting, for convenience, on the first day of every calendar month. Thus, the menstrual cycle is reset.

The Mirena IUS also plays a vital role in preventing PMS-like symptoms as it performs its function of protecting the endometrium without significant systemic absorption. A recent study has shown a 50% decrease in hysterectomies in our practice since the introduction of the Mirena IUS in 1995.[21] With its profound effect on menorrhagia and the possibility of less progestogenic side-effects, Mirena looks a very promising component of PMS treatment in the future.

Hormone implants are not licensed in all countries and are unsuitable for women who may wish to discontinue treatment easily in order to become pregnant. Oestradiol patches are an alternative and our original double-blind, cross-over study used 200 mcg of oestradiol patch twice weekly.[25] This produced plasma oestradiol levels of 800 pmol/l and suppressed luteal phase progesterone and ovulation. Once again, this treatment was better than placebo in every symptom cluster of PMS. and is now our treatment of choice in severe PMS.

Subsequently, a randomised, but uncontrolled, observational study from our PMS clinic indicated that PMS sufferers could have the same beneficial response to 100 mcg patches as they do with the 200 mg dose. They also have fewer symptoms of breast discomfort, bloating and there is less anxiety from the patient or general practitioner about high-dose oestrogen therapy.[26] The 21-day progesterone assays in the patients receiving 100 mcg showed low anovulatory levels prompting the intriguing question that even this moderate dose might reliably suppress ovulation and be contraceptive. Clearly, a great deal of work must be done before we can suggest that this treatment is effective birth control; however, it is of great importance because many young women on this therapy for PMS will be pleased if it also was an effective contraceptive. This is a study which needs to be conducted.

The original studies outlined in this paper are all scientifically valid, placebo-controlled trials showing a considerable improvement in PMS symptoms with oestrogens. Although this treatment is used by most gynaecologists in the UK, its value has not been exploited by psychiatrists anywhere in the world. We believe that the benefit of this therapy in severe PMS is due to the inhibition of ovulation but there is probably also a central, mental, tonic effect. Klaiber et al.,[2] in their study of high-dose Premarin showed this and our other psycho-endocrine studies of climacteric depression[27] and post-natal depression[28] have shown the benefit of high-dose transdermal oestrogens for these conditions, which is not related to, or dependent upon, suppression of ovulation.

Ultimately, there are some women who, after treatment with oestrogens and Mirena coils, will prefer to have a hysterectomy in order to remove all cycles with a virtual guarantee of improvement of symptoms. This should not be seen as a failure, or even treatment of last resort, as it does carry many other advantages.[29] It is important that these women who have had a hysterectomy and bilateral salpingo-oophorectomy have effective replacement therapy, ideally with replacement of the ovarian androgens. Implants of oestradiol 50 mg and testosterone 100 mg are an ideal route and combination of hormones for this long-term therapy post-hysterectomy with a continuation rate of 90% at 10 years.[21] We have unpublished data of 47 such patients who have had a hysterectomy, bilateral salpingo-oophorectomy and implants of oestradiol and testosterone for severe PMS who have gone through many years of treatment with transdermal oestrogens and cycle progestogens or Mirena coil. The symptoms are removed in all patients and all but one was 'very satisfied' with the outcome.

POSTNATAL DEPRESSION

Postnatal depression is another example of depression being caused by fluctuations of sex hormones and having the potential to be treated effectively by hormones. It is a common condition which affects 10–15% of women following childbirth and may persist for over a year in 40% of those affected. There does seem to be a lack of any overall influence of psychosocial background factors in determining vulnerability to this postpartum disorder although it can be recurrent.

Although common, the disease is often not reported to the healthcare professional, particularly the general practitioner or the visiting midwife, as the exhaustion and depression is regarded as normal. Indeed, the symptoms of postnatal depression may be confused with the normal sequelae of childbirth. The symptoms can consist of depressed mood with lack of pleasure with the baby or any interest in her surroundings. There may be sleep disturbance, either insomnia or hypersomnia. There may be loss of weight, loss of energy and certainly loss of libido together with agitation, retardation and feelings of worthlessness or guilt. Frequent thoughts of death and suicide are common.

Postnatal depression is not more common after a long labour, difficult labour, caesarean section, separation from the baby after birth, nor is it determined by education or socio-economic group. The only environmental factor which seems to be important is the perceived amount of support given by the partner. There is no doubt that the first 6 or more months after delivery can be an exhausting time, full of anxiety and insecurity in mothers with the new responsibility of the baby. Even allowing for that, there does seem to be a clear hormonal aspect to this condition.

Postnatal depression is severe and more prolonged in women who are lactating and lower oestradiol levels are found in depressed women following delivery than with controls. It is probable that the low oestradiol levels with breast feeding and the higher incidence of depression are related in a causative way.

We studied the effect of high-dose transdermal oestrogens in this condition in an attempt to close the circle of studies treating this triad of hormone responsive depressions – premenstrual depression, climacteric depression and postnatal depression. This was a double-blind, placebo-controlled trial of 60 women with major depression which began within 3 months of childbirth and persisted for up to 18 months postnatally.[28] They had all been resistant to antidepressants and the diagnosis of postnatal depression was made by two psychiatrists who are expert in the field. We excluded breast feeding women from the study. They were given either placebo patches or transdermal oestradiol patches 200 mcg daily for 3 months without any added progestogen. After 3 months, cyclical Duphaston 10 mg daily was added for 12 days each month. The women were assessed monthly by a self-rating of depressive symptoms on the Edinburgh postnatal depression score, (EPDS) and by clinical psychiatric interview. Both groups were severely depressed with a mean EPDS score of 21.8 before treatment. During the first month of therapy, the women who received oestrogen improved rapidly and to a greater extent than controls. None of the other factors, age, psychiatric, obstetric or gynaecological history, severity and duration of current episode of depression and concurrent antidepressant medication influenced the response to treatment.

The study showed that the mean EPDS score was less with the active group at 1 month and then maintained for 8 months and that the percentage with EPDS scores over 14, (diagnostic of postnatal depression) was reduced by 50% at 1 month and 90% at 5 months. This was much better than the placebo response.

Not only did this study show that transdermal oestrogens were effective for the treatment of postnatal depression but a subsequent study by Lawrie et al.[30] showed that depot-progestogen was worse than placebo causing deterioration in the severity of postnatal depression. Thus we have again the picture of the mood elevating effect of oestrogens and the depressing effect of progestogen.

An uncontrolled study showed similar improvements using sublingual oestradiol in 23 women with major postnatal depression.[31] These women had plasma levels of 79.0 pmol/l before the treatment with sublingual oestradiol. The oestradiol levels were 342 pmol/l at 1 week and 480 pmol/l at 8 weeks.

There was improvement in 12 out of the 23 patients at 1 week and, after 2 weeks, there was recovery in 19 of the 23 patients. The mean Montgomery Asberg depression rating scale was 40.7 before treatment, 11 at 1 week and 2 at 8 weeks. At the end of the second week of treatment, the MADRS scores were compatible with clinical recovery in 19 out of the 23 patients. This study stressed the rapidity of response to the oestradiol therapy and this was our observation also. However, it must be stressed that this is an uncontrolled study in women with a very low, almost postmenopausal, level of oestradiol. Another placebo-controlled study is required together with information about bleeding patterns to support or refute our original paper.[28]

It would support the hormonal pathogenesis of this condition if we could mimic postnatal depression by hormonal manipulation. This was done by a study by Bloch *et al.*[42] who studied 16 women, 8 with a history of postnatal depression. They induced hypogonadism with leuprolide acetate and stimulated pregnancy by 'add-back' supraphysiological doses of oestradiol and progesterone for 8 weeks and then withdrawing both steroids. Five of the eight women with a history of postnatal depression and none of the women without a prior history developed significant mood symptoms during the withdrawal period.

This study supported the view that there was an involvement of the reproductive hormones, oestradiol and progesterone, in the development of postpartum depression in a specific group of women. Furthermore, the study showed that women with a history of postpartum depression are differentially sensitive to the mood destabilising effects of gonadal steroids.

CLIMACTERIC DEPRESSION

Like many aspects of depression in women, the diagnosis of climacteric depression and its treatment remains controversial. This may be because there is no real evidence of an excess of depression occurring after the menopause, nor any evidence that oestrogens help postmenopausal depression or what used to be called 'involutional melancholia'. This is quite true and indeed many women with long-standing depression improve considerably when the periods stop. This is because the depression created by premenstrual syndrome, heavy painful periods, menstrual headaches and the exhaustion that attend excess blood loss disappears. Therefore, the longitudinal studies of depression carried out by many psychologists, particularly those as notable as Hunter,[33] have shown no peak of depression in a large population of menopausal women. Randomised studies have also shown no significant improvement in depressed postmenopausal women.[34]

The depression that occurs in women around the time of the menopause is at its worst in the 2 or 3 years before the periods stop. This, of course, is perimenopausal depression and is no doubt related to premenstrual depression as it becomes worse with age and with falling oestrogen levels.

The earliest placebo-controlled study which defined the precise menopausal syndrome showed that oestrogens helped hot flushes, night sweats and vaginal dryness. They also had a mood elevating effect.[35] This work was further supported by that of Campbell and Whitehead[36] who used Premarin and by the study of Montgomery *et al.*[23] using higher dose oestradiol implants. This study of 90 peri- and postmenopausal women with depression showed considerable improvement in the treatment group compared with placebo but only in the perimenopausal women. There is no improvement in the depression in the postmenopausal women with this treatment when compared with placebo. This effect is not transient and we have shown that the improvement in depression is maintained even at 23 months. By this stage, the placebo patients had dropped out and there was no placebo group in the study.

Psychiatric opinion regarding the therapeutic potential of oestrogens in the treatment of depressed perimenopausal women is now becoming more favourable, particularly in the US. Soares et al.[37] studied 50 such women, 26 with major depressive disorder, 11 with dysthymic depression and 30 with minor depressive illness. They treated them with 100 mcg oestradiol patches in a 12-week placebo-controlled study. There was a remission of depression in 17 out of 25 of the treatment patients (68%) and only 5 out of the 25 placebo patients (20%). This improvement occurred regardless of the DSM-IV diagnosis.

Rasgon et al.[38] studied 16 perimenopausal women with unipolar major depressive disorder for an 8-week period in an open protocol trial comparing low-dose 0.3 mg Premarin to Fluoxetine daily. There was a greater response with oestrogen alone. All but two of the total patients responded but the response was greater in the oestrogen therapy patients; it was significant that the reduction of depression scores began rapidly after the first week of treatment.

More recently, Harlow et al.[39] studied a large number, (976) of perimenopausal women with a history of major depression and those without. The patients with the history of depression had higher FSH levels and lower oestradiol levels at enrolment to the study and those women with a history of antidepressant medication had 3 times the rate of early menopause. A similar excess rate was found in perimenopausal women who had had a history of severe depression.

It is re-assuring for 'menopausologists' to read the recent views of some psychiatrists[39] that 'periods of intense hormonal fluctuations have been associated with the heightened prevalence and exacerbation of underlying psychiatric illness, particularly the occurrence of premenstrual dysphoria, puerperal depression and depressive treatment during the perimenopause. It is speculated that sex steroids such as oestrogens, progestogens, (sic), testosterone and DHEA exert a significant modulation of brain functioning. There are preliminary, although promising data on the use of oestradiol, (particularly transdermal oestradiol to alleviate depression during the menopause.' Neuropsychiatrists have also conceded that 'there is a clear need to examine the necessary duration of HRT for neuroprotection to decrease a woman's risk for depression, cognitive dysfunction and development of Alzheimer's disease'.[40]

PROGESTOGEN INTOLERANCE

These women having moderately high-dose oestrogen therapy must, of course, have cyclical progestogen if they still have a uterus in order to prevent irregular bleeding and endometrial hyperplasia. The problem is that women with hormone-responsive depression enjoy a mood elevating effect with oestrogens but this is attenuated by the necessary progestogen.[41] This hormone can produce depression, tiredness, loss of libido, irritability, breast discomfort – in fact, all of the symptoms of premenstrual syndrome, particularly in women with a history or previous history of PMS. A randomised trial of norethisterone against placebo in oestrogenised hysterectomised women, previously referred to, clearly shows this and in fact the paper was subtitled a 'A model for the causation of PMS'.[22]

If women become depressed with 10–12 days of progestogen, it may be necessary to halve the dose, decrease the duration or change the progestogen used.[42] It is our policy to shorten the duration of progestogen routinely in women with hormone-responsive depression because adverse side-effects with any gestogen are almost invariable. We would, therefore, use transdermal oestrogens either 100 mcg or 200 mcg of an oestradiol patch or a 50 mg oestradiol implant and then reset menstrual bleeding by prescribing Norethisterone 5 mg for the first 7 days of each calendar month. This will produce a regular bleed on about day 10 or 11 of each calendar month.

Should heavy withdrawal bleeds occur, the duration of progestogen can be extended to the more orthodox 12 days. At this stage, many women would prefer to have a Mirena system inserted so there will be reduced bleeding (and eventual amenorrhoea in 40–50%) nor any need to take oral progestogen with its side effects. An alternative to Mirena would be vaginal progesterone pessaries or gel to minimise systemic progestogenic side effects. It is usual for women at this stage, who are aware of the benefits of oestrogens and the problems of their menstrual cycles, to request hysterectomy and bilateral salpingo-oophorectomy with the use of unopposed oestradiol and often testosterone.[43]

CONCLUSIONS

Oestrogen therapy has been shown to be effective for the treatment of postnatal depression, premenstrual depression and perimenopausal depression, the triad of hormone responsive mood disorders. Transdermal oestradiol, 100 mcg or 200 mcg patches, producing plasma levels of 300 pmol/l and 600 pmol/l, respectively, are the optimum therapy. These patients often require plasma levels of more than 600 pmol/l for efficacy as there does appear to be a dose-response effect. In non-hysterectomised women, cyclical progestogen is usually added for endometrial protection. The most effective long-term medical therapy is oestradiol patches or an implant of oestradiol with the Mirena intra-uterine system. The Mirena minimises systemic PMS-like side-effects, thus maximising efficacy. Consideration should also be given to the addition of testosterone for depression, libido and energy, particularly where patients have only partially responded to oestrogen therapy alone. Ultimately, a hysterectomy plus bilateral salpingo-oophorectomy and implants with oestradiol and testosterone may be requested.

The effect of oestrogen on the central nervous system, particularly mood and depression, remains a controversial area. However, there are now considerable data for the psychotherapeutic benefits of oestrogens in the triad of hormone-responsive depressive disorders. It is re-assuring that an increasing number of psychiatrists now accept that there is a place for gynaecological intervention in the management of these depressive disorders.[44] Research should continue in this area to ensure that in the future clinicians consider using oestrogen, not just antidepressants, when women present with a hormone-responsive psychiatric illness.[45]

References

1 Panay N, Studd JWW. The psychotherapeutic effects of oestrogens. Gynecol Endocrinol 1998; (5): 353–365

2 Klaiber EL, Broverman DM, Vogel W, Kobayashi Y. Estrogen therapy for severe persistent depressions in women. Arch Gen Psychiatry 1979; 36: 550–559

3 Kruijver FP, Balesar R, Espila AM, Unmehopa UA, Swaab DF. Estrogen-receptor beta distribution in the human hypothalamus: similarities and differences with ER alpha distribution. J Comp Neurol 2003; 466: 251–277

4 Crowley WR. Effects of ovarian hormones on norepinephrine and dopamine turnover in individual hypothalamic and extrahypothalamic nuclei. Neuroendocrinology 1982; 34: 3816

5 Sherwin B. Hormones, mood and cognitive functioning in postmenopausal women. Obstet Gynecol 1996; 87: 20–26

6 Maudsley H. Sex in mind and education. Fortnightly Review, 1874

7 Battey R. Battey's operation – its matured results. Transactions of the Georgia Medical Association, 1873

8 Longo LD. The rise and fall of Battey's operation: a fashion in surgery. Bull Hist Med 1979; 53: 244–267

9 Frank RT. The hormonal basis of premenstrual tension. Arch Neurol Psychiatry 1931; 26: 1053–1057

10 Greene R, Dalton K. The premenstrual syndrome. BMJ 1953; I: 1007–1014

11 Studd JWW. Premenstrual tension syndrome. BMJ 1979; I: 410

12 Backstrom T, Boyle H, Baird DT. Persistence of symptoms of premenstrual tension in hysterectomized women. Br J Obstet Gynaecol 1981; 88: 530–536.

13 Studd JWW. Prophylactic oophorectomy at hysterectomy. Br J Obstet Gynaecol 1989; 96: 506–509

14 Leather AT, Studd JWW, Watson NR, Holland EFN. The treatment of severe premenstrual syndrome with goserelin with and without 'add-back' estrogen therapy: a placebo-controlled study. Gynecol Endocrinol 1999; 13: 48–55

15 Leather AT, Studd JWW, Watson NR, Holland EFN. The prevention of bone loss in young women treated with GNRH analogues with 'add back' oestrogen therapy. Obstet Gynecol 1993; 81: 104–107

16 Di Carlo C, Palomba S, Tommaselli GA et al. Use of leuprolide acetate plus tibolone in the treatment of severe premenstrual syndrome. Fertil Steril 2001; 76: 850–852

17 Sundstrom I, Myberg S, Bixo M, Hammarback S, Backstrom T. Treatment of premenstrual syndrome with gonadotropin-releasing hormone agonist in a low dose regimen. Acta Obstet Gynecol Scand 1999; 78: 891–899

18 O'Brien PM, Abukhalil IE. Randomized controlled trial of the management of premenstrual syndrome and premenstrual mastalgia using luteal phase-only danazol. Am J Obstet Gynecol 1999; 180: 18–23

19 Greenblatt RB, Asch RH, Mahesh VB, Bryner JR. Implantation of pure crystalline pellets of estradiol for conception control. Am J Obstet Gynecol 1977; 127: 520–527

20 Magos AL, Studd JWW. The premenstrual syndrome. In: Studd JWW ed. Progress in Obsterics and Gynaecology, vol. 4. Edinburgh:Churchill Livingstone, 1984; 334–350

21 Studd JWW, Domoney C, Khastgir G. The place of hysterectomy in the treatment of menstrual disorders. In: Disorders of the Menstrual Cycle, vol 29. London: RCOG Press, 2000; 313-322

22 Magos AL, Brewster E, Singh R, O'Dowd T, Brincat M, Studd JWW. The effects of norethisterone in postmenopausal women on oestrogen replacement therapy: a model for the premenstrual syndrome. Br J Obstet Gynaecol 1986; 93: 1290–1296.

23 Bjorn I, Backstrom T. Drug related negative side-effects is a common reason for poor

compliance in hormone replacement therapy. Maturitas 1999; 32: 77–86

24 Panay N, Studd JWW. Progestogen intolerance and compliance with hormone replacement therapy in menopausal women. Hum Reprod Update 1997; 3: 159–171

25 Watson NR, Studd JWW, Savvas M, Garnett T, Baber R J. Treatment of severe premenstrual syndrome with oestradiol patches and cyclical oral norethisterone. Lancet 1989; I: 730–732

26 Smith RNH, Studd JWW, Zambleera D, Holland EFN. A randomised comparison over 8 months of 100 mcgs and 200mcg twice weekly doses in the treatment of severe premenstrual syndrome. Br J Obstet Gynaecol 1995; 102: 475–484

27 Montgomery JC, Brincat M, Tapp A et al. Effect of oestrogen and testosterone implants on psychological disorders in the climacteric. Lancet 1987; I: 297–299

28 Gregoire AJP, Kumar R, Everitt B, Henderson A, Studd JWW. Transdermal oestrogen for treatment of severe postnatal depression. Lancet 1996; I: 930–933

29 Khastgir G, Studd JWW. Patients' outlook, experience and satisfaction with hysterectomy, bilateral oophorectomy and subsequent continuation of hormone replacement therapy. Am J Obstet Gynecol 2000; 183: 1427–1433

30 Lawrie TA, Hofmeyr GJ, De Jager M, Burke M, Paikei B. A double blind randomised placebo controlled study of postnatal norethisterone enanthate: the effect on postnatal depression and hormones. Br J Obstet Gynaecol 1998; 105: 1082–1090

31 Ahokas A, Kaukoranta J, Wahlbeck K. Oestrogen deficiency in severe postpartum depression. Successful treatment with sublingual physiologic 17 Beta oestradiol a preliminary study. J Clin Psychiatry 2001; 62: 332–336

32 Bloch M, Schmidt PJ, Danaceau M, Murphy J, Nieman L, Rubinow DR. Effects of denerbal steroids in women with a history of postpartum depression. Am J Psychiatry 2000; 57: 924–930

33 Hunter MS. Depression and the menopause. BMJ 1996; 313: 1217–1218

34 Morrison MF, Kallan MJ, Ten Have T, Katz I, Tweedy K, Battistini M. Lack of efficacy of estradiol for depression in postmenopausal women: a randomized controlled trial. Biol Psychiatry 2004; 55: 406–412

35 Utian M. The true clinical features of postmenopause and oophorectomy and their response to oestrogen therapy. South Afr Med J 1972; 46: 732–737

36 Campbell S, Whitehead M. Oestrogen therapy and the menopausal syndrome. Clin Obstet Gynaecol 1977; 4: 31–47

37 Soares CN, al Maida OP, Joffe E, Cohen LS. Efficacy of oestradiol for the treatment of depressive disorders in perimenopausal women: a double blind randomised placebo controlled trial. Arch Gen Psychiatry 2001; 58: 529–534

38 Rasgon NL, Altshuler LL, Fairbanks LA et al. Estrogen replacement therapy in the treatment of major depressive disorder in perimenopausal women. J Clin Psychiatry 2002; 63 (Suppl 7): 545–548

39 Harlow BL, Wise LA, Otto MW, Soares CN, Cohen LS. Depression and its influence on reproductive endocrine and menstrual cycle markers associated with perimenopause: The Harvard Study of Moods and Cycles. Arch Gen Psychiatry 2003; 60: 29–36

40 Miller KJ. The other side of estrogen replacement therapy: outcome study results of mood improvement in estrogen users and nonusers. Curr Psychiatry Report 2003; 5: 439–444

41 Smith RN, Holland ES, Studd JWW. The symptomatology of progestogen intolerance. Maturitas 1994; 18: 87–91.

42 Panay N, Studd JWW. Progestogen intolerance and compliance with hormone replacement therapy in menopausal women. Human Reprod Update 1997; 3: 159–171

43 Watson NR, Studd JWW, Savvas M, Bayber R. The longterm effects of oestrogen implant therapy for the treatment of premenstrual syndrome. Gynecol Endocrinol 1990; 4: 99–107

44 Schmidt PJ. Mood, depression and reproductive hormones in the menopausal transition. Am J Med 2005; 118(Suppl 2): 54–58

45 Studd JWW, Panay N. Hormones and depression in women. Climacteric 2004; 7: 338–346

Jorma Paavonen

Vestibulitis – conservative treatment or surgery?

Vulvar pain syndrome, or vulvodynia, is an emerging and largely ignored pain syndrome. Vulva clinics have been established in many countries and vulvodynia has also become popular in the media.[1] Vulvodynia affects the quality of life of many women. Patients with vulvodynia suffer from either allodynia (hypersensitivity to touch) which causes dyspareunia, *i.e.* vulvar vestibulitis syndrome (VVS), or constant vulvar pain.[2]

BACKGROUND

Excessive sensitivity or hyperesthesia of the vulva was first described in 1889 by Skene, and again by Thomas and Munde in 1891, and by Kelly in 1928.[3,4] In 1980, the International Society for the Study of Vulvar Disease (ISSVD) Task Force defined vulvodynia as 'a chronic burning discomfort in the vulva with multiple causes'. The term VVS was introduced by Friedrich in 1987.[5] Three criteria for the diagnosis of VVS were proposed – entry dyspareunia, vestibular erythema, and a positive swab test (light pressure with a cotton tipped swab induces severe pain).

The term vulvodynia was introduced by Tovell and Young in 1978,[6] and again by McKay in 1983.[7] VVS has also been called vestibular adenitis, focal vulvitis, or vestibulodynia.[8,9]

Constant vulvodynia has also been called dysesthetic vulvodynia, essential vulvodynia, referred nerve root pain, or pudendal neuralgia.[4] It has many features characteristic of neuropathic pain syndrome.

CLASSIFICATION OF VULVAR PAIN

The most recent ISSVD terminology and classification of vulvar pain was developed in 2003.[10] In this classification, the term vulvodynia is used.

Jorma Paavonen MD
Professor, Department of Obstetrics and Gynecology, University of Helsinki, Haartmaninkatu 2, 00290
Helsinki, Finland. E-mail: jorma.paavonen@hus.fi

'Generalised' specifies involvement of the whole vulva, and 'localised' specifies involvement of a portion of the vulva such as vestibule. 'Unprovoked' means that the discomfort occurs spontaneously and 'provoked' means that the discomfort is triggered by physical contact. The term 'vestibulitis' has been eliminated from the most recent ISSVD terminology and replaced by the term 'provoked vulvodynia'. It is hoped that the 2003 ISSVD terminology and classification will be acceptable to those involved in the management of patients with vulvar pain. Its use may augment the understanding of vulvar pain. In this article, the terms 'vestibulitis' and 'dysesthetic vulvodynia' are still used.

PREVALENCE

Prevalence studies suggest that up to 15% of women have suffered of vulvodynia at some point.[11] A recent survey in a community setting in the UK showed a prevalence of 2.8–9.3%.[8] In the US, 16% of women have experienced chronic vulvar burning.[1] Many women chose not to seek treatment even though the symptoms limited sexual activity and quality of life. Many of those who sought treatment had seen three or more different physicians. In the US, about 4% of a total of 36 million physicians' visits for chronic pain by women are caused by vulvodynia. Age range extends from adolescents to old women in their eighties.[12] In general, patients with VVS are younger than patients with dysesthetic vulvodynia. VVS is as common among Caucasian than among African-American women, and even more common among Hispanic women.[13,14] A history of sexual abuse is rare among women with vulvodynia.[12]

SYMPTOMS AND SIGNS

Vulvar pain is described as burning, stinging, rawness, or stabbing which is difficult to localise.[15,16] Vulvar pain differs from itching and precludes a scratch response. Women with VVS do not have constant pain. Women with primary VVS have never been able to tolerate introital touch without pain.[17] Women with secondary VVS have had normal sexual activity without pain until VVS developed.[17] On the other hand, patients with dysesthetic vulvodynia complain of constant pain. The simple test for VVS requires only a cotton-tipped swab. Vestibular point tenderness at the crypt next to the hymenal ring can be demonstrated in the posterior vestibulum, anterior vestibulum, or both. Sensitivity to touch may be intolerable making gynaecological examination impossible. Pain perceived on light touch is totally out of proportion. This allodynia means that the sensation perceived (*i.e.* pain) differs from that applied (*i.e.* touch). Small, reddened areas may be present at the sites of maximum point tenderness. Vaginal mucosa appears normal and wet mount examination usually shows normal lactobacilli, normal hormonal effects, and few white cells excluding vaginitis.

Many patients with vulvodynia complain of low-back pain, or symptoms consistent with overactive bladder, interstitial cystitis, irritable bowel syndrome, or even fibromyalgia.[12] Many patients also suffer of depression.

Vaginismus, or pelvic floor muscle (PFM) instability is another important sign.[18–20] The longer VVS has persisted, the more severe the vaginismus may be.

DIAGNOSIS

Diagnosis of vulvodynia is always based on medical history (introital dyspareunia), signs (point tenderness, often vestibular erythema), and exclusion of vulvovaginal infections or dermatoses. Introital dyspareunia can be classified into mild (dyspareunia present most of the time, does not prevent sexual intercourse), moderate (dyspareunia always present, intercourse sometimes possible), or severe (dyspareunia totally prohibits intercourse).[21] Patients complaining vulvar pruritus are not likely to have vulvodynia. Patients with dysesthetic vulvodynia usually show normal findings on gynaecological examination.

HISTOPATHOLOGY

Vestibular biopsies from VVS cases show mild-to-severe, non-specific, chronic inflammation involving mucosa and periglandular tissue,[22,23] although not all studies have demonstrated inflammation.[24] Routine biopsy is not needed for the diagnosis of VVS, but may be necessary to exclude other vulvar pathologies. Immunohistochemical studies of the peripheral nerve supply of the vestibular mucosa have shown an increased density of intra-epithelial nerve endings and epithelial nerve fibre proliferation in papillary dermis.[25–27] A correlation between the degree of mucosal inflammation and nerve fibre proliferation has been demonstrated.[28,29] The cause of the increased density of nerve fibres in VVS is unknown, but could be attributed to an increased presence of neural growth factors. Clearly, better understanding the pathogenesis of VVS is needed.

AETIOPATHOGENESIS

The aetiology of vulvodynia is unknown which reflects the lack of systematic high quality studies. Most studies have been small, descriptive, case-control studies subject to bias and confounding. Selected suspected risk factors or risk markers are shown in Table 1. Prolonged use of oral contraceptives from an early age increases the risk for vulvodynia.[30] Lower mechanical pain threshold in the posterior vestibulum has been demonstrated in oral contraceptive users

Table 1 Suspected risk factors or risk markers for vulvodynia

- Recurrent or persistent vulvovaginal candidiasis
- Human papillomavirus (HPV) infection
- Contact allergy
- Oral contraceptive use
- Vulvar trauma or injury
- Childhood sexual abuse
- High urinary oxalate concentration
- Psychosexual anxiety
- Herpes simplex virus (HSV) infection
- Autoimmune reaction

as compared to controls.[31] Oral contraceptive use may induce morphological changes and atrophy in the vestibular mucosa which, in turn, may influence the pain threshold. Nerve endings may be more superficial if the epithelium is thinner in oral contraceptive users.

Specific viral or bacterial infections, such as human papillomavirus (HPV), herpes simplex virus (HSV), cytomegalovirus (CMV), or *Chlamydia trachomatis* do not cause VVS. At least 12 small studies have looked at the prevalence of HPV DNA in the vestibular tissue of VVS patients with the prevalence ranging from 0% to 100% suggesting no role for HPV.[32] Prolonged treatment with antimycotics is not helpful suggesting that vulvodynia is not caused by yeast infection.[33] However, vulvodynia may first appear after any severe infection suggesting a pathogen connection.[34] VVS may be an autoimmune disease although this remains to be proven.

NATURAL HISTORY

The longer the history, the less likely is spontaneous recovery. Symptoms have often persisted for several years, in some cases greater than 10 years. However, natural history studies of VVS do not exist. VVS and dysesthetic vulvodynia may represent a continuum of the same pain syndrome, but more studies of the natural history are needed.

PSYCHOLOGICAL ASPECTS

The absence of signs on clinical examination often leads healthcare providers to state that vulvodynia is psychosomatic. VVS is poorly recognised by general practitioners and even by gynaecologists.[8] Vulvodynia patients, like most patients with chronic pain syndrome, are distressed and depressed.[2] Sexual dysfunction and chronic pain is often a mystery, causes low self-image, anxiety and isolation, difficulty in sleeping, and negative thinking. Based on limited studies, there is no evidence that women with vulvodynia differ from control women regarding specific psychosocial characteristics.[35]

TREATMENT

Dysesthetic vulvodynia

Treatment of neuropathic pain syndromes including dysesthetic vulvodynia is relatively straightforward with drugs used for painful sensory neuropathy.[36] Tricyclic antidepressants block re-uptake of serotonin and noradrenalin and presumably relieve pain by inhibition of the sodium channel. Most patients with dysesthetic vulvodynia respond and achieve at least 50% reduction in pain. However, benefits can be outweighed by adverse effects. The next drug of choice is an anticonvulsant, gabapentin or pregabalin structurally related to γ-aminobutyric acid (GABA), neurotransmitters that play a role in pain transmission and calcium channel modulation.[37] Sometimes, a combination of two drugs, for instance amitriptyline and pregabalin, may be more effective and cause less adverse effects than either drug alone. Selective serotonin re-uptake

Table 2 Conservative therapies used in the management of vulvar vestibulitis syndrome

- Topical oestrogen cream
- Topical lidocain gel
- Topical corticosteroid cream
- Topical cromolyn cream
- Topic non-steroidal anti-inflammatory drug cream
- Topical podofyllotoxin application
- Topical capsaicin cream (0.025%)
- Local injections of interferon alpha
- Local injection of bethamethasone with bupivacain
- Prolonged use of antifungals
- Behavioural therapy
- Physical therapy with biofeedback
- Acupuncture
- Local injections of botulinum toxin

inhibitors (SSRI) are not as effective as tricyclic agents or anticonvulsants against neuropathic pain.

Vulvar vestibulitis syndrome

Conservative management

Many drugs or therapeutic procedures have been used in the conservative management of VVS with highly variable success (Table 2). Only one randomised, controlled trial has been reported.[38] Initial evaluation should include re-assurance and exclusion of other causes of dyspareunia or vulvar pain. If vaginismus is present, a biofeedback pelvic musculature training programme should be recommended. This is often successful, and many women may be able to resume intercourse after a few months.[39,40] Figure 1 shows a simple pragmatic algorithm used in our Vulva Clinic for the management of patients with VVS. Accordingly, refractory cases are evaluated for vestibulectomy.

Surgical management

Vestibulectomy in the treatment of refractory VVS was first described by Woodruff et al.[41] in 1981. Vestibulectomy showed a significant decrease in symptoms (complete response, partial response, or both) in 89% of a total of 646 cases.[42] Since 1995, we have systematically used vestibulectomy in refractory VVS cases using the original technique. Briefly, a horse-shoe shaped area of the vestibulum and inner labial fold is excised as one block followed by dissection of corresponding posterior vaginal wall proximally to a distance of 4–5 cm. The vaginal mucosa is then easily advanced replacing the excised vestibular area and approximated and sutured to the perineum using interrupted sutures. As shown in Table 3, 88% of the patients had satisfactory long-term outcome. Thus, a high success rate can be achieved with proper

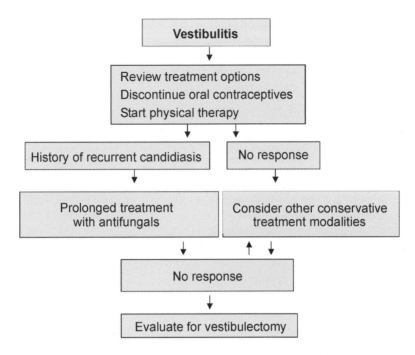

Fig. 1 Algorithm for the management of patients with vulvar vestibulitis syndrome.

surgical technique. Compared to the other available treatment modalities, vestibulectomy provides the best results in the most refractory cases. However, so far, vestibulectomy has been considered as the 'last resort' for patients with severe refractory VVS who fail to respond to conservative management.

Comparative studies of surgical versus non-surgical management
One randomised comparison of cognitive-behavioural therapy, electro-myographic biofeedback therapy, and vestibulectomy among 78 women with VVS showed that all three treatment groups improved significantly from pretreatment to 6-month follow-up, as measured by pain reduction and sexual function although vestibulectomy was more effective than the other two.[38]

RESEARCH PRIORITIES

Better understanding of the pathogenesis of vulvodynia is necessary for the development of new treatment modalities. Research priorities include epidemiological studies to identify risk factors or risk markers for vulvodynia, definition of the role of specific microbial pathogens as triggers in the aetiopathogenesis of vulvodynia, and randomised trials of surgical versus conservative treatment of VVS.

CONCLUSIONS

Vulvodynia is a distressing and debilitating disorder which is poorly understood and poorly managed. The lack of consistent terminology is confusing. The

Table 3 Long-term outcome of vestibulectomy: a case series

•	Total number of patients	34
•	History of dyspareunia pre-operatively (years)	6.4 (range, 2–28)
•	Duration of postoperative follow-up (years)	3.9 (range, 1–5.9)
•	Current age (years)	34 (range 22-47)
•	Married	15 (44%)
•	General health status (scale range 0–100)	79 (range, 50–100)
•	Same male sexual partner	19/33 (58%)
•	Delivered vaginally	7/33 (21%)
•	Any dyspareunia present	6 (17%)
•	Frequency of sexual intercourse (last month)	3.3 (range, 0–20)
•	Complaints of vaginal dryness	5 (14%)
•	VAS pre-operatively (scale range 0–10)	8.9 (range, 7–10)
•	VAS currently (scale range 0–10)	2.9 (range, 0–10)
•	Mean reduction of VAS	6.0
•	Positive swab test – anterior vestibulum	11/31 (33%)
•	Positive swab test – posterior vestibulum	3/31 (9%)
•	Overall response complete/partial	30/34 (88%)
•	Would choose operation again	32/34 (94%)

VAS, Visual analogue scale.

management of classic dysesthetic vulvodynia is straightforward using drugs effective against chronic neuropathic pain. However, vulvar vestibulitis syndrome (VVS) remains a therapeutic challenge. A pragmatic approach is recommended since VVS may resolve with time. In refractory cases, vestibulectomy has proven effective although the evidence is based mostly on small descriptive studies. Comparative studies of conservative versus surgical management of VVS are needed.

References

1 Vulvodynia: Towards understanding a pain syndrome. Proceedings from a workshop April 14–15, 2003. National Institute of Health, Pub. No. 04-5462, April 2004
2 Lotery HE, McClure N, Galask RP. Vulvodynia. Lancet 2004; 363: 1058–1060
3 Bohm-Starke N. Vulvar vestibulitis syndrome: Pathophysiology of the vestibular mucosa. Unpublished thesis, Stockholm 2001
4 Baggish MS, Miklos R. Vulvar pain syndrome: a review. Obstet Gynecol Surv 1995; 50: 618–627
5 Friedrich Jr EG. Vulvar vestibulitis syndrome. J Reprod Med 1987; 32: 110–114
6 Tovell MM, Young Jr AW. Classification of vulvar diseases. Clin Obstet Gynecol 1978; 21: 955–961
7 McKay M. Burning vulva syndrome, report of the ISSVD taskforce. J Reprod Med 1984; 29: 457
8 Munday P, Buchan A. Vulvar vestibulitis is a common and poorly recognized cause of dyspareunia. BMJ 2004; 328: 1214–1215
9 Bornstein J, Zarfati D, Goldshmid N, Stolar Z, Lahat N, Abramovici H. Vestibulodynia – a subset of vulvar vestibulitis or a novel syndrome? Am J Obstet Gynecol 1997; 177: 1439–1443

10 Moyal-Barracco M, Lynch PJ. 2003 ISSVD Terminology and classification of vulvodynia. J Reprod Med 2004; 49: 772–777

11 Goetsch MF. Vulvar vestibulitis: Prevalence and historic features in a general gynecologic practice population. Am J Obstet Gynecol 1991; 164: 1609–1616

12 Gordon AS, Panahian-Jand M, McComb F, Melegari C, Sharo S. Characteristics of women with vulvar pain disorders: responses to a web-based survey. J Sex Marital Ther 2003; 29: 45–58

13 Harlow BL, Stewart EG. A population-based assessment of chronic unexplained vulvar pain: have we underestimate the prevalence of vulvodynia? JAMA 2003; 58: 82–88

14 Adanu RMK, Haefner HK, Reed BD. Vulvar pain in women attending a general medical clinic in Accra, Ghana. J Reprod Med 2005; 50: 130–134

15 Paavonen J. Diagnosis and treatment of vulvodynia. Ann Med 1995; 27: 175–181

16 Paavonen J. Vulvodynia – a complex syndrome of vulvar pain. Acta Obstet Gynecol Scand 1995; 74: 243–247

17 Goetsch MF. Vulvar vestibulitis. Contemp Obstet Gynecol 1999; 10: 56–65

18 Glazeer HI, Rodge G, Swencionis C, Herz R, Yvonne AW. Treatment of vulvar vestibulitis syndrome with electromyographic biofeedback of pelvic floor musculature. J Reprod Med 1995; 40: 283–290

19 McKay E, Kaufman RH, Doctor U, Berkova Z, Glazer H, Redko V. Treating vulvar vestibulitis with electromyographic biofeedback of pelvic floor musculature. J Reprod Med 2001; 46: 337–342

20 Bergeron S, Brown C, Lord M-J, Oala M, Binik YM, Khalifé S. Physical therapy for vulvar vestibulitis syndrome: a retrospective study. J Sex Marital Ther 2002; 28: 183–192

21 Marinoff SC, Turner MLC. Vulvar vestibulitis syndrome. Dermatol Clin 1992; 10: 435–444

22 Chadha S, Gianotten WL, Drogendijk AC et al. Histopathologic features of vulvar vestibulitis. Int J Gynecol Pathol 1998; 17: 7–11

23 Prayson RA, Stoler MH, Hart WR. Vulvar vestibulitis. A histopathologic study of 36 cases, including human papillomavirus in situ hybridization analysis. Am J Surg Pathol 1995; 19: 154–160

24 Lundqvist EN, Hofer PA, Olofsson JI, Sjöberg I. Is vulvar vestibulitis an inflammatory condition? A comparison of histological findings in affected and healthy women. Acta Dermatol Venerol 1997; 77: 319–322

25 Halperin R, Zehavi S, Vaknin Z, Ben-Ami I, Pansky M, Schneider D. The major histopathologic characteristics in the vulvar vestibulitis syndrome. Gynecol Obstet Invest 2005; 59: 75–79

26 Slone S, Reynolds L, Gall S et al. Localization of chromogranin, synaptophysin, serotonin, and CXCR2 in neuroendocrine cells of the minor vestibular glands: an immunohistochemical study. Int J Gynecol Pathol 1999; 18: 360–365.

27 Tympanidis P, Terenghi G, Dowd P. Increased innervation of the vulval vestibule in patients with vulvodynia. Br J Dermatol 2003; 148: 1021–1027

28. Bohm-Starke N, Hilliges M, Falconer C, Rylander E. Increased intraepithelial innervation in women with vulvar vestibulitis syndrome. Gynecol Obstet Invest 1998; 46: 256–260

29 Weström LV, Willén R. Vestibular nerve fiber proliferation in vulvar vestibulitis syndrome. Obstet Gynecol 1998; 91: 572–576

30 Bouchard C, Brisson J, Fortier M, Morin C, Blanchette C. Use of oral contraceptive pills and vulvar vestibulitis: a case-control study. Am J Epidemiol 2002; 156: 254–261

31 Bohm-Starke N, Johannesson UJ, Hilliges M, Rylander E, Torebjörk E. Decreased mechanical pain threshold in the vestibular mucosa of women using oral contraceptives: a contributing factor in vulvar vestibulitis? J Reprod Med 2004; 49: 888–892

32 Morin C, Bouchard C, Brisson J, Fortier M, Blanchette C, Meisels A. Human papillomaviruses and vulvar vestibulitis. Obstet Gyneocol 2000; 95: 683–687

33 Bornstein J, Livnat G, Stolar Z, Abramovici H. Pure versus complicated vulvar vestibulitis: a randomized trial of fluconazole treatment. Gynecol Obstet Invest 2000; 50: 194–197

34 Benoist C, Mathis D. The pathogen connection. Nature 1998; 394: 227–228

35 Van Lankveld JJDM, Philomeen TH, Weijenborg M, Ter Kuile MM. Psychological profiles of and sexual function in women with vulval vestibulitis and their partners. Obstet Gynecol 1996; 88: 65–70

36 Mendell JR, Sahenk Z. Painful sensory neuropahty. N Engl J Med 2003; 348: 1243–1255

37 Backonja M, Beydoun A, Edwards KR *et al*. Gabapentin for the symptomatic treatment of painful neuropathy in patients with diabetes mellitus. JAMA 1998; 280: 1831–1836

38 Bergeron S, Binik YM, Khalifé S *et al*. A randomized comparison of group cognitive-behavioral therapy, surface electromyographic biofeedback, and vestibulectomy in the treatment of dyspareunia resulting from vulvar vestibulitis. Pain 2001; 91: 297–306

39 Jernfors V, Rekonen S, Paavonen J. Physical therapy in the management of dyspareunia and vulvar vestibulitis syndrome. Abstract #280. The 34th Nordic Congress of Obstetrics and Gynecology, June 12–15, 2004, Helsinki, Finland

40 De Oliveira Bernardes N, Bahamondes L. Intravaginal electrical stimulation for the treatment of chronic pelvic pain. J Reprod Med 2005; 50: 267–272

41 Woodruff JD, Genadry R, Poliakoff S. Treatment of dyspareunia and vaginal outlet distortions by perineoplasty. Obstet Gynecol 1981; 57: 750–754

42 Bornstein J, Zarfati D, Goldik Z, Abramovici H. Vulvar vestibulitis: physical or psychosexual problem? Obstet Gynecol 1999; 93: 876–880

Index

N.B. English and American spellings were used throughout this book according to the preference of the author(s). However, the index has followed English spellings.

Progress in Obstetrics and Gynaecology
Edited by John Studd

Contents of Volume 15

First published 2003

ISBN 0 443 072221
ISSN 0261 0140

Progress in Obstetrics and Gynaecology
Edited by John Studd

Contents of Volume 14

ISBN 0 443 064075
ISSN 0261 0140